Clinical Pediatric Nephrology

Clinical Pediatric Nephrology

Editor: Regenia Billups

AMERICAN
MEDICAL PUBLISHERS
www.americanmedicalpublishers.com

AMERICAN
MEDICAL PUBLISHERS
www.americanmedicalpublishers.com

Cataloging-in-Publication Data

Clinical pediatric nephrology / edited by Regenia Billups.
p. cm.
Includes bibliographical references and index.
ISBN 979-8-88740-002-0
1. Pediatric nephrology. 2. Pediatric nephrology--Diagnosis. 3. Pediatric nephrology--Treatment.
4. Kidneys--Diseases. I. Billups, Regenia.
RJ476.K5 C55 2023
618.926 1--dc23

American Medical Publishers,
41 Flatbush Avenue,
1st Floor, New York,
NY 11217, USA

ISBN 979-8-88740-002-0 (Hardback)

Contents

Preface

A branch of medicine concerned with the diagnosis and treatment of kidney diseases is called nephrology. Pediatrics refers to the study and practice of childcare for infants, children and adolescents. Pediatric nephrology is a sub-specialty of nephrology that deals with the treatment of acute and chronic diseases that affect renal function, blood pressure, and fluid and electrolyte disorders in children. The common symptoms of kidney conditions include foamy urine, loss of appetite, severe swelling around the eye, blood clots, etc. Urine examination is the most common and direct test to assess kidney problems. In some cases, blood tests for checking the concentration of hemoglobin, platelets, calcium, urea, or creatinine in the blood are also used to assess kidney problems. Imaging techniques such as ultrasonography, computed axial tomography (CT) and magnetic resonance imaging (MRI) are also used to diagnose the structural abnormalities in the kidneys. This book includes some of the vital pieces of works being conducted across the world, on various topics related to pediatric nephrology. It will serve as a reference to a broad spectrum of readers.

After months of intensive research and writing, this book is the end result of all who devoted their time and efforts in the initiation and progress of this book. It will surely be a source of reference in enhancing the required knowledge of the new developments in the area. During the course of developing this book, certain measures such as accuracy, authenticity and research focused analytical studies were given preference in order to produce a comprehensive book in the area of study.

This book would not have been possible without the efforts of the authors and the publisher. I extend my sincere thanks to them. Secondly, I express my gratitude to my family and well-wishers. And most importantly, I thank my students for constantly expressing their willingness and curiosity in enhancing their knowledge in the field, which encourages me to take up further research projects for the advancement of the area.

Editor

1

Human Papillomavirus Vaccination in Male and Female Adolescents Before and After Kidney Transplantation: A Pediatric Nephrology Research Consortium Study

Corina Nailescu [1], Raoul D. Nelson [2], Priya S. Verghese [3], Katherine E. Twombley [4], Aftab S. Chishti [5], Michele Mills [6], John D. Mahan [7], James E. Slaven [8] and Marcia L. Shew [1]*

[1] Department of Pediatrics, Indiana University, Riley Hospital for Children, Indianapolis, IN, United States, [2] Department of Pediatrics, University of Utah, Primary Children's Hospital, Salt Lake City, UT, United States, [3] Department of Pediatrics, University of Minnesota Masonic Children's Hospital, Minneapolis, MN, United States, [4] Department of Pediatrics, Medical University of South Carolina Children's Hospital, Charleston, SC, United States, [5] Department of Pediatrics, Kentucky Children's Hospital, University of Kentucky, Lexington, KY, United States, [6] Department of Pediatrics, C. S. Mott Children's Hospital, University of Michigan, Ann Arbor, MI, United States, [7] Department of Pediatrics, Nationwide Children's Hospital, The Ohio State University, Columbus, OH, United States, [8] Department of Biostatistics, Indiana University, Indianapolis, IN, United States

****Correspondence:***
Corina Nailescu
cnailesc@iu.edu

Background: Kidney transplant (KT) recipients have higher incidence of malignancies, including Human Papillomavirus (HPV)-associated cancers. Thus, HPV vaccines may have an important role in preventing HPV-related disease in this population; however, immunogenicity and safety data are lacking.

Objective: To examine the immunological response and tolerability to HPV vaccination in pediatric KT recipients compared to future KT candidates.

Methods: The quadrivalent HPV vaccine was administered to girls and boys age 9–18 recruited from seven centers part of the Pediatric Nephrology Research Consortium. Subjects were recruited for three groups: (1) *CKD:* chronic kidney disease stages 3, 4, and 5 not on dialysis; (2) *Dialysis;* (3) *KT* recipients. The outcome consisted of antibody concentrations against HPV 6, 11, 16, and 18. Geometric mean titers (GMTs) and seroconversion rates were compared. Vaccine tolerability was assessed.

Results: Sixty-five participants were recruited: 18 in the CKD, 18 in the dialysis, and 29 into the *KT* groups. KT patients had significantly lower GMTs after vaccination for all serotypes. The percentages of subjects who reached seroconversion were overall lower for the *KT* group, reaching statistical significance for HPV 6, 11, and 18. Comparing immunosuppressed subjects (anyone taking immunosuppression medications, whether KT recipient or not) with the non-immunosuppressed participants, the former had significantly lower GMTs for all the HPV serotypes and lower seroconversion rates for HPV 6, 11, and 18. KT females had higher GMTs and seroconversion rates for certain serotypes. There were no adverse events in either group.

Conclusions: HPV vaccine was well-tolerated in this population. Pediatric KT recipients had in general lower GMTs and seroconversion rates compared to their peers with CKD or on dialysis. Immunosuppression played a role in the lack of seroconversion. Our results emphasize the importance of advocating for HPV vaccination prior to KT and acknowledge its safety post transplantation. Future studies are needed to investigate the effect of a supplemental dose of HPV vaccine in KT recipients who do not seroconvert and to evaluate the long-term persistence of antibodies post-KT.

Keywords: HPV—human papillomavirus, vaccination, kidney transplantation, chronic kidney disease, dialysis, pediatric

INTRODUCTION

Solid organ transplant (SOT) recipients are at increased risk for malignancies in both pediatric and adult populations (1–3), with an elevated risk of dying of their cancer, even after adjustment for stage and treatment (4). Pediatric and adult kidney transplant (KT) recipients carry similar risk and malignancies are third most common cause of mortality within this population (5, 6). Specifically, female KT recipients have an increased risk of cervical cancer up to 14-fold, vulvar cancer up to 50-fold and anal cancers up to 100-fold (7, 8). In addition, male SOT recipients have an increased risk for penile cancers (9). Human papillomavirus (HPV) 16 and to a much lesser extent HPV 18 are responsible for the majority of these cancers (10). In addition, HPV 16 is also responsible for a large proportion of oral pharyngeal cancers (11). Not only that HPV infections are the most prevalent sexually transmitted infections in the US (12), but non-carcinogenic HPV types, HPV 6 and 11, can be associated with genital warts and can be difficult to treat in the face of immunosuppression (13). Immunosuppressed individuals, including transplant recipients, have higher rates of HPV infections (14–16), greater likelihood of persistent infections (17, 18) and higher rates of HPV clinical disease, including cancer (9, 19, 20). Thus, preventing HPV infections in this population is critical. HPV-related vaccine trials have been shown to prevent HPV infection in immunocompetent individuals when the vaccine is given prior to viral exposure (21). In addition, more recent studies have demonstrated a true reduction in abnormal Pap smears and cervical cancers with use of HPV vaccine (22, 23). Because HPV is sexually transmitted and often acquired soon after the onset of sexual activity (24), vaccination should ideally occur before sexual debut.

The efficacy and safety of the HPV vaccine in certain immunocompromised populations, such as pediatric chronic kidney disease (CKD), dialysis and KT recipients, has not been well-studied. This is a population at increased risk for infections and HPV related sequelae; in addition, they appear to also be at high risk for not getting vaccinated due to lack of data and less immediate concerns about sexual activity when ill and awaiting transplant, as has been shown in other patients with severe chronic illnesses (25, 26). The goal of this study was to examine the immunological response and tolerability of the quadrivalent HPV vaccine in both female and male pediatric patients with CKD, on dialysis and with a KT. The primary hypothesis was that all these populations will mount an immune response to the vaccine. Our secondary hypothesis was that pediatric patients with CKD 3, 4, 5 and on dialysis, therefore future KT candidates, will respond to the HPV vaccination better than the KT recipients.

MATERIALS AND METHODS

Study Population

Males and females ages 9–18 years were recruited from seven collaborating large medical centers in the Pediatric Nephrology Research Consortium: Riley Hospital for Children in Indianapolis, IN, Primary Children's Hospital in Salt Lake City, UT, Medical University of South Carolina Children's Hospital in Charleston, SC, University of Minnesota Masonic Children's Hospital in Minneapolis, MN, Kentucky Children's Hospital in Lexington, KY, C.S. Mott Children's Hospital in Ann Arbor, MI and Nationwide Children's Hospital in Columbus, OH. Subjects were recruited in three cohorts:

- Group 1 (CKD) included patients with CKD stages 3 [glomerular filtration rate (GFR) 30–59 mL/min per 1.73 m^2], 4 (GFR 15–29 mL/min per 1.73 m^2) or 5 not on dialysis (GFR <15 mL/min/1.73 m^2, but not on dialysis).
- Group 2 (Dialysis) included patients on either chronic hemodialysis or peritoneal dialysis.
- Group 3 (KT) included patients who had received a KT at least 6 months prior to enrollment, in keeping with the recommendations of the American Society of Transplantation that inactivated vaccines may be resumed 3–6 months after a SOT (27).

Exclusion criteria were: pregnancy (self-reported), post-transplant lymphoproliferative disorder, active infectious diseases, fever, bleeding disorders, having received blood products in the past 6 months and hypersensitivity to any of the vaccine components.

Study Design

All participants who met eligibility criteria and who had not been vaccinated against HPV were approached within the dialysis units or clinics by a study coordinator at each site. Study

Abbreviations: SOT, solid organ transplant; KT, kidney transplant; HPV, human papilloma virus; CKD, chronic kidney disease; GFR, glomerular filtration rate; eGFR, estimated GFR calculated using the modified Schwartz formula (0.413 × height in cm/serum creatinine in mg/dL); T1, time 1 (day 1 of enrollment prior to dose 1 of the vaccine administration); T2, time 2 (one month after vaccine series was completed); VRC, vaccination report card; AEs, adverse events; SD, standard deviation; IQR, interquartile range.

coordinators discussed the study and consent was obtained from the parent/guardian and assent from the participant. Medical records were used to abstract age, gender, race, and estimated GFR (eGFR) using the modified Schwartz formula (0.413 × height in cm/serum creatinine in mg/dL). For the CKD 3, 4, 5 and dialysis patients, it was documented whether they were on immunosuppression medications for their respective primary kidney diseases. The rationale for doing so was to perform sub-analyses to determine whether patients on immunosuppression medications (including KT recipients, but also patients with CKD 3, 4, and 5 taking immunosuppression medications to treat their primary disease) had a weaker immune response to the HPV vaccine compared to the rest. In addition, for KT patients, type of donor (living vs. deceased), number of transplants and time since most recent transplant were recorded. HPV quadrivalent vaccine (Gardasil®, Merck & Co., Inc.) was administered to each study participant per protocol according to the Advisory Committee on Immunization Practices recommendations at the time (28). Dose 1 of the HPV vaccine was administered to each study participant on day 1 of enrollment, after obtaining a baseline blood sample for antibody testing. Dose 2 was targeted to be administered at month 2 and dose 3 at month 6. The minimum interval between dose 1 and 2 of the vaccine was 4 weeks. The minimum recommended interval between dose 2 and 3 of the vaccine was 12 weeks. No subject received dose 2 or 3 more than 4 weeks later than initially targeted date. The Institutional Review Board of each participating center approved the study.

Outcomes

The primary outcome was the antibody response to each of the four HPV serotypes contained within the vaccine (6, 11, 16, 18). Serum was collected from all subjects on day 1 of enrollment prior to dose 1 of the vaccine administration [Time 1 (T1)] and at month 7 (or 1 month after vaccine series was completed) [Time 2 (T2)]. Anti-HPV responses were measured using a competitive Luminex Immunoassay performed by PPD Vaccines and Biologics (Wayne, PA) and expressed as geometric mean titers (GMTs). A participant was considered to have seroconverted if no antibody titers were found at enrollment and antibody levels post immunization were above the sero-status cutoffs for HPV types 6, 11, 16, and 18, as determined by the assay developer (GMTs $\geq$ 20, $\geq$16, $\geq$20, and $\geq$24 mM units/mL, respectively).

Secondary analyses evaluated the potential effect of other variables on antibody response to the HPV vaccine, such as age, gender, race, eGFR and use of immunosuppression medications. Within the transplanted group, donor type (living vs. deceased), number of transplants and time from transplant were also evaluated.

In addition, although the sample size was small, data was collected regarding safety of the HPV vaccine in this patient population, since it has not been well-studied. All subjects received a vaccination report card (VRC) after each vaccine dose administration. On the VRC, the parent/guardian was asked to record the subject's oral evening temperature daily for 5 days. In addition, injection-site and systemic adverse events (AEs) for a total of 15 days after each vaccination were recorded by parent/guardian. For injection-site erythema and swelling, subjects were instructed by the VRC to measure an injection-site reaction at its greatest width ("maximum size") from edge to edge in maximum units ranging from 0 to >7 inches (17.5 cm) on the VRC, rounding up to the next unit if in between 2 units [each unit on the VRC measured ~1 inch (2.5 cm)]. For all AEs, subjects were instructed by the VRC to estimate the severity of AEs as mild (awareness of symptom but easily tolerated), moderate (discomfort enough to cause interference with usual activities), or severe (incapacitating with inability to work or do usual activity). Serious AEs were collected for the whole duration of the study regardless of causality and were followed for outcome. In addition, for KT recipients, data was specifically collected on any biopsy-proven acute rejection episodes after T1 up to 6 months after the last dose of the vaccine administration.

Statistical Analyses

Basic demographic and clinical characteristics are presented as means [standard deviations (SD)] for age, median [interquartile range (IQR)] for eGFR due to non-linearity, and frequencies (percentages) for categorical variables (sex, race, use of immunosuppression medications), with analyses comparing groups performed with ANOVA, Kruskal–Wallis, and Chi-Square tests, respectively. The two main outcomes of serotiter and seroconversion were assessed to determine if there were significant differences between groups at T2. Serotiter values were analyzed using Kruskal–Wallis non-parametric tests and seroconversion proportions using Fisher's Exact tests, with descriptive statistics being given as medians (IQRs) and frequencies (percentages), respectively. Pairwise comparisons were made for serotiter levels using a Bonferroni adjusted *p*-0.0167 to control for inflated type I error rates. Similar analyses, for demographics and the two outcome variables, were also performed comparing those who were on immunosuppression medications vs. those who were not, with similar analyses, using Student's *t*-tests, Wilcoxon rank-sum tests, and Fisher's Exact tests. All analyses were performed using SAS v9.4 (SAS Institute, Cary, NC) and all analytic assumptions were verified. Non-inferiority analyses were also performed, but all were non-significant due to the extremely low power due to our small sample size (results not presented).

RESULTS

A total of 72 subjects were enrolled: 28 from Riley Hospital for Children in Indianapolis; 15 from Primary Children's Hospital in Salt Lake City; 9 from University of Minnesota Masonic Children's Hospital in Minneapolis; 9 from Medical University of South Carolina Children's Hospital in Charleston; 5 from Kentucky Children's Hospital in Lexington; 5 from C.S. Mott Children's Hospital in Ann Arbor; 1 from Nationwide Children's Hospital in Columbus. A total of 65 participants completed the study: 18 participants in the CKD group, 18 participants in the dialysis group and 29 participants in the KT group (7 subjects were excluded for either not receiving all three doses of the vaccine or for not doing both serology collections). The average age of enrollment was 13.6 years (SD 2.6) and little

TABLE 1 | Demographics and renal status at enrollment*.

	Overall (n = 65)	CKD (n = 18)	Dialysis (n = 18)	Transplant (n = 29)	p-value**
Age [years; mean (SD)]	13.6 (2.6)	12.9 (2.7)	14.9 (2.5)	13.2 (2.4)	0.055
Sex [Male; N (%)]	34 (54.8)	12 (70.6)	4 (25.0)	18 (62.1)	0.018
Race [N (%)]					
Asian	2 (3.2)	0 (0)	2 (12.5)	0 (0)	0.006
Black	11 (17.5)	2 (11.1)	2 (12.5)	7 (24.1)	
Hispanic	9 (14.3)	2 (11.1)	6 (37.5)	1 (3.5)	
White	41 (65.1)	14 (77.8)	6 (37.5)	21 (72.4)	
Use of immunosuppression medications [N (%)]	38 (61.3)	1 (5.9)	8 (50.0)	29 (100)	<0.001
eGFR [mL/min/1.73 m^2] [median (IQR)]	31.6 (12.8, 61.9)	30.0 (20.6, 31.6)	9.6 (6.6, 11.2)	63.1 (45.7, 85.6)	<0.001

*Values are means (standard deviation) for age, frequencies (percentages) for categorical variables, and median (IQR) for eGFR; **p-values are from ANOVA, Fisher's Exact, and Kruskal–Wallis tests, respectively. Frequencies may not add to column totals due to missing data.*

TABLE 2 | Antibody responses to HPV vaccine (GMTs)—continuous variable by groups*.

	CKD (n = 18)	Dialysis (n = 18)	Transplant (n = 29)	p-value**
HPV 6[#]	869 (128, 1739); 539.67	217.5 (137, 326); 205.37	115 (12, 590); 113.16	0.016
HPV 11	1694.5 (622, 2740); 1208.30	431.5 (180, 996); 370.08	83 (13, 675); 110.13	0.001
HPV 16	5639.5 (934, 9189); 4390.79	1581.5 (436, 3404); 1709.62	436 (74, 4316); 508.43	0.011
HPV 18	1406.5 (150, 5121); 1039.62	331.5 (69, 622); 266.45	52 (9, 497); 91.30	0.004

*Values are medians (IQRs); mean GMTs at T2. **p-values are from Kruskal–Wallis non-parametric tests. #HPV 6 analyses had sample sizes of 17, 16 and 29, respectively, as those who were not naïve at baseline were excluded for that particular outcome's analysis. Post-hoc pairwise comparisons were made with Wilcoxon rank-sum tests, using a p-value of 0.017 for significance to control for inflated type I error rate; pairwise comparisons indicate the significant associations are driven by the difference between CKD and KT groups, although CKD and dialysis groups were also different for HPV type 11.*

over one half were males (N = 34, 54.8%). The majority of participants were white (N = 41, 65.1%) or black (N = 11, 17.5%). **Table 1** compares the demographics of the three groups with differences demonstrated among the three groups in regards to sex, race, eGFR and use of immunosuppression medications. All the KT patients were taking immunosuppression medications; in addition, some of the patients in the other two groups were also taking immunosuppression medications to treat the immune-mediated diseases leading to CKD or dialysis). Within the KT group (n = 29) the median (range) time since first transplant was 3.9 years (3.6, 10.5), about half (51.9%) had received a kidney from a living donor, one individual had had two transplants; two KT recipients reported events of rejection during the study enrollment.

All participants were seronegative for all four of the vaccine HPV types at enrollment, except for three participants who were not naïve for HPV 6, and thus excluded from serotiter and seroconversion analyses for that particular HPV type only. Serotiters for all HPV types were detected post-vaccination at T2, with KT patients having significantly lower GMTs for all serotypes; pairwise comparisons indicated the significant associations were driven by the difference between CKD and KT groups, although CKD and dialysis groups were also different for HPV type 11 (**Table 2**). Examination of the seroconversion rates based on manufacturer cutoffs showed significant heterogeneity between the groups (**Table 3**). The seroconversion rates post-vaccination were significantly lower for the transplanted group for three of the serotypes (HPV 6, 11, and 18). Although not statistically different, seroconversion rates were also lower for the HPV 16 serotype.

All variables found to be different among the three treatment groups were examined directly with the two outcome variables, GMTs at T2 and seroconversion. Age, sex, race, and eGFR were found to have no association with GMTs at T2 or actual seroconversion. However, when only the KT population was examined, being a female KT-recipient was associated with greater GMTs at T2 for HPV 6 and 11 only (p = 0.020 and 0.046, respectively) and with higher seroconversion rates for HPV 18 only (90.9 vs. 44.4% for females and males, respectively; p = 0.020). Although statistically significant, this is difficult to interpret clinically with the inconsistencies among the various HPV types and small numbers for multiple analyses.

Comparing subjects who were using immunosuppression medications (including KT recipients, as well as CKD 3,

TABLE 3 | Seroconversion rates—categorical variable by groups*.

	CKD ($n = 18$)	Dialysis ($n = 18$)	Transplant ($n = 29$)	*p*-value**
HPV 6#	17 (100)	15 (93.8)	21 (72.4)	0.017
HPV 11	18 (100)	16 (88.9)	20 (69.0)	0.010
HPV 16	18 (100)	17 (94.4)	26 (89.7)	0.570
HPV 18	17 (94.4)	15 (83.3)	18 (62.1)	0.032

*Values are frequencies (percentages) of participants who seroconverted, defined as being HPV naïve at T1 and having GMTs ≥20, ≥16, ≥20 and ≥24 milli-Merck units/mL for HPV types 6, 11, 16, and 18, respectively at T2. **p-values are from Fisher's Exact tests. #HPV 6 analyses had sample sizes of 17, 16, and 29, respectively as those who were not naïve at baseline were excluded for that particular outcome's analysis.*

TABLE 4 | Comparison between subjects who used immunosuppression medications vs. subjects not on immunosuppression medications*.

	Immuno suppression medications use ($n = 38$)	No Immuno suppression medication use ($n = 24$)	*p*-value**
Age [years; mean (SD)]	13.5 (2.4)	13.6 (3.1)	0.904
Sex [Male; *N* (%)]	19 (50.0)	14 (60.9)	0.440
Race [*N* (%)]			
Asian	1 (2.6)	1 (4.2)	0.030
Black	9 (23.7)	2 (8.3)	
Hispanic	2 (5.3)	7 (29.2)	
White	26 (68.4)	14 (58.3)	
eGFR [mL/min/1.73 m^2] [median (IQR)]	56.7 (20.4, 69.4)	21.4 (9.8, 31.1)	<0.001
GMTs at T2 [median (IQR)]			
HPV 6#	120 (19, 564)	362.5 (140.5, 1216)	0.005
HPV 11	121 (13, 675)	1247 (522, 2028.5)	<0.001
HPV 16	436 (89, 3404)	4751.5 (1829, 9091)	<0.001
HPV 18	50 (9, 497)	963.5 (396, 4243.5)	<0.001
Seroconversion [*N* (%)]			
HPV 6#	26 (74.3)	24 (100)	0.008
HPV 11	27 (71.1)	24 (100)	0.004
HPV 16	34 (89.5)	24 (100)	0.151
HPV 18	24 (63.2)	23 (95.8)	0.005

*Values are means (standard deviation) for age; frequencies (percentages) for sex, race, and seroconversion; median (IQR) for eGFR and for GMTs. **p-values are from Student's t-test, Fisher's Exact tests, and Wilcoxon tests, respectively. Frequencies may not add to column totals due to missing data. The total number of subjects in this analysis was 38 + 24 = 62, as opposed to 65 subjects in the other analyses. This is due to missing medication information from the data collection forms on three subjects. #HPV 6 analyses had sample sizes of 35 and 24, respectively, as those who were not naïve at baseline were excluded for that particular outcome's analysis.*

4, and 5 on immunosuppression medications to treat their primary kidney conditions) vs. not, the immunosuppression medication-using group had significantly lower serotiters for all four HPV serotypes at T2 and lower seroconversion rates for HPV 6, 11, and 18 (**Table 4**). The immunosuppression medications used in the transplant population included prednisone, tacrolimus, cyclosporine A and mycophenolate mofetil. The immunosuppression medications used to treat the primary kidney diseases in the CKD and dialysis patients included prednisone, tacrolimus, mycophenolate mofetil and azathioprine. Unlike in the KT population, when the male vs. female differences were examined specifically in the immunosuppression medication-using group, no differences were seen.

Within the transplant population, neither the donor type, neither time since transplant, nor the number of transplants, made any difference in terms of GMTs at T2 or seroconversion rates.

As for the AEs, they were minimal, limited to only mild local reactions. Two patients underwent acute rejection episodes within 6 months following the last dose of the vaccine. However, upon review of chart data, these events were considered to be likely related to medication non-adherence.

DISCUSSION

American Society of Transplantation recommends that HPV vaccine be given to all SOT candidates and recipients in the recommended age-group (27). However, the efficacy and tolerability of the HPV vaccine in such populations, as well as the optimal timing to do so, are not completely understood. Our results demonstrated that the HPV vaccine was well-tolerated and an adequate immune response for all four HPV types was observed with CKD and dialysis patients. However, the immune response was slightly lower within the transplanted population and immunosuppressant medications had an effect on lack of seroconversion. HPV vaccine acceptance by patients and their parents/guardians has always been problematic even in the general population (29, 30) and probably more so in these specific groups, where data is scant (26). Our study provides further evidence that patients who are likely to need a KT in the future respond best to the HPV vaccine pre-transplantation, while with CKD or on dialysis. As the majority of causes of end-stage renal disease in pediatrics are congenital diseases in which the kidney function slowly deteriorates over time, pediatric nephrologists often have the advantage of being able to better plan a KT (whether preemptive or not) considering multiple aspects, including vaccinations, compared to their adult nephrologist colleagues (26). This study showed that girls and boys with CKD and on dialysis had stronger immunologic responses to the HPV vaccine compared to those who were already transplanted. Therefore, this study should help pediatric nephrologists and pediatricians in their work with patients and families to pursue and complete the administration of HPV vaccine ideally prior to transplant whenever possible, but also post-transplant in cases where it was not given prior to KT. Is is to be noted that in 2015 the Advisory Committee on Immunization Practices (ACIP) recommended the 9-valent HPV vaccine (9vHPV) (Gardasil 9, Merck and Co., Inc.) as an alternative to the quadrivalent vaccine (31). The 9-valent vaccine was found to be safe, provided more extensive serotype coverage and it was even found to be cost-saving when compared with the quadrivalent vaccine, therefore it is currently more widely used (31). Our study was initiated well before 2015, hence the use of the quadrivalent vaccine.

It is important for the HPV vaccine to be given before HPV infection is acquired, meaning before the onset of sexual activity (28). This is the rationale behind the fact that the HPV vaccine is recommended to be given at 11–12 years of age, although it can be administered starting at age 9 (28). In the US, the proportion of males who reported having sexual intercourse before age 13 years varied from 5 to 25% across metropolitan sites (32), hence the need to vaccinate at a young age, designed to capture most teenagers before becoming sexually active. In our study, the onset of sexual activity was not assessed out of concerns that in a multisite trial, the investigators could not assure patient confidentiality relative to their parents/caregivers for all participants. However, obtaining this information in future studies would be helpful in assessing clinical risk and outcomes in patients with chronic diseases (33, 34). In children with CKD and on dialysis, contrary to what was believed in the past, recent cohort studies have shown that growth and sexual maturation are only slightly delayed compared to healthy subjects (35). Although there is lack of specific data, given the circumstances, it is plausible that adolescents with CKD or on dialysis are not far behind from their peers in terms of their onset of sexual activity. It is therefore of concern that in our study the mean age of subjects was 13.6 (SD 2.6), meaning that our patient population was vaccinated on average later than the recommended age.

Our study showed for the first time both in boys and girls that overall, transplant patients had a decreased response to the HPV vaccine compared to CKD and dialysis patients, likely related to their state of medication-induced immunosuppression. However, specifically for HPV 16, seroconversion rates were not found to be significantly lower for KT patients and neither were they found to be lower for patients taking immunosuppression medications. Although power may have biased this result, it is also somewhat reassuring since the majority of HPV cancers are associated with type 16. At the very least, the data supports ongoing vaccination in this group due to the fact that the majority of individuals did effectively respond to the vaccine. Review of literature revealed that the first studies to look into HPV vaccine responses in immunosuppressed populations was in HIV-positive cohorts, which showed promising results, as 95–100% of the subjects demonstrated seroconversion (36–38). Thus, seroconversion was not much lower than in healthy populations (39). Surprisingly, the first study of the immunogenicity of the HPV vaccine in SOT recipients was done in a cohort of 47 adults (females and males) and reported much lower rates of seroconversion: 63.2, 68.4, 63.2, and 52.6% for HPV 6, 11, 16, and 18, respectively (40). Somewhat similarly, in pediatrics, a study of a cohort of 57 patients (females only) aged 9–21 years old with CKD, on dialysis, or post-KT, showed that among patients with transplants, the percentages achieving seropositivity were significantly lower compared to CKD and dialysis patients: 63.6, 63.6, and 72.7% for HPV 6, 11, and 18, respectively (41). Our study included both girls and boys age 10 to 16 with CKD, on dialysis, or post-KT and showed lower seroconversion rates: 72.4, 69.0, and 62.1% for HPV 6, 11, and 18, respectively, in transplant patients, thus demonstrating similar results for the first time in boys, as well.

In this study, it is likely that the entire population was affected by varying levels of immunosuppression, regardless of the study group. Indeed, patients with CKD and more so the ones on dialysis have been shown to have various degrees of immunosuppression, whether caused by defects in neutrophil function, antigen processing, cell-mediated immunity, or antibody-mediated immunity (42, 43). Antibody responses to certain vaccines have been found to be attenuated in this patient population for certain vaccines, such as the measles, mumps and rubella (44). On the contrary, for other vaccines immune responses have been found to be similar to the general population (45). In the case of HPV vaccine, a study on pediatric and adult patients with CKD 4, 5, and on dialysis showed 98.2, 100, 100, and 98.2% serocoversion for HPV genotypes 6, 11, 16, and 18, respectively (46). These values are comparable to the data generated in healthy adult women large populations, which reported 99.7, 99.5, 99.7, and 99.2% seropositivity for HPV genotypes 6, 11, 16, and 18, respectively (39). Our study also reported robust immune responses in the CKD and dialysis pediatric patients. Although there was a non-statistically significant tendency to less robust responses for dialysis patients compared to CKD, this was probably explained by the fact that half of the dialysis patients were on immunosuppressive medications for their kidney conditions. In addition, we have found no difference in terms of HPV vaccine responses between patients on hemodialysis vs. peritoneal dialysis in our study population (data not presented). It is likely that being on anti-rejection medications creates a more profound state of immunosuppression in transplant recipients than the immune dysregulation seen in CKD or while on dialysis, since KT patients had less robust immune responses to the HPV vaccine in our study. Likewise, patients with CKD or on dialysis who were on immunosuppression medications for their primary kidney diseases, which are in fact similar to anti-rejection medications, also demonstrated poorer seroconversion rates.

It is possible that girls and boys who are KT recipients respond differently to the HPV vaccine. The quadrivalent HPV vaccine was approved in the US in 2006 for use in girls/women only. Subsequently, in 2009, the indication was extended to boys/men as well. The few studies that compared the seroconversion rates to HPV vaccine between males and females in the general population have not shown any differences (47, 48). Our study showed that overall there were no differences between males and females in terms of HPV antibody responses. However, when data was analyzed specifically for the KT recipients, male subjects had lower GMTs at T2 for HPV 6 and 11 (but not 16 or 18) and lower seroconversion rates for HPV 18 (but not for HPV6, HPV11, or HPV16) compared to females. Although statistically significant, this is difficult to interpret clinically with the inconsistencies among the various HPV types and small numbers for multiple analyses. Interestingly enough, unlike in the KT population, when the male vs. female differences were examined specifically in the immunosuppression medication-using group, no differences were seen. Sex-based differences in immune function and responses to vaccination have been described before, where females typically developed higher antibody responses and experienced more adverse reactions following vaccination than males for bacillus Calmette-Guerin, measles, mumps, rubella, yellow fever and influenza vaccines

(49, 50). In addition, men SOT recipients have a higher incidence of malignancies, also suggesting the fact that SOT men could become more immunosuppressed than women when treated with anti-rejection medications (51). In any event, the fact that male KT recipients tend to have lower antibody titers and seroconversion rates for certain serotypes following HPV vaccination, while of uncertain significance, still raises questions about optimal vaccination strategies specifically in this patient population, which has been already shown to also have lower vaccination rates compared to females (52).

AEs reported were similar to those noted in prior studies, limited to minor vaccine local skin reactions. Two patients underwent acute rejection episodes within 6 months following dose 3 of the HPV vaccine. In 2014, a study initiated HPV vaccination in 14 pediatric KT recipients; unfortunately six of them developed acute rejection shortly after the initiation of the vaccine series, which lead to an early termination of the study (53). In contrast, in 2016, only two of the 23 pediatric KT recipients of HPV vaccination were reported to have acute rejection episodes (41). In our patient population, we report a similar acute rejection burden; upon chart review, it was felt that our two cases of acute rejection were related to medication non-adherence, as opposed to vaccine administration.

We acknowledge that our study has certain limitations. Like in many pediatric SOT studies, our study was limited by its small sample size. Unfortunately three subjects were missing information on medication use in the data collection form and some were not complete, thus impairing our ability to analyze the effect of specific immunosuppresion medications. Indeed, for specific vaccinations, for example influenza vaccination in KT recipients, it has been demonstrated that different imunosuppression regimens can influence the immune response (54). In addition, our study lacked long-term follow up, as we did not look into long-term HPV-vaccine induced antibody persistence post-transplantation; other studies suggested that there was a decline in titers over time (40). Lastly, we were unable to determine factors beyond immunosuppression that may play a role in preventing seroconversion in transplant recipients. However, this is the largest and the only multicenter study that examined the humoral response to the HPV vaccine in both girls and boys with KTs, compared to CKD and on dialysis. It is also the first study that compared the humoral response between girls and boys in these populations. In addition, we included only data for the subjects who were HPV naïve at baseline, had complete data in terms of antibody titers and completed the entire three dose vaccination series.

In conclusion, this study addresses the immune response to the HPV vaccine in pediatric KT recipients, CKD and dialysis patients, as well as its safety. The HPV vaccine was well-tolerated in these populations. Pediatric KT recipients had in general lower GMTs and seroconversion rates compared to their peers in the CKD and dialysis groups. In addition, immunosuppression (either due to the need to address immune-mediated diseases of the native kidneys or to prevent rejection in KT) played a role in the lack of seroconversion. Our results emphasize the importance of advocating for HPV vaccination prior to KT and acknowledge its safety post transplantation. However, questions still remain. Specifically, studies to identify factors associated with the lack of seroconversion in KT recipients are needed for targeted interventions. In addition, future studies should investigate the effect of a supplemental dose of HPV vaccine in KT recipients who do not seroconvert. It would also be important to evaluate the long-term persistence of antibodies post-KT and the possible need for re-immunization post-KT.

ETHICS STATEMENT

The studies involving human participants were reviewed and approved by Indiana University Office of Research Administration Institutional Board Review. Written informed consent to participate in this study was provided by the participants' legal guardian/next of kin.

AUTHOR CONTRIBUTIONS

CN generated the hypothesis, obtained funding, designed the study, recruited subjects at her institution, interpreted data, and wrote the manuscript. RN, PV, KT, AC, MM, and JM had solutions for improving design, recruited subjects at their respective institutions, and corrected the manuscript. JS analyzed and presented data, while also helping CN and MS write the statistics paragraph and interpret data. MS mentored and helped CN in all of the above endeavors.

ACKNOWLEDGMENTS

We thank Dr. Alfred Saah for the careful review of the manuscript.

REFERENCES

1. Kitchlu A, Dixon S, Dirk JS, Chanchlani R, Vasilevska-Ristovska J, Borges K, et al. Elevated risk of cancer after solid organ transplant in childhood: a population-based cohort study. *Transplantation.* (2019) 103:588–96. doi: 10.1097/TP.0000000000002378
2. Yanik EL, Smith JM, Shiels MS, Clarke CA, Lynch CF, Kahn AR, et al. Cancer risk after pediatric solid organ transplantation. *Pediatrics.* (2017) 139:e20163893. doi: 10.1542/peds.2016-3893
3. Hall EC, Pfeiffer RM, Segev DL, Engels EA. Cumulative incidence of cancer after solid organ transplantation. *Cancer.* (2013) 119:2300–8. doi: 10.1002/cncr.28043
4. D'Arcy ME, Coghill AE, Lynch CF, Koch LA, Li J, Pawlish KS, et al. Survival after a cancer diagnosis among solid organ transplant recipients in the United States. *Cancer.* (2019) 125:933–42. doi: 10.1002/cncr.31782
5. Smith JM, Martz K, Blydt-Hansen TD. Pediatric kidney transplant practice patterns and outcome benchmarks, 1987-2010: a report of the North American pediatric renal trials and collaborative studies. *Pediatr Transplant.* (2013) 17:149–57. doi: 10.1111/petr.12034
6. Awan AA, Niu J, Pan JS, Erickson KF, Mandayam S, Winkelmayer WC, et al. Trends in the causes of death among kidney transplant recipients in the United States (1996-2014). *Am J Nephrol.* (2018) 48:472–81. doi: 10.1159/000495081
7. Hinten F, Meeuwis KA, van Rossum MM, de Hullu JA. HPV-related (pre)malignancies of the female anogenital tract in

renal transplant recipients. *Crit Rev Oncol Hematol.* (2012) 84:161–80. doi: 10.1016/j.critrevonc.2012.02.008

8. Liao JB, Fisher CE, Madeleine MM. Gynecologic cancers and solid organ transplantation. *Am J Transplant.* (2019) 19:1266–77. doi: 10.1111/ajt.15292
9. Madeleine MM, Finch JL, Lynch CF, Goodman MT, Engels EA. HPV-related cancers after solid organ transplantation in the United States. *Am J Transplant.* (2013) 13:3202–9. doi: 10.1111/ajt.12472
10. Smith JS, Lindsay L, Hoots B, Keys J, Franceschi S, Winer R, et al. Human papillomavirus type distribution in invasive cervical cancer and high-grade cervical lesions: a meta-analysis update. *Int J Cancer.* (2007) 121:621–32. doi: 10.1002/ijc.22527
11. Antonsson A, Neale RE, Boros S, Lampe G, Coman WB, Pryor DI, et al. Human papillomavirus status and p16(INK4A) expression in patients with mucosal squamous cell carcinoma of the head and neck in Queensland, Australia. *Cancer Epidemiol.* (2015) 39:174–81. doi: 10.1016/j.canep.2015.01.010
12. Satterwhite CL, Torrone E, Meites E, Dunne EF, Mahajan R, Ocfemia MC, et al. Sexually transmitted infections among US women and men: prevalence and incidence estimates, 2008. *Sex Transm Dis.* (2013) 40:187–93. doi: 10.1097/OLQ.0b013e318286bb53
13. Komlos KF, Kocjan BJ, Kosorok P, Luzar B, Meglic L, Potocnik M, et al. Tumor-specific and gender-specific pre-vaccination distribution of human papillomavirus types 6 and 11 in anogenital warts and laryngeal papillomas: a study on 574 tissue specimens. *J Med Virol.* (2012) 84:1233–41. doi: 10.1002/jmv.23318
14. Orlando G, Bianchi S, Fasolo MM, Mazza F, Frati ER, Rizzardini G, et al. Cervical Human Papillomavirus genotypes in HIV-infected women: a cross-sectional analysis of the VALHIDATE study. *J Prev Med Hyg.* (2017) 58:E259–e65. doi: 10.15167/2421-4248/jpmh2017.58.4.804
15. Long ME, Chantigian PDM, Weaver AL. Cervical cytology and histology after solid organ transplant: a longitudinal cohort study. *J Low Genit Tract Dis.* (2018) 22:362–6. doi: 10.1097/LGT.0000000000000414
16. Veroux M, Corona D, Scalia G, Garozzo V, Gagliano M, Giuffrida G, et al. Surveillance of human papilloma virus infection and cervical cancer in kidney transplant recipients: preliminary data. *Transplant Proc.* (2009) 41:1191–4. doi: 10.1016/j.transproceed.2009.03.015
17. Berkhout RJ, Bouwes Bavinck JN, ter Schegget J. Persistence of human papillomavirus DNA in benign and (pre)malignant skin lesions from renal transplant recipients. *J Clin Microbiol.* (2000) 38:2087–96.
18. Pietrzak B, Mazanowska N, Ekiel AM, Durlik M, Martirosian G, Wielgos M, et al. Prevalence of high-risk human papillomavirus cervical infection in female kidney graft recipients: an observational study. *Virol J.* (2012) 9:117. doi: 10.1186/1743-422X-9-117
19. Meeuwis KA, Melchers WJ, Bouten H, van de Kerkhof PC, Hinten F, Quint WG, et al. Anogenital malignancies in women after renal transplantation over 40 years in a single center. *Transplantation.* (2012) 93:914–22. doi: 10.1097/TP.0b013e318249b13d
20. Busnach G, Piselli P, Arbustini E, Baccarani U, Burra P, Carrieri MP, et al. Immunosuppression and cancer: a comparison of risks in recipients of organ transplants and in HIV-positive individuals. *Transplant Proc.* (2006) 38:3533–5. doi: 10.1016/j.transproceed.2006.10.144
21. Guerra FM, Rosella LC, Dunn S, Wilson SE, Chen C, Deeks SL. Early impact of Ontario's human papillomavirus (HPV) vaccination program on anogenital warts (AGWs): A population-based assessment. *Vaccine.* (2016) 34:4678–83. doi: 10.1016/j.vaccine.2016.08.020
22. Niccolai LM, Meek JI, Brackney M, Hadler JL, Sosa LE, Weinberger DM. Declines in Human Papillomavirus (HPV)-associated high-grade cervical lesions after introduction of HPV vaccines in connecticut, United States, 2008-2015. *Clin Infect Dis.* (2017) 65:884–9. doi: 10.1093/cid/cix455
23. Arbyn M, Xu L. Efficacy and safety of prophylactic HPV vaccines. a Cochrane review of randomized trials. *Expert Rev Vaccines.* (2018) 17:1085–91. doi: 10.1080/14760584.2018.1548282
24. Collins S, Mazloomzadeh S, Winter H, Blomfield P, Bailey A, Young LS, et al. High incidence of cervical human papillomavirus infection in women during their first sexual relationship. *BJOG.* (2002) 109:96–8. doi: 10.1111/j.1471-0528.2002.01053.x
25. Castellino SM, Allen KE, Pleasant K, Keyes G, Poehling KA, Tooze JA. Suboptimal uptake of human papillomavirus (HPV) vaccine in survivors of childhood and adolescent and young adult (AYA) cancer. *J Cancer Surviv* (2019) 13:730–8. doi: 10.1007/s11764-019-00791-9
26. Fox TG, Nailescu C. Vaccinations in pediatric kidney transplant recipients. *Pediatr Nephrol.* (2019) 34:579–91. doi: 10.1007/s00467-018-3953-z
27. Danziger-Isakov L, Kumar D. Vaccination in solid organ transplantation. *Am J Transplant.* (2013) 13 (Suppl. 4):311–7. doi: 10.1111/ajt.12122
28. Centers for Disease Control and Prevention (CDC). Recommendations on the use of quadrivalent human papillomavirus vaccine in males–Advisory Committee on Immunization Practices (ACIP), 2011. *MMWR Morb Mortal Wkly Rep.* (2011) 60:1705–8.
29. Dempsey AF, Patel DA. HPV vaccine acceptance, utilization and expected impacts in the U.S.: Where are we now? *Hum Vaccin.* (2010) 6:715–20. doi: 10.4161/hv.6.9.12730
30. Donahue KL, Stupiansky NW, Alexander AB, Zimet GD. Acceptability of the human papillomavirus vaccine and reasons for non-vaccination among parents of adolescent sons. *Vaccine.* (2014) 32:3883–5. doi: 10.1016/j.vaccine.2014.05.035
31. Petrosky E, Bocchini JA Jr, Hariri S, Chesson H, Curtis CR, Saraiya M, et al. Use of 9-valent human papillomavirus (HPV) vaccine: updated HPV vaccination recommendations of the advisory committee on immunization practices. *MMWR Morb Mortal Wkly Rep.* (2015) 64:300–4.
32. Lindberg LD, Maddow-Zimet I, Marcell AV. Prevalence of sexual initiation before Age 13 years among male adolescents and young adults in the United States. *JAMA Pediatr.* 2019. doi: 10.1001/jamapediatrics.2019.0458
33. Gambadauro P, Carli V, Hadlaczky G, Sarchiapone M, Apter A, Balazs J, et al. Correlates of sexual initiation among European adolescents. *PloS ONE.* (2018) 13:e0191451. doi: 10.1371/journal.pone.0191451
34. Kahn NF, Halpern CT. Associations between patterns of sexual initiation, sexual partnering, and sexual health outcomes from adolescence to early adulthood. *Arch Sex Behav.* (2018) 47:1791–810. doi: 10.1007/s10508-018-1176-9
35. Franke D, Winkel S, Gellermann J, Querfeld U, Pape L, Ehrich JH, et al. Growth and maturation improvement in children on renal replacement therapy over the past 20 years. *Pediatr Nephrol.* (2013) 28:2043–51. doi: 10.1007/s00467-013-2502-z
36. Wilkin T, Lee JY, Lensing SY, Stier EA, Goldstone SE, Berry JM, et al. Safety and immunogenicity of the quadrivalent human papillomavirus vaccine in HIV-1-infected men. *J Infect Dis.* (2010) 202:1246–53. doi: 10.1086/656320
37. Levin MJ, Moscicki AB, Song LY, Fenton T, Meyer WA, 3rd, Read JS, et al. Safety and immunogenicity of a quadrivalent human papillomavirus (types 6, 11, 16, and 18) vaccine in HIV-infected children 7 to 12 years old. *J Acquir Immune Defic Syndr.* (2010) 55:197–204. doi: 10.1097/QAI.0b013e3181de8d26
38. Weinberg A, Song LY, Saah A, Brown M, Moscicki AB, Meyer WA, 3rd, et al. Humoral, mucosal, and cell-mediated immunity against vaccine and nonvaccine genotypes after administration of quadrivalent human papillomavirus vaccine to HIV-infected children. *J Infect Dis.* (2012) 206:1309–18. doi: 10.1093/infdis/jis489
39. Brown DR, Garland SM, Ferris DG, Joura E, Steben M, James M, et al. The humoral response to Gardasil over four years as defined by total IgG and competitive Luminex immunoassay. *Hum Vaccin.* (2011) 7:230–8. doi: 10.4161/hv.7.2.13948
40. Kumar D, Unger ER, Panicker G, Medvedev P, Wilson L, Humar A. Immunogenicity of quadrivalent human papillomavirus vaccine in organ transplant recipients. *Am J Transplant.* (2013) 13:2411–7. doi: 10.1111/ajt.12329
41. Nelson DR, Neu AM, Abraham A, Amaral S, Batisky D, Fadrowski JJ. Immunogenicity of human papillomavirus recombinant vaccine in children with CKD. *Clin J Am Soc Nephrol.* (2016) 11:776–84. doi: 10.2215/CJN.09690915
42. Chonchol M. Neutrophil dysfunction and infection risk in end-stage renal disease. *Semin Dial.* (2006) 19:291–6. doi: 10.1111/j.1525-139X.2006.00175.x
43. Dalrymple LS, Go AS. Epidemiology of acute infections among patients with chronic kidney disease. *Clin J Am Soc Nephrol.* (2008) 3:1487–93. doi: 10.2215/CJN.01290308
44. Schulman SL, Deforest A, Kaiser BA, Polinsky MS, Baluarte HJ. Response to measles-mumps-rubella vaccine in children on dialysis. *Pediatr Nephrol.* (1992) 6:187–9. doi: 10.1007/BF00866312

45. Fadrowski JJ, Furth SL. Varicella zoster virus: vaccination and implications in children with renal failure. *Expert Rev Vaccines.* (2004) 3:291–8. doi: 10.1586/14760584.3.3.291
46. Praditpornsilpa K, Kingwatanakul P, Deekajorndej T, Rianthavorn P, Susantitaphong P, Katavetin P, et al. Immunogenicity and safety of quadrivalent human papillomavirus types 6/11/16/18 recombinant vaccine in chronic kidney disease stage IV, V and VD. *Nephrol Dial Transplant.* (2017) 32:132–6. doi: 10.1093/ndt/gfv444
47. Block SL, Nolan T, Sattler C, Barr E, Giacoletti KE, Marchant CD, et al. Comparison of the immunogenicity and reactogenicity of a prophylactic quadrivalent human papillomavirus (types 6, 11, 16, and 18) L1 virus-like particle vaccine in male and female adolescents and young adult women. *Pediatrics.* (2006) 118:2135–45. doi: 10.1542/peds.2006-0461
48. Ferris D, Samakoses R, Block SL, Lazcano-Ponce E, Restrepo JA, Reisinger KS, et al. Long-term study of a quadrivalent human papillomavirus vaccine. *Pediatrics.* (2014) 134:e657–65. doi: 10.1542/peds.2013-4144
49. Klein SL, Marriott I, Fish EN. Sex-based differences in immune function and responses to vaccination. *Trans R Soc Trop Med Hyg.* (2015) 109:9–15. doi: 10.1093/trstmh/tru167
50. Furman D, Hejblum BP, Simon N, Jojic V, Dekker CL, Thiebaut R, et al. Systems analysis of sex differences reveals an immunosuppressive role for testosterone in the response to influenza vaccination. *Proc Natl Acad Sci USA.* (2014) 111:869–74. doi: 10.1073/pnas.1321060111
51. Bhat M, Mara K, Dierkhising R, Watt KDS. Immunosuppression, race, and donor-related risk factors affect de novo cancer incidence across solid organ transplant recipients. *Mayo Clin Proc.* (2018) 93:1236–46. doi: 10.1016/j.mayocp.2018.04.025
52. Choi Y, Eworuke E, Segal R. What explains the different rates of human papillomavirus vaccination among adolescent males and females in the United States? *Papillomavirus Res.* (2016) 2:46–51. doi: 10.1016/j.pvr.2016.02.001
53. Gomez-Lobo V, Whyte T, Kaufman S, Torres C, Moudgil A. Immunogenicity of a prophylactic quadrivalent human papillomavirus L1 virus-like particle vaccine in male and female adolescent transplant recipients. *Pediatr Transplant.* (2014) 18:310–5. doi: 10.1111/petr.12226
54. Nailescu C, Xu X, Zhou H, Hall H, Wilson AC, Leiser JD, et al. Influenza vaccine after pediatric kidney transplant: a Midwest Pediatric Nephrology Consortium study. *Pediatr Nephrol.* (2011) 26:459–67. doi: 10.1007/s00467-010-1729-1

2

Pediatric Immunization Practices in Nephrotic Syndrome: An Assessment of Provider and Parental Knowledge

Cheryl L. Tran[1], David T. Selewski[2], Gia J. Oh[3], Jonathan P. Troost[4], Susan F. Massengill[5], Samhar I. Al-Akash[6], Shefali Mahesh[7], Rasheda Amin[8,9], Isa F. Ashoor[10], Rahul Chanchlani[11], Mahmoud Kallash[12], Robert P. Woroniecki[13] and Debbie S. Gipson[14]*

[1] Division of Pediatric Nephrology, Department of Pediatrics, Mayo Clinic, Rochester, MN, United States, [2] Division of Pediatric Nephrology, Department of Pediatrics, Medical University of South Carolina, Charleston, SC, United States, [3] Division of Nephrology, Department of Pediatrics, Stanford University, Stanford, CA, United States, [4] Michigan Institute for Clinical and Health Research, University of Michigan, Ann Arbor, MI, United States, [5] Levine Children's Hospital at Atrium Health, Charlotte, NC, United States, [6] Driscoll Children's Hospital, Corpus Christi, TX, United States, [7] Division of Nephrology and Dialysis, Akron Children's Hospital, Akron, OH, United States, [8] Pediatric Specialists of Virginia, Fairfax, VA, United States, [9] Department of Pediatrics, George Washington University, Washington, DC, United States, [10] Division of Nephrology, Department of Pediatrics, Louisiana State University, New Orleans, LA, United States, [11] Division of Pediatric Nephrology, Department of Pediatrics, McMaster University, Hamilton, ON, Canada, [12] Division of Nephrology, Nationwide Children's Hospital, Columbus, OH, United States, [13] Division of Pediatric Nephrology and Hypertension, Stony Brook Children's Hospital and Renaissance School of Medicine, Stony Brook, NY, United States, [14] Division of Pediatric Nephrology, Department of Pediatrics, University of Michigan, Ann Arbor, MI, United States

***Correspondence:**
Cheryl L. Tran
tran.cheryl2@mayo.edu*

Background: Children with nephrotic syndrome (NS) are at high risk for vaccine-preventable infections due to the immunological effects from the disease and concurrent treatment with immunosuppressive medications. Immunizations in these patients may be deferred due to their immunosuppressive treatment which may increase the risk for vaccine-preventable infections. Immunization practices in children with NS continue to vary among pediatric nephrologists. This raises the question of whether children with NS are receiving the recommended vaccinations at appropriate times. Therefore, it is critical to understand the practices and patient education provided by physicians to patients on the topic of vaccinations.

Methods: After informed consent, parents/guardians of 153 pediatric patients (<18 years old) diagnosed with NS from 2005 to 2018 and 50 pediatric nephrologists from 11 participating centers completed anonymous surveys to evaluate immunization practices among pediatric nephrologists, assess the vaccine education provided to families of children with NS, assess the parental knowledge of immunization recommendations, and assess predictors of polysaccharide pneumococcal vaccine adherence. The Advisory Committee on Immunization Practices (ACIP) Immunization 2019 Guideline for those with altered immunocompetence was used to determine accuracy of vaccine knowledge and practices.

Results: Forty-four percent of providers self-reported adherence to the ACIP guidelines for inactive vaccines and 22% to the guidelines for live vaccines. Thirty-two percent of parents/guardians reported knowledge that aligned with the ACIP guidelines for inactive vaccines and 1% for live vaccines. Subjects residing in the Midwest and provider recommendations for vaccines were positive predictors of vaccine adherence ($p < 0.001$ and p 0.02, respectively).

Conclusions: Vaccine recommendation by medical providers is paramount in vaccine adherence among pediatric patients with NS. This study identifies potential educational opportunities for medical subspecialty providers and family caregivers about immunization recommendations for immunosuppressed patients.

Keywords: nephrotic syndrome, children, immunization, immunosuppression, education

INTRODUCTION

Nephrotic syndrome (NS) is caused by renal diseases that affect the permeability of the glomerular filtration barrier resulting in massive proteinuria, including immunoglobulins and complement proteins (1–4). Given the immunological effects from the disease and concurrent treatment with immunosuppressive medications, children with NS are at high risk for severe bacterial infections, especially with encapsulated bacteria (5). *Streptococcus pneumoniae* is a common encapsulated bacterial pathogen that is known to cause serious infections in children with NS (6, 7). Given the risk for this infectious pathogen, the pneumococcal polysaccharide vaccine (PPSV 23) has been specifically recommended for pediatric patients with certain medical conditions/diseases (i.e., NS, chronic renal failure, and immunosuppression medications). This susceptibility to infection extends beyond bacterial infections and includes serious viral infections such as Varicella, which can result in severe disseminated infections in immunocompromised hosts.

Children with NS have a high burden of healthcare utilization with a mean charge per hospitalization of $26,500 that exceeds many other chronic illnesses (8). Gipson et al. evaluated hospitalization costs in a cohort of children with NS and clearly showed that serious complications of NS, including infection, occur commonly and increase healthcare costs. In this study, 16% of 9,934 discharges in 2006 and 2009 had at least one severe complication (pneumonia, sepsis, peritonitis, thromboembolism, or diabetes) attributable to NS or its treatment. Infection-related complications were the most common including pneumonia, sepsis, or peritonitis. In 2019, Carpenter et al. investigated the prevalence of infection and venous thromboembolism in hospitalized pediatric patients with NS (9). This group demonstrated high rates of infection in hospitalized pediatric NS patients, with *Streptococcus pneumoniae* being the most common pathogen. Appreciating the infectious susceptibility associated with nephrotic syndrome is critical since improved vaccination practices would potentially aid in the prevention of many of these infections (10, 11).

This raises the question of whether children with NS are receiving the recommended vaccinations at appropriate times. A critical first step in this process is to understand the practices and patient education provided by physicians to patients on the topic of vaccinations. The aims of this are: (1) evaluate the immunization practices among pediatric nephrologists, (2) assess the education provided to families of children with NS by the pediatric nephrology providers, (3) assess the parental knowledge and understanding of these immunization recommendations, and (4) assess predictors of PPSV 23 adherence.

Abbreviations: ACIP, Advisory Committee on Immunization Practices; AAP, American Academy of Pediatrics; CDC, Center for Disease Control; NS, nephrotic syndrome; PPSV 23, pneumococcal polysaccharide vaccine; PCP, primary care provider.

METHODS

Parents/guardians of pediatric patients (<18 years old) diagnosed with NS from 2005 to 2018 from 11 institutions in the Pediatric Nephrology Research Consortium and Kidney Research Network participated in the study. Patient inclusion criteria were children <18 years old with primary NS diagnosed between 2005 and 2018 who were seen in the pediatric nephrology practice at the participating center on at least one occasion. All pediatric nephrologists at the participating study centers were also included in the study. A parent/guardian survey was distributed, and a separate pediatric nephrology provider survey was distributed to pediatric nephrologists at each center. This study was performed in line with the principles of the Declaration of Helsinki. Institutional Review Boards of each participating center approved the study. Consent and assent were obtained per institutional guidelines.

Survey and Measures

The parent/guardian survey contained 24 questions which were created by the authors and included demographic data, immunosuppression history, parental knowledge of immunization recommendations and their intent to follow the recommendations, and potentially vaccine-preventable hospitalizations for infections. The provider survey contained 21 questions which were created by the authors and included demographic data, provider immunization recommendation practices, knowledge of the current immunization guidelines, and hospitalizations for infections at any time during their practice that may have been vaccine-preventable. Family caregivers/study coordinators provided redacted copies of patient immunization records. Validation studies of self-administered surveys have shown this type of survey methodology to be a promising tool across medical disciplines (12–14). Surveys were self-administered by the families and providers in the clinic office. The surveys are provided in the **Supplementary Material 1, 2**.

The Advisory Committee on Immunization Practices (ACIP) Recommended Child and Adolescent Immunization Schedule was used to determine accuracy of parent and provider knowledge of current immunization guidelines (**Figure 1**) (15). In brief summary, the ACIP recommends inactive vaccines for any pediatric patient who is not receiving immunosuppression

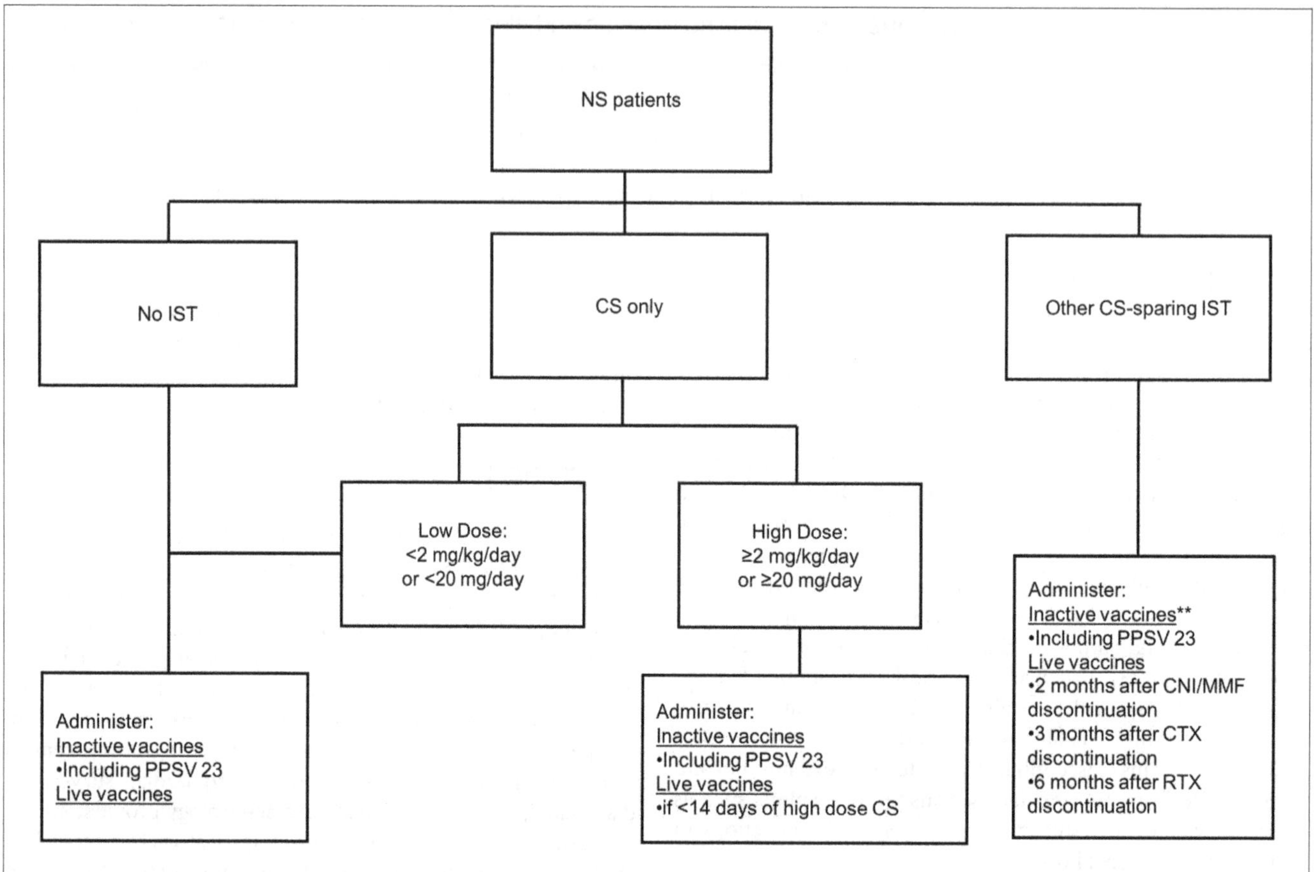

FIGURE 1 | Flow diagram of abbreviated vaccine guidelines. Information for this was adapted from the Advisory Committee on Immunization Practices 2019 vaccine guidelines. Abbreviations: NS, nephrotic syndrome; IST, immunosuppression; CS, corticosteroids; PPSV 23, polysaccharide pneumococcal vaccine; CNI, calcineurin inhibitor; MMF, mycophenolate mofetil; CTX, cyclophosphamide; RTX, rituximab. **Defer 6 months after RTX discontinuation, or administer if no finite endpoint for RTX and assess titers after discontinuation of RTX.

medications as well as those on most immunosuppression therapies. There is an exception to consider deferring inactive vaccines for 6 months after receiving B-cell depleting therapy, or may consider administration of inactive vaccines while receiving B-cell depleting therapy with assessment of titers after discontinuation of the B-cell depleting agent. With regards to live vaccines, the ACIP recommends administration of live vaccines in patients who are not on immunosuppression therapy; patients who have received <14 days of high dose corticosteroids; and patients who have been off of Calcineurin inhibitors (CNI)/Mycophenolate Mofetil (MMF) for 2 months, off of cytotoxic agents (i.e., Cyclophosphamide) for 3 months, and off of B-cell depleting agents (i.e., Rituximab) for 6 months. A more detailed summary of this guideline is provided in **Supplementary Material 3.**

Patient demographic variables included state of residence, patient age, race, parent/guardian level of education, and household income. Provider demographic variables included institution, type of practice (academic vs. private), type of subspecialty training (Pediatric Nephrology, Internal Medicine-Pediatric Nephrology, or Internal Medicine Nephrology), and percent effort allocated to clinical care.

Statistical Analysis

Descriptive statistics included frequencies for categorical variables and mean ± standard deviation (SD) or median (IQR) for continuous variables, as appropriate. Fischer's exact tests were used to compare knowledge and guidelines across regions, and evaluate predictors of PPSV 23 vaccination. Multivariable logistic regression was used to test independent predictors of PPSV 23 vaccination. Variables with unadjusted $p < 0.2$ entered a multivariable model and were removed in descending order until all remaining terms were significant. For all analyses, $p \leq 0.05$ were considered statistically significant.

RESULTS

Study Population Demographics

Between November 2015 and December 2018, 175 pediatric patients diagnosed with NS between January 2005 and December 2018, from 11 North American centers, were eligible for the study, of which 153 parents/guardians of pediatric subjects consented to the study and completed the anonymous survey (parent/guardian response rate 87.4%). Fifty-eight pediatric nephrologists at participating centers were provided an

TABLE 1a | Demographic description of pediatric nephrotic syndrome subject population.

Variable	NS subject study participants $n = 153$
Current Age (y), n (%)	
0–5	46 (30)
6–11	70 (46)
12–22	37 (24)
Age at Diagnosis (y), n (%)	
0–5	117 (76)
6–11	30 (20)
12–18	6 (4)
Race, n (%)	
Asian/Pacific Islander	21 (14)
Black/African American	27 (18)
Hispanic/Latino	25 (16)
Native American	4 (3)
White/Caucasian	62 (40)
Other	14 (9)
Region of care, n (%)	
Coastal	28 (18)
Midwest	64 (42)
South	61 (40)
Highest level of parent education, n (%)	
No schooling to 8th grade	3 (2)
Some high school to high school graduate	30 (20)
Some college, college graduate, or vocational training	87 (57)
Some postgraduate work to postgraduate degree	30 (20)
Decline to answer	3 (2)
Household annual income, n (%)	
<$25,000	32 (21)
$25,000–$39,999	22 (14)
$40,000–$49,999	7 (5)
$50,000–$74,999	15 (10)
$75,000–$99,999	20 (13)
>$100,000	44 (29)
Decline to answer	13 (8)
Immunosuppression exposure, n (%)	
Calcineurin inhibitor	94 (61)
Cyclophosphamide	19 (12)
Mycophenolate mofetil	55 (36)
Prednisone	143 (93)
Rituximab	23 (15)
Other	3 (2)
None	2 (1)
Number of times seen by pediatric nephrology provider in the past year	
Once	9 (6)
2–3 times	63 (41)
≥4 times	81 (53)

TABLE 1b | Demographic description of pediatric nephrology provider population.

Variable	Pediatric nephrology provider participants $n = 50$
Region, n (%)	
Coastal	12 (24)
Midwest	21 (42)
South	17 (34)
Type of practice, n (%)	
Academic	43 (86)
Private	4 (8)
Both academic & private	3 (6)
Type of subspecialty training, n (%)	
Pediatric nephrology	47 (94)
Internal medicine-pediatric nephrology	3 (6)
Provider percent effort, median (IQR)	
Clinical care to pediatric patients	70 (55–86)
Clinical care to adult patients	0 (0)
Administration	4 (0–20)
Research	5 (0–16)
Education	5 (0–10)

anonymous survey, of which 50 (86.2%) completed the survey. All subjects were stratified by region [Coastal (3 centers), Midwest (4 centers), and South (4 centers)]. Due to the small number of study centers on either coast, the current study grouped these centers into one "Coastal" region to avoid identifying a single site and its study participants.

At study enrollment (**Table 1a**), the median age at NS diagnosis was 3 years of age (IQR 2-5); nearly half of the pediatric patients (46%) were 6–11 years of age at study enrollment; 40% were White; majority of parents/guardians had some post high school education (77%); and nearly all pediatric patients had exposure to immunosuppression (99%). In the pediatric nephrology provider population (**Table 1b**), the majority practiced in an academic setting (86%); majority trained specifically in Pediatric Nephrology (94%); and all provided care to pediatric patients with the median percent effort allocated to clinical care of 70% (IQR 55–86%).

Pediatric Nephrology Provider Vaccine Recommendations

Table 2 displays the pediatric nephrology provider recommendations for inactive vaccines. All providers indicated that they provide recommendations for inactive vaccines to patients. Eighty-two percent recommended inactive vaccines while off of steroids and in remission, and 78% recommended inactive vaccines on low dose steroids. However, only 44% recommended inactive vaccines while on high dose steroids with 58% recommending inactive vaccines when off of other immunosuppressive medications. Only 44% recommended inactive vaccines at any time regardless of immunosuppression status. Overall, 56% of providers had at least one response inconsistent with guidelines.

Table 3 displays the pediatric nephrology provider recommendations for live vaccines. Of the 50 providers surveyed, only 1 (2%) indicated they did not provide live vaccine recommendations to patients. Seventy-eight percent recommended live vaccines while off steroids and in remission; however, only 30% recommended live vaccines while on low dose steroids. All providers recommended avoiding live vaccines while on daily high dose steroids, and 76% recommended

TABLE 2 | Provider inactive vaccine recommendation.

Inactive immunizations	Total $N = 50$ (%)	Coastal $N = 12$ (%)	Midwest $N = 21$ (%)	South $N = 17$ (%)	Fischer's exact p
I do not provide recommendations regarding INACTIVE immunizations	0 (0)	0 (0)	0 (0)	0 (0)	–
I provide/recommend when the patient is...					
a. Off steroids and in remission	41 (82)	10 (83)	16 (76)	15 (88)	0.73
b. On low dose (every other day) steroids	39 (78)	10 (83)	17 (81)	12 (71)	0.75
c. On daily high dose steroids	22 (44)	5 (42)	7 (33)	10 (59)	0.28
d. Off other immunosuppressive medications (i.e., cyclosporine, tacrolimus, mycophenolate mofetil, cyclophosphamide, rituximab)	29 (58)	9 (75)	9 (43)	11 (65)	0.18
I would not alter the immunization schedule for INACTIVE immunizations in patients with NS. They can receive them at any time	22 (44)	5 (42)	7 (33)	10 (59)	0.28
I would never provide an INACTIVE immunization to a NS patient regardless of therapy or remission status	0 (0)	0 (0)	0 (0)	0 (0)	–
All responses consistent with guidelines	22 (44)	5 (42)	7 (33)	10 (59)	0.28

Data are shown as number (percent).
NS, nephrotic syndrome.

receiving live vaccines while off other immunosuppressive medication. Overall, only 22% of provider's responses were in complete agreement with the ACIP guidelines for live vaccines. The main deviance from the ACIP guidelines was with respect to low dose steroids. Of the 39 providers that did not follow guidelines, 35 (90%) indicated they would not recommend live vaccines while on low dose steroids.

Pediatric NS Parent/Guardian Vaccine Knowledge

Table 4 shows the parent/guardian knowledge of recommended inactive vaccines. Out of 153 respondents, 13% indicated that no one told them when it was acceptable to receive inactive immunizations. Of the remaining, only 48% indicated that inactive vaccines could be administered while off steroids and in remission with 38% indicating that inactive vaccines could be given on low dose steroids. Only 33% indicated that inactive vaccines could be administered while on high dose steroids with 33% indicating that inactive vaccines could be given when off other immunosuppressive medications. Overall, 32% of parents/guardian responses suggested understanding of immunization practices that aligned with ACIP guidelines for inactive vaccines.

Table 5 shows the parent/guardian knowledge of recommended live vaccines. Twenty percent of parents/guardians indicated that no one told them when it was acceptable to receive live immunizations. Of the remaining, 27% indicated that live vaccines could be administered while off steroids and in remission; 8% indicated that live vaccines could be given while on low dose steroids; and 4% of parents/guardians indicated that live vaccines could be administered on high dose steroids. Twenty-one percent indicated that live vaccines could be administered when off other immunosuppression medications. Overall, 1% of parent/guardian responses suggested an understanding of current live vaccination best practices.

Pediatric NS Patient Immunization Status Validation and Predictors

One-hundred and 52 parents/guardians of pediatric NS subjects (99%) indicated that their child had been vaccinated and one pediatric NS subject (1%) had never been vaccinated. Records of vaccinations were available from 141 (93%) participants for validation of immunization status. Immunization status was considered up to date if the subject received all ACIP recommended vaccines based on immunosuppression status, age at time of survey, and vaccine release date. One-hundred and twenty-two subjects (87%) were up to date on the recommended vaccines. Fifty-three percent received the 7-valent pneumococcal vaccine, 71% received the 13-valent pneumococcal vaccine, and 48% received the PPSV 23.

Subjects residing in the Midwest was a positive predictor of subjects receiving the PPSV 23 ($p < 0.001$). Additionally, receiving immunization recommendations from the pediatric nephrology provider was a positive predictor of subjects receiving the PPSV 23 as well (p 0.02) (**Table 6**). Multivariable logistic regression of the differences in **Table 6** revealed that region and immunization recommendations were independent predictors of vaccinations. Those in the Coastal region were less likely to be vaccinated than the Midwest (OR = 0.30 95% CI = 0.13–0.66) and those with recommendations from the pediatric nephrologist were more likely to be vaccinated than those without recommendations (OR = 1.95 95% CI = 1.05–3.63) (**Table 7**). When provider responses were reviewed, providers in the Coastal region were less likely to review immunization records on a periodic basis ($p < 0.01$) and were more likely to state that they were unsure if they would recommend the

TABLE 3 | Provider live vaccine recommendation.

Live immunizations	Total $N = 50$ (%)	Coastal $N = 12$ (%)	Midwest $N = 21$ (%)	South $N = 17$ (%)	Fischer's exact p
I do not provide recommendations regarding LIVE immunizations	1 (2)	0 (0)	1 (5)	0 (0)	0.99
I provide/recommend when the patient is...					
a. Off steroids and in remission	39 (78)	9 (75)	17 (81)	13 (76)	0.91
b. On low dose (every other day) steroids	15 (30)	3 (25)	7 (33)	5 (29)	0.93
c. On daily high dose steroids	0 (0)	0 (0)	0 (0)	0 (0)	–
d. Off other immunosuppressive medications (i.e., cyclosporine, tacrolimus, mycophenolate mofetil, cyclophosphamide, rituximab)	38 (76)	10 (83)	15 (71)	13 (76)	0.91
I would not alter the immunization schedule for LIVE immunizations in patients with NS. They can receive them at any time	0 (0)	0 (0)	0 (0)	0 (0)	–
I would never provide a LIVE immunization to a NS patient regardless of therapy or remission status	0 (0)	0 (0)	0 (0)	0 (0)	–
All responses consistent with guidelines	11 (22)	3 (25)	5 (24)	3 (18)	0.83

Data are shown as number (percent).
NS, nephrotic syndrome.

TABLE 4 | Parent inactive vaccine recommendation.

Inactive immunizations	Total $N = 153$ N (%)	Coastal $N = 28$ N (%)	Midwest $N = 64$ N (%)	South $N = 61$ N (%)	Fischer's exact p
No one ever told me when it was ok to receive INACTIVE immunizations.	20 (13)	6 (21)	4 (6)	10 (16)	0.07
I was told it was OK to receive INACTIVE immunizations when my child is...					
a. Off steroids and in remission	74 (48)	12 (43)	39 (61)	23 (38)	0.03
b. On Low dose (every other day) steroids	58 (38)	8 (29)	30 (47)	20 (33)	0.15
c. On daily high dose steroids	50 (33)	8 (29)	24 (38)	18 (30)	0.57
d. Off other immunosuppressive medications (i.e., cyclosporine, tacrolimus, mycophenolate mofetil, cyclophosphamide, rituximab)	51 (33)	7 (25)	24 (38)	20 (33)	0.56
I was told that my child could receive INACTIVE immunizations at any time regardless of type of medication or remission status.	49 (32)	7 (25)	24 (38)	18 (30)	0.47
I was told that my child could never receive INACTIVE immunizations.	0 (0)	0 (0)	0 (0)	0 (0)	–
Parent had correct knowledge of guidelines	49 (32)	7 (25)	24 (38)	18 (30)	0.47

Data are shown as number (percent).

PPSV23 if the patient had previously received the 7-valent pneumococcal conjugate vaccine (PCV) or PCV-13 (p 0.03) (**Supplementary Material 4**).

DISCUSSION

While there have been published studies investigating vaccine practices and vaccine adherence patterns, these studies have evaluated the medical provider population alone or the parent population alone. Our study investigates both the subspecialty medical provider and parent population from the same institution and region simultaneously. This study demonstrates gaps in vaccine knowledge of both pediatric nephrology providers and parents of children with NS who are immunosuppressed.

The decision to vaccinate a child can be influenced by parental knowledge, parental understanding of the benefits of vaccination, provider knowledge, and other complex factors related to their child's underlying disease and treatment. Deficiencies in vaccinations directly impact the health of the individual child and of the larger pediatric community if herd protection is not achieved due to poor vaccine adherence. Children most at risk for severe vaccine-preventable infections are those who are immunocompromised, which includes children with NS.

TABLE 5 | Parent live vaccine recommendation.

Live immunizations	Total N = 153 N (%)	Coastal N = 28 N (%)	Midwest N = 64 N (%)	South N = 61 N (%)	Fischer's exact p
No one ever told me when it was ok to receive LIVE immunizations.	30 (20)	10 (36)	9 (14)	11 (18)	0.05
I was told it was OK to receive LIVE immunizations when my child is...					
a. Off steroids and in remission	41 (27)	6 (21)	21 (33)	14 (23)	0.37
b. On low dose (every other day) steroids	12 (8)	0 (0)	9 (14)	3 (5)	0.05
c. On daily high dose steroids	6 (4)	0 (0)	4 (6)	2 (3)	0.56
d. Off other immunosuppressive medications (i.e., cyclosporine, tacrolimus, mycophenolate mofetil, cyclophosphamide, rituximab)	32 (21)	2 (7)	21 (33)	9 (15)	0.007
I was told that my child could receive LIVE immunizations at any time regardless of type of medication or remission status.	5 (3)	0 (0)	4 (6)	1 (2)	0.27
I was told that my child could never receive LIVE immunizations.	18 (12)	5 (18)	7 (11)	6 (10)	0.57
Parent had correct knowledge of guidelines	1 (1)	0 (0)	0 (0)	1 (2)	0.58

Data are shown as number (percent).

The Center for Disease Control (CDC), ACIP, and the Committee on Infectious Diseases of the American Academy of Pediatrics (AAP) release an updated recommended immunization schedule for healthy children annually (16). This immunization schedule is available to medical providers online (http://www.cdc.gov/vaccines/recs/schedules/child-schedule.htm). In addition to the yearly updated recommendations, health care providers should be aware of guidelines for vaccinating immunocompromised patients, which are readily available online (https://www.cdc.gov/vaccines/hcp/acip-recs/general-recs/immunocompetence.html and https://www.cdc.gov/vaccines/schedules/downloads/child/0-18yrs-child-combined-schedule.pdf). Despite these guidelines and published comprehensive reviews outlining vaccine guidelines in various immunosuppressed states, there remains a discrepancy in vaccine practices among pediatric nephrologists in the management of children with NS on immunosuppressive therapy (17–19).

The discrepancy in vaccine practice amongst providers and low compliance in following ACIP guidelines is likely multifactorial. It could be in part due to the provider's misinterpretation of vaccine guidelines due to the complex immunosuppression regimens that these NS patients may require, or the provider's disagreement of vaccination guidelines based on anecdotal experience with NS relapses and/or belief that immunosuppressed patients may not mount a robust vaccine response. In this study, only 44% of provider responses were in complete alignment with the ACIP guidelines for inactive vaccines and 22% for live vaccines. The CDC general principles for those with altered immunocompetence, state that inactivated vaccines could be deferred during a time of immunosuppression since vaccines may be less effective during this period. However, if an inactivated vaccine is given during the time that a patient is immunosuppressed, then the inactive vaccine may need to be repeated when immune function has improved. Yet, the CDC guidelines emphasize the need for immunocompromised patients to receive certain inactive conjugated and polysaccharide-based vaccines (i.e., pneumococcal vaccines, *Haemophilus influenzae* type b, and meningococcal vaccines) due to the increased risk for disease if the vaccine is withheld. Live vaccines are typically deferred until immune function has improved due to the risk of uninhibited growth of the attenuated live virus or bacteria in those with altered immunocompetence (20–23). It is clear that the vaccine guidelines for those who are immunosuppressed can be nuanced.

Since 80% of pediatric patients with new onset NS are steroid-sensitive and eventually taper off of steroid therapy, some pediatric nephrologists may opt to withhold vaccines until these patients have return of immune function to help mount a more effective response to the vaccine (24). In our study, 44% of the pediatric nephrologists surveyed reported withholding inactive vaccines when a NS patient is on any dose of steroids due to concern that the patient may not mount an immune response. Ten percent of the pediatric nephrologists surveyed observed a NS relapse after immunization administration. However, published studies have demonstrated vaccine efficacy in NS patients who are immunosuppressed. Aoun and Ulinski exhibited good serologic response to the PPSV 23 in children with NS on high dose prednisone in the short term and in the long term (25). They also demonstrated that the long term pneumococcal antibody response was not impacted by other immunosuppressive agents (26). Hsu et al. demonstrated good vaccine efficacy of the pneumococcal vaccine in children with NS on high dose steroids and no differences in rate of NS relapse (27). In addition, other inactive polysaccharide-based vaccines, such as meningococcal C conjugate vaccine has not been shown to be associated with increased NS relapses (28). Other studies have demonstrated that the Varicella vaccine has been well-tolerated in children with NS and highly immunogenic in those on low-dose, every other day prednisone (29, 30). Despite these groups demonstrating vaccine efficacy without differences in

TABLE 6 | Pediatric NS patient PPSV 23 vaccine adherence and predictors*.

Variable	N (% NS children vaccinated to PPSV 23)	N (% NS children unvaccinated to PPSV 23)	Fischer's exact *p*
Parent income (*N* = 125)			0.30
<$25,000 (*n* = 29)	17 (58.6)	12 (41.4)	
$25,000–39,999 (*n* = 19)	8 (42.1)	11 (57.9)	
$40,000–49,999 (*n* = 7)	14 (57.1)	3 (42.9)	
$50,000–74,999 (*n* = 15)	11 (73.3)	4 (26.7)	
$75,000–99,999 (*n* = 18)	10 (55.6)	8 (44.4)	
≥$100,000 (*n* = 37)	15 (40.5)	22 (59.4)	
Parent education (*N* = 134)			0.07
No schooling to 8th grade (*n* = 2)	2 (100)	0 (0)	
Some high school to high school graduate (*n* = 25)	10 (40)	15 (60)	
Some college, college graduate, or vocational training (*n* = 82)	47 (57.3)	35 (42.7)	
Some postgraduate work to postgraduate degree (*n* = 25)	9 (36)	16 (64)	
Race (*N* = 135)			0.83
White (*n* = 53)	28 (52.8)	25 (47.1)	
Black (*n* = 25)	12 (48)	13 (52)	
Hispanic (*n* = 24)	14 (58.3)	10 (41.7)	
Asian (*n* = 17)	8 (47.1)	9 (52.9)	
Native American (*n* = 4)	1 (25)	3 (75)	
Other (*n* = 12)	5 (41.7)	7 (58.3)	
Region (*N* = 135)			<0.001
Coastal (*n* = 17)	1 (5.9)	16 (94.1)	
Midwest (*n* = 58)	38 (65.5)	20 (34.4)	
South (*n* = 60)	29 (48.3)	31 (51.7)	
Number of times seen by pediatric nephrology provider in the past year (*N* = 135)			0.99
Once	4 (44.4)	5 (55.6)	
2–3 times	28 (50.9)	27 (49.1)	
≥4 times	36 (50.7)	35 (49.3)	
Immunization recommendations provided by Pediatric nephrologist (*N* = 118)			0.02
Yes (*n* = 100)	55 (55)	45 (45)	
No (*n* = 18)	4 (22.2)	14 (77.8)	

NS, nephrotic syndrome; PPSV 23, polysaccharide pneumococcal vaccine 23-valent.
**Excluded the following from analysis: (1) Centers in Coastal region without vaccine records to validate PPSV 23 status, (2) Pediatric NS subjects who were unable to receive the PPSV 23 due to age eligibility, (3) Parents/guardians who declined to answer in the parent income and parent education variables, and (4) Parents/guardians who answered "I am not sure" in Immunization recommendations provided by pediatric nephrologist variable.*

NS relapse rates, there has been a wide variation of vaccine practices as evidenced by two studies conducted in 1993 and 2001 (17, 18). Our study similarly observed varied vaccine practices by providers, which translates to the gap in parental knowledge and understanding of the timing of vaccine administration in their children with NS as seen in the parental/guardian survey responses.

NS can be a difficult disease to treat especially in patients who have a steroid-dependent, frequently-relapsing, or steroid-resistant clinical course. These patients may have no or very brief periods of time off of immunosuppression medications to keep the disease in control. As a result, opportunities to vaccinate with inactive and/or live vaccines become limited if providers choose to withhold immunizations until full recovery of immune function. Withholding vaccines in this high-risk population can lead to an increased risk of vaccine-preventable disease (9). It is known that infection is a common trigger for NS relapses which can result in the need for hospitalization to help manage the complications of the relapse, thus leading to significantly higher hospitalization charges (8).

Factors associated with immunization adherence have been studied by various groups. Our group specifically evaluated the adherence to PPSV23 administration since it is recommended by the ACIP for pediatric patients with NS and immunosuppressed states. Cost of vaccines, lack of parental knowledge of the benefits of vaccines, and lack of vaccine recommendation by medical providers has been reported to adversely impact immunization adherence (31, 32). Our study similarly showed that provider vaccine recommendations were associated with vaccine adherence to PPSV 23. However, we did not investigate

TABLE 7 | Adjusted logistic regression model of PPSV 23 vaccine (Complete case analysis $n = 110$).

Variable	Odds ratio [95% confidence interval]	*p*-value
Region		0.01
Coastal	0.30 [0.13–0.66]	0.003
Midwest	Reference	Reference
South	0.56 [0.24–1.30]	0.18
Immunization recommendations provided by pediatric nephrologist		0.04
Yes	1.95 [1.05–3.63]	0.04
No	Reference	Reference

PPSV 23, polysaccharide pneumococcal vaccine 23-valent.

the cost of vaccines as a potential factor of immunization adherence in this survey study. Schuller et al. demonstrated an increased likelihood of vaccination if the child's caregiver received higher education, lived in the Northeast, had private insurance, and was of Hispanic race among US children (33). We found that subjects residing in the Midwest were more likely to receive the PPSV 23, which may be due to a higher number of participating study sites in the Midwest region compared to other regions surveyed in North America for our study, and therefore the Midwest region may be more representative than a region with fewer sites. Additionally, parent income, level of parent education, and race were not positive predictors of subjects receiving the PPSV 23 in the current study. The differences in the factors associated with vaccines adherence in our study compared to other published studies may also be explained by our small sample size. Our study also evaluated other possible contributing factors to vaccine adherence including the ability of the subspecialty clinic to provide vaccines (i.e., pneumococcal vaccine) and the communication of vaccine recommendations from the pediatric nephrology provider to the patient's primary care provider (PCP). Seventy-six percent of providers indicated that their subspecialty clinic can administer pneumococcal vaccines. The remaining providers who do not have this capability may defer the responsibility of vaccinations to the PCP. Ninety-two percent of providers indicated that they communicate their vaccine recommendations to their patient's PCP with a letter as the most common modality of communication.

The current study demonstrates the need for a more uniform vaccine practice in the pediatric NS population among pediatric nephrologists, which will in turn better educate and help parents/guardians understand the importance of vaccination and when it is appropriate for their child to receive certain vaccines.

Limitations and Strengths

The limitations of this study include the heterogeneity of survey responses among the parent/guardian cohort and pediatric nephrology providers with regards to knowledge of the ACIP guidelines. The discrepant responses amongst both groups could be explained by comprehension and communication between parent and provider or alternatively by survey interpretation. Since the surveys were anonymous for both cohorts, we were unable to associate the parent/guardian and provider response resulting in the inability to directly correlate responses. While this study evaluated the communication of vaccine recommendations from pediatric nephrologist to PCP, an assessment of the knowledge and practice of the patient's PCP was not evaluated which could have identified another area for improvement of vaccine adherence in this cohort. Lastly, the small sample size of this study may have played a role in the differences in factors associated with vaccine adherence compared to other published studies.

The strengths of this study include the high response rate. This study also investigated the immunization knowledge from both pediatric nephrology providers and parent/guardians of children with NS simultaneously from their shared institutions, which helped to evaluate for any institution/region-specific immunization practices.

CONCLUSION

Our findings support the growing evidence that vaccine recommendation by medical providers is paramount in vaccine adherence among pediatric patients with NS. The disparate survey responses among the pediatric nephrology providers and parents/guardians likely reflect the individual interpretations of the ACIP guidelines by the medical providers and possibly their anecdotal experiences with treatment of NS. Additionally, some pediatric nephrology practices do not have the capability to administer certain vaccines (i.e., PPSV 23) and therefore rely on vaccinations through the patient's PCP. Ensuring primary care establishment with a PCP as well as being a champion to clarify and communicate vaccination provisioning guidance with the patient's PCP may help to improve vaccine adherence. Future studies assessing the knowledge and practice of vaccine recommendations by PCPs for pediatric patients with NS may also highlight other areas for improvement of vaccine adherence such as communication between healthcare providers to assure vaccinations occur in a timely and complete fashion in the child's primary care office. Lastly, it is important that the ACIP immunization guidelines are reviewed by the pediatric nephrologist and primary care physicians yearly to be informed of any change in the immunization practice recommendations for those with altered immune competence.

ETHICS STATEMENT

The studies involving human participants were reviewed and approved by each participating center. Written informed consent to participate in this study was provided by the participants' legal guardian/next of kin.

AUTHOR CONTRIBUTIONS

Data analysis was performed by JT and CT. All authors read and approved the final manuscript, contributed to the study conception, design, and data collection.
Grant Number: UL1TR002240) for the Michigan Institute for Clinical and Health Research.

ACKNOWLEDGMENTS

We are indebted to the patients and families who graciously participated in this research. We express our thanks to all the site coordinators who assisted with patient/provider identification, enrollment, and data collection.

REFERENCES

1. Peterson PA, Berggard I. Urinary immunoglobulin components in normal, tubular, and glomerular proteinuria: quantities and characteristics of free light chains, IgG, IgA, and fcgamma fragment. *Eur J Clin Invest.* (1971) 1:255–64.
2. Giangiacomo J, Cleary TG, Cole BR, Hoffsten P, Robson AM. Serum immunoglobulins in the nephrotic syndrome. A possible cause of minimal-change nephrotic syndrome. *N Engl J Med.* (1975) 293:8–12.
3. Anderson DC, York DL, Rose G, Smith CW. Assessment of serum factor B. serum opsonins, granulocyte chemotaxis, and infection in nephrotic syndrome of children. *J Infect Dis.* (1979) 140:1–11.
4. Ballow M, Kennedy TL, Gaudio KM, Siegel NJ, McLean RH. Serum hemolytic factor D values in children with steroid-responsive idiopathic nephrotic syndrome. *J Pediatr.* (1982) 100:192–6.
5. Uncu N, Bülbül M, Yildiz N, Noyan A, Koşan C, Kavukçu S, et al. Primary peritonitis in children with nephrotic syndrome: results of a 5-year multicenter study. *Eur J Pediatr.* (2010). 169:73–6. doi: 10.1007/s00431-009-0989-x
6. Speck WT, Dresdale SS, McMillan RW. Primary peritonitis and the nephrotic syndrome. *Am J Surg.* (1974) 127:267–9.
7. Gorensek MJ, Lebel MH, Nelson JD. Peritonitis in children with nephrotic syndrome. *Pediatrics.* (1988) 81:849–56.
8. Gipson DS, Messer KL, Tran CL, Herreshoff EG, Samuel JP, Massengill SF, et al. Inpatient health care utilization in the United States among children, adolescents, and young adults with nephrotic syndrome. *Am J Kidney Dis.* (2013) 61:910–7. doi: 10.1053/j.ajkd.2012.12.025
9. Carpenter SL, Goldman J, Sherman AK, Selewski DS, Kallash M, Tran CL, et al. Association of infections and venous thromboembolism in hospitalized children with nephrotic syndrome. *Pediatr Nephrol.* (2019). 34:261–7. doi: 10.1007/s00467-018-4072-6
10. Fiore AE, Levine OS, Elliott JA, Facklam RR, Butler JC. Effectiveness of pneumococcal polysaccharide vaccine for preschool-age children with chronic disease. *Emerg Infect Dis.* (1999) 5:828–31.
11. Overturf GD. American academy of pediatrics. Committee on infectious diseases. Technical report: prevention of pneumococcal infections, including the use of pneumococcal conjugate and polysaccharide vaccines and antibiotic prophylaxis. *Pediatrics.* (2000) 106:367–76. doi: 10.1542/peds.106.2.367
12. Muntner P, Woodward M, Carson AP, Judd SE, Levitan EB, Mann DM, et al. Development and validation of a self-assessment tool for albuminuria: results from the reasons for geographic and racial differences in stroke (REGARDS) study. *Am J Kidney Dis.* (2011) 58:196–205. doi: 10.1053/j.ajkd.2011.01.027
13. Chehab G, Sander O, Richter J, Acar H, Vordenbäumen S, Brinks R, et al. Validation and evaluation of the German brief index of lupus damage (BILD)–a self-reported instrument to record damage in systemic lupus erythematosus. *Lupus.* (2013) 22:1050–5. doi: 10.1177/0961203313500369
14. Andy UU, Harvie HS, Smith AL, Propert KJ, Bogner HR, Arya LA. Validation of a self-administered instrument to measure adherence to anticholinergic drugs in women with overactive bladder. *Neurourol Urodyn.* (2015) 34:424–8. doi: 10.1002/nau.22605
15. ACIP. https://www.cdc.gov/vaccines/schedules/hcp/imz/child-adolescent.html. 2019.
16. Robinson CL, Bernstein H, Poehling K, Romero JR, Szilagyi P. Advisory committee on immunization practices recommended immunization schedule for children and adolescents aged 18 years or younger-United States 2020. *MMWR Morb Mortal Wkly Rep.* (2020) 69:130–2. doi: 10.15585/mmwr.mm6905a3
17. Schnaper HW. Immunization practices in childhood nephrotic syndrome: a survey of North American pediatric nephrologists. *Pediatr Nephrol.* (1994) 8:4–6.
18. Shroff A, Frank R, Vergara M, Gauthier B, Trachtman H. Prevention of serious bacterial infections in new-onset nephrotic syndrome: a survey of current practices. *Clin Pediatr.* (2002) 41:47–9. doi: 10.1177/000992280204100110
19. Banerjee S, Dissanayake PV, Abeyagunawardena AS. Vaccinations in children on immunosuppressive medications for renal disease. *Pediatr Nephrol.* (2016) 31:1437–48. doi: 10.1007/s00467-015-3219-y
20. Sixbey JW. Routine immunizations and the immunosuppressed child. *Adv Pediatr Infect Dis.* (1987) 2:79–114.
21. Davis LE, Bodian D, Price D, Butler IJ, Vickers JH. Chronic progressive poliomyelitis secondary to vaccination of an immunodeficient child. *N Engl J Med.* (1977) 297:241–5.
22. Ninane J, Grymonprez A, Burtonboy G, Francois A, Cornu G. Disseminated BCG in HIV infection. *Arch Dis Child.* (1988) 63:1268–9.
23. Lu Y, Bousvaros A. Varicella vaccination in children with inflammatory bowel disease receiving immunosuppressive therapy. *J Pediatr Gastroenterol Nutr.* (2010) 50:562–5. doi: 10.1097/MPG.0b013e3181bab351
24. Lombel RM, Gipson DS, Hodson EM. Treatment of steroid-sensitive nephrotic syndrome: new guidelines from KDIGO. *Pediatr Nephrol.* (2013) 28:415–26. doi: 10.1007/s00467-012-2310-x
25. Aoun B, Wannous H, Azéma C, Ulinski T. Polysaccharide pneumococcal vaccination of nephrotic children at disease onset-long-term data. *Pediatr Nephrol.* (2010) 25:1773–4. doi: 10.1007/s00467-010-1492-3
26. Ulinski T, Leroy S, Dubrel M, Danon S, Bensman A. High serological response to pneumococcal vaccine in nephrotic children at disease onset on high-dose prednisone. *Pediatr Nephrol.* (2008) 23:1107–13. doi: 10.1007/s00467-008-0782-5
27. Hsu K, Pelton S, Karumuri S, Heisey-Grove D, Klein J. Population-based surveillance for childhood invasive pneumococcal disease in the era of conjugate vaccine. *Pediatr Infect Dis J.* (2005). 24:17–23. doi: 10.1097/01.inf.0000148891.32134.36
28. Taylor B, Andrews N, Stowe J, Hamidi-Manesh L, Miller E. No increased risk of relapse after meningococcal C conjugate vaccine in nephrotic syndrome. *Arch Dis Child.* (2007). 92:887–9. doi: 10.1136/adc.2006.105247
29. Quien RM, Kaiser BA, Deforest A, Polinsky MS, Fisher M, Baluarte HJ. Response to the varicella vaccine in children with nephrotic syndrome. *J Pediatr.* (1997) 131:688–90.
30. Furth SL, Arbus GS, Hogg R, Tarver J, Chan C, Fivush BA. Varicella vaccination in children with nephrotic syndrome: a report of the Southwest pediatric nephrology study group. *J Pediatr.* (2003) 142:145–8. doi: 10.1067/mpd.2003.37
31. How CH, Phua See Chun P, Shafi F, Jakes RW. Parental knowledge, attitudes and perception of pneumococcal disease and pneumococcal conjugate vaccines in Singapore: a questionnaire-based assessment. *BMC Public Health.* (2016) 16:923. doi: 10.1186/s12889-016-3597-5
32. Low MSF, Tan H, Hartman M, Tam CC, Hoo C, Lim J, et al. Parental perceptions of childhood seasonal influenza vaccination in Singapore: a cross-sectional survey. *Vaccine.* (2017) 35:6096–02. doi: 10.1016/j.vaccine.2017.09.060
33. Schuller KA, Probst JC. Factors associated with influenza vaccination among US children in 2008. *J Infect Public Health.* (2013) 6:80–8. doi: 10.1016/j.jiph.2012.12.001

3

Positive Response to One-Year Treatment With Burosumab in Pediatric Patients With X-Linked Hypophosphatemia

*Silvia Martín Ramos [1], Marta Gil-Calvo [2], Virginia Roldán [3], Ana Castellano Martínez [3] and Fernando Santos [1,4,5]**

[1] Hospital Universitario Central de Asturias, Oviedo, Spain, [2] Hospital Clínico Universitario de Santiago, Santiago de Compostela, Spain, [3] Hospital Universitario Puerta del Mar, Cádiz, Spain, [4] Instituto de Investigación Sanitaria del Principado de Asturias, Oviedo, Spain, [5] Universidad de Oviedo, Oviedo, Spain

***Correspondence:**
Fernando Santos
fsantos@uniovi.es

X-linked hypophosphatemia (XLH) causes significant burden in pediatric patients in spite of maintained treatment with phosphate supplements and vitamin D derivatives. Administration of burosumab has shown promising results in clinical trial but studies assessing its effect in the everyday practice are missing. With this aim, we analyzed the response to one-year treatment with burosumab, injected subcutaneously at 0.8 mg/kg every 2 weeks, in five children (three females) aged from 6 to 16 years, with genetically confirmed XLH. Patients were being treated with phosphate and vitamin D analogs until the beginning of burosumab treatment. In all children, burosumab administration led to normalization of serum phosphate in association with marked increase of tubular reabsorption of phosphate and reduction of elevated serum alkaline phosphatase levels. Baseline height of patients, from −3.56 to −0.46 SD, increased in the three prepubertal children (+0.84, +0.89, and +0.16 SD) during burosumab treatment. Growth improvement was associated with reduction in body mass index (−1.75, −1.47, and −0.17 SD, respectively), suggesting a salutary effect of burosumab on physical activity and body composition. Burosumab was well-tolerated, mild local pain at the injection site and transient and mild headache following the initial doses of burosumab being the only reported undesirable side effects. No patient exhibited hyperphosphatemia, progression of nephrocalcinosis, worsening of metabolic control or developed hyperparathyroidism. Mild elevation of serum PTH present at the beginning of treatment in one patient 4 was not modified by burosumab administration. These results indicate that in the clinical setting, beyond the strict conditions and follow-up of clinical trials, burosumab treatment for 1 year exerts positive effects in pediatric patients with XLH without major adverse events.

Keywords: X-linked hypophosphatemia (XLH), rickets, burosumab, FGF23, hypophosphatemia, vitamin D, children

INTRODUCTION

X-linked hypophosphatemic rickets (XLH) is a monogenic disorder that follows a Mendelian dominant inheritance (OMIM 307800) and it is the most common hereditary form of rickets (1).

XLH is caused by loss of function of the gene *PHEX* (2), a phosphate regulating gene with homologies to endopeptidases, leading to elevated circulating levels of fibroblast growth factor

23 (FGF23), renal wasting of phosphate and defective renal production of 1,25-dihydroxyvitamin D (3).

Although XLH is characterized by a broad phenotypical expression, active lesions of rickets, subsequent bone deformities and disharmonic growth retardation are major manifestations of the disease in the pediatric age. Dental abscesses and mineralization defects in teeth are also common findings (1).

Classical medical treatment of XLH is based on the oral administration of phosphate supplements and 1-hydroxy metabolites of vitamin D, given chronically, at least until the end of body growth (4). This therapy usually heals the active radiological lesions of rickets and improves growth but does not normalize serum phosphate, does not avoid major clinical manifestations of the disease, does not result in the achievement of a normal final adult height and entails the risk of potential undesirable side effects such as nephrocalcinosis or hyperparathyroidism (5, 6).

The development of burosumab, a humanized monoclonal antibody for FGF23 is a promising treatment in patients with XLH (7). Preliminary clinical trials indicate that burosumab improves renal tubular phosphate reabsorption, serum phosphorus levels, linear growth, and physical function and reduces pain and the severity of rickets in children with XLH (8, 9). However, very limited data on pediatric patients with XLH treated with burosumab are available. Thus, to know the efficacy and safety of burosumab treatment in the everyday clinical setting we here present five children with genetically confirmed XLH receiving the drug for more than a year.

PATIENTS AND METHODS

Patients younger than 18 years of age with XLH genetically confirmed and on treatment with burosumab for more than a year were identified in three Spanish hospitals. All patients received burosumab subcutaneously at a dose of 0.8 mg/kg every 2 weeks, after an initial dose of 0.4 mg/kg. Phosphate supplements and 1-hydroxy derivatives of vitamin D administration were withdrawn 2 weeks before the beginning of burosumab.

After informed consent, the medical records of these patients were reviewed. The following data were collected from the basal visit, immediately before starting burosumab, and, when available, from each of the outpatient clinic visits during the period of burosumab treatment: height, weight, and clinical manifestations including adverse effects potentially related with the administration of burosumab; fasting serum concentrations of phosphate, alkaline phosphatase, calcium, 1,25-dihydroxyvitamin D and intact parathyroid hormone (PTH); urine calcium/creatinine ratio, tubular phosphate reabsorption (TPR) and tubular maximum reabsorption of phosphate for glomerular filtration rate (TmP/GFR) were calculated. Radiological findings as well as the presence of nephrocalcinosis or dental impairment were also collected.

Somatometric measurements, including height, weight, and body mass index (BMI), were expressed in absolute values and as standard deviation (SD) score of Spanish reference growth charts for age and sex. The profile of the several biochemical variables measured was drawn using absolute values except for alkaline phosphatase whose values were expressed as percentage of the initial one because of the wide dispersion of the results in the different hospitals.

The protocol was approved by *Comité de Ética de la Investigación con Medicamentos del Principado de Asturias (SP no 38/18)*. All subjects gave written informed consent in accordance with the Declaration of Helsinki.

RESULTS

Table 1 shows baseline characteristics of the patients before starting burosumab treatment. Hypophosphatemia associated to urinary wasting of phosphate, relatively low values of 1,25-dihydroxyvitamin D and elevated alkaline phosphatase levels all support the diagnosis of XLH, confirmed by the mutation found in the *PHEX* gene. Serum concentrations of calcium and 25-hydroxyvitamin D were normal (not shown). Serum intact PTH levels were also normal except in patient 4 who had a mild elevation (upper normal reference value 65 pg/mL).

Response to burosumab assessed by the biochemical profiles of serum phosphate, serum alkaline phosphatase and renal reabsorption of phosphate is graphically shown in **Figure 1**. The dose of burosumab did not need to be modified and was kept at 0.8 mg/kg every 2 weeks as originally planned. Serum phosphate normalized in all patients, in patient 1 after a transient worsening of hypophosphatemia immediately following the first burosumab dose. The normalization of serum phosphate was associated to greater renal phosphate reabsorption as shown by increases in TRP and TmP/GFR.

Growth of patients is shown in **Table 2**. Height improved in three out of the five children and remained unchanged in two who were pubertal females of 13 and 16 years of age. Weight and BMI decreased, particularly in those children who exhibited greater increase in height SDS, or remained unchanged.

As for the unsuitable effects of burosumab, no patient developed new radiological lesions, nephrocalcinosis or dental problems during the period of burosumab treatment. The patients had been receiving conventional treatment of XLH and did not have active radiological lesions of rickets. As for nephrocalcinosis, it was already present in one patient before starting treatment with burosumab and the kidney ultrasounds did not worsen during burosumab treatment. No patient developed new findings of nephrocalcinosis after 1 year of burosumab treatment. Likewise, no adverse effects potentially related with burosumab were reported except for mild local pain at the injection site (1 patient) and transient and mild headache following the initial doses of burosumab (1 patient). Patient 4 had elevation of PTH at the beginning of treatment. None of the four remaining patients developed hyperparathyroidism, serum PTH concentrations increasing in all of them but within the normal range.

DISCUSSION

This manuscript supports the efficacy and safety of burosumab administered to pediatric patients with XLH in the everyday clinical setting, beyond the strict monitoring conditions of clinical trials (8, 9). This is important because, as stated in a recently published evidence-based guideline for the

TABLE 1 | Clinical, genetic, and biochemical findings in five children with X-linked hypophosphatemia at the moment of starting treatment with burosumab, after withdrawal of administration of vitamin D derivatives and phosphate supplements at least 2 weeks before.

	Patient 1	Patient 2	Patient 3	Patient 4	Patient 5
Age (years)	7	6	16	13	13
Sex	Female	Male	Female	Male	Female
PHEX gene mutation and zigosity	c.871C>T; p.Arg291Ter Heterozygous	c.670C>T; p.Gln224Ter Hemizygous	c. 1936_?del; p.Asp646_?del Heterozygous	c.1079+1G>A; splicing Hemizygous	c.1735G>A; p.Gly579Arg Heterozygous
Serum phosphate (mg/dL)	2.2	2.6	1.7	2.3	1.7
Serum AP (U/L)	504	425	516	1093	605
Serum 1,25(OH)$_2$D (pg/mL)	15.9	36.6	22.0	13.4	23.0
Serum PTH (pg/mL)	34	19	22	83	40
TRP (%)	61	54	32	85	80
TmP/GFR (mg/dL)	0.90	1.40	0.54	1.99	1.36
Height in cm (SD)	119.9 (−0.53)	105.0 (−2.4)	143.5 (−2.89)	129.7 (−3.56)	154.2 (−0.46)
Skeletal findings	Leg bowing Hyperlordosis	Leg bowing	Leg bowing	Leg bowing Scaphocephaly	Leg bowing
Dental abnormalities	No	No	No	Dental abscesses	Dental abscesses

AP, alkaline phosphatase; PTH, parathyroid hormone; 1,25(OH)$_2$D, 1,25-dihydroxyvitamin D; TRP, tubular reabsorption of phosphate; TmP/GFR, tubular maximum reabsorption of phosphate for glomerular filtration rate.

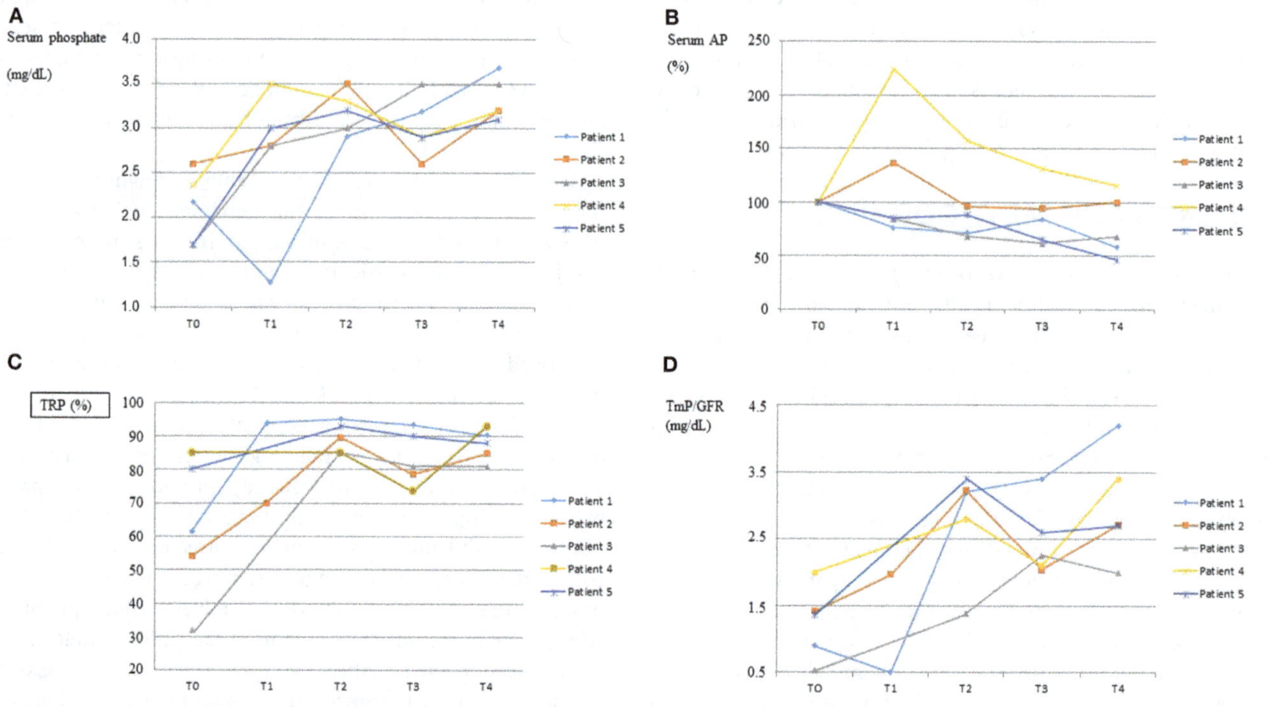

FIGURE 1 | Response to burosumab. The course over time of serum phosphate, serum alkaline phosphatases (AP), tubular reabsorption of phosphate (TRP) and tubular maximum reabsorption of phosphate for glomerular filtration rate (TmP/GFR) are shown in graphs **(A–D)**, respectively, for each patient. On the "x" axis, T0 indicates baseline values, immediately before starting burosumab treatment, and T1–T4 indicate values every 3–4 months on burosumab treatment. X ± SD values for T0 and T4 were as follows. Serum Phosphate (mg/dL): 2.10 ± 0.39 and 3.33 ± 0.24; Serum AP (U/L): 628 ± 267 and 525 ± 419; TRP (%): 62.5 ± 21.3 and 87.4 ± 4.7; TmP/GFR (mg/dL): 1.26 ± 0.53 and 2.99 ± 0.83.

diagnosis and management of XLH (10), recommendations on the use of burosumab cannot be conclusive because the available information is based on the results of trials testing the drug in children with severe XLH (10). We here report that treatment with burosumab for 1 year at a subcutaneous dose of 0.8 mg/kg/14 days results in normalization of serum phosphate, decrease of serum alkaline phosphatase, elevation of serum 1,25-dihydroxyvitamin D, and

TABLE 2 | Effect of 1 year burosumab treatment on growth in five children with X-linked hypophosphatemia.

	Patient 1	Patient 2	Patient 3	Patient 4	Patient 5
Height in cm (SD)	130.0 (0.31)	115.4 (−1.51)	144.5 (−2.92)	136.0 (−3.4)	155.6 (−0.76)
Height Δ (SD)	+0.84	+0.89	−0.03	+0.16	−0.30
Weight in kg (SD)	33 (0.79)	27.2 (0.37)	46 (−1.22)	43.7 (−1.14)	53.5 (−0.02)
Weight Δ (SD)	−0.97	−0.39	−0.11	−0.07	−0.18
BMI in kg/m^2 (SD)	19.53 (0.84)	20.42 (1.66)	22.03 (0.14)	23.63 (0.64)	22.27 (0.37)
BMI Δ (SD)	−1.75	−1.47	−0.08	−0.17	−0.02

BMI, body mass index; Δ, SD change during burosumab treatment.

marked improvement of tubular reabsorption of phosphate in five pediatric patients with genetically confirmed XLH after interruption of classical treatment with phosphate supplements and vitamin D derivatives. It is of note that TRP (%) of patients 4 and 5 were within the expected range for a child with normal serum phosphate concentrations but TRP should be much higher (above 90–95%) in the presence of marked hypophosphatemia such as that found in these two patients, below 2.5 mg/dl in both.

Burosumab induced a positive effect on growth in three out of the five children, as demonstrated by a marked increase of height SDS at the end of the 1-year treatment period. In these patients the amelioration of height was noticeably higher than that found by Carpenter et al. (8) in their trial after 64 weeks of treatment. XLH exerts a marked adverse effect on growth (11) and final adult height of pediatric patients with XLH is usually low, even if they have received conventional treatment since diagnosis (12) or growth hormone (13) at infancy or early childhood. Our findings indicate that the growth promoting action of burosumab does not occur in growth retarded pubertal XLH patients, regardless its positive effects on phosphate metabolism. The two patients (patient 1 and 2) with the greater height SD increase during burosumab treatment were those of younger age (7 and 6 years), suggesting the convenience of early administration of burosumab, before puberty. It also supports the assumption that the impairment of growth in XLH is not entirely dependent on hypophosphatemia and rachitic bone lesions (11, 14) so that growth retardation may persist in spite of improvement in mineral metabolism. The characterization of growth response to burosumab needs to be investigated in further studies involving greater number of patients and longer follow-ups.

It is interesting to note that BMI markedly decreased in patients 1 and 2. These patients underwent the greatest improvement in height and, although, unfortunately, our study does not provide quantitatively measured objective data on musculoskeletal function (15), this positive effect on weight and body composition likely resulted from the higher physical activity of children, a fact disclosed by the patients' parents in the clinical interviews. Likewise, families reported the interruption of frequent oral doses of phosphate as an appreciable benefit linked to the new treatment. Burosumab also exerted a beneficial effect on radiological osseous abnormalities although no specific score to quantify bone deformity and/or legs' bowing was used.

Burosumab was well-tolerated and no serious undesirable effects were detected. Headache and local injection-site reactions reported by one of our patients have been notified in the literature in approximately 60% of children treated with burosumab (16). No patient exhibited hyperphosphatemia, progression of nephrocalcinosis, worsening of metabolic control or developed hyperparathyroidism. Mild elevation of serum PTH present at the beginning of treatment in patient 4 was not modified by burosumab administration.

In summary, this study shows the efficacy and safety of burosumab administered for 1 year in the clinical management and follow-up of pediatric patients with XLH. Additional studies are necessary to assess the influence of burosumab on the long-term outcome of these patients and to define the criteria for its use.

ETHICS STATEMENT

The studies involving human participants were reviewed and approved by Comité de Ética de la Investigación con Medicamentos del Principado de Asturias (SP n° 38/18). Written informed consent to participate in this study was provided by the participants' legal guardian/next of kin. Written informed consent was obtained from the minor(s)' legal guardian/next of kin for the publication of any potentially identifiable images or data included in this article.

AUTHOR CONTRIBUTIONS

SM designed the data chart, obtained patient's information from the medical records, analyzed the data, drew the figures, and contributed to writing the manuscript. MG-C, VR, and AC obtained patients' information from the medical records, revised and corrected the data presentation, and the manuscript. FS designed the study, revised and corrected the data presentation and contributed to writing the different versions of the manuscript.

ACKNOWLEDGMENTS

Partly supported by Kyowa Kirin & Fundación Nutrición y Crecimiento.

REFERENCES

1. Bitzan M, Goodyer PR. Hypophosphatemic rickets. *Pediatr Clin N Am.* 66:179–207. doi: 10.1016/j.pcl.2018.09.004
2. Francis F, Hennig S, Korn B, Reinhardt R, de Jong P, Poustka A, et al. A gene (PEX) with homologies to endopeptidases is mutated in patients with X-linked hypophosphatemic rickets. The HYP Consortium. *Nat Genet.* (1995) 11:130–6. doi: 10.1038/ng1095-130
3. Carpenter TO. The expanding family of hypophosphatemic syndromes. *J Bone Miner Metab.* (2012) 30:1–9. doi: 10.1007/s00774-011-0340-2

4. Carpenter TO, Imel EA, Holm IA, Jan de Beur SM, Insogna KL. A clinician's guide to X-linked hypophosphatemia. *J Bone Miner Res.* (2011) 26:1381–8. doi: 10.1002/jbmr.340
5. Linglart A, Biosse-Duplan M, Briot K, Chaussain C, Esterle L, Guillaume-Czitrom S, et al. Therapeutic management of hypophosphatemic rickets from infancy to adulthood. *Endocr Connect.* (2014) 3:R13–30. doi: 10.1530/EC-13-0103
6. Skrinar A, Dvorak-Ewell M, Evins A, Macica C, Linglart A, Imel EA, et al. The lifelong impact of X-linked hypophosphatemia: results from a burden of disease survey. *J Endocr Soc.* (2019) 3:1321–34. doi: 10.1210/js.2018-00365
7. Kinoshita Y, Fukumoto S. X-linked hypophosphatemia and FGF23-related hypophosphatemic diseases: prospect for new treatment. *Endocr Rev.* (2018) 39:274–91. doi: 10.1210/er.2017-00220
8. Carpenter TO, Whyte MP, Imel EA, Boot AM, Högler W, Linglart A, et al. Burosumab therapy in children with X-linked hypophosphatemia. *N Engl J Med.* (2018) 378:1987–98. doi: 10.1056/NEJMoa1714641
9. Imel EA, Glorieux FH, Whyte MP, Munns CF, Ward LM, Nilsson O, et al. Burosumab versus conventional therapy in children with X-linked hypophosphataemia: a randomised, active-controlled, open-label, phase 3 trial. *Lancet.* (2019) 39:2416–242. doi: 10.1016/S0140-6736(19)30654-3
10. Haffner D, Emma F, Eastwood DM, Duplan MB, Bacchetta J, Schnabel D, et al. Clinical practice recommendations for the diagnosis and management of X-linked hypophosphataemia. *Nat Rev Nephrol.* (2019) 15:435–55. doi: 10.1038/s41581-019-0152-5
11. Fuente R, Gil-Peña H, Claramunt-Taberner D, Hernández O, Fernández-Iglesias A, Alonso-Durán L, et al. X-linked hypophosphatemia and growth. *Rev Endocr Metab Disord.* (2017) 18:107–15. doi: 10.1007/s11154-017-9408-1
12. Zivičnjak M, Schnabel D, Billing H, Staude H, Filler G, Querfeld U, et al. Age-related stature and linear body segments in children with X-linked hypophosphatemic rickets. *Pediatr Nephrol.* (2011) 26:223–31. doi: 10.1007/s00467-010-1705-9
13. Meyerhoff N, Haffner D, Staude H, Wühl E, Marx M, Beetz R, et al. Effects of growth hormone treatment on adult height in severely short children with X-linked hypophosphatemic rickets. *Pediatr Nephrol.* (2018) 33:447–56. doi: 10.1007/s00467-017-3820-3
14. Santos F, Fuente R, Mejia N, Mantecon L, Gil-Peña H, Ordoñez FA. Hypophosphatemia and growth. *Pediatr Nephrol.* (2013) 28:595–603. doi: 10.1007/s00467-012-2364-9
15. Saraff V, Schneider J, Colleselli V, Ruepp M, Rauchenzauner M, Neururer S, et al. Sex-, age-, and height-specific reference curves for the 6-min walk test in healthy children and adolescents. *Eur J Pediatr.* (2015) 174:837–40. doi: 10.1007/s00431-014-2454-8
16. Lyseng-Williamson KA. Burosumab in X-linked hypophosphatemia: a profile of its use in the USA. *Drugs Ther Perspect.* (2018) 34:497–506. doi: 10.1007/s40267-018-0560-9

Function of miR-24 and miR-27 in Pediatric Patients With Idiopathic Nephrotic Syndrome

Fen-fen Ni [1], Guang-lei Liu [2], Shi-lei Jia [1], Ran-ran Chen [1], Li-bing Liu [1], Cheng-rong Li [1], Jun Yang [3]* and Xiao-Jie Gao [1]**

[1] Department of Nephrology, Shenzhen Children's Hospital, Shenzhen, China, [2] The Fifth Affiliated (Zhuhai) Hospital of Zunyi Medical University, Zhuhai, China, [3] Department of Immunology, Shenzhen Children's Hospital, Shenzhen, China

***Correspondence:**
Cheng-rong Li
chengrongli0755@163.com
Jun Yang
shenzhen81111@163.com
Xiao-Jie Gao
gxj0824@hotmail.com

Purpose: We investigated the pathogenesis of idiopathic nephrotic syndrome (INS) by measuring the effects two specific miRNAs on Th2 cells in children with this disease.

Methods: After informed consent, we enrolled 20 children with active INS before steroid initiation, 20 children with INS in remission after steroid therapy, and 20 age-matched healthy controls. Flow cytometry was used to measure the levels of Th2 cells and a cytometric bead array was used to measure the levels of IgE, interleukin (IL)−4, and IL-13. RT-PCR was used to measure the levels of miR-24 and miR-27 in $CD4^{+}TCD25^{-}$ cells. PBMCs were isolated using Ficoll density gradient centrifugation, and transfected with different mimic or inhibitor miRNAs. RT-PCR was used to measure the expression of different RNAs, and flow cytometry was used to determine the percentage of Th2 cells.

Results: Relative to healthy controls, children with active INS had higher percentages of Th2 cells ($P < 0.05$), but there was no significant difference in controls and children in remission. The plasma levels of IgE, IL-4, and IL-13 were significantly increased in children with active INS ($P < 0.05$). There were lower levels of miR-24 and miR-27 in children with active non-atopic INS ($P < 0.05$). Transfection experiments indicated that upregulation of each miRNA decreased the percentage of Th2 cells and the level of IL-4 ($P < 0.05$), and down-regulation of each miRNA had the opposite effects ($P < 0.05$).

Conclusion: Children with active INS, with or without atopy, had higher levels of IgE, possibly related to their higher levels of IL-13 and IL-4 due to a drift toward Th2 cells. miR-24 and miR-27 suppressed the expression of Th2 cells and have a critical function regulating Th2 cell expression in INS.

Keywords: idiopathic nephrotic syndrome, miR-24, Th2 cells, IL-4, IL-13, miR-27

INTRODUCTION

Idiopathic nephrotic syndrome (INS) is the most common renal disease in children, and a main cause of chronic renal failure in children from China (1). The clinical manifestations of INS are proteinuria, low level of plasma albumin, hyperlipidemia, and edema. The prevalence is greatest in preschool children who are 3–5 years-old. About 80–90% of patients with kidney disease who are under 10 years-old have minimal change disease (MCD), a common cause of INS (2). However, the specific etiology and mechanism of INS in children remain unclear. Previous studies showed that

INS is associated with immune system dysfunctions, including humoral immune disorders, T cell subset dysfunction, and abnormal secretion of cytokines, especially due to T cell dysfunction (3–8).

T helper type 2 (Th2) cells, which mainly produce IL-4, IL-5, and IL-13, play a major role in responses to parasitic infections and allergic inflammatory diseases (9–11). A seminal 1959 study reported an association of pollen sensitivity with seasonal proteinuria, and that about 30% of children with INS had atopic manifestations, such as allergic rhinitis and idiopathic dermatitis (12). Subsequent studies confirmed elevated levels of immunoglobulin E (IgE) during the active phase of INS (13–15), but it is unknown whether the increased levels of IgE in these children are pathogenic or coincidental.

Previous researchers proposed a "two hit" hypothesis for the pathogenesis of INS. The "first hit" occurs when microbial products, allergens, or T-cell cytokines (such as IL-13) damage the glomeruli, resulting in the overexpression of CD80 by podocytes and temporary proteinuria (16–18). In normal settings, regulatory cytokines produced by T regulatory cells (Tregs) terminate the CD80 overexpression, so that the proteinuria is transient and mild (18–20). However, a "second hit" occurs when MCD is present, and this leads to a failure to block CD80 expression by podocytes due to a disruption of autoregulatory responses in Tregs or even in the podocytes themselves. After this second hit, CD80 expression remains continuously elevated, leading to nephrotic syndrome (20). Th2 related cytokines such as IL-13, which stimulates IgE-mediated responses, can promote proteinuria in patients with MCD because it can directly induce CD80 expression in podocytes (13–15, 18). Recent studies found increased levels of IL-13 and IL-4 during the active phase of INS, and that IL-13 functions in the pathogenesis of kidney disease (13–15, 18), but the mechanisms responsible for the increased level of IL-13 are still unclear. Several studies also reported that Th2 cells were over-active in INS (8, 18, 21, 22), but the mechanisms leading to over-activation of these cells are also unknown. Studies of these topics may help to elucidate the role of altered immune responses in the pathogenesis of INS.

MicroRNAs (miRNAs) are short (20–23 nucleotides) non-coding RNAs that can alter the expression of targeted genes (23, 24). In particular, a specific miRNA binds to the 3′-untranslated region (3′-UTR) of its target mRNA, and this is followed by inhibition of translation or increased mRNA degradation (23, 24). Initially, most studies of miRNAs were in the field of oncology, but recent studies have also examined their role in kidney disease (25, 26). For example, several studies showed that multiple miRNAs can inhibit the differentiation and function of Th2 cells (27–29). In 2016, researchers studying allergies found that miR-24 and miR-27 also inhibited the function of Th2 by inhibiting the production of cytokines such as IL-4 (28, 29). However, the effects of these two miRNAs on Th2 expression in patients with active INS, and their specific mechanisms need further study.

Atopic patients have abnormally increased proportions Th2 cells and related factors (9–11). However, it is not clear whether these alterations in children with INS are related to atopy and the pathogenesis of nephropathy. Thus, we systematically measured the dynamics of multiple cytokines, miR-24, and miR-27 in the regulation of Th2 cell differentiation during the active and remission phases of INS, and measured changes in the number and function of Th2 cells isolated from children with non-atopic INS under conditions of altered miRNA expression. Our general purpose was to clarify the role of immune system alterations in the pathogenesis of INS, and to identify potential therapeutic targets and new ideas for the treatment of kidney disease.

PATIENTS AND METHODS

Subjects

Forty children with INS (23 males and 17 females; median age: 38 months; age range: 22–92 months) were enrolled as patients and were divided into two groups: before steroid initiation (11 males and nine females; median age: 35 months; age range: 22–84 months) and after steroid therapy (12 males and eight females; median age: 41 months; age range: 26–92 months). There were also 20 healthy volunteers of similar age (11 males and nine females; median age: 31.3 months; age range: 25–105 months) enrolled as controls (Ctrl) who visited the hospital for physical exams.

All patients were examined at Shenzhen Children's Hospital from September 2015 to October 2016. The inclusion criteria were diagnosis of INS based on the 2010 criteria determined using evidence-based diagnosis and treatment guidelines for common kidney diseases in children from China (30). The 40 children were divided into four groups: an active phase (first-onset) group with atopic constitution (AA, $n = 6$), an active phase group with non-atopic constitution (ANA, $n = 14$), a remission group with atopic constitution (ReA, $n = 6$), and a remission group with non-atopic constitution (ReNA, $n = 14$). Atopy was diagnosed based on family history, the presence of relevant symptoms (asthma, recurrent urticaria, eczema, and allergic rhinitis), and elevated serum IgE concentration. The results of the skin-prick tests were positive for all atopic children. Prednisone therapy was initiated at a dose of 2 mg/kg/day. All patients were steroid-sensitive, had negative test results for urinary protein within 4 weeks of treatment, completed the treatment protocol, and received no other immunosuppressants. In addition, none of the patients had a secondary kidney disease (secondary nephrotic syndrome, nephrotic syndrome, congenital kidney disease, etc.) and none had other systemic visceral syndromes. Blood samples were collected for analysis before steroid initiation in the active NS group and 4 weeks after steroid discontinuation in the remission group.

All parents or legal guardians provided informed consent prior to study enrollment, and the study was performed after approval by the local Medical Ethics Committee.

Blood Samples

Venous blood was collected from patients and healthy controls in EDTA tubes. Then, Ficoll density gradient centrifugation was used to isolate peripheral blood mononuclear cells (PBMCs) for analysis by flow cytometry. Plasma samples were collected after centrifugation and were frozen (at −80°C) prior to using the cytometric bead array (CBA; kit no. 11363D, Dynal, Invitrogen, USA) for isolation of $CD4^{+}CD25^{-}$ T cells). Cell purity was based on a threshold of 97% from flow cytometry. Cell activity (determined using the trypan blue exclusion assay) was based on a threshold of 95%.

Extraction of Total RNA Extraction and Synthesis of cDNA

Total RNA (including miRNAs) samples were isolated from $CD4^{+}CD25^{-}$ T cells using the miRNeasy Mini Kit (Qiagen, Germany) according to the manufacturer's instructions. Following confirmation of purity (average OD_{260nm}/OD_{280nm} = 1.98), cDNA was synthesized using oligo-dT primers and RevertAid™ H Minus reverse transcriptase (Fermentas, Lithuania). The miScript II RT kit (Qiagen) was used for synthesis of miRNA cDNAs. Negative controls (no first-strand synthesis) were synthesized using reverse transcription without reverse transcriptase.

LightCycler Real-Time PCR

The level of IL-4 was determined using real-time PCR with the Quantitect™ SYBR green PCR Kit (Takara, Japan) and a LightCycler® 2.0 (Roche Molecular Biochemicals, Switzerland). The primers were: 5′-TCATTTTCCCTCGGTTTCAG-3′ (forward) and 5′- ATAGGTGTCGATTTGCAGTG-3′ (reverse). Real-time PCR with the miScript SYBR Green PCR Kit (Qiagen) and the LightCycler® 2.0 were used to quantitate the levels of miR-24 and miR-27. The primers were synthesized from recommendations in the miRNA miScript Primer Assay (Qiagen). The second derivative maximum method was used to identify the crossing point (Cp) with LightCycler software version 3.5.30 (Roche Molecular Biochemicals). After normalization using Relative Quantification Software version 1.0 (Roche Molecular Biochemicals), the levels of the PCR products were presented relative to those of *GAPDH* (target genes) or *U6* (miRNAs).

Flow Cytometry Analysis of Th2 Cells

To measure expression of cytoplasmic markers of Th2 cells, cells were cultured in a 37°C/5% CO_2 incubator, with ionomycin (250 ng/mL; SigmaAldrich), PMA (25 ng/mL; Sigma-Aldrich), and monensin (20 ng/mL; eBio-science, San Diego, CA, USA) added as stimulation for 24 h. Then, cells were stained for different markers, and were fixed and permeabilized using the Cytofix/Cytoperm kit (eBioscience). The cells were stained with specific antibodies (or corresponding isotype-matched controls) and then analyzed using a FACS Canto II flow cytometer (BD Biosciences, Mississauga, ON, Canada). Staining with the fixable viability stain 450 (FVS450, BD Biosciences) was used to determine viability. Validated antibodies (CD3-eFour450A, CD8-FITC, and IL-4-PE) were purchased from eBioscience.

CBA Detection of Plasma IgE, IL-4, and IL-13

A CBA kit (e Bioscience) was used to measure the plasma levels of IgE, IL-4, and IL-13. Each sample was measured twice.

Cell Transfection and Culture

The roles of miR-24 and miR-27 in Th2 cells were examined using transfection experiments in PBMCs. First, PBMCs were isolated from healthy controls or patients using Ficoll density gradient centrifugation. Then mimics (Ctrl-m, miR-24-m, or miR-27-m) or inhibitors (Ctrl-i, miR-24-i, or miR-27-i) from RiboBio (Guangzhou, China) were transfected into the PBMCs using the riboFECT CP Transfection Kit (Guangzhou, China). Cells were cultured in RPMI-1640 medium (Gibco, CA, USA) that was supplemented with 15% fetal calf serum (Gibco, CA, USA) and maintained at 37°C/5% CO_2 in 24-well plates (3×10^6 cells per mL). Cells were then harvested for flow cytometry and RT-PCR analyses.

Statistical Analysis

Statistical analyses were performed using SPSS software for Windows version 13.0 (SPSS Inc., USA). Data are expressed as means ± standard deviations. For comparisons of multiple groups, a one-way analysis of variance was used. For comparison of two groups, Student's *t*-test was used. *P*-values below 0.05 were considered significant.

RESULTS

Patients With Atopic and Non-atopic INS Have Increased Serum IgE Levels

We first measured the plasma levels of IgE in the five different groups using a CBA (**Figure 1**). Analysis of IgE concentration indicated significantly greater levels in the AA group (1350.67 ± 837.39 IU/mL, $P < 0.05$) and the ANA group (441.01 ± 357.45 IU/mL, $P < 0.05$) than in the Ctrl group (57.76 ± 48.25 IU/mL). In addition, the AA group had higher levels of IgE than the other groups (all $P < 0.05$). Compared with the ANA group, the Ctrl, ReNA (62.97 ± 27.31 IU/mL), and ReA (237.75 ± 95.15 IU/mL) groups had significantly reduced levels of IgE (all $P < 0.05$). However, the ReA and ReNA groups had no significant difference ($P > 0.05$).

Patients With Active Phase INS Have Over-Expression of Th2 Cells and Associated Cytokines

We quantified the Tregs from whole blood samples in the five groups using flow cytometry (**Figures 2A,B**). The percentage of peripheral Th2 cells in the AA group (5.60% ± 1.21) and the ANA group (4.23% ± 0.92) were significantly greater than in the Ctrl group (3.29% ± 1.02, both $P < 0.05$). As with IgE, there was no significant difference between the ReA (3.60% ± 0.78) and ReNA (3.40% ± 0.64) groups ($P > 0.05$). Also as with IgE, the AA group had a higher percentage of Th2 cells than all other groups (all $P < 0.05$).

We then measured the plasma levels of IL-4 and IL-13 in all five groups using CBA (**Figures 2C,D**). Relative to the control group, the AA group had higher levels of IL-4 (66.66 pg/mL ± 43.85 vs. 23.29 pg/mL ± 13.91, $P < 0.05$) and IL-13 (65.15 pg/mL ± 16.50 vs. 15.66 pg/mL ± 8.16, $P < 0.05$). Also relative to the control group, the ANA group had higher levels of IL-4 (37.04 pg/mL ± 17.39 vs. 23.29 pg/mL ± 13.91, $P < 0.05$)

and IL-13 (33.15 pg/mL ± 14.09 vs. 15.66 pg/mL ± 8.16, $P < 0.05$). However, there was no significant difference between the ReA and ReNA groups in these cytokines (IL-4: 35.91 pg/mL ± 15.75 vs. 23.73 pg/mL ± 11.71, $P > 0.05$; IL-13: 22.33 pg/mL ± 8.87 vs. 16.53 pg/mL ± 7.76, $P > 0.05$). Compared with the AA group, all other groups had significantly decreased levels of both cytokines (all $P < 0.05$).

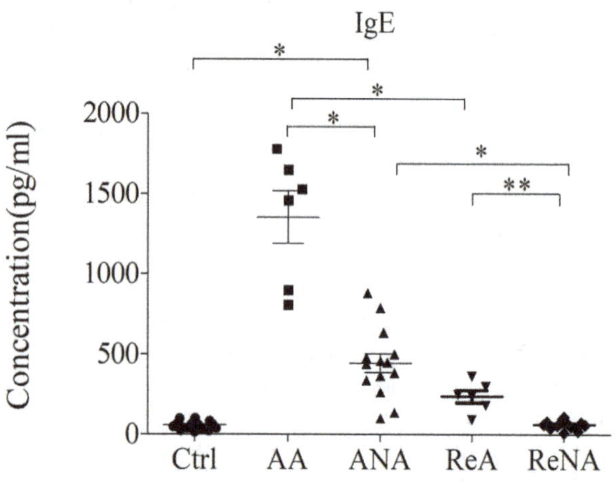

FIGURE 1 | Children with atopic and non-atopic INS have increased serum levels of IgE. Here and below: all data are shown as means ± SDs; $^*P < 0.05$ and $^{**}P > 0.05$; and abbreviations are healthy control (Ctrl, $n = 20$), active phase atopic (AA, $n = 6$), active phase non-atopic (ANA, $n = 14$), remission phase atopic (ReA, $n = 6$), and remission phase non-atopic (ReNA, $n = 14$).

Patients With Non-atopic INS Have Altered Expression of miR-24 and miR-27

Previous research showed that miR-24 and miR-27 affected Th2 cell expression. Because we identified increased expression of Th2 cells in the ANA group, we also determined whether these miRNAs were also decreased (**Figure 3**). The results showed that the levels of miR-24 and miR-27 were significantly lower in the ANA group than in the Ctrl group (both $P < 0.05$; **Table 1**). The levels of these two miRNAs were greater in the ReNA group than in the ANA group, but not up to the levels in the Ctrl group ($P < 0.05$).

miR-24 and miR-27 Suppress the Expression of Th2 Cells and IL-4

We further examined the relationship between miR-24, miR-27, and Th2 cells by transfection of PBMCs isolated from healthy volunteers and INS patients with ANA using six different miRNAs: negative control (Ctrl-m); miR-24 mimic (miR-24-m); miR-27 mimic (miR-27-m); miRNA inhibitor negative control (Ctrl-i); miR-24 inhibitor (miR-24-i); or miR-27 inhibitor

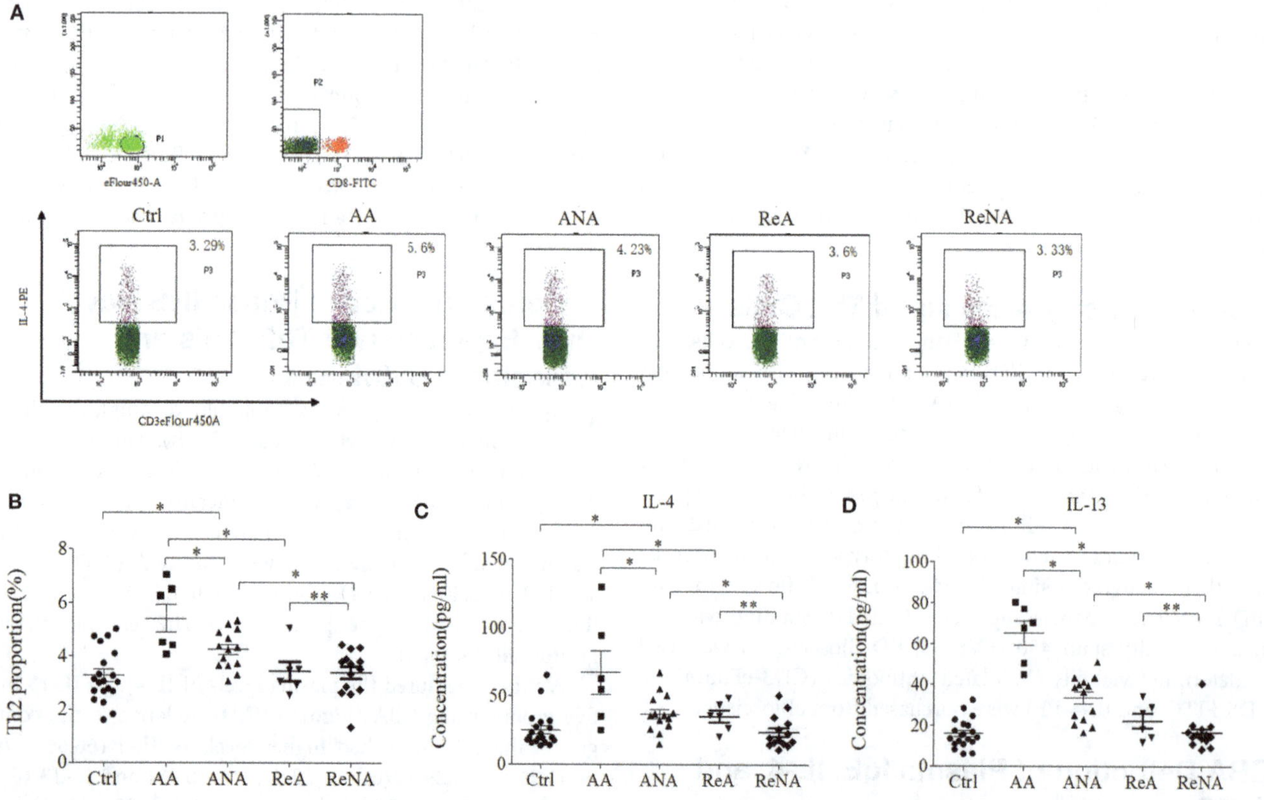

FIGURE 2 | Children with INS have increased levels of Th2 cells and Th2-related cytokines. **(A)** Flow cytometric analysis of Th2 cells. **(B)** Percentages of Th2 cells. **(C)** Plasma concentrations of IL-4. **(D)** Plasma concentrations of IL-13. $^*P < 0.05$ and $^{**}P > 0.05$.

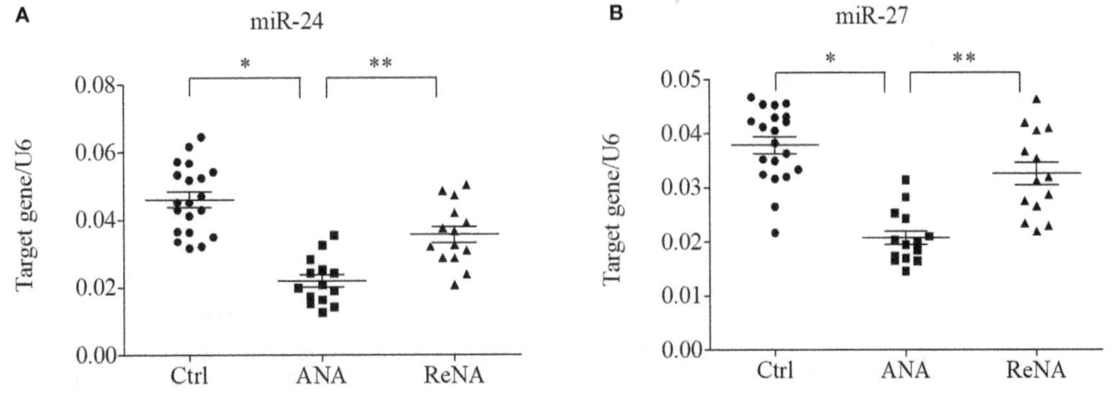

FIGURE 3 | Children with INS have reduced expression of miR-24 and miR-27 in $CD4^+CD25^-$ T cells. Expression of miRNAs (relative to U6) were determined by real-time PCR. **(A)** Expression levels of miR-24. **(B)** Expression levels of miR-27. **P* < 0.05 and ***P* > 0.05.

TABLE 1 | Expression of miR-24 and miR-27 in patients with non-atopic INS and healthy controls.

	Ctrl ($n = 20$)	ANA ($n = 14$)	ReNA ($n = 14$)
miR-24	$(46.03 \pm 10.08)\times10^{-3}$	$(21.84 \pm 6.86)\times10^{-3a}$	$(35.59 \pm 9.10)\times10^{-3b}$
miR-27	$(37.83 \pm 6.83)\times10^{-3}$	$(20.72 \pm 4.93)\times10^{-3a}$	$(32.55\pm7.86)\times10^{-3b}$

Values are expressed as mean ± SD.
[a]P < 0.05 for one-way ANOVA vs. Ctrl group.
[b]P < 0.05 for one-way ANOVA vs. ANA group.
Ctrl, healthy control; ANA, active phase non-atopic; ReNA, remission phase non-atopic.

(miR-27-i). The results showed that up-regulation of miR-24 (**Figures 4A,B**) and miR-27 (**Figures 5A,B**) reduced the percentage of Th2 cells (**Figures 4C,D, 5C,D**) and the expression of IL-4 mRNA (**Figures 4E,F, 5E,F**). In agreement, down regulation of miR-24 (**Figures 6A,B**) and miR-27 (**Figures 7A,B**), increased the percentage of Th2 cells (**Figures 6C,D, 7C,D**) and the expression of IL-4 mRNA (**Figures 6E,F, 7E,F**).

DISCUSSION

A large body of evidence has demonstrated that the immune system may play a crucial role in INS (3), although the pathogenic details of this disease remain mostly unknown. Previous research suggested that INS may be due to an abnormal T cell response or the dysregulation of T lymphocytes (3–8). MCD is the most common cause of INS (1, 2, 18, 19), and Th2 cells play an important role in many allergic and inflammatory diseases (9–11, 27, 31). More than 60 years ago, Hardwicke et al. reported an association of seasonal proteinuria with pollen sensitivity (12). Patients with MCD often have allergy-like symptoms, such as bronchial asthma, allergic rhinitis, atopic dermatitis, and urticaria. Some studies also confirmed that patients with INS may have increased levels of serum IgE, especially children with INS recurrence (13–15, 18). However, the causal relationship between the increased serum level of IgE or atopy and the pathogenesis of INS remains uncertain. The present study confirms that children in the active phase of INS with or without atopy had increased plasma levels of IgE compared with healthy controls, and they also had higher levels than children in the remission phase of INS. Among children in remission, the IgE levels of non-atopic children were nearly normal, but the IgE levels of atopic children were high. Thus, children with atopic and non-atopic INS have increased serum levels of IgE. However, further investigations of the underlying cytokine regulatory network are needed to more completely understand the relationship between INS and IgE production.

Th2 cells secrete IL-13 and IL-4, and this can promote the production of IgE in B cells (9–11). In particular, IL-13 induces a change from expression of IgM to IgE in B cells, and also induces podocytes to increase their synthesis of CD80. Increased CD80 expression by podocytes is associated with proteinuria (13–15, 18). Elevated levels of IL-13 are present in the urine and serum of patients who have kidney disease, and are also associated with a proteinuria (13–15, 18). These previous studies thus suggest that IL-13 functions in the pathogenesis of kidney disease, but the mechanism responsible for the increased IL-13 level is still unclear. Recent studies reported that Th2-related factors, IL-13 and IL-4, have increased levels in patients with active INS (13–15, 18). Other studies noted that patients with INS have increased proportions of Th2 cells (8, 18, 21, 22), but it was uncertain whether this alteration contributed to the pathogenesis of INS. This led us to examine the expression of Th2 cells in peripheral blood and the plasma concentrations of IL-13 and IL-4 in patients with different INS disease states. Our results demonstrated significantly increased levels of Th2 cells, IL-13, and IL-4 in patients with active phase INS with or without atopy. These results thus suggest that the proteinuria and increased IgE levels that occur during the active phase of INS, regardless of the presence of atopy, might be due to the increased levels of IL-13 and IL-4, which were caused by a drift toward Th2 cells. However, the mechanism responsible for this drift toward Th2 cells needs further study to elucidate the role of the immune system in the pathogenesis of INS.

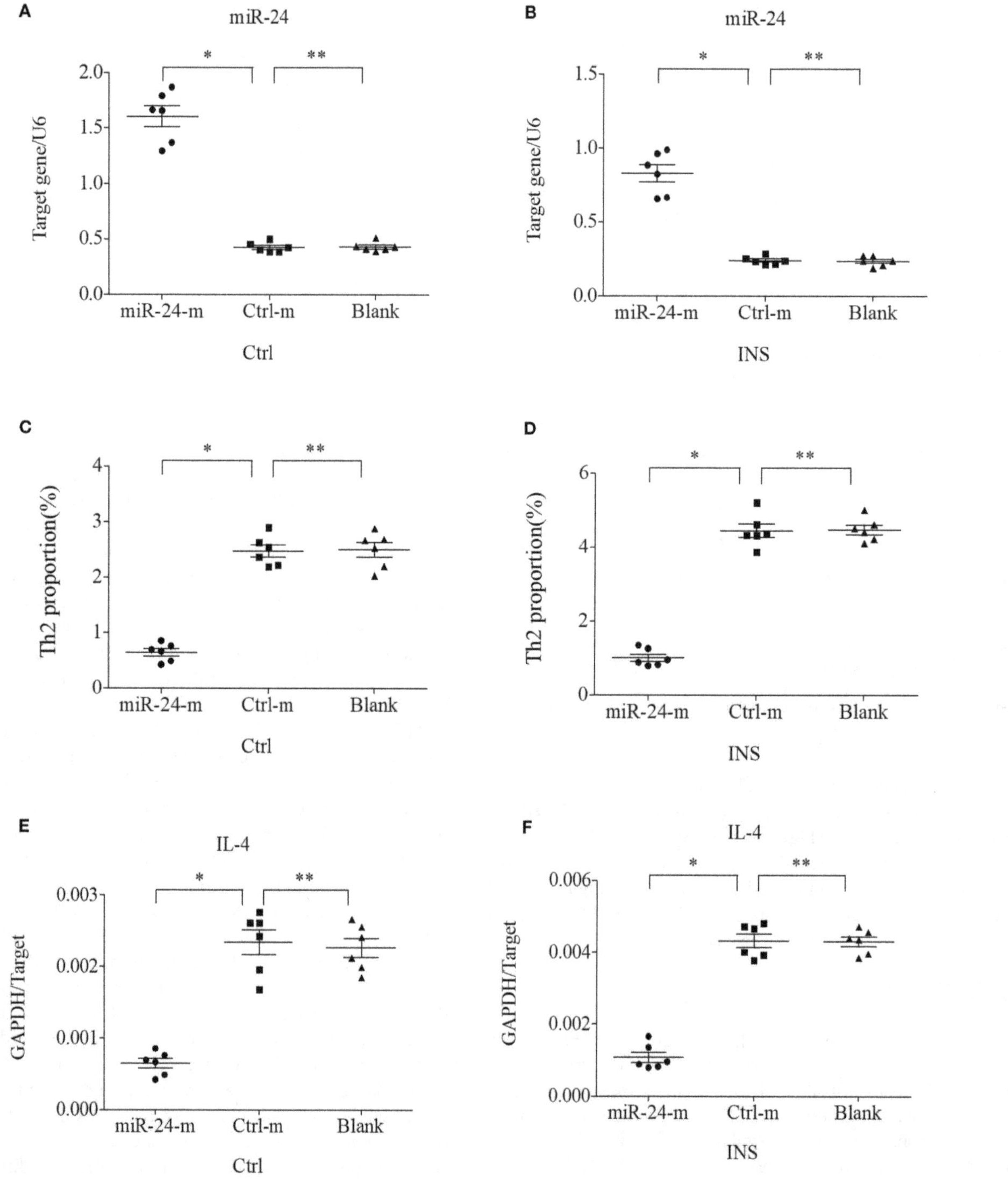

FIGURE 4 | Up-regulation of miR-24 in PBMCs from controls and INS patients **(A,B)** reduces the percentage of Th2 cells **(C,D)** and the expression of IL-4 mRNA **(E,F)**. Here and in **Figures 5–7**: expression of miRNAs (relative to U6) and IL-4 (relative to GAPDH) were determined by real-time PCR; ANA ($n = 6$), Crtl ($n = 6$); and abbreviations are Ctrl-m (miRNA negative control), miR-24-m/miR-27-m (miR-24/miR-27 mimic), Ctrl-i (miRNA inhibitor [negative control]), and miR-24-i/miR-27-i (miR-24/miR-27 inhibitor). $^{*}P < 0.05$ and $^{**}P > 0.05$.

miRNAs are subtle "master controllers" of gene expression, and function in the pathogenesis of many human diseases, especially chronic and multifactorial diseases (23, 24). Previous studies reported that some specific miRNAs were abnormally expressed in patients with various allergic and autoimmune diseases, such as asthma, systemic lupus erythematosus (SLE),

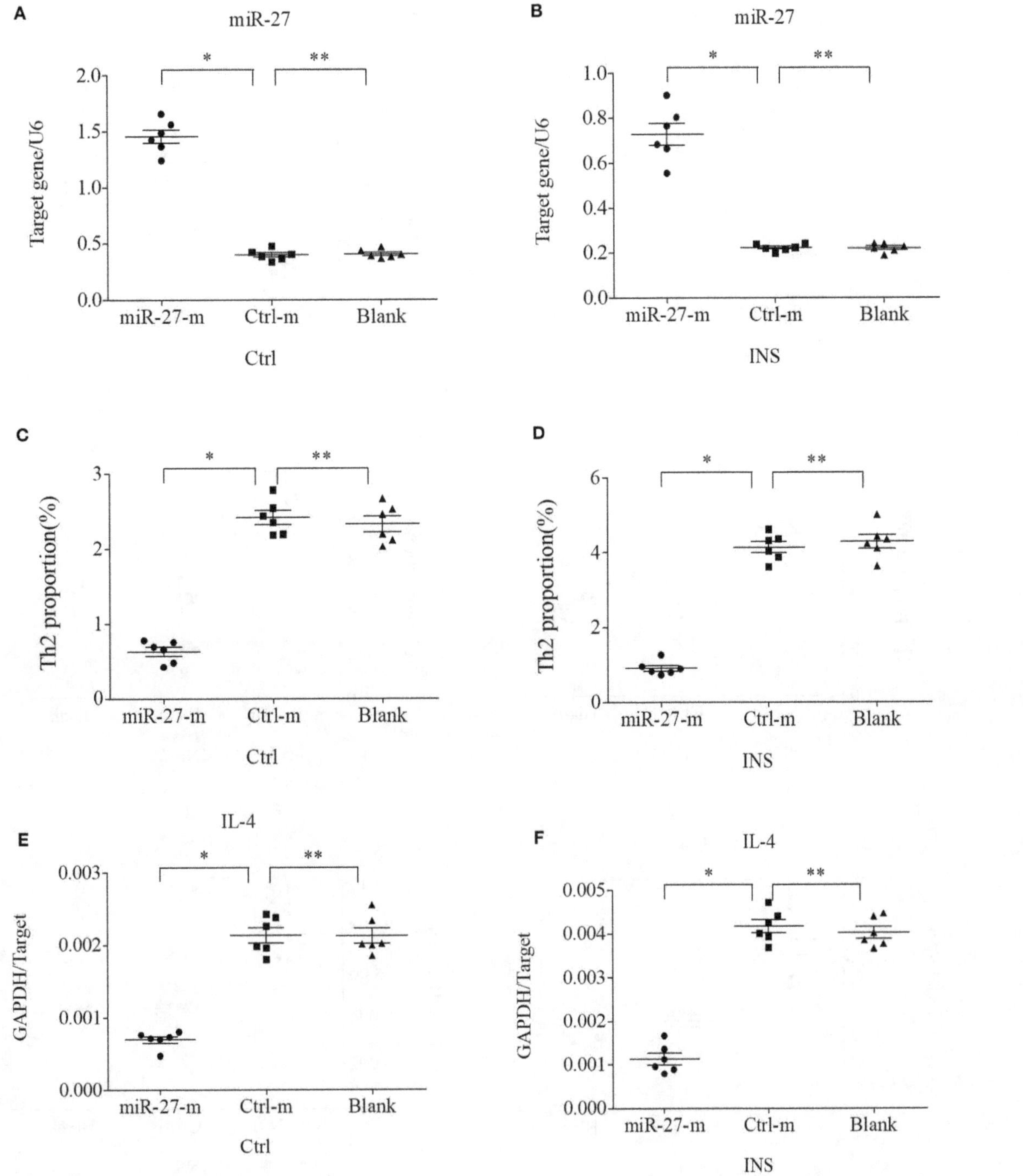

FIGURE 5 | Up-regulation of miR-27 in PBMCs from controls and INS patients **(A,B)** reduces the percentage of Th2 cells **(C,D)** and the expression of IL-4 mRNA **(E,F)**. $^{*}P < 0.05$ and $^{**}P > 0.05$.

and lupus nephritis, and that their expression also increased with disease activity (27, 32, 33). Other specific miRNAs are important for Th2 cell proliferation, differentiation, and immune function (27–29). In particular, miR-24 and miR-27 suppress allergic inflammation and target a network of regulators of Th2 cell-associated cytokine production (28, 29). Thus, the abnormal increase of Th2 cells and its related factor IL-13 in children with INS is not related to atopy, but is related to the pathogenesis of nephropathy. However, it is unclear whether alterations in the levels of different miRNAs lead to alterations in Th2 expression in patients with active INS. Therefore, we determined the expression of miR-24 and miR-27 and examined their possible

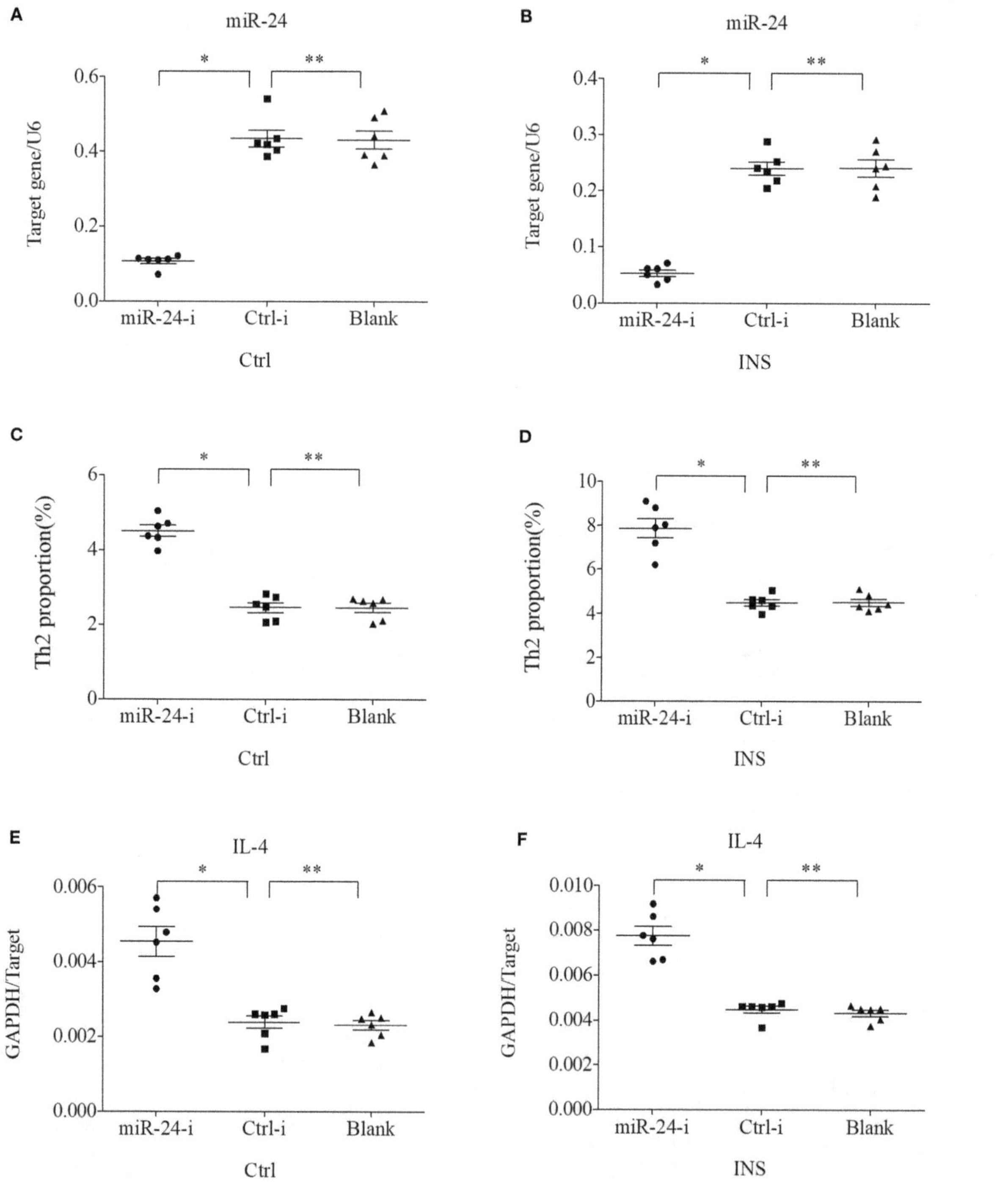

FIGURE 6 | Down regulation of miR-24 in PBMCs from controls and INS patients **(A,B)** increases the percentage of Th2 cells **(C,D)** and the expression of IL-4 mRNA **(E,F)**. $^{*}P < 0.05$ and $^{**}P > 0.05$.

role in regulating Th2 cell differentiation. Our results clearly showed that these two miRNAs had low expression in pediatric patients with active non-atopic INS. This suggests that the drift toward Th2 cells might be related to the low expression of these miRNAs in these children.

To verify this hypothesis, we first isolated PBMCs from healthy controls and children with non-atopic INS. Then, we transfected these cells with miR-24 or miR-27 mimics to increase expression, or with miR-24 or miR-27 inhibitors to reduce expression. The results showed that the percentage

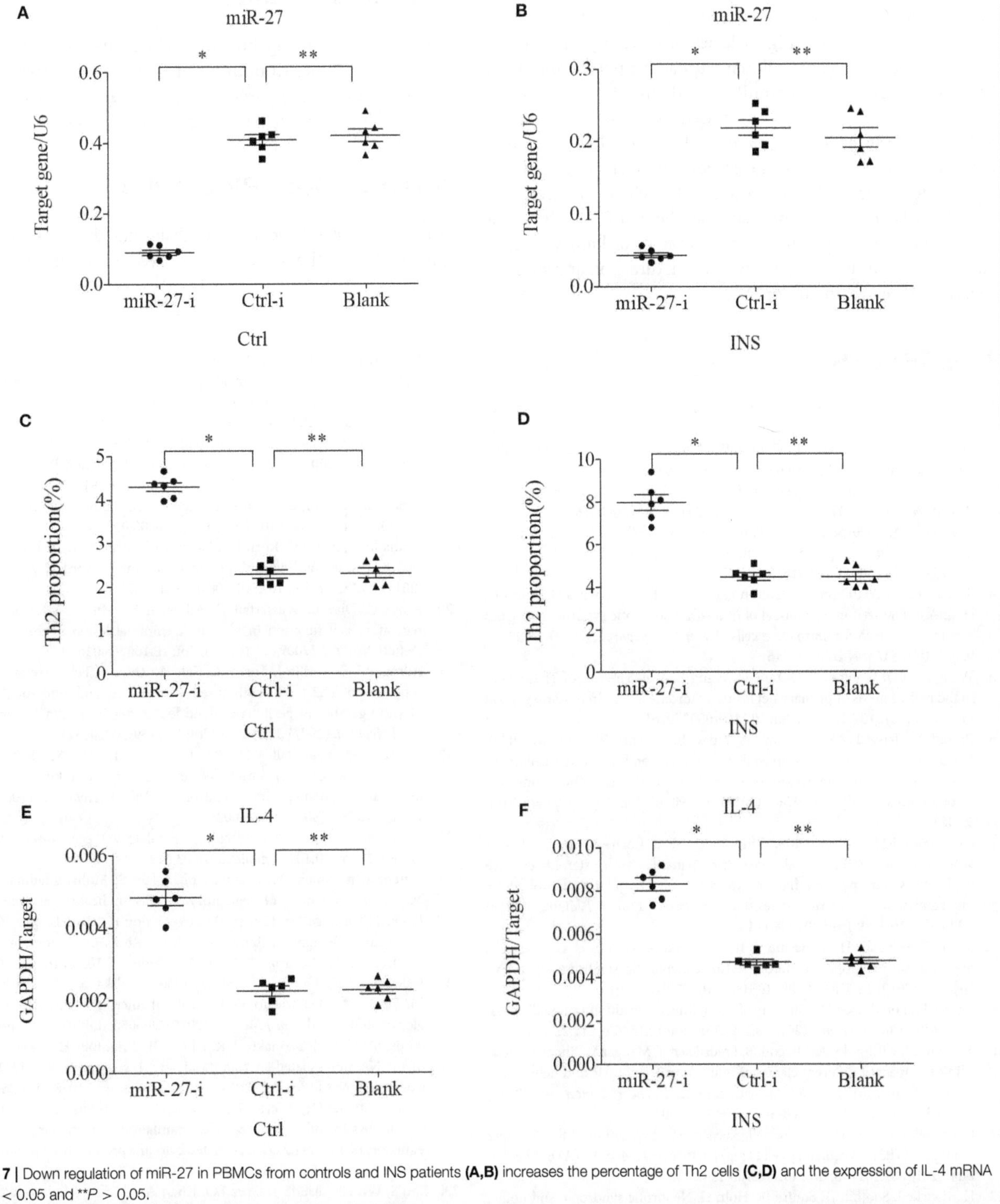

FIGURE 7 | Down regulation of miR-27 in PBMCs from controls and INS patients **(A,B)** increases the percentage of Th2 cells **(C,D)** and the expression of IL-4 mRNA **(E,F)**. $^{*}P < 0.05$ and $^{**}P > 0.05$.

of Th2 cells and the level of IL-4 decreased when the levels of these miRNAs was increased. In agreement, the percentage of Th2 cells and the expression of IL-4 increased when the levels of these miRNAs was decreased. These results support our initial hypothesis that miR-24 and miR-27 reduce the percentage of Th2 cells, and suggest they might play an important role in Th2 expression during active INS.

In conclusion, our results indicate that the Th2 related-cytokine IL-13 is related to the pathogenesis of kidney disease but is not related to atopy, although the mechanisms responsible for the increased level of this cytokine remain unclear. Our results also indicate that pediatric patients with active phase INS that is either atopic or non-atopic have higher levels of IgE, and this might be related to their higher levels of IL-13 and IL-4 due to a drift toward Th2 cells. Children with active phase non-atopic INS had reduced levels of miR-24 and miR-27, an increased percentage of Th2 cells, and an increased level of IL-4, and this led to IL-13 over-expression and increased IgE levels. In other words, these two miRNAs suppress the expression of Th2 cells and play an important role in the drift toward Th2 cells in children with active INS. Therefore, we speculate that these miRNAs should be considered as potential targets for treatment of kidney disease. Our research thus provides a new research direction and suggests a possible novel treatment for INS.

ETHICS STATEMENT

The studies involving human participants were reviewed and approved by Ethics Committee of Shenzhen Children's Hospital. Written informed consent to participate in this study was provided by the participants' legal guardian/next of kin.

AUTHOR CONTRIBUTIONS

All authors listed have made a substantial, direct and intellectual contribution to the work, and approved it for publication.

REFERENCES

1. Yang JY, Yao Y, Chinese Society of Pediatric Nephrology. Analysis of 1,268 patients with chronic renal failure in childhood: a report from 91 hospitals in China from 1990 to 2002. *Zhonghua Er Ke Za Zhi.* (2004) 42:724–30. doi: 10.3760/j.issn:0578-1310.2004.10.002
2. Vivarelli M, Massella L, Ruggiero B, Emma F. Minimal change disease. *Clin J Am Soc Nephrol.* (2017) 12:332–45. doi: 10.2215/CJN.05000516
3. Colucci M, Corpetti G, Emma F, Vivarelli M. Immunology of idiopathic nephrotic syndrome. *Pediatr Nephrol.* (2018) 33:573–84. doi: 10.1007/s00467-017-3677-5
4. Sellier-Leclerc AL, Duval A, Riveron S, Macher MA, Deschenes G, Loirat C, et al. A humanized mouse model of idiopathic nephrotic syndrome suggests a pathogenic role for immature cells. *J Am Soc Nephrol.* (2007) 18:2732–9. doi: 10.1681/ASN.2006121346
5. Wang L, Li Q, Wang L, Li C, Yang H, Wang X, et al. The role of Th17/IL-17 in the pathogenesis of primary nephrotic syndrome in children. *Kidney Blood Press Res.* (2013) 37:332–45. doi: 10.1159/000350161
6. Prasad N, Jaiswal AK, Agarwal V, Yadav B, Sharma RK, Rai M, et al. Differential alteration in peripheral T-regulatory and T-effector cells with change in P-glycoprotein expression in Childhood Nephrotic Syndrome: a longitudinal study. *Cytokine.* (2015) 72:190–6. doi: 10.1016/j.cyto.2014.12.028
7. Guimarães FTL, Ferreira RN, Brito-Melo GEA, Rocha-Vieira E, Pereira WF, Pinheiro SVB, et al. Pediatric patients with steroid-sensitive nephrotic syndrome have higher expression of T regulatory lymphocytes in comparison to steroid-resistant disease. *Front Pediatr.* (2019) 7:114. doi: 10.3389/fped.2019.00114
8. Kanai T, Shiraishi H, Yamagata T, Ito T, Odaka J, Saito T, et al. Th2 cells predominate in idiopathic steroid-sensitive nephrotic syndrome. *Clin Exp Nephrol.* (2010) 14:578–83. doi: 10.1007/s10157-010-0330-z
9. Raphael I, Forsthuber TG. Stability of T-cell lineages in autoimmune diseases. *Expert Rev Clin Immunol.* (2012) 8:299–301. doi: 10.1586/eci.12.22
10. Tosolini M, Kirilovsky A, Mlecnik B, Fredriksen T, Mauger S, Bindea G, et al. Clinical impact of different classes of infiltrating T cytotoxic and helper cells (Th1, th2, treg, th17) in patients with colorectal cancer. *Cancer Res.* (2011) 71:1263–71. doi: 10.1158/0008-5472.CAN-10-2907
11. Chapoval S, Dasgupta P, Dorsey NJ, Keegan AD. Regulation of the T helper cell type 2 (Th2)/T regulatory cell (Treg) balance by IL-4 and STAT6. *J Leukoc Biol.* (2010) 87:1011–8. doi: 10.1189/jlb.1209772
12. Hardwicke J, Soothill JF, Squire JR, Holti G. Nephrotic syndrome and pollen hypersensitivity. *Lancet.* (1959) 1:500–2. doi: 10.1016/S0140-6736(59)91026-8
13. Mishra OP, Teli AS, Singh U, Abhinay A, Prasad R. Serum immunoglobulin E and interleukin-13 levels in children with idiopathic nephrotic syndrome. *J Trop Pediatr.* (2014) 60:467–71. doi: 10.1093/tropej/fmu040
14. Hossain A. Serum IgE level in relapsing idiopathic nephrotic syndrome in children. *Urol Nephrol Open Access J.* (2019) 7:238. doi: 10.15406/unoaj.2019.07.00238
15. Mishra OP, Ibrahim N, Usha, Das BK. Serum immunoglobulin E in idiopathic nephrotic syndrome. *J Trop Pediatr.* (2004) 50:149–52. doi: 10.1093/tropej/50.3.149
16. Garin EH, Diaz LN, Mu W, Wasserfall C, Araya C, Segal M, et al. Urinary CD80 excretion increases in idiopathic minimal-change disease. *J Am Soc Nephrol.* (2009) 20:260–6. doi: 10.1681/ASN.2007080836
17. Reiser J, Mundel P. Danger signaling by glomerular podocytes defines a novel function of inducible B7-1 in the pathogenesis of nephrotic syndrome. *J Am Soc Nephrol.* (2004) 15:2246–8. doi: 10.1097/01.ASN.0000136312.46464.33
18. Abdel-Hafez M, Shimada M, Lee PY, Johnson RJ, Garin EH. Idiopathic nephrotic syndrome and atopy: is there a common link? *Am J Kidney Dis.* (2009) 54:945–53. doi: 10.1053/j.ajkd.2009.03.019
19. Shimada M, Araya C, Rivard C, Ishimoto T, Johnson RJ, Garin EH. Minimal change disease: a "two-hit" podocyte immune disorder? *Pediatr Nephrol.* (2011) 26:645–9. doi: 10.1007/s00467-010-1676-x
20. Araya C, Diaz L, Wasserfall C, Atkinson M, Mu W, Johnson R, et al. T regulatory cell function in idiopathic minimal lesion nephrotic syndrome. *Pediatr Nephrol.* (2009) 24:1691–8. doi: 10.1007/s00467-009-1214-x
21. Adrogue HE, Borillo J, Torres L, Kale A, Zhou C, Feig D, et al. Coincident activation of Th2 T cells with onset of the disease and differential expression of GRO-gamma in peripheral blood leukocytes in minimal change disease. *Am J Nephrol.* (2007) 27:253–61. doi: 10.1159/000101371
22. Araya CE, Wasserfall CH, Brusko TM, Mu W, Segal MS, Johnson RJ, et al. A case of unfulfilled expectations. Cytokines in idiopathic minimal lesion nephrotic syndrome. *Pediatr Nephrol.* (2006) 21:603–10. doi: 10.1007/s00467-006-0026-5
23. Phiwpan K, Zhou X. MicroRNAs in regulatory T cells. *Cancer Lett.* (2018) 423:80–5. doi: 10.1016/j.canlet.2018.03.012
24. Soltanzadeh-Yamchi M, Shahbazi M, Aslani S, Mohammadnia-Afrouzi M. MicroRNA signature of regulatory T cells in health and autoimmunity. *Biomed Pharmacother.* (2018) 100:316–23. doi: 10.1016/j.biopha.2018.02.030
25. Trionfini P, Benigni A, Remuzzi G. MicroRNAs in kidney physiology and disease. *Nat Rev Nephrol.* (2015) 11:23–33. doi: 10.1038/nrneph.2014.202
26. Nalewajska M, Gurazda K, Styczyńska-Kowalska E, Marchelek-Myśliwiec M, Pawlik A, Dziedziejko V. The role of microRNAs in selected forms of glomerulonephritis. *Int J Mol Sci.* (2019) 20:5050. doi: 10.3390/ijms20205050
27. Simpson LJ, Patel S, Bhakta NR, Choy DF, Brightbill HD, Ren X, et al. A microRNA upregulated in asthma airway T cells promotes TH2 cytokine production. *Nat Immunol.* (2014) 15:1162–70. doi: 10.1038/ni.3026
28. Pua HH, Steiner DF, Patel S, Gonzalez JR, Ortiz-Carpena JF, Kageyama R, et al. MicroRNAs 24 and 27 suppress allergic inflammation and target a network of regulators of T helper 2 cell-associated cytokine production. *Immunity.* (2016) 44:821–32. doi: 10.1016/j.immuni.2016.01.003
29. Cho S, Wu CJ, Yasuda T, Cruz LO, Khan AA, Lin LL, et al. miR-23∼27∼24 clusters control effector T cell differentiation and function. *J Exp Med.* (2016) 213:235–49. doi: 10.1084/jem.20150990
30. Subspecialty Group of Nephrology, Society of Pediatrics, Chinese Medical Association. Evidence-based guidelines on diagnosis and treatment of childhood common renal diseases. (I) Evidence-based guideline on diagnosis and treatment of steroid-sensitive, relapsing/steroid-dependent nephrotic syndrome (for trial implementation). *Zhonghua Er Ke Za Zhi.* (2009) 47:167–70. doi: 10.3760/cma.j.issn.0578-1310.2009.03.003
31. Nakayama T, Hirahara K, Onodera A, Endo Y, Hosokawa H, Shinoda K, et al. Th2 cells in health and disease. *Annu Rev Immunol.* (2017) 35:53–84. doi: 10.1146/annurev-immunol-051116-052350

32. Honarpisheh M, Köhler P, von Rauchhaupt E, Lech M. The involvement of microRNAs in modulation of innate and adaptive immunity in systemic lupus erythematosus and lupus nephritis. *J Immunol Res.* (2018) 2018:4126106. doi: 10.1155/2018/4126106

33. Stypińska B, Paradowska-Gorycka A. Cytokines and microRNAs as candidate biomarkers for systemic lupus erythematosus. *Int J Mol Sci.* (2015) 16:24194–218. doi: 10.3390/ijms161024194

5

Genetic Testing for Steroid-Resistant-Nephrotic Syndrome in an Outbred Population

*Jennifer D. Varner[1,2], Megan Chryst-Stangl[1,2], Christopher Imokhuede Esezobor[3], Adaobi Solarin[4], Guanghong Wu[1,2], Brandon Lane[1,2], Gentzon Hall[1,2], Asiri Abeyagunawardena[5], Ayo Matory[1], Tracy E. Hunley[6], Jen Jar Lin[7], David Howell[8] and Rasheed Gbadegesin[1,2]**

[1] Division of Nephrology, Departments of Pediatrics and Medicine, Duke University Medical Center, Durham, NC, United States, [2] Duke Molecular Physiology Institute, Duke University Medical Center, Durham, NC, United States, [3] Department of Pediatrics, College of Medicine of the University of Lagos, Lagos, Nigeria, [4] Department of Pediatrics, Lagos State University Teaching Hospital, Ikeja, Nigeria, [5] Department of Pediatrics, University of Peradeniya, Peradeniya, Sri Lanka, [6] Division of Nephrology, Department of Pediatrics, Vanderbilt University, Nashville, TN, United States, [7] Department of Pediatrics, Wake Forest Baptist Medical Center, Winston Salem, NC, United States, [8] Department of Pathology, Duke University Medical Center, Durham, NC, United States

***Correspondence:**
Rasheed Gbadegesin
rasheed.gbadegesin@duke.edu

Background: Steroid-resistant nephrotic syndrome (SRNS) is a leading cause of end-stage kidney disease in children and young adults. Despite advances in genomic science that have led to the discovery of >50 monogenic causes of SRNS, there are no clear guidelines for genetic testing in clinical practice.

Methods: Using high throughput sequencing, we evaluated 492 individuals from 181 families for mutations in 40 known SRNS genes. Causative mutations were defined as missense, truncating, and obligatory splice site variants with a minor allele frequency <1% in controls. Non-synonymous variants were considered pathogenic if determined to be deleterious by at least two *in silico* models. We further evaluated for differences in age at disease onset, family history of SRNS or chronic kidney disease, race, sex, renal biopsy findings, and extra-renal manifestations in subgroups with and without disease causing variants.

Results: We identified causative variants in 40 of 181 families (22.1%) with SRNS. Variants in *INF2*, *COL4A3*, and *WT1* were the most common, accounting for over half of all causative variants. Causative variants were identified in 34 of 86 families (39.5%) with familial disease and 6 of 95 individuals (6.3%) with sporadic disease (χ^2 $p < 0.00001$). Family history was the only significant clinical predictor of genetic SRNS.

Conclusion: We identified causative mutations in almost 40% of all families with hereditary SRNS and 6% of individuals with sporadic disease, making family history the single most important clinical predictors of monogenic SRNS. We recommend genetic testing in all patients with SRNS and a positive family history, but only selective testing in those with sporadic disease.

Keywords: focal segmental glomerulosclerosis, genetic testing, monogenic disease, podocyte, steroid-resistant nephrotic syndrome

BACKGROUND

Nephrotic syndrome (NS) is a clinical syndrome characterized by massive proteinuria, hypoalbuminemia, peripheral edema, and hyperlipidemia. It may be complicated by venous thromboembolism, cardiovascular disease, and increased risk of infections due to loss of immunoglobulins (1, 2). With an annual incidence of 2–7 per 100,000 and a prevalence rate of 16 per 100,000, NS is the most common glomerular disease in children and adults (2–4).

The initial response to corticosteroid treatment is the most important clinical predictor of long-term prognosis (5, 6). The majority of patients with steroid-resistant nephrotic syndrome (SRNS) will progress to end-stage kidney disease (ESKD) within 5–10 years of diagnosis (7, 8). In addition, SRNS accounts for >10% of all cases of children with ESKD and is the most prevalent diagnosis among children receiving maintenance dialysis (1, 9' 10).

The two most common histopathologic changes seen on renal biopsy are minimal change disease (MCD) and focal segmental glomerulosclerosis (FSGS) (1). MCD is the most common histopathological finding in children, but the prevalence of FSGS is increasing (11). Under light microscopy, there are no notable changes in MCD, but electron microscopy demonstrates microvillus transformation and impaired podocyte foot process adherence to the glomerular basement membrane (12). Patients with FSGS have segmental scarring of the glomeruli that progresses over time. While 95% of patients with MCD achieve remission after 8 weeks of corticosteroid treatment, only 20% with FSGS have a complete response to steroids (2).

The precise molecular pathophysiology of SRNS remains unclear, but it is understood to be caused by podocyte dysfunction or loss, leading to dysfunction of the charge- and size-selective glomerular filtration barrier (3, 12). The glomerular filtration barrier consists of three layers- a fenestrated capillary endothelium, the glomerular basement membrane, and podocytes with interdigitating foot processes connected by a slit diaphragm. In healthy tissue, the podocyte excludes the filtration of albumin and other macroproteins (13). Changes in the podocyte architecture lead to increased permeability and the resultant proteinuria seen in NS. MCD is characterized by reversible changes to the podocyte architecture without podocyte loss (12). Conversely, FSGS is characterized by podocyte depletion; 20-40% podocyte loss leads to segmental scarring, which in turn causes glomerular enlargement and further podocyte depletion (12).

Early studies of congenital NS led to the discovery of mutations in *NPHS1* (which encodes the podocyte protein nephrin) as a cause of early onset SRNS (14). Advances in genomic technologies over the past 20 years, including the advent of next-generation sequencing, have led to the discovery of >50 genes associated with SRNS (10, 15). The vast majority of these genes code for proteins located in the glomerular filtration barrier, specifically within the podocyte and slit diaphragm, hence SRNS is regarded as a podocytopathy (3, 15).

Single-gene (monogenic) causes of kidney disease account for a minority of cases, with an estimated prevalence between 5 and 30% (7, 15–18). Despite technological advances allowing for easier and more cost-effective detection of monogenic kidney disease, the likelihood of identifying a genetic cause decreases with increasing age of disease onset (19, 20). Mutations in autosomal recessive genes tend to present early in childhood. Autosomal dominant genes tend to have varying degrees of penetrance and severity and typically present later in childhood or into adulthood (4, 8, 21).

The clinical utility of genetic testing in NS is evolving, but there are no clear guidelines for clinical practice. Recommended testing criteria have included testing all patients with SRNS vs. only those with early-onset SRNS, patients with extra-renal manifestations, patients with a family history of NS or consanguineous background or all patients with NS prior to biopsy or completion of steroid treatment (4, 8, 9, 17, 21, 22). Many recommendations are based on studies of cohorts enriched for monogenic disease, such as those with congenital or infantile NS or cohorts with high rates of consanguinity. In this study, we sought to use high throughput sequencing to determine the prevalence of mutations in 40 known SRNS genes and to identify which clinical characteristics were associated with high probability of identifying genetic SRNS in a heterogeneous population with low rates of consanguinity.

METHODS

Human Participants

This study was approved by the institutional review board of Duke University Medical Center and the institutional review boards of all collaborating sites. Written informed consent was obtained from study participants and from the parents of participants under the age of 18. Patients were enrolled from 1998 to 2017 after obtaining informed consent. Subjects in this international cohort were enrolled from multiple centers in the United States, Canada, New Zealand, United Kingdom, Nigeria, and Sri Lanka. Eligible participants in this study included patients with a clinical diagnosis of nephrotic syndrome defined as proteinuria >40 mg/m^2/h, hypoalbuminemia, and edema or patients with biopsy-proven FSGS or MCD. Clinical records of all subjects were reviewed for age at diagnosis of disease, biopsy reports, race, sex, full family history, and presence or absence of extra-renal manifestations suggestive of syndromic disease. Additional data were gathered on treatment course, including response to initial corticosteroid therapy and history of recurrence of NS following kidney transplant.

Preliminary Genomic Sequencing

Eligible families were analyzed by direct sequencing of candidate genes, linkage analysis, and next generation sequencing methods including whole-exome sequencing (WES) and podocyte-exome sequencing. Sequencing and variant analysis were performed as previously described (23–29).

Targeted Sequencing of Custom Amplicons

DNA from the probands of families who had not undergone genetic sequencing prior to April of 2017 and those in whom no causative variant was identified by prior methods were analyzed using targeted sequencing of custom amplicons (TSCA). One hundred eighty-one families with SRNS in whom no causal variant was previously identified and four control subjects with a known causative mutation (positive controls) were analyzed using TSCA. Using Illumina Design Studio (Illumina Inc., San Diego, CA), 1,528 amplicons 250 bp in length were designed and selected to cover all coding regions and 5′ untranslated regions of 45 known SRNS genes and NS risk genes. The library preparation was performed at the Duke Molecular Physiology Institute using Illumina TrueSeq kit. Genomic sequencing was performed by the Duke Center for Genomic and Computational Biology on the Illumina NextSeq 500 platform, mid-output, with 150 bp paired-end reads according to the manufacturer's guidelines. The average genomic coverage was 932×. Sequence reads were aligned to the GRCH37/hg19 human reference genome using BWA-MEM. Using internal quality control metrics for each sample, variants with poor quality were removed. Effects were predicted using SNPEff and the Ensembl Variant Effect Predictor, and variants with an effect of "INTRON," "INTRAGENIC," "UTR_3_PRIME," and "UTR_5_PRIME," or no effect reported were removed.

Causative Variant Calling

Five sequenced genes (*PLCG2, APOL1, MYH9, HLA-DQA1,* and *COL4A5*) were excluded from this analysis; four are risk alleles (*PLCG2, APOL1, MYH9, HLA-DQA1*) and one (*COL4A5*) is associated with X-linked disease. We evaluated TSCA data for causative variants in the remaining 40 known SRNS genes (**Supplementary Table S1**, **Figure 1**). We removed all variants with a minor allele frequency ≥1%, synonymous variants, and intronic variants except for those at obligatory splice site regions. The remaining variants included nonsynonymous variants, truncating variants, and obligatory splice site variants.

For the ten autosomal dominant genes screened by TSCA (*INF2, COL4A4, COL4A3, ACTN4, ANLN, TRPC6, WT1, CD2AP, ARHGAP24,* and *LMX1B*), we filtered for heterozygous variants. For the remaining 30 autosomal recessive genes, we filtered first for homozygous variants. In patients with potential compound heterozygous variants (i.e., two or more heterozygous variants in a single gene) further variant analysis was performed only on those in whom parental DNA was available.

All potential disease-causing variants identified by WES, candidate gene sequencing, and TSCA were confirmed by Sanger sequencing. All sequence variants were analyzed using Sequencher™ software (Gene Codes Corp., Ann Arbor, MI, United States). For patients with potential compound heterozygous variants identified by TSCA, Sanger sequencing was also performed on the parents to determine whether variants were present on a single chromosome (cis) or alternate chromosomes (trans).

The confirmed variants were evaluated using three *in silico* software models [PolyPhen-2 (30), SIFT (31), and MutationTaster (32)] to determine the effect of amino acid changes. Those found to be deleterious by at least two models were considered to be pathogenic.

Statistical Analysis

Continuous variables are expressed as median and interquartile range. Comparisons between categorical variables were made using the chi-square test, and $p < 0.05$ was considered significant.

RESULTS

Cohort Description

Our study cohort was comprised of 492 patients from 181 families with SRNS with a low prevalence of consanguinity (**Table 1**). The majority of the families (150 of 181, 82.9%) were enrolled from the United States.

Eighty-six families (47.5%) had a family history of SRNS or chronic kidney disease (CKD). Sixty-five of these families (75.6%) had an autosomal dominant pattern of inheritance, defined as ≥2 affected individuals in two or more generations. Twenty-one families (24.4%) had an autosomal recessive pattern of inheritance, defined as ≥2 affected individuals in a single generation. Ninety-five individuals were enrolled who had no family history of SRNS or CKD. These individuals were classified as having sporadic disease.

The male-to-female ratio of our cohort was 1.5:1. The median age at diagnosis was 12 years (range 1–61 years). Fifty-eight percent of the cohort were white non-Hispanic, and 25.4% were black. Renal biopsy results were available for the probands of 153 families. FSGS was the most common histological finding and was present in 109 cases. MCD was present on 26 renal biopsies.

Identification of Causative Variants

We evaluated results from whole-exome sequencing, candidate gene sequencing, and targeted sequencing of custom amplicons to identify variants in 40 genes known to cause SRNS. We detected causative variants in 40 of 181 families (22.1%) in 12 known SRNS genes (**Supplementary Table S2**). Variants in *INF2* (12 families), *COL4A3* (5 families) and *WT1* (4 families) were the most common and accounted for 55% of all identified causative variants.

We detected 38 distinct variants in 12 of 40 known SRNS genes (**Supplementary Table S2**). Nineteen of these variants have been previously reported and can be found in public databases. Thirteen novel variants were first discovered in this cohort and have been reported by our group (23–29). We identified eight likely disease-causing variants by TSCA, including six novel variants in five known SRNS genes (*WT1, ACTN4, INF2, TRPC6,* and *NPHS2*) (**Table 2**, **Figure 2**). There were no compound heterozygous variants confirmed by TSCA.

Clinical Factors Associated With Mutation

Causative variants were identified in 34 families (39.5%) with a family history of disease, compared to only six individuals (6.3%) with sporadic disease (**Table 3**). This difference was statistically significant (χ^2 28.93, $p < 0.0001$). The difference in the mutation detection rate between patients with an autosomal dominant pattern of inheritance (29 of 65 families) and those

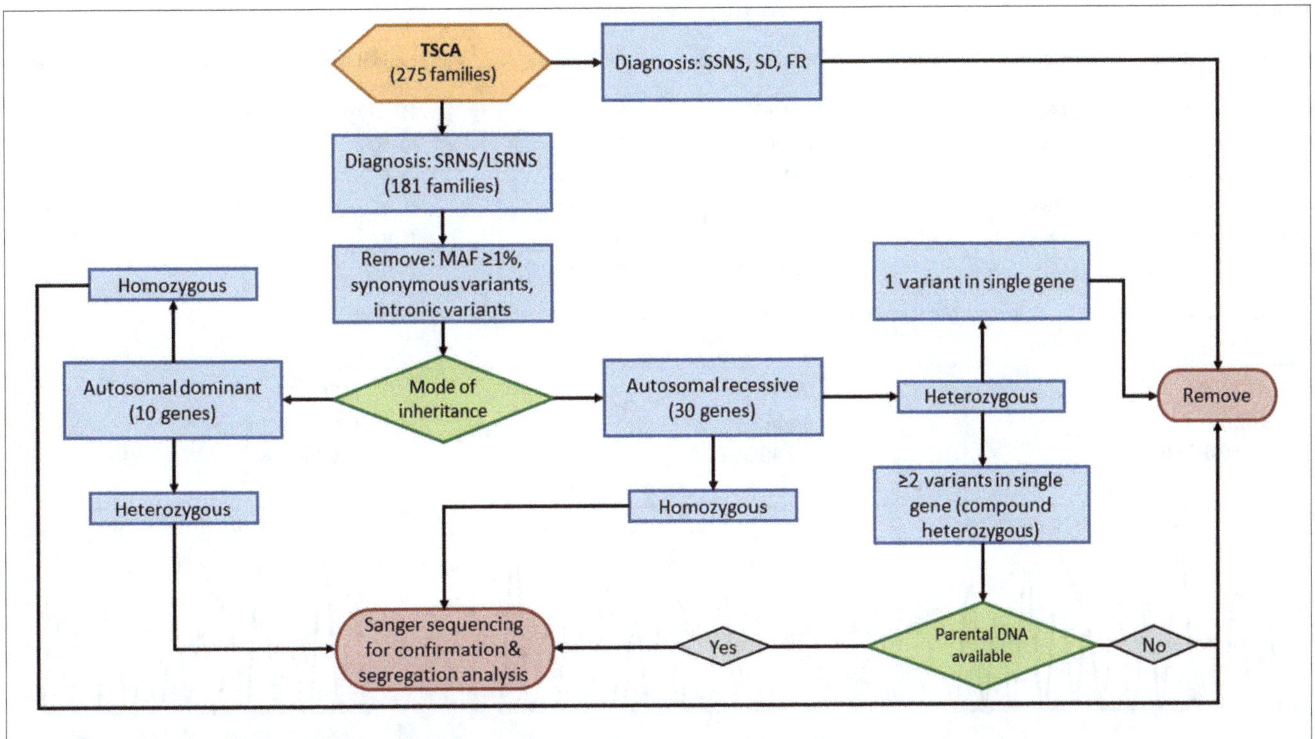

FIGURE 1 | Filtering parameters for variants identified by targeted sequencing of custom amplicons.

TABLE 1 | Demographics of 181 families with familial and sporadic SRNS.

Characteristic	Autosomal dominant	Autosomal recessive	Sporadic	Full cohort
Age at onset (median in years) [interquartile range]	23 [15]	20 [19]	6 [10]	12 [19.5]
SEX				
Male (%)	22 (33.8)	15 (71.4)	55 (57.9)	92 (50.8)
Female (%)	43 (66.2)	6 (28.6)	40 (42.1)	89 (49.2)
RACE				
White, Non-hispanic	41	17	48	106 (58.6)
Black	17	3	26	46 (25.4)
Hispanic	6	0	14	20 (11.0)
Other	1	1	7	9 (5.0)
HISTOLOGY				
FSGS	39	14	56	109 (60.2)
MCD	4	1	21	26 (14.4)
Other	1	1	16	18 (10.0)
No biopsy (includes ESKD)	21	5	2	28 (15.5)
US sample (%)	48 (73.8)	15 (71.4)	87 (91.6)	150 (82.9)

Age at onset and race are defined by the proband in each family.

with an autosomal recessive inheritance (5 of 21 families) was not significant (χ^2 2.87, $p = 0.09$). There was no significant difference in mutation detection rate based on race (white vs. non-white χ^2 2.77, $p = 0.10$), country of origin (US vs. non-US χ^2 0.41, $p = 0.52$), sex (χ^2 1.43, $p = 0.23$), or renal biopsy findings (FSGS vs. MCD χ^2 0.25, $p = 0.61$).

DISCUSSION

Due to a lack of population-based studies, the prevalence of monogenic SRNS in children with SRNS is unknown.. However, data from different cohorts suggest that the prevalence varies between 5 and 30%, depending on the population being studied; higher prevalence rates are generally found in populations with high rates of consanguinity and populations with founder mutations in different genes (33–35).

Prior investigations into the prevalence of monogenic disease have been performed on cohorts selected to enhance the likelihood of identifying monogenic NS. In a large international study of patients with SRNS that showed a 30% prevalence of monogenic NS, fewer than 20% of families were from the United States, and many were from regions with a high degree of consanguinity (16). A more recent study from the longitudinal Nephrotic Syndrome Study Network (NEPTUNE) identified an overall prevalence of only 4.2% in US patients with sporadic disease (33).

Our study was designed to provide guidelines for clinical practice in the United States by screening a cohort that is generalizable to the US population. More than 80% of the 181 families enrolled in this study were from the US, with a low rate of consanguinity. There was no significant difference in the rate of mutation detection between the US and non-US subgroups. Furthermore, family history was collected from all participants

TABLE 2 | Six novel variants in known SRNS genes identified by targeted sequencing of custom amplicons.

Family	Race	Country	Gene	Protein change	Inheritance	Age at onset (yr)	Renal biopsy	Diagnosis
6,511	White	USA	*WT1*	p.T416A	AD	31–35	FSGS	SRNS
6,586	White	USA	*WT1*	p.C393Y	AD	46–50	FSGS	SRNS
6,725	White	USA	*NPHS2*	p.Y162X	Sporadic	1–5	FSGS	SRNS
34,262	White	USA	*ACTN4*	p.D874N	Sporadic	6–10	FSGS	SRNS
34,462	Black	USA	*INF2*	p.E249X	AD	6–10	FSGS	SRNS
40,015	Hispanic	USA	*TRPC6*	p.G39fsX41	Sporadic	6–10	MCD	SRNS

AD, autosomal dominant; FSGS, focal segmental glomerulosclerosis; MCD, minimal change disease; SRNS, steroid-resistant nephrotic syndrome.

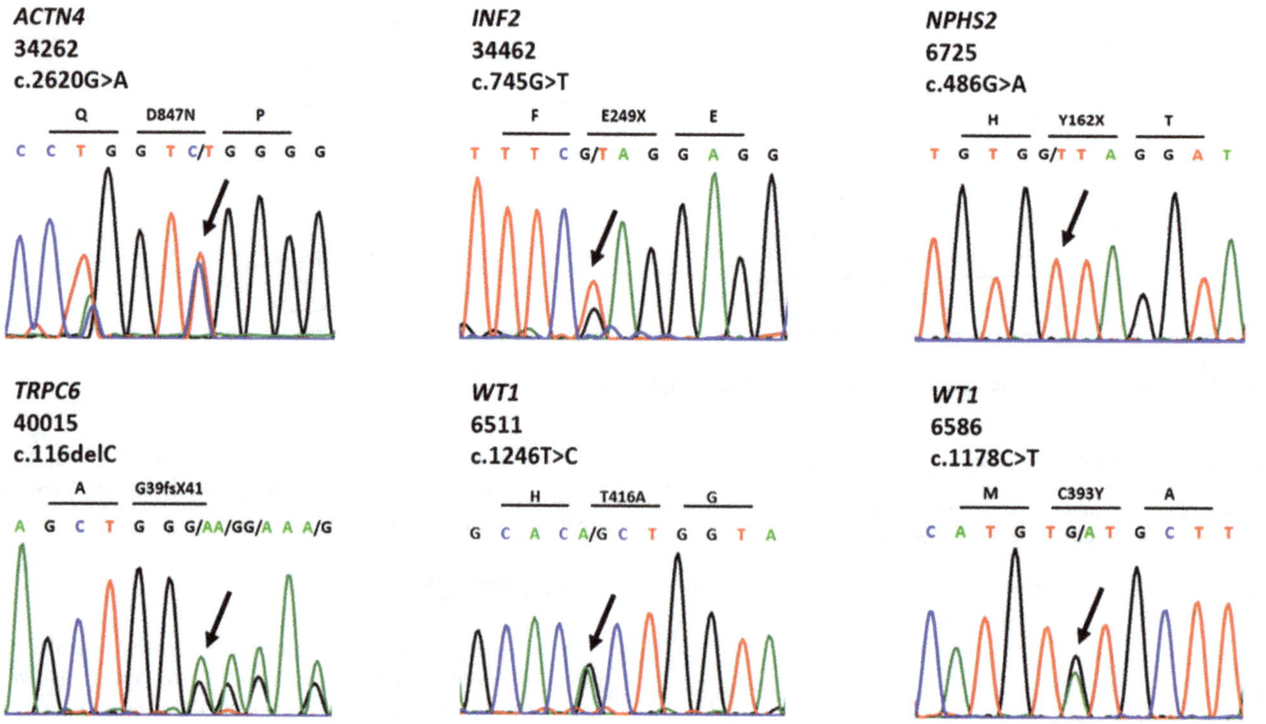

FIGURE 2 | Chromatograms for novel variants identified by targeted sequencing of custom amplicons.

of our study, thus allowing for analysis of patterns of inheritance and mutation detection rates in familial vs. sporadic disease.

We detected causative mutations in 22.1% of our study cohort (40 of 181 families), comprised of 38 distinct variants in 12 known SRNS genes. The majority of these were autosomal dominant genes, possibly due to the large proportion of families with autosomal dominant disease in our cohort or due to decreased prevalence of homozygous autosomal recessive mutations in an outbred population. Six of the variants identified by TSCA are novel, including three variants in exons not covered by most SRNS gene panels.

Genetic testing has the potential to provide extremely useful information when utilized in the correct context. There are currently no guidelines for the use of genetic testing for SRNS in clinical practice in the United States and other countries. Our study suggests that clinicians should consider genetic testing as they would any other diagnostic test; by determining if the test is likely to aid in clinical diagnosis, if the test would change the approach to therapy or if the test would provide clinicians with additional information to discuss the short and long term prognosis of the disease (22). Advantages of establishing molecular diagnosis in patients with SRNS include: (i) better disease definition, (ii) well-informed discussions of short- and long-term prognosis, (iii) selection of appropriate kidney donors to protect both the donor and recipient, (iv) better prediction of post-transplant outcomes, and (v) improved interpretation of clinical trials as they apply to a given patient.

Although the advent of high throughput sequencing has accelerated the pace of gene discovery in SRNS, the amount of data produced requires analytical resources that are often outside the scope of reasonable clinical practice. Consequently, there is a need for guidelines for the use of next-generation sequencing strategies in clinical practice. Typical gene panels are limited to a few genes and often do not include all coding regions of

TABLE 3 | Clinical characteristics of 40 families in whom disease-causing mutations were identified compared to those in whom no causative mutation was found.

Characteristic	Mutation *n*(%)	No mutation *n*(%)	*p*-value
Sex			0.23
Male	17 (18.5)	75 (81.5)	
Female	23 (25.8)	66 (74.2)	
Race			0.09
White, non-hispanic	28 (26.4)	78 (73.6)	
Other	12 (16.0)	63 (84.0)	
Family history			<0.00001
Yes	34 (39.5)	52 (60.5)	
No	6 (6.3)	89 (93.7)	
Histopathology			0.61
MCD	5 (19.2)	21 (80.8)	
FSGS	26 (23.9)	83 (76.1)	
Sample origin			0.52
US	32 (21.3)	118 (78.7)	
Non-US	8 (26.7)	22 (73.3)	

these genes. A benefit of massively parallel high throughput sequencing such as that employed in this and other recent studies is an increased chance of detecting a causative mutation. Whole-exome sequencing covers all regions of the genome and allows for the identification of known and novel mutations as well as the possible identification of new candidate genes. However, it produces a massive amount of data, identifying on average 2,000–4,000 non-synonymous variants with a MAF <1%. This amount of data requires significant effort to interpret results (9). Targeted high throughput sequencing such as TSCA limits the volume of data compared to WES, while still allowing for sequencing of all coding regions of candidate genes.

For clinical decision making, clinicians must certainly consider their own patient population. It has been demonstrated that patients with NS who live in regions with higher rates of consanguinity show a higher prevalence of monogenic disease due in part to the increased likelihood of homozygous variants in autosomal recessive genes (36). Studies conducted outside of the US on the large PodoNet Registry cohort (www.podonet.org) have demonstrated the prognostic value of genetic testing in this population (34, 35). Parameters for genetic testing should therefore be different for different patient populations (36).

In order to provide clinical guidelines for genetic testing in US patients with SRNS, we evaluated our cohort for characteristics that were associated with the identification of a monogenic cause of SRNS. We identified causative mutations in almost 40% of families with a family history of SRNS or CKD compared to only 6% of patients with SRNS and no family history, a difference that was highly significant and makes a positive family history of SRNS or CKD the single most important clinical predictor of mutation amongst patients with SRNS. Although more variants were identified in patients with presumed autosomal dominant disease (45%) compared to autosomal recessive disease (24%) this difference was not statistically significant. We acknowledge that, because there were more families with dominant inheritance in this cohort, it is possible that there was some bias leading to an increased number of detected mutations in autosomal dominant genes and families with dominant inheritance. There were no other clinical factors associated with mutation identification in this cohort. We therefore conclude that a positive family history of SRNS or CKD, regardless of the pattern of inheritance, should be a primary consideration in determining whether genetic testing is warranted.

One limitation to our study was the identification of compound heterozygotes through TSCA. Current methods do not identify on which chromosome a variant is located, meaning that compound heterozygous traits cannot be classified as cis or trans, and thus requiring sequencing of parental DNA. For this reason, it is possible that some compound heterozygous mutations were missed in our cohort. New sequencing technologies are in development that will allow for this distinction in future high throughput targeted sequencing and may increase findings. In addition, because this is a retrospective study, some components of the history and follow-up were limited for some patients. Information regarding age of disease onset or diagnosis was missing for some families, as were details of extra-renal manifestations suggestive of syndromic disease. Statistical analysis could therefore not be performed for these two clinical parameters.

In conclusion, our data show that a family history of SRNS or CKD is the single most important clinical predictor of mutation in patients in a US population. We therefore recommend genetic testing in all patients with SRNS and a family history of SRNS or CKD. In patients with no family history (i.e., those with sporadic NS), steroid-resistance is insufficient as a sole criterion for genetic testing and we do not recommend universal testing in these patients. There is still a need for a larger population-based study to develop a robust algorithm for genetic testing in patients with SRNS.

ETHICS STATEMENT

This study was carried out in accordance with the recommendations of the Institutional Review Board of Duke University with written informed consent from all adult subjects and from the parents of all subjects under 18 years of age. All subjects gave written informed consent in accordance with the Declaration of Helsinki. The protocol was approved by the Institutional Review Board of Duke University and the Institutional Review Boards of all collaborating sites.

AUTHOR CONTRIBUTIONS

JV gathered clinical data, performed experiments, analyzed data, and prepared the manuscript. RG and DH conceived, designed, and supervised the study. RG and GH edited the manuscript. MC-S and AM performed experiments, and MC-S analyzed genomic data. DH, RG, GW, BL, and GH provided laboratory support and conceptual advice. RG, CE, AS, AA, TH, and JL gathered clinical data and biological samples. All authors discussed results and commented on the manuscript and provided approval for this paper.

ACKNOWLEDGMENTS

This study was supported by the National Institutes of Health and National Institute of Diabetes and Digestive and Kidney Disease (NIDDK) grant 5R01DK098135 and 5R01DK094987. RG and JV are recipients of the Doris Duke Clinical Research Mentorship award. GH is a recipient of the American Society of Nephrology/Harold Amos Medical Faculty Development Award and an NIDDK grant 5K08DK111940. We would like to thank the personnel of the genomics core at the Duke Molecular Physiology Institute (DMPI) and all families involved in the Duke Genetics of Nephrotic Syndrome project.

REFERENCES

1. Niaudet P. Steroid-resistant idiopathic nephrotic syndrome in children. In: Avner ED, Harmon WE, Niaudet P, editors. *Pediatric Nephrology*. Philadelphia, PA: Lilppincott Williams & Wilkins (2004). p. 557–73.
2. Eddy AA, Symons JM. Nephrotic syndrome in childhood. *Lancet* (2003) 362:629–39. doi: 10.1016/s0140-6736(03)14184-0
3. Hall G, Gbadegesin RA. Translating genetic findings in hereditary nephrotic syndrome: the missing loops. *Am J Physiol Renal Physiol.* (2015) 309:F24–8. doi: 10.1152/ajprenal.00683.2014
4. Becherucci F, Mazzinghi B, Provenzano A, Murer L, Giglio S, Romagnani P. Lessons from genetics: is it time to revise the therapeutic approach to children with steroid-resistant nephrotic syndrome? *J Nephrol.* (2016) 29:543–50. doi: 10.1007/s40620-016-0315-4
5. The primary nephrotic syndrome in children. Identification of patients with minimal change nephrotic syndrome from initial response to prednisone. a report of the international study of kidney disease in children. *J Pediatr.* (1981) 98:561–4.
6. Nephrotic syndrome in children: prediction of histopathology from clinical and laboratory characteristics at time of diagnosis. a report of the international study of kidney disease in children. *Kidney Int.* (1978) 13:159–65.
7. Giglio S, Provenzano A, Mazzinghi B, Becherucci F, Giunti L, Sansavini G, et al. Heterogeneous genetic alterations in sporadic nephrotic syndrome associate with resistance to immunosuppression. *J Am Soc Nephrol.* (2015) 26:230–6. doi: 10.1681/asn.2013111155
8. Preston R, Stuart HM, Lennon R. Genetic testing in steroid-resistant nephrotic syndrome: why, who, when and how? *Pediatr. Nephrol.* (2017). doi: 10.1007/s00467-017-3838-6. [Epub ahead of print].
9. Vivante A, Hildebrandt F. Exploring the genetic basis of early-onset chronic kidney disease. *Nat Rev Nephrol.* (2016) 12:133–46. doi: 10.1038/nrneph.2015.205
10. Rheault MN, Gbadegesin RA. The genetics of nephrotic syndrome. *J Pediatr Genet.* (2016) 5:15–24. doi: 10.1055/s-0035-1557109
11. Bonilla-Felix M, Parra C, Dajani T, Ferris M, Swinford RD, Portman RJ, et al. Changing patterns in the histopathology of idiopathic nephrotic syndrome in children. *Kidney Int.* (1999) 55:1885–90. doi: 10.1046/j.1523-1755.1999.00408.x
12. Wiggins RC. The spectrum of podocytopathies: a unifying view of glomerular diseases. *Kidney Int.* (2007) 71:1205–14. doi: 10.1038/sj.ki.5002222
13. Grahammer F, Schell C, Huber TB. The podocyte slit diaphragm–from a thin grey line to a complex signalling hub. *Nat. Rev. Nephrol.* (2013) 9:587–98. doi: 10.1038/nrneph.2013.169
14. Kestila M, Lenkkeri U, Mannikko M, Lamerdin J, McCready P, Putaala H, et al. Positionally cloned gene for a novel glomerular protein–nephrin–is mutated in congenital nephrotic syndrome. *Mole Cell.* (1998) 1:575–82.
15. Bierzynska A, McCarthy HJ, Soderquest K, Sen ES, Colby E, Ding WY, et al. Genomic and clinical profiling of a national nephrotic syndrome cohort advocates a precision medicine approach to disease management. *Kidney Int.* (2017) 91:937–47. doi: 10.1016/j.kint.2016.10.013
16. Sadowski CE, Lovric S, Ashraf S, Pabst WL, Gee HY, Kohl S, et al. A single-gene cause in 29.5% of cases of steroid-resistant nephrotic syndrome. *J Am Soc Nephrol.* (2015) 26:1279–89. doi: 10.1681/asn.2014050489
17. Warejko JK, Tan W, Daga A, Schapiro D, Lawson JA, Shril S, et al. Whole exome sequencing of patients with steroid-resistant nephrotic syndrome. *Clin J Am Soc Nephrol.* (2018) 13:53–62. doi: 10.2215/cjn.04120417
18. Buscher AK, Konrad M, Nagel M, Witzke O, Kribben A, Hoyer PF, et al. Mutations in podocyte genes are a rare cause of primary FSGS associated with ESRD in adult patients. *Clin Nephrol.* (2012) 78:47–53. doi: 10.5414/CN107320
19. Santin S, Bullich G, Tazon-Vega B, Garcia-Maset R, Gimenez I, Silva I, et al. Clinical utility of genetic testing in children and adults with steroid-resistant nephrotic syndrome. *Clin J Am Soc Nephrol.* (2011) 6:1139–48. doi: 10.2215/cjn.05260610
20. Hinkes BG, Mucha B, Vlangos CN, Gbadegesin R, Liu J, Hasselbacher K, et al. Nephrotic syndrome in the first year of life: two thirds of cases are caused by mutations in 4 genes (NPHS1, NPHS2, WT1, and LAMB2). *Pediatrics* (2007) 119:e907–19. doi: 10.1542/peds.2006-2164
21. Brown EJ, Pollak MR, Barua M. Genetic testing for nephrotic syndrome and FSGS in the era of next-generation sequencing. *Kidney Int.* (2014) 85:1030–8. doi: 10.1038/ki.2014.48
22. Gbadegesin RA, Winn MP, Smoyer WE. Genetic testing in nephrotic syndrome–challenges and opportunities. *Nat Rev Nephrol.* (2013) 9:179–84. doi: 10.1038/nrneph.2012.286
23. Winn MP, Conlon PJ, Lynn KL, Farrington MK, Creazzo T, Hawkins AF, et al. A mutation in the TRPC6 cation channel causes familial focal segmental glomerulosclerosis. *Science* (2005) 308:1801–4. doi: 10.1126/science.11 06215
24. Akilesh S, Suleiman H, Yu H, Stander MC, Lavin P, Gbadegesin R, et al. Arhgap24 inactivates Rac1 in mouse podocytes, and a mutant form is associated with familial focal segmental glomerulosclerosis. *J Clin Invest.* (2011) 121:4127–37. doi: 10.1172/jci46458
25. Gbadegesin RA, Lavin PJ, Hall G, Bartkowiak B, Homstad A, Jiang R, et al. Inverted formin 2 mutations with variable expression in patients with sporadic and hereditary focal and segmental glomerulosclerosis. *Kidney Int.* (2012) 81:94–9. doi: 10.1038/ki.2011.297
26. Gbadegesin RA, Hall G, Adeyemo A, Hanke N, Tossidou I, Burchette J, et al. Mutations in the gene that encodes the F-actin binding protein anillin cause FSGS. *J Am Soc Nephrol.* (2014) 25:1991–2002. doi: 10.1681/asn.2013090976
27. Malone AF, Phelan PJ, Hall G, Cetincelik U, Homstad A, Alonso AS, et al. Rare hereditary COL4A3/COL4A4 variants may be mistaken for familial focal segmental glomerulosclerosis. *Kidney Int.* (2014) 86:1253–9. doi: 10.1038/ki.2014.305
28. Hall G, Gbadegesin RA, Lavin P, Wu G, Liu Y, Oh EC, et al. A novel missense mutation of Wilms' Tumor 1 causes autosomal dominant FSGS. *J Am Soc Nephrol.* (2015) 26:831–43. doi: 10.1681/asn.2013101053
29. Phelan PJ, Hall G, Wigfall D, Foreman J, Nagaraj S, Malone AF, et al. Variability in phenotype induced by the podocin variant R229Q plus a single pathogenic mutation. *Clin Kidney J.* (2015) 8:538–42. doi: 10.1093/ckj/sfv063
30. Adzhubei IA, Schmidt S, Peshkin L, Ramensky VE, Gerasimova A, Bork P, et al. A method and server for predicting damaging missense mutations. *Nat Methods* (2010) 7:248–9. doi: 10.1038/nmeth0410-248
31. Sim NL, Kumar P, Hu J, Henikoff S, Schneider G, Ng PC. SIFT web server: predicting effects of amino acid substitutions on proteins. *Nucleic Acids Res.* (2012) 40:W452–7. doi: 10.1093/nar/gks539
32. Schwarz JM, Cooper DN, Schuelke M, Seelow D. MutationTaster2: mutation prediction for the deep-sequencing age. *Nat Methods* (2014) 11:361–2. doi: 10.1038/nmeth.2890
33. Sampson MG, Gillies CE, Robertson CC, Crawford B, Vega-Warner V, Otto EA, et al. Using population genetics to interrogate the monogenic nephrotic syndrome diagnosis in a case cohort. *J Am Soc Nephrol.* (2016) 27:1970–83. doi: 10.1681/asn.2015050504

34. Trautmann A, Schnaidt S, Lipska-Zietkiewicz BS, Bodria M, Ozaltin F, Emma F, et al. Long-term outcome of steroid-resistant nephrotic syndrome in children. *J Am Soc Nephrol.* (2017) 28:3055–65. doi: 10.1681/asn.2016101121
35. Trautmann A, Bodria M, Ozaltin F, Gheisari A, Melk A, Azocar M, et al. Spectrum of steroid-resistant and congenital nephrotic syndrome in children: the PodoNet registry cohort. *Clin J Am Soc Nephrol.* (2015) 10:592–600. doi: 10.2215/cjn.06260614
36. Al-Hamed MH, Al-Sabban E, Al-Mojalli H, Al-Harbi N, Faqeih E, Al Shaya H, et al. A molecular genetic analysis of childhood nephrotic syndrome in a cohort of Saudi Arabian families. *J Hum Genet.* (2013) 58:480–9. doi: 10.1038/jhg.2013.27

6

A Rare Presentation of NSAID-Induced Secondary Membranous Nephropathy in a Pediatric Patient

Siddharth Shah[1], M. Asope Elder[1] and Jessica Hata[2]*

[1] *Department of Pediatrics, Norton Children's and University of Louisville, Louisville, KY, United States,* [2] *Department of Pathology, Norton Children's and University of Louisville, Louisville, KY, United States*

Correspondence:
Siddharth Shah
siddharth.shah@louisville.edu

Background: Membranous nephropathy (MN) is a common cause of nephrotic syndrome in adults, but it is responsible for <5% of nephrotic syndrome cases in children. MN has primary and secondary forms. Secondary MN is caused by viral infections, autoimmune diseases like lupus, or drugs. Non-steroid anti-inflammatory drug (NSAID)-induced secondary MN is rarely described in the pediatric population. Thus, the clinical presentation and time to recovery are vastly unknown in the pediatric subgroup.

Clinical Presentation: We report a case of a 15-year-old female who presented with acute onset of nephrotic range proteinuria, significant hypoalbuminemia, hyperlipidemia, and lower extremity edema related to the presence of nephrotic syndrome. She had a history of ibuprofen use periodically for 6 months before presentation because of menstrual cramps and intermittent lower abdominal pain. After the presentation, we performed a renal biopsy that reported stage 1–2 MN, likely secondary. The phospholipase A2 receptor (PLA2R) antibody on the blood test and PLA2R immune stain on the renal biopsy sample were negative. We performed a comprehensive evaluation of the viral and immune causes of secondary MN, which was non-revealing. She had stopped ibuprofen use subsequent to the initial presentation. She was prescribed ACE inhibitor therapy. After 6 months of ACE inhibitor treatment, the proteinuria had resolved.

Conclusion: Proteinuria can last for several weeks when NSAID induces secondary MN and nephrotic syndrome. With the widespread use of NSAIDs prevalent in the pediatric community, further studies are needed to evaluate and study the role of NSAIDs in this condition.

Keywords: NSAID, membranous nephropathy, proteinuria, nephrotic syndrome, ACE inhibitor

INTRODUCTION

Membranous nephropathy (MN) is a rare cause of nephrotic syndrome in the pediatric population and contributes to <5% of childhood nephrotic syndrome cases (1). Primary MN is a renal-specific autoimmune glomerular disease characterized by proteinuria, primarily mediated by antibodies against phospholipase A2 receptor (PLA2R). It is characterized by specific histological findings on renal biopsy, such as a pathognomic "spike pattern" of the glomerular basement membrane on light microscopy (LM); positive PLA2R immunostaining, IgG and complement C3 distributed in a delicate granular pattern distributed across a subepithelial portion of glomeruli on immunofluorescence microscopy (IFM); and electron-dense deposits confined to the subepithelial space on electron microscopy (EM), with the absence of mesangial deposits (2, 3). Secondary MN has previously been shown to be caused by viral infections (e.g., Hepatitis B, Hepatitis C, or HIV), autoimmune conditions (e.g., lupus), drugs (e.g., penicillamine, gold, or NSAIDs), hematological malignancies, and solid organ tumors (1, 2). The histological findings of secondary MN can vary depending on the cause, and PLA2R immunostaining is negative (2). Primary MN is a more common form of MN in adults in the literature review, comprising ~80% of total MN cases, but secondary MN may be more common in children (1). Due to the rarity of secondary MN in the pediatric population and the lack of controlled studies, there are no reliable treatment guidelines or predictions of outcomes for this condition.

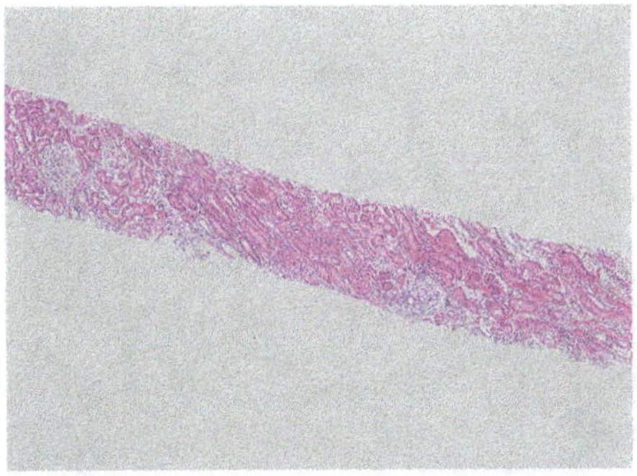

FIGURE 1 | H&E, 4X: The renal biopsy shows glomeruli with normal cellularity and no significant tubular atrophy or interstitial fibrosis.

PATIENT INFORMATION

We report the case of a 15-year-old female (weight 68.3 kg, BMI of 22.56) who presented with acute onset bilateral lower extremity edema and fatigue. She had gained nine pounds of weight at presentation compared to her previous weight 1 month earlier. She denied using any medications, except she said she had been taking ibuprofen at high doses (1,600–2,400 mg/day) intermittently for the past 6 months because of menstrual cramps and intermittent lower abdominal pain. She rejected any illicit substance use and was living at home with her parents and sibling.

CLINICAL FINDINGS

The comprehensive metabolic panel suggested the presence of hyponatremia, with a serum sodium level of 132 meq/L (reference range: 135–145 meq/L), and significant hypoalbuminemia, with a serum albumin level of 2.4 g/dL (reference range: 3.6–5.1 g/dL). Renal function was normal, based on blood urea nitrogen (BUN) of 11 mg/dL (reference range: 4–20 mg/dL) and serum creatinine of 0.5 mg/dL (reference range: 0.5–1 mg/dL). The complete blood count was acceptable, with a WBC count of 13.62 $\times$ 10^3/uL, hemoglobin of 12.4 g/dL, and a platelet count of 407 $\times$ 10^3/uL. The serum lipid profile was abnormal, with a total cholesterol level of 366 mg/dL (reference range: <170 mg/dL) and elevated serum LDL of 249 mg/dL (reference range: <110 mg/dL). The urine dipstick showed +3 protein and was negative for blood. The random urine albumin-to-creatinine ratio was high: 5,229 mcg/mg of creatinine (reference normal <30 mcg/mg of creatinine). The renal ultrasound was normal.

DIAGNOSTIC ASSESSMENT

A clinical diagnosis of nephrotic syndrome was made based on hypoalbuminemia, hyperlipidemia, and heavy proteinuria. Although minimal change disease (MCD) is a common cause of nephrotic syndrome in pediatric patients, the risk of focal segmental glomerulosclerosis (FSGS) increases when the onset of nephrotic syndrome occurs in late childhood or adolescence (4).

Our patient was 15 years of age at presentation; hence, an early renal biopsy was performed to determine the cause. The glomeruli appeared normal overall on light microscopy (LM), and there were no "spikes" or "holes" in the glomerular basement membrane (**Figures 1**, **2**). There was no significant tubular atrophy, interstitial inflammation or interstitial fibrosis. Even though MN is rare among pediatric patients, primary MN was in the differential given the patient's age. We performed PLA2R immunostain on renal biopsy specimens to differentiate primary and secondary MN as there are differences in treatment in these two conditions. On immunofluorescence microscopy (IFM), the PLA2R immunostain was negative, but there was positive mesangial and glomerular diffuse capillary loop staining for IgG, kappa, and lambda (**Figure 3**). There was also positive staining for segmental granular mesangial C1q. Further, we saw negative staining for IgA and C3, and there was no full-house pattern on IFM, which made lupus less likely as a plausible diagnosis. Electron microscopy (EM), revealed the presence of mesangial and diffuse subepithelial electron-dense deposits (**Figures 4**, **5**). There were no tubule-reticular bodies (as seen with lupus), and podocytes were effaced on EM. Given the presence of subepithelial electron-dense deposits and diffuse capillary loop staining for IgG, a diagnosis of MN was made (1). However, the classical findings of primary MN, such as a "spike pattern" of the glomerular basement membrane, C3 staining on immunofluorescence, and positive PLA2R staining, were absent, leading to an increased possibility of secondary MN. Additionally, there was an additional presence of mesangial electron-dense deposits and positive C1q staining, which is reported with cases of secondary MN (1, 2). Viral and immune studies were performed to evaluate the causes of secondary MN and found to be non-revealing (**Table 1**). Based on the above findings and the patient's history of high- dose ibuprofen use, the diagnosis of NSAID-induced secondary MN was made.

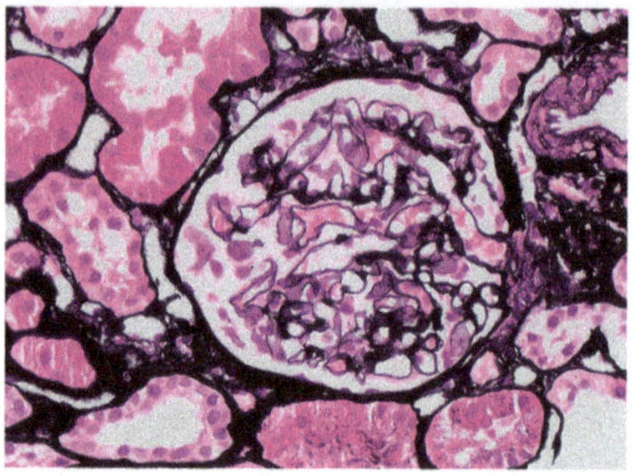

FIGURE 2 | Jones Silver, 40X: The glomerulus lacks well-developed "spikes" or "holes".

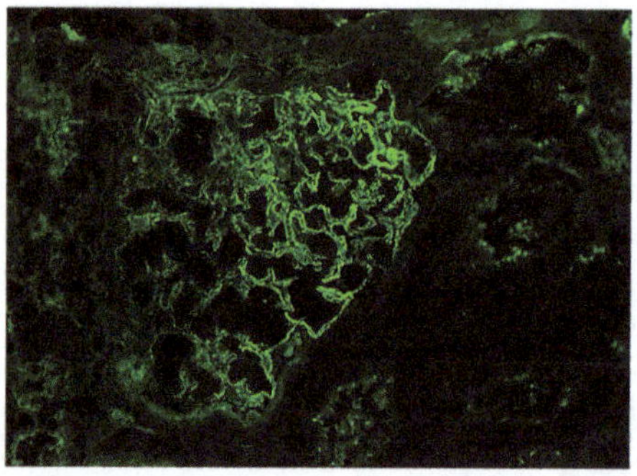

FIGURE 3 | IgG, 40X: The glomerulus demonstrates mesangial and diffuse global, granular capillary loop staining.

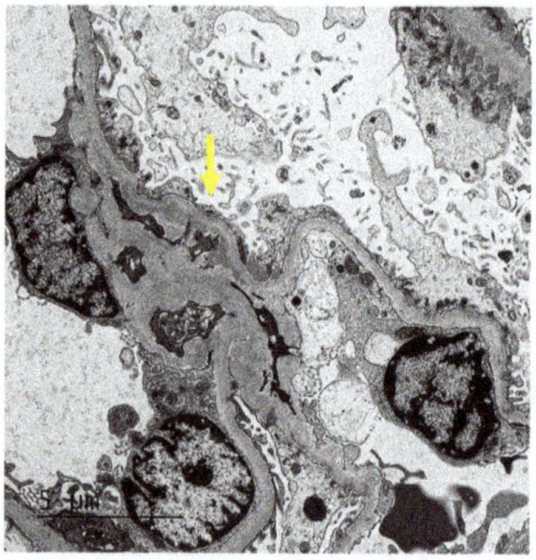

FIGURE 4 | EM: The glomerulus demonstrates mesangial (arrow) and segmental small subepithelial electron-dense deposit.

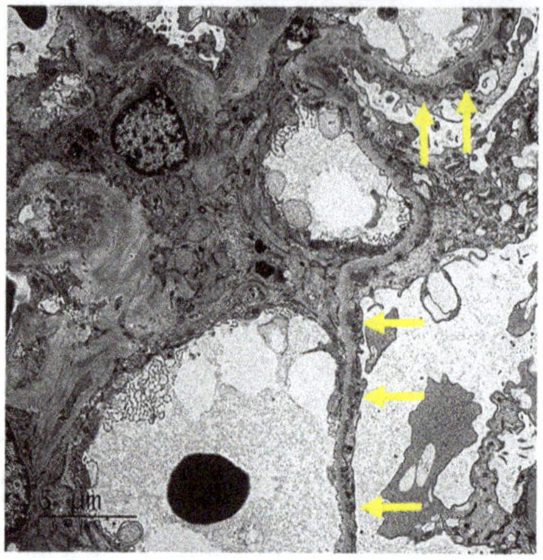

FIGURE 5 | EM: The glomerulus demonstrates mesangial and segmental small subepithelial electron-dense deposit (arrows).

TABLE 1 | Viral and immunological studies.

Test	Result	Reference/ normal
Rheumatoid factor (RF)	<14 IU/ml	< 14 IU/ml
Thyroid stimulating hormone (TSH)	3.78 u(iU)/mL	0.470–4.680 u(iU)/mL
Immunoglobulin G (IgG)	488 mg/dL	500–1,590 mg/dL
Antinuclear antibody (ANA) screen	Negative	Negative
Complement C3	217 mg/dL	83–193 mg/dL
Complement C4	43 mg/dL	15–57 mg/dL
Hepatitis panel (Hepatitis A IgM, Hepatitis B surface Ag, Hepatitis B core Ab, Hepatitis C antibody)	Negative	Negative
HIV screen	Negative	Negative
Cytomegalovirus PCR	Negative	Negative
Epstein-Barr virus PCR	Negative	Negative
Serum protein electrophoresis	Normal	
Serum phospholipase A2 receptor antibody (PLA2R)	Negative	Negative

THERAPEUTIC ASSESSMENT

Our patient stopped using NSAIDs after the initial presentation. She was also initially started on steroids (prednisone) because of her presentation with nephrotic syndrome and based on the available pediatric literature review, but they were weaned over 4 weeks because of a lack of improvement of proteinuria and a strong suspicion of secondary MN (1). Because of the lack of data on treatment options for NSAID-induced secondary MN in pediatric patients, we reviewed the available literature on adult patients, where the treatment varies and includes no treatment, ACE inhibitor use, and steroid use (5–7). Apparently, proteinuria can last for several weeks after stopping NSAIDs in NSAID-induced secondary MN (2, 6). We initiated treatment with an ACE inhibitor and monitored the improvement in proteinuria.

FOLLOW-UP AND OUTCOMES

The swelling on extremities improved in 6–8 weeks, while the patient's serum albumin level took 4 months to return to the

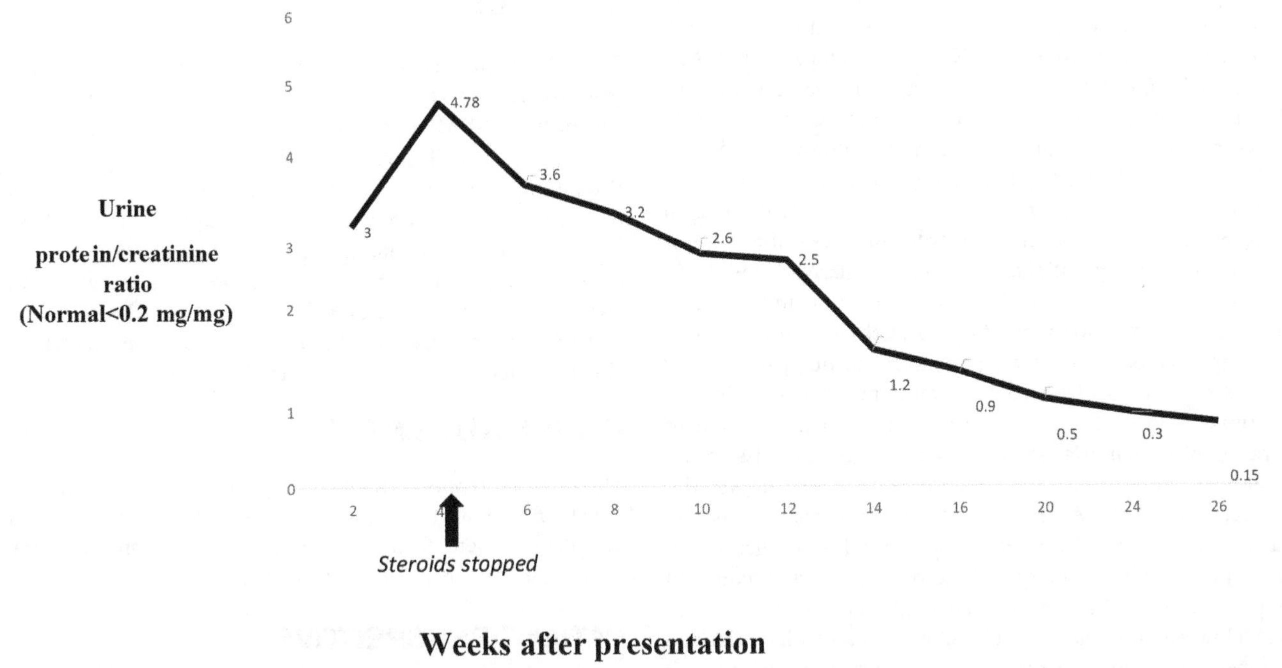

FIGURE 6 | Trends in proteinuria on ACE inhibitor therapy.

normal range after the initial presentation. The proteinuria took over 6 months to resolve completely (**Figure 6**). She had dizziness on 10 mg/day lisinopril, and dose had to be reduced to 7.5 mg/day. Lisinopril was stopped 6 months after presentation. She continues to be in remission and has had no episodes of relapse or significant proteinuria 1 year after presentation.

DISCUSSION

NSAIDs are widely used in the pediatric population to treat pain or fever, and their side effects on kidneys are often not well-recognized. The absence of evident symptoms often leads to a delay in the diagnosis of NSAID-induced kidney disease (8). NSAIDs cause acute kidney injury (AKI) secondary to pre-renal vasoconstriction, acute tubular necrosis (ATN), or acute tubulointerstitial nephritis (ATIN) (8). In hypovolemic states, the production of prostaglandins is upregulated to maintain renal blood flow. NSAIDs inhibit the cyclooxygenase (COX) enzyme, which affects the biosynthesis of prostaglandins, leading to pre-renal vasoconstriction, pre-renal AKI, and ATN in association with hypovolemia (9). It also leads to ATIN and enlargement of kidneys due to an immuno-allergic reaction (8). In terms of nephrotic syndrome, both MCD and MN have been reported with NSAID use (10). MN has been reported with all NSAIDs, including selective COX-2 inhibitors (2, 5). The exact mechanism of NSAID-induced secondary MN is unknown. Different theories have been proposed, including COX inhibition, glomerular deposition of antigens that bind to NSAIDs, or NSAIDs triggering autoimmune reaction against antigens in the glomerular filtration barrier (2, 10).

The duration of NSAID treatment prior to the development of MN is highly variable, from a few weeks to a few months, but there is a rapid development of nephrotic-range proteinuria or presentation with nephrotic syndrome at disease onset (2). Because the symptoms of hypoalbuminemia and edema may be more apparent in NSAID-induced MN, an early renal biopsy is often performed, and this also explains the early stage of MN (stage I or II) often seen on renal biopsies in these patients (2). Our patient also had stage I–II MN on renal biopsy. Since NSAIDs can cause nephrotic syndrome with both MCD and MN presentation, the presence of electron-dense subepithelial deposits and podocyte effacement on EM and the absence of interstitial inflammatory infiltrates on LM are characteristic findings of NSAID-induced MN. In contrast, interstitial infiltrates typically present in NSAID-induced MCD (10). Because of the absence of interstitial infiltrates, renal function can be generally normal in patients with NSAID-induced MN, as also seen in our patient (10). The absence of interstitial infiltrates on renal biopsy could also explain the normal kidney sizes and the lack of enlarged kidneys seen in our patient on renal ultrasound. The lack of a classical "spike" pattern on LM, the absence of PLA2R immune-stain on IFM and negative serum PLA2R antibody screen, and the mesangial presence of deposits along with sub-epithelial deposits on EM led to increased suspicion of secondary MN, as seen in previous reports (1, 2).

A previous retrospective case series published before the availability of PLA2R immune-stain diagnosed the presence of NSAID-induced MN when patients had early-stage I–II MN on renal biopsy; the patients were concurrently taking NSAIDs at the presentation of nephrotic syndrome, and other causes of MN were not detected (6). This series identified 13 adult patients with NSAID-induced MN, and the duration of NSAID use ranged from 1 to 36 months prior to disease onset, the duration of symptoms, such as edema, ranged from 1 to 24 weeks, and treatment ranged from the withdrawal of NSAIDs to further steroid or ACE inhibitor use (6). Interestingly, the time for improvement of proteinuria (as evaluated by 24-h urine protein <1 g) ranged from 9 to 40 weeks after disease presentation among patients who were regularly followed (6). Our patient was treated with an ACE inhibitor and regularly followed, but proteinuria lasted for 26 weeks after presentation. The improvement criteria for proteinuria in our patient were more stringent, as observed by a random urine protein and creatinine ratio <0.2, and this may have also explained the longer duration of proteinuria. Once the patient was in remission, no relapse was observed, in line with previous reports of NSAID-induced MN (2, 6). A randomized controlled trial comparing the anti-proteinuric effects of lisinopril and losartan treatment for 27 patients with primary MN showed a significant reduction in proteinuria in both groups after 12 months of follow-up (11). However, the role of ACE inhibitors in secondary MN and whether they help to decrease the duration of proteinuria or change the natural course of the disease after stopping NSAIDs needs to be further studied.

There are occasional pediatric case reports of drug-induced secondary MN from pencillamine, but the use of such medicines is now decreasing while NSAID use remains prevalent (12). To the best of our knowledge, this report is one of the initial comprehensive case reports on NSAID- induced MN and its outcome in a pediatric patient, as the literature regarding this topic is limited in this population. Our patient had some unique features on renal biopsy that may provide more insight into this challenging condition.

CONCLUSION

NSAIDs are widely used in children and adolescents and can lead to side effects on kidneys, which often go unrecognized. The diagnosis of NSAID-induced secondary MN is challenging and requires a proper laboratory work-up and histological testing. Proteinuria can last for several weeks, even after the resolution of edema in this condition. Further studies are needed to better understand the natural history and long-term outcomes of NSAID-induced secondary membranous nephropathy. More awareness is needed regarding the effects of NSAIDs on kidneys, and their careful use would help to decrease the incidence of NSAID-induced nephrotic syndrome in children.

ETHICS STATEMENT

The case report was reviewed and approved by the Institutional review Board at Louisville, KY, USA. We obtained written informed consent from the parent to publish any potentially identifiable data included in this report.

PATIENT PERSPECTIVE

Note from Father:

Yes, as a father I can say that for me and her mother it was very hard to come to terms with the fact that something wrong had happened just because of a simple over the counter medication. It took us aback and made us nervous.

AUTHOR CONTRIBUTIONS

SS was the primary pediatric nephrologist involved in diagnosing and treating the patient's presentation with nephrotic syndrome. MA was the pediatric resident involved in the care of the patient. JH was the pathologist involved in examining the renal biopsy sample and diagnosing membranous nephropathy. All authors contributed to the article and approved the submitted version.

REFERENCES

1. Menon S, Valentini RP. Membranous nephropathy in children: clinical presentation and therapeutic approach. *Pediatr Nephrol.* (2010) 25:1419–28. doi: 10.1007/s00467-009-1324-5
2. Moroni G, Ponticelli C. Secondary membranous nephropathy. A narrative review. *Front Med (Lausanne).* (2020) 7:611317. doi: 10.3389/fmed.2020.611317
3. Couser WG. Primary membranous nephropathy. *Clin J Am Soc Nephrol.* (2017) 12: 983–97. doi: 10.2215/cjn.11761116
4. Srivastava T, Simon SD, Alon US. High incidence of focal segmental glomerulosclerosis in nephrotic syndrome of childhood. *Pediatr Nephrol.* (1999) 13:13–8. doi: 10.1007/s0046700 50555
5. Tattersall J, Greenwood R, Farrington K. Membranous nephropathy associated with diclofenac. *Postgrad Med J.* (1992) 68:392–3. doi: 10.1136/pgmj.68.799.392
6. Radford MG, Jr., Holley KE, Grande JP, Larson TS, Wagoner RD, Donadio JV, et al. Reversible membranous nephropathy associated with the use of nonsteroidal anti-inflammatory drugs. *JAMA.* (1996) 276:466–9.
7. Nawaz FA, Larsen CP, Troxell ML. Membranous nephropathy and nonsteroidal anti- inflammatory agents. *Am J Kidney Dis.* (2013) 62:1012–7. doi: 10.1053/j.ajkd.2013.03.045
8. Clavé S, Rousset-Rouvière C, Daniel L, Tsimaratos M. The invisible threat of non-steroidal anti-inflammatory drugs for kidneys. *Front Pediatr.* (2019) 7:520. doi: 10.3389/fped.2019.00520
9. Patzer L. Nephrotoxicity as a cause of acute kidney injury in children. *Pediatr Nephrol.* (2008) 23:2159–73. doi: 10.1007/s00467-007-0721-x
10. Mérida E, Praga M. NSAIDs and nephrotic syndrome. *Clin J Am Soc Nephrol.* (2019) 14:1280–2 doi: 10.2215/cjn.08090719
11. Kosmadakis G, Filiopoulos V, Georgoulias C, Tentolouris N, Michail S. Comparison of the influence of angiotensin-converting enzyme inhibitor lisinopril and angiotensin II receptor antagonist losartan in patients with idiopathic membranous nephropathy and nephrotic syndrome. *Scand J Urol Nephrol.* (2010) 44:251–6. doi: 10.3109/00365591003667351
12. Locard-Bisot S, Cochat P, Gilly J, Parchoux B, Colon S, Rousson A, et al. Membranous glomerulonephritis in children: 20 cases. *Pediatrie.* (1990) 45:527–32.

7

Prevalence of Bladder and Bowel Dysfunction in Toilet-Trained Children with Urinary Tract Infection and/or Primary Vesicoureteral Reflux

Jitendra Meena, Georgie Mathew, Pankaj Hari, Aditi Sinha and Arvind Bagga*

Division of Nephrology, Department of Pediatrics, ICMR Center for Advanced Research in Nephrology, All India Institute of Medical Sciences, New Delhi, India

Correspondence:
Pankaj Hari
pankajhari@hotmail.com

Introduction: Urinary tract infection (UTI) in children leads to renal scarring in 10–15% of patients. Urinary tract anomalies and bladder and bowel dysfunction (BBD) are documented risk factors for recurrent UTIs. Estimates of baseline prevalence of BBD in children with UTI will help the clinician in the management strategy. Hence, a systematic review and meta-analysis was conducted to estimate the pooled prevalence of BBD.

Methods: MEDLINE, EMBASE, and CENTRAL (Cochrane Central Register of Controlled Trials) databases were searched for articles related to UTI, primary vesicoureteral reflux (VUR), and BBD. We included studies that provided prevalence of BBD in toilet-trained patients aged 1–18 years with UTI and/or VUR. BBD was defined based on clinical history or questionnaire or urodynamic studies. Two authors independently reviewed, assessed, and abstracted data from studies. Pooled prevalence was calculated based on a random effects model.

Results: Forty-three studies fulfilling the eligibility criteria were selected from a total of 1,731 studies. Among patients presenting with UTI without primary VUR, pooled prevalence of BBD was 41% (95% CI: 26–55; nine studies, 920 patients, I^2 = 96.0%), whereas its prevalence in patients with primary VUR was 49% (43–56; 30 studies, 5,060 patients, I^2 = 96.0%). Weighting by the study design and quality did not affect the prevalence. In patients with primary VUR, prevalence of BBD was higher in females (53%; 42–65) than in males (44%; 15–73). In studies where urodynamic study was used for the diagnosis of BBD, prevalence was 63%. The presence of BBD in patients with primary VUR increased risk of recurrent UTIs [relative risk (RR): 2.1; 1.7–2.5]. In five studies that reported separate data on constipation, pooled prevalence of constipation was 27% (16–37).

Conclusion: Almost half of the patients with primary VUR have BBD, and its presence increases the risk of recurrent UTIs. Trends of high BBD prevalence were also observed in patients presenting with UTI without VUR. These prevalence estimates suggest that all toilet-trained children presenting with UTI with or without VUR should be assessed for BBD, which will help in their further management.

Keywords: dysfunctional elimination syndrome, vesicoureteral reflux, voiding dysfunction, constipation, urinary tract infection

INTRODUCTION

Rationale

Urinary tract infections (UTIs) are one of the most commonly encountered infections in childhood and may lead to long-term sequelae in a proportion of patients (1, 2). Whereas, presence of urinary tract anomalies is a known risk factor for recurrent UTIs in children, risk of recurrence is also influenced by age, gender, and bladder and bowel dysfunction (BBD) (3, 4). The term BBD is used to describe the spectrum of lower urinary tract symptoms accompanying bowel disturbance in the form of constipation and/or encopresis (4). BBD has also been reported as one of the important risk factors for recurrent UTIs in children. The risk of UTI is higher in patients with BBD and primary vesicoureteral reflux (VUR) than in patients with only VUR (5). Presence of BBD delays resolution of VUR and increases risk of UTI following reimplantation (6, 7). BBD has also been reported to impact the rate of breakthrough UTIs in patients with VUR who are on continuous antibiotic prophylaxis (5). As the presence of BBD in patients with UTI affects long-term outcomes, early recognition, and treatment are essential (6). In patients with UTI, variable prevalence (18–54%) of BBD has been reported in previous studies. Knowledge about the baseline prevalence of BBD in toilet-trained children presenting with UTI with or without primary VUR will help clinician in planning the management strategy for these patients (8). We performed a systematic review and meta-analysis to provide pooled estimates of prevalence of BBD in patients presenting with UTI and/or primary VUR.

Objective

The aim of this study was to determine the prevalence of BBD in toilet-trained children with UTI with or without primary VUR.

Research Question

What is the prevalence of BBD in toilet-trained children with UTI with or without primary VUR?

MATERIALS AND METHODS

Study Design

A systematic review and meta-analysis was performed by review of observational and interventional trials published between January 1980 and December 2018.

Participants, Interventions, and Comparators

All published data during 1980–2018 were searched for prevalence of BBD in toilet-trained children with UTIs with or without primary VUR. No interventions or comparators were assessed.

Search Strategy

Protocol for the study was published (PROSPERO: CRD42019127086) and conducted in accordance with the Meta-analysis Of Observational Studies in Epidemiology guidelines (9). Two authors (JM and GM) independently performed literature search in MEDLINE, EMBASE, and CENTRAL (Cochrane Central Register of Controlled Trials) for original articles published, between January 1980 and December 2018. Search strategy design included patients aged 1–18 years with UTI and/or primary VUR. Search strategy was based on four basic groups of terminology: study population (pediatric/children/adolescent) and terms related to or describing the BBD, UTI, and VUR. Terminologies used for literature search were as follows: Bladder bowel dysfunction, dysfunctional elimination syndrome, dysfunctional voiding, lower urinary tract dysfunction, enuresis, urinary incontinence, urgency, overactive bladder, constipation, encopresis, fecal incontinence, vesicoureteral reflux, urinary tract infection, pyelonephritis, cystitis, pediatric, children, adolescent, prevalence, and incidence. Specific search strategies were created for each search engine by using MeSH term and terms described above (**Supplementary Table 1**). Electronic search was also supplemented by hand search of bibliographies of the included studies and relevant review articles.

Data Sources, Study Selection, and Data Extraction

Predefined criteria were used for final selection of studies included in the review. All observational studies and controlled trials were included in this review if they (i) reported data on BBD prevalence in patients aged 1–18 years with UTI and/or primary VUR and (ii) defined BBD based on clinical history or questionnaire or urodynamic studies (UDSs). Conference abstracts were also included if they provided sufficient information on sample size, methods of data collection, case definition, and prevalence of BBD. Studies were excluded if they reported (i) BBD prevalence in 10 or less patients; (ii) patients with neurological abnormalities that affect normal functioning of bladder and bowel, or secondary VUR; (iii) non-toilet-trained children; and (iv) in languages other than English. A well-structured, standardized proforma was used for data extraction. Data included information for risk of bias assessment of the study, prevalence of BBD, author name, year of publication, journal, study setting and design, study population, baseline demographic characteristics, details of intervention, and control group (in case of randomized controlled trials), case definition of BBD, and recurrence of UTI. Any disagreement between two reviewers was resolved through discussion with the third author (PH).

Statistical Analysis and Quality Assessment

The authors independently assessed the quality of articles using the Cochrane risk bias tool for randomized controlled trials. Quality of observation studies was assessed by using a risk of bias assessment tool developed by Hoy et al. for prevalence studies (10). We reviewed full-text articles to determine the following: (i) whether study participants are a close representation of true population; (ii) whether the method used for selection of the study participants was appropriate; (iii) whether data were directly collected from patients and their response rate; (iv) whether acceptable case definition and tool were used for defining BBD and UTI; and (v) whether appropriate numerator and denominator were used for calculating prevalence of BBD. Disagreement between two authors in assessment of risk of bias was resolved by the third author (PH).

Meta-analysis was performed using Stata version 14. We pooled data from individual studies using random effects model with assumption that BBD prevalence would be variable across the studies. Forest plots represent studies in order of year of publication. Heterogeneity in studies was explored by inspection of forest plot as well as using chi-square test on Cochran's *Q* statistics. Study heterogeneity was assessed by using the Higgins and Thompson I^2 method (11). The I^2 heterogeneity was categorized as follows: 0–50% low, 50–75% moderate, and >75% considerable heterogeneity. Sensitivity analyses were undertaken to investigate the individual study influence and the studies using only low risk of bias. A subgroup analysis was performed to explain heterogeneity and calculate prevalence of BBD by sex, study design (controlled trials and prospective and retrospective observation studies), and method of assessment.

RESULTS

Search Results

A total of 1,731 articles were identified through the search strategy in all databases (PubMed 667, EMBASE 525, and CENTRAL 539). There were 1,319 articles after removing 412 duplicates, and 105 of these articles were assessed as potentially relevant, for the systematic review, by screening through the title and abstract. Among these, 80 were full-text original articles, whereas the rest 25 were conference abstracts (**Figure 1**). We also screened the reference list of the full-text articles, but no additional article was identified through this process. Finally, 43 studies comprising 6,627 patients were selected for this review (**Table 1**).

Study Selection and Characteristics

On the basis of patients enrolled, we categorized studies into two groups: (i) nine studies of patients with UTI and without primary VUR (5, 17, 24–26, 28, 31, 43, 53) and (ii) 30 studies of patients with primary VUR (12–16, 18–23, 27, 29, 30, 32–35, 37–42, 44–47, 49–52, 54). Three studies were included in the final systematic review as they reported data on rates of recurrence of UTI (15, 22, 45), and one study by Chung et al. provided data on constipation (50).

Prevalence of Bladder and Bowel Dysfunction Among Patients With Urinary Tract Infection Without Primary Vesicoureteral Reflux

A total of nine studies comprising of 920 patients reported prevalence of BBD in toilet-trained children presenting with UTI without VUR (5, 17, 24–26, 28, 31, 43, 53). The pooled prevalence of BBD in patients with UTI was 41% (95% CI: 26–55%) (**Figure 2**). Owing to high heterogeneity ($I^2 = 95.99\%$), random effects estimates were used. Three studies reported separate data on prevalence of BBD in girls, at 41% (95% CI: 25–58%). None of the studies provided separate information on prevalence of BBD in boys. On a subgroup analysis, the prevalence of BBD was higher (51%, 10–93%) in prospective studies as compared with retrospective studies (35%, 21–49%).

Prevalence of Bladder and Bowel Dysfunction Among Patients With Primary Vesicoureteral Reflux

Thirty studies comprising 5,060 patients reported prevalence of BBD in patients with primary VUR (14–16, 18–23, 27, 29, 30, 32–35, 37–42, 44–47, 49–52, 54–58). The pooled prevalence of BBD was 49% (95% CI: 43–56%) (**Figure 3**). In this group of studies, the heterogeneity was also high ($I^2 = 96\%$). Separate data for prevalence of BBD for boys were reported in five studies, with pooled prevalence of 44% (95% CI: 15–73%). Seven studies reported data for girls with BBD prevalence of 53% (95% CI: 42–65%). In studies with high risk of bias, the prevalence of BBD was high (71%), as compared with that in studies with low-to-moderate risk of bias (45% and 48%). No difference in BBD prevalence was observed when comparing prospective with retrospective studies. In eight studies that used UDS, the pooled prevalence of BBD was 63% (95% CI: 56–70%; $I^2 = 52.8\%$).

Risk of Recurrence of Urinary Tract Infection in Patients With Bladder and Bowel Dysfunction

Seven studies of patients with primary VUR explored the relationship between recurrence of UTI and BBD (15, 18, 19, 22, 37, 45, 47). A meta-analysis of these studies using random effects estimate showed that in the presence of BBD, the risk of recurrent UTIs was increased two-fold, as compared with that in patients without BBD (RR: 2.01; 95% CI: 1.47–2.74, $I^2 = 57.3\%$)

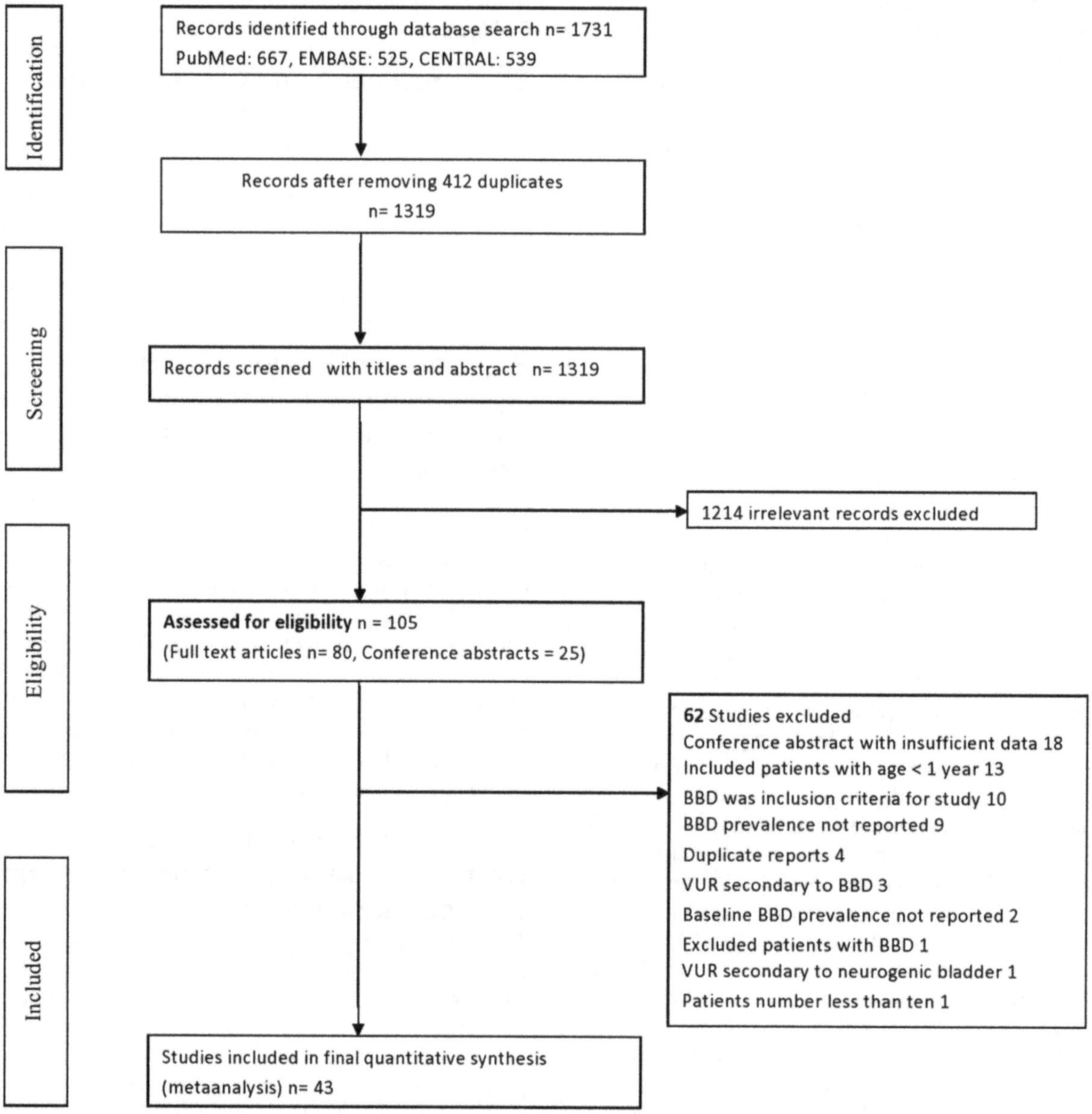

FIGURE 1 | Systematic review flow diagram for selection of studies.

(**Figure 4**). One study in patients with UTI without primary VUR reported that the presence of BBD did not significantly increase the risk of UTI (RR: 1.07, 95% CI: 0.51–2.23).

Prevalence of Constipation

Two studies on patients with UTI showed that the pooled prevalence of constipation was 30% (95% CI: 25–36%) (24). Data for constipation were reported in 972 patients with primary VUR across seven studies (18, 21, 40, 47, 49, 50, 52). Pooled prevalence of constipation from these seven studies was 27% (95% CI: 16–37%).

Risk of Bias

Quality of studies was assessed based on Cochrane risk bias tool for randomized trials, and a modified tool by Hoy et al. was used for observational studies (10). Based on these tools, seven studies were at high risk of bias, 17 at moderate risk of bias, and 15 at low risk of bias, whereas in four studies, risk of bias could not be assessed owing to insufficient information (**Table 1**).

DISCUSSION

Summary of the Main Findings

Patients with bladder dysfunction are at increased risk of bowel dysfunction and vice versa. Anatomical and function interaction that leads to this increase risk has been well-established. BBD is an important risk factor for UTI in children, more so in the ones who are toilet trained. In a meta-analysis, the American Urological Association (AUA) guideline for the management of

TABLE 1 | Basic characteristics of studies included in the systematic review.

References	Country	Study design	Risk of bias assessment	Study group	Sample size
Taylor et al. (12)	USA	Prospective	3	VUR	37
Seruca (13)	Portugal	Prospective and retrospective	3	VUR	43
Snodgrass et al. (14)	USA	Cross sectional	1	VUR	70
van Gool et al. (15)	USA	Prospective	1	VUR	310
Lipski et al. (16)	USA	Retrospective	2	VUR	30
David et al. (17)	France	Retrospective	3	UTI	30
Koff et al. (18)	USA	Prospective	1	VUR	143
Snodgrass et al. (19)	USA	Prospective	1	VUR	128
Trsinar et al. (20)	Slovenia	Prospective	2	VUR	94
Soygür et al. (21)	Turkey	Prospective	1	VUR	62
Willemsen et al. (22)	Netherlands	Prospective	1	VUR	102
Capozza et al. (23)	Italy	Prospective	1	VUR	180
Barroso et al. (24)	Brazil	Prospective	1	UTI	45
Mazzola et al. (25)	Switzerland	Retrospective	3	UTI	141
Vlajkovic et al. (20)	Yugoslavia	Prospective	1	VUR	74
Shaikh et al. (26)	USA	Prospective	1	UTI	123
Chen et al. (27)	USA	Retrospective	1	VUR	1721
Mingin et al. (28)	USA	Retrospective	2	UTI	12
Lavelle et al. (29)	USA	Prospective	2	VUR	52
Im et al. (30)	Korea	Retrospective	2	VUR	56
Colen et al. (31)	USA	Retrospective	2	UTI	132
Szymanik-Grzelak et al. (32)	Poland	Not clear	Unclear	VUR	150
Higham-Kessler et al. (33)	USA	Retrospective	2	VUR	80
Yucel et al. (34)	USA	Retrospective	2	VUR	92
Izquierdo and Luque Mialdea (35)	Spain	Prospective	2	VUR	63
Williams (36)	USA	Retrospective	Unclear	VUR	82
Sillén (37)	Sweden	Prospective	1	VUR	148
Whittam et al. (38)	USA	Retrospective	2		295
Altobelli et al. (39)	Italy	Retrospective	1	VUR	138
Hong et al. (40)	USA	Prospective	1	VUR	298
Palcic et al. (41)	Croatia	Retrospective	Unclear	VUR	92
Giuseppe et al. (42)	Italy	Retrospective	3	VUR	78
Öztürk et al. (43)	Not known	Not clear	Unclear	UTI	192
Akhavan et al. (44)	USA	Retrospective	2	VUR	78
Alexander et al. (45)	USA	Retrospective cohort	2	VUR	225
Heckler et al. (46)	USA	Prospective	2	VUR	169
Hoberman et al. (47)	USA	Randomized controlled trial	1	VUR	126
Cetin (48)	Turkey	Not clear	3	UTI	188
Chang et al. (49)	Taiwan	Retrospective	2	VUR	34
Chung et al. (50)	Korea	Retrospective	3	VUR	90
Arlen et al. (51)	USA	Retrospective	2	VUR	222
Shaikh et al. (5)	USA	Prospective	1	UTI	57
Sharif-Rad et al. (52)	Iran	Retrospective	1	VUR	225

Risk of bias assessment (Low = 1, moderate = 2, High = 3).

primary VUR showed that the presence of BBD significantly delayed resolution of VUR (7). In children presenting with UTI, who already possess a risk factor like primary VUR, the presence of BBD further increases risk of breakthrough UTI even while on antibiotic prophylaxis (5). Two recent studies support the notion that BBD predisposes patients for recurrence of UTI and increases risk of renal scarring as well (3, 5). Recently, a reanalysis of data from the RIVUR trial by Wang et al. showed that antibiotic prophylaxis is more beneficial in the group of patients with BBD compared with those without it (8). Hence,

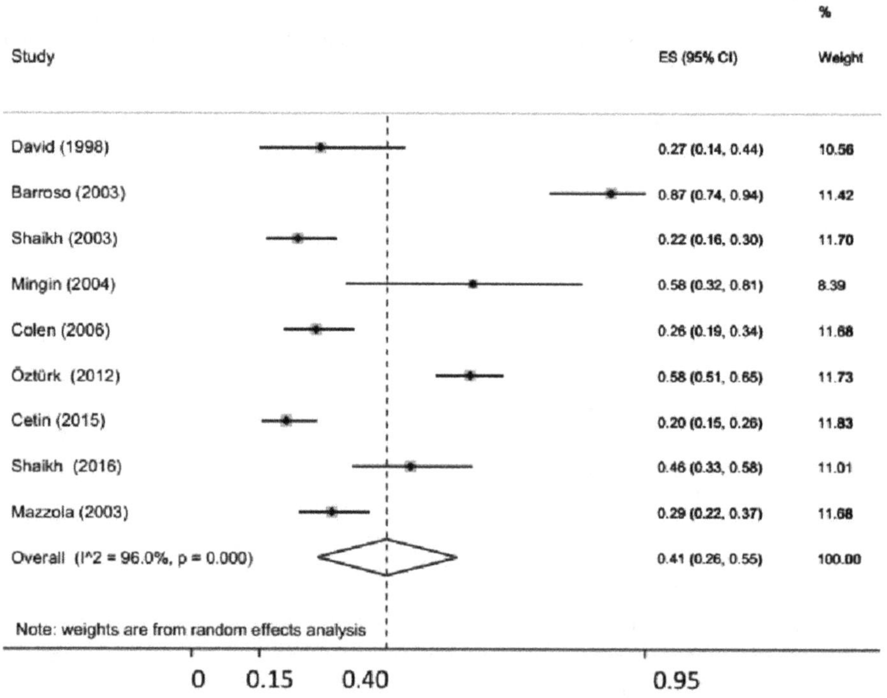

FIGURE 2 | Prevalence of bladder dysfunction in children with urinary tract infection (UTI) without primary vesicoureteral reflux (VUR).

it is of paramount importance to assess children presenting with UTI for BBD even in the presence of other anatomical risk factors before deciding management strategy. In this review, we found that prevalence of BBD is slightly higher in patients with primary VUR than in patients with UTI without VUR. Within primary VUR, cohort girls had higher prevalence of BBD than boys. When BBD is assessed by more invasive tools like UDS, almost two-thirds of patients with primary VUR were detected to have BBD. In the present meta-analysis, we also found that the presence of BBD increases risk of recurrence of UTI by almost two times in patients with primary VUR. Functional constipation was documented in almost one-third of the patients with either VUR or UTI. Prevalence of BBD in patients with UTI without VUR is clearly higher, in the present meta-analysis, than in the general population of school-going children (20%) (55). This higher prevalence of BBD in children with UTI than the general population might point toward a strong association between BBD and UTI.

We found higher prevalence of BBD in patients with primary VUR than did a meta-analysis in the 2010 guideline for management of VUR by the AUA. In the meta-analysis by AUA, pooled prevalence of BBD in 15 studies was 31%. We used a predefined strategy for selection of the studies, which resulted in inclusion of different studies compared with those included in the meta-analysis by AUA. We also found that BBD is more common in girls with VUR, which could explain higher risk of breakthrough UTI in girls. Gaither et al. also reported higher risk of BBD in girls (56). Prevalence of BBD in patients with primary VUR, in the present meta-analysis, has varied from 18 to 91% (14–16, 18–23, 27, 29, 30, 32–35, 37–42, 44–47, 49–52, 54–58). This large variation in prevalence is likely due to multiple factors, which include characteristics of study population, study design, intervention, and assessment tool used for BBD. The largest randomized trial (RIVUR) in patients with primary VUR reported almost similar prevalence of BBD (56%) as in the present meta-analysis.

The relationship between VUR, BBD, and recurrent UTIs is complex and not so well-understood. A previous report from Shaikh et al. showed that patients with both VUR and BBD have the highest rate of recurrent UTIs than have patients with only VUR or BBD (5). This meta-analysis underscores the same fact and showed almost two-fold higher risk of recurrent UTIs in patients with coexisting VUR and BBD than in patients with VUR alone. Reanalysis of RIVUR trial showed that a subgroup of patients with both VUR and BBD had the most benefit from antibiotic prophylaxis. Significant reduction in recurrent UTIs following successful management of BBD with urotherapy has been reported, which again suggests a strong role of BBD in recurrence of UTI (57, 58). Hence, evaluation for BBD is essential while planning management for patients with primary VUR.

Prevalence of functional constipation was reported to be 9.5% in healthy children in a recent systematic review (59). In our review, prevalence of constipation was almost three times higher in children with or without VUR, suggesting that BBD is an important risk factor for UTI in toilet-trained children. A systematic review reported that 37–64% patients with functional constipation have lower urinary tract symptoms, hinting toward the association of BBD.

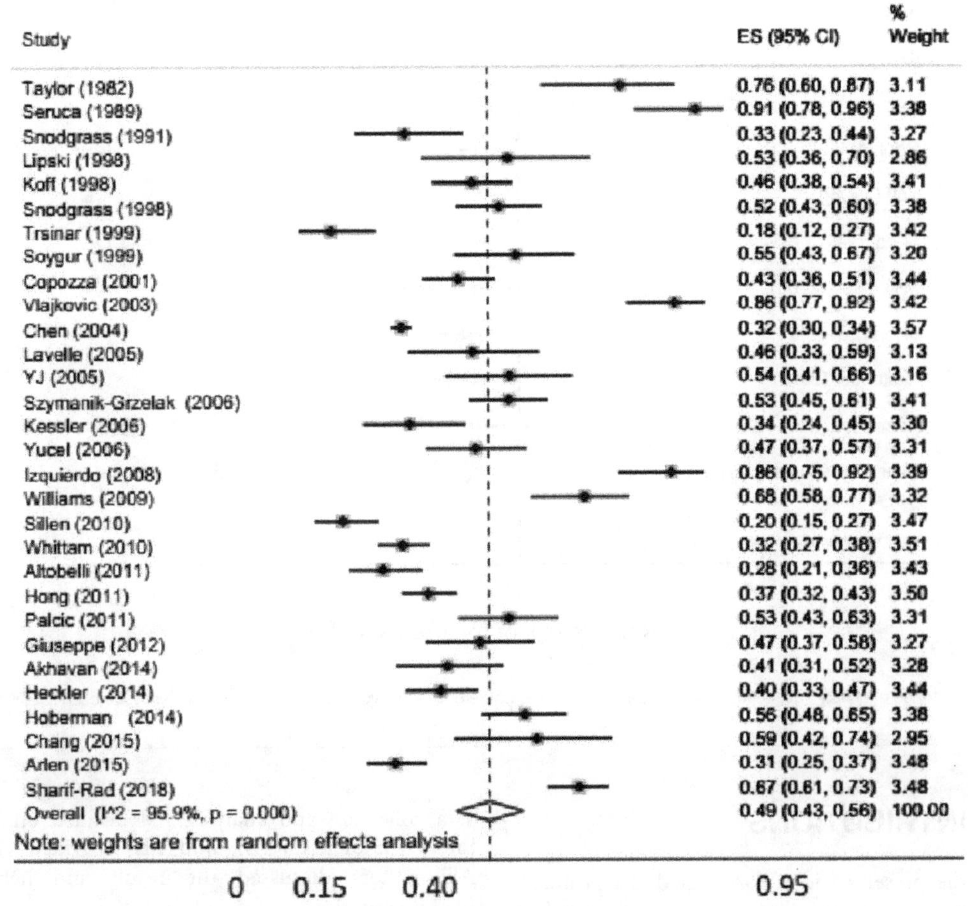

FIGURE 3 | Prevalence of bladder dysfunction in children with primary vesicoureteral reflux (VUR).

Limitations and Strengths

There are few limitations of our systematic review. Large heterogeneity for final pooled prevalence could be considered a limitation; however, because there is no existing standardized diagnostic criterion to define BBD in children, we had to use all previous studies that provided data for BBD prevalence using various definitions. Second, the large heterogeneity could be because studies with all kinds of study design have been used in the present review, although in the sensitivity analysis, we could not find any major difference in various subgroups. Third, we had to exclude many studies that included infants, as these children aged < 1 year are likely to be non-toilet trained and because diagnosing BBD in them is difficult. This exclusion criterion was defined *a priori*. Finally, we had limited our search to English-language databases only; hence, it might have resulted in exclusion of few studies published in non-English languages.

This systematic review has several strengths. First, we followed a rigorous methodology that included a comprehensive search of three major databases of medical literature, predefined protocol for study selection process, data extraction, and a statistical analysis that was registered in PROSPERO. We provided estimated pooled prevalence of BBD separately, in children with UTI only without VUR and other cohort of patients with primary VUR. We also showed that in patients with VUR, prevalence of BBD is higher in girls, which could explain higher number of recurrent UTIs in girls. Finally, we also assessed relative risk of recurrence of UTI in patients with both VUR and BBD and with VUR alone.

CONCLUSIONS

In summary, this systematic review of currently available literature shows that BBD is common in toilet-trained children presenting with UTI with or without primary VUR. A subgroup meta-analysis also shows that functional constipation is common in these children, with almost every third child affected with it. We also found that the presence of both BBD and VUR doubles the risk of recurrence of UTI; hence, all children presenting with UTI should be carefully evaluated for presence of BBD and managed accordingly. As BBD is an important risk factor for UTI recurrence, in future, intervention trials for patients with primary VUR should be stratified as per presence of BBD.

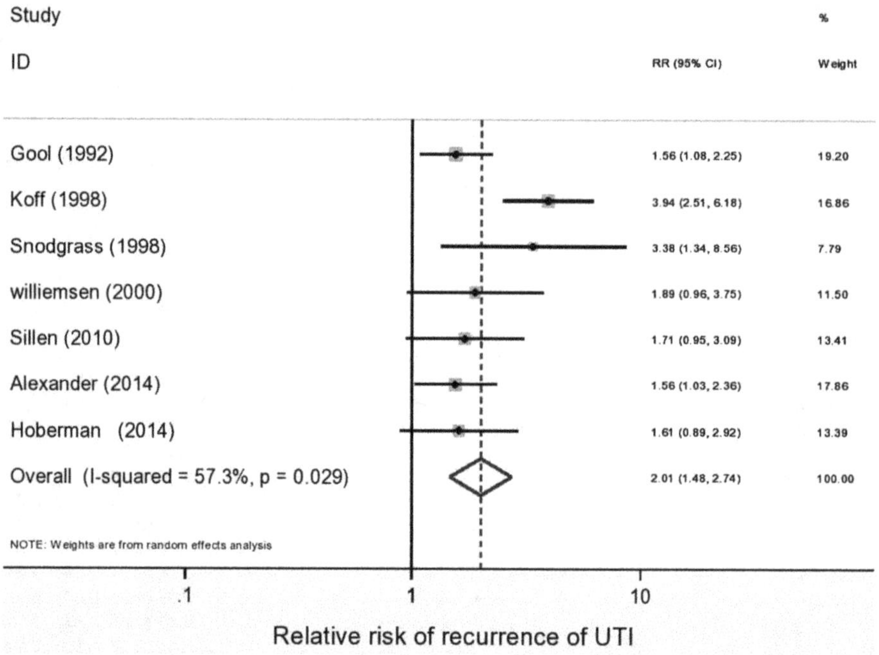

FIGURE 4 | Risk of recurrence of urinary tract infection (UTI) in patients with vesicoureteral reflux (VUR) and bladder and bowel dysfunction (BBD) compared with patients without BBD.

AUTHOR CONTRIBUTIONS

JM conceived of the presented idea, formulated the protocol, and wrote the manuscript. JM and GM did independent data collection and analysis. PH decided on conflicting data interpretation. AS, AB, and PH provided critical feedback. All authors discussed the result and helped shape the final manuscript.

REFERENCES

1. Shaikh N, Morone NE, Bost JE, Farrell MH. Prevalence of urinary tract infection in childhood: a meta-analysis. *Pediatr Infect Dis J.* (2008) 27:302–8. doi: 10.1097/INF.0b013e31815e4122
2. Shaikh N, Craig JC, Rovers MM, Da Dalt L, Gardikis S, Hoberman A, et al. Identification of children and adolescents at risk for renal scarring after a first urinary tract infection: a meta- analysis with individual patient data. *JAMA Pediatr.* (2014) 168:893–900. doi: 10.1001/jamapediatrics.2014.637
3. Keren R, Shaikh N, Pohl H, Gravens-Mueller L, Ivanova A, Zaoutis L, et al. Risk factors for recurrent urinary tract infection and renal scarring. *Pediatrics.* (2015) 136:e13–21. doi: 10.1542/peds.2015-0409
4. Conway PH, Cnaan A, Zaoutis T, Henry BV, Grundmeier RW, Keren R. Recurrent urinary tract infections in children: risk factors and association with prophylactic antimicrobials. *JAMA.* (2007) 298:179–86. doi: 10.1001/jama.298.2.179
5. Shaikh N, Hoberman A, Keren R, Gotman N, Docimo S, Mathews R, et al. Recurrent urinary tract infections in children with bladder and bowel dysfunction. *Pediatrics.* (2016) 137:e20152982. doi: 10.1542/peds.2015-2982
6. Yang S, Chua ME, Bauer S, Wright A, Brandström P, Hoebeke P, et al. Diagnosis and management of bladder bowel dysfunction in children with urinary tract infections: a position statement from the International Children's Continence Society. *Pediatr Nephrol.* (2018) 33:2207–19. doi: 10.1007/s00467-017-3799-9
7. Peters CA, Skoog SJ, Arant BS, Copp HL, Elder JS, Hudson RG, et al. Summary of the AUA guideline on management of primary vesicoureteral reflux in children. *J Urol.* (2010) 184:1134–44. doi: 10.1016/j.juro.2010.05.065
8. Wang ZT, Wehbi E, Alam Y, Khoury A. A reanalysis of the RIVUR trial using a risk classification system. *J Urol.* (2018) 199:1608–14. doi: 10.1016/j.juro.2017.11.080
9. Stroup DF, Berlin JA, Morton SC, Olkin I, Williamson GD, Rennie D, et al. Meta-analysis of observational studies in epidemiology: a proposal for reporting. Meta-analysis Of Observational Studies in Epidemiology (MOOSE) group. *JAMA.* (2000) 283:2008–12. doi: 10.1001/jama.283.15.2008
10. Hoy D, Brooks P, Woolf A, Blyth F, March L, Bain C, et al. Assessing risk of bias in prevalence studies: modification of an existing tool and evidence of interrater agreement. *J Clin Epidemiol.* (2012) 65:934–9. doi: 10.1016/j.jclinepi.2011.11.014
11. Higgins JPT, Thompson SG. Quantifying heterogeneity in a meta-analysis. *Stat Med.* (2002) 21:1539–58. doi: 10.1002/sim.1186
12. Taylor CM, Corkery JJ, White RH. Micturition symptoms and unstable bladder activity in girls with primary vesicoureteric reflux. *Br J Urol.* (1982) 54:494–8. doi: 10.1111/j.1464-410X.1982.tb13573.x
13. Seruca H. Vesicoureteral reflux and voiding dysfunction: a prospective study. *J Urol.* (1989) 142 (2 Pt 2):494–8; discussion 501. doi: 10.1016/S0022-5347(17)38794-3
14. Snodgrass W. Relationship of voiding dysfunction to urinary tract infection and vesicoureteral reflux in children. *Urology.* (1991) 38:341–4. doi: 10.1016/0090-4295(91)80148-Z
15. van Gool JD, Hjälmås K, Tamminen-Möbius T, Olbing H. Historical clues to the complex of dysfunctional voiding, urinary tract infection and vesicoureteral reflux. The International Reflux Study in Children. *J Urol.* (1992) 148(5 Pt 2):1699–702. doi: 10.1016/S0022-5347(17)37006-4
16. Lipski BA, Mitchell ME, Burns MW. Voiding dysfunction after bilateral extravesical ureteral reimplantation. *J Urol.* (1998) 159:1019–21. doi: 10.1016/S0022-5347(01)63826-6
17. David C, Dacher JN, Monroc M, Eurin D, Le Dosseur P. [Retrograde cystography after a first episode of acute pyelonephritis in the child and adolescent]. *J Radiol.* (1998) 79:133–7.

18. Koff SA, Wagner TT, Jayanthi VR. The relationship among dysfunctional elimination syndromes, primary vesicoureteral reflux and urinary tract infections in children. *J Urol.* (1998) 160(3 Pt 2):1019–22. doi: 10.1016/S0022-5347(01)62686-7
19. Snodgrass W. The impact of treated dysfunctional voiding on the nonsurgical management of vesicoureteral reflux. *J Urol.* (1998) 160:1823–5. doi: 10.1016/S0022-5347(01)62425-X
20. Trsinar B, Cotic D, Oblak C. Possible causes of unsuccessful endoscopic collagen treatment of vesicoureteric reflux in children. *Eur Urol.* (1999) 36:635–9. doi: 10.1159/000020059
21. Soygür T, Arikan N, Yeşilli C, Gögüş O. Relationship among pediatric voiding dysfunction and vesicoureteral reflux and renal scars. *Urology.* (1999) 54:905–8. doi: 10.1016/S0090-4295(99)00291-5
22. Willemsen J, Nijman RJ. Vesicoureteral reflux and videourodynamic studies: results of a prospective study. *Urology.* (2000) 55:939–43. doi: 10.1016/S0090-4295(00)00549-5
23. Capozza N, Patricolo M, Lais A, Matarazzo E, Caione P. Endoscopic treatment of vesico-ureteral reflux: twelve years' experience. *Urol Int.* (2001) 67:228–31. doi: 10.1159/000050993
24. Barroso U Jr, Barroso DV, Jacobino M, Vinhaes AJ, Macedo A Jr, Srougi M. Etiology of urinary tract infection in scholar children. *Int Braz J Urol.* (2003) 29:450–4. doi: 10.1590/S1677-55382003000500012
25. Mazzola BL, von Vigier RO, Marchand S, Tönz M, Bianchetti MG. Behavioral and functional abnormalities linked with recurrent urinary tract infections in girls. *J Nephrol.* (2003) 16:133–8.
26. Shaikh N, Hoberman A, Wise B, Kurs-Lasky M, Kearney D, Naylor S, et al. Dysfunctional elimination syndrome: is it related to urinary tract infection or vesicoureteral reflux diagnosed early in life? *Pediatrics.* (2003) 112:1134–7. doi: 10.1542/peds.112.5.1134
27. Chen JJ, Mao W, Homayoon K, Steinhardt GF. A multivariate analysis of dysfunctional elimination syndrome, and its relationships with gender, urinary tract infection and vesicoureteral reflux in children. *J Urol.* (2004) 171:1907–10. doi: 10.1097/01.ju.0000120288.82950.a2
28. Mingin GC, Hinds A, Nguyen HT, Baskin LS. Children with a febrile urinary tract infection and a negative radiologic workup: factors predictive of recurrence. *Urology.* (2004) 63:562–5; discussion 565. doi: 10.1016/j.urology.2003.10.055
29. Lavelle MT, Conlin MJ, Skoog SJ. Subureteral injection of Deflux for correction of reflux: analysis of factors predicting success. *Urology.* (2005) 65:564–7. doi: 10.1016/j.urology.2004.09.068
30. Im YJ, Jeon HJ, Han SW. The impact of voiding dysfunction on vesicoureteral reflux and renal scars. *Korean J Urol.* (2005) 46:897. doi: 10.3978/j.issn.2223-4683.2012.06.09
31. Colen J, Docimo SG, Stanitski K, Sweeney DD, Wise B, Brandt P, et al. Dysfunctional elimination syndrome is a negative predictor for vesicoureteral reflux. *J Pediatr Urol.* (2006) 2:312–5. doi: 10.1016/j.jpurol.2006.01.013
32. Szymanik-Grzelak H, Sladowska J, Panczyk-Tomaszewska M, Sekowska R, Roszkowska-Blaim M. [Voiding dysfunction in children with vesicoureteral reflux]. *Przegl Lek.* (2006) 63 (Suppl. 3):142–5.
33. Higham-Kessler J, Reinert SE, Snodgrass WT, Hensle TW, Koyle MA, Hurwitz RS, et al. A review of failures of endoscopic treatment of vesicoureteral reflux with dextranomer microspheres. *J Urol.* (2007) 177:710–4; discussion 714–715. doi: 10.1016/j.juro.2006.09.082
34. Yucel S, Ates M, Erdogru T, Baykara M. Dysfunctional elimination syndrome in three generations of one family: might it be hereditary? *Urology.* (2004) 64:1231.e15–17. doi: 10.1016/j.urology.2004.06.034
35. Izquierdo RM-C, Luque Mialdea R. [Evaluation of the lower urinary tract function in pediatric patients with primary vesicoureteral reflux]. *Arch Esp Urol.* (2008) 61:191–207.
36. Williams H, Roelof BA, Venkatesan K, Steinhardt G. The impact of subureteral injection of Deflux for vesicoureteral reflux on children with voiding dysfunction. *J Urol.* (2009) 181:4. doi: 10.1016/S0022-5347(09)60633-9
37. Sillén U. Bladder dysfunction and vesicoureteral reflux. *Adv Urol.* (2008) 2008:815472. doi: 10.1155/2008/815472
38. Whittam BM, Thomasch JR, Makari JH, Tanaka ST, Thomas JC, Pope JC, et al. Febrile urinary tract infection after ureteroneocystostomy: a contemporary assessment at a single institution. *J Urol.* (2010) 183:688–92. doi: 10.1016/j.juro.2009.10.039
39. Altobelli E, Buscarini M, Nappo SG, Nguyen HT, Caione P. Urodynamics investigation on children with vesicoureteral reflux identifies overactive bladder and poor compliance in those with voiding dysfunction. *Pediatr Surg Int.* (2011) 27:517–22. doi: 10.1007/s00383-010-2822-z
40. Hong YK, Onal B, Diamond DA, Retik AB, Cendron M, Nguyen HT. Robot-assisted laparoscopic excision of symptomatic retrovesical cysts in boys and young adults. *J Urol.* (2011) 186:2372–8. doi: 10.1016/j.juro.2011.07.113
41. Palcic I, Strizic H, Cvitkovic RA. Urodynamic findings in children with vesicoureteral reflux after three years of age. *Pediatr Nephrol.* (2011) 26:1697. doi: 10.1007/s00467-011-1958-y
42. Giuseppe M, Chia L, Valeria M, Alessandro P. The outcome of children with VUR and voiding dysfunction managed with urotherapy. *Neurourol Urodyn.* (2012) 31(Suppl. 1):S22. doi: 10.1002/nau.22259
43. Öztürk BB, Özcakar B, Kavaz A, Ekim M, Yalcinkaya F. Voiding dysfunction in patients with urinary tract infection. *Pediatr Nephrol.* (2012) 27:9 doi: 10.1007/s00467-012-2232-7
44. Akhavan A, Avery D, Lendvay TS. Robot-assisted extravesical ureteral reimplantation: outcomes and conclusions from 78 ureters. *J Pediatr Urol.* (2014) 10:864–8. doi: 10.1016/j.jpurol.2014.01.028
45. Alexander SE, Arlen AM, Storm DW, Kieran K, Cooper CS. Bladder volume at onset of vesicoureteral reflux is an independent risk factor for breakthrough febrile urinary tract infection. *J Urol.* (2015) 193:1342–6. doi: 10.1016/j.juro.2014.10.002
46. Heckler AM, Sung J, Watters S, Martinez Acevedo A, Conlin M, Skoog S. The long-term incidence of urinary tract infection after endoscopic management of vesicoureteral reflux. *Urology.* (2014) 83:1383–7. doi: 10.1016/j.urology.2013.12.045
47. Hoberman A, Greenfield S, Mattoo T, Keren R, Mathews R, Pohl H, et al. Antimicrobial prophylaxis for children with vesicoureteral reflux. *N Engl J Med.* (2014) 370:2367–76. doi: 10.1056/NEJMoa1401811
48. Cetin N, Sav NM, Yildiz B. The prevalence of constipation, enuresis and voiding dysfunction symptoms in children with uncomplicated recurrent urinary tract infection. *Pediatric Nephrol.* (2015). 30:1596.
49. Chang S-J, Tsai L-P, Hsu C-K, Yang SS. Elevated postvoid residual urine volume predicting recurrence of urinary tract infections in toilet-trained children. *Pediatr Nephrol.* (2015) 30:131–7. doi: 10.1007/s00467-014-3009-y
50. Chung JM, Park CS, Lee SD. Postoperative ureteral obstruction after endoscopic treatment for vesicoureteral reflux. *Korean J Urol.* (2015) 56:533–9. doi: 10.4111/kju.2015.56.7.533
51. Arlen AM, Cooper CS, Leong T. Role of body mass index in school-aged children with lower urinary tract dysfunction: does weight classification predict treatment outcome? *J Pediatr Urol.* (2017) 13:454.e1–454.e5. doi: 10.1016/j.jpurol.2017.03.033
52. Sharifi-Rad L, Ladi-Seyedian S-S, Amirzargar H, Kajbafzadeh A-M. Pelvic floor electromyography and urine flow patterns in children with vesicoureteral reflux and lower urinary tract symptoms. *Int Braz J Urol.* (2018) 44:1207–14. doi: 10.1590/s1677-5538.ibju.2018.0401
53. Tuygun C, Sertcelik N, Bakirtas H, Cakici H, Cetin K, Imamoglu AM. Usefulness of a new dysfunctional voiding and incontinence scoring system in predicting treatment effect in children with voiding dysfunction. *Urol Int.* (2007) 79:76–82. doi: 10.1159/000102919
54. Vlajković M, Ilić S, Bogićević M, Rajić M, Ristić L, Petronijević V, et al. Radionuclide voiding patterns in children with vesicoureteral reflux. *Eur J Nucl Med Mol Imaging.* (2003) 30:532–7. doi: 10.1007/s00259-002-1077-x
55. Vaz GT, Vasconcelos MM, Oliveira EA, Ferreira AL, Magalhães PG, Silva FM, et al. Prevalence of lower urinary tract symptoms in school-age children. *Pediatr Nephrol.* (2012) 27:597–603. doi: 10.1007/s00467-011-2028-1
56. Gaither TW, Cooper CS, Kornberg Z, Baskin LS, Copp HL. Risk factors for the development of bladder and bowel dysfunction. *Pediatrics.* (2018) 141:e20172797. doi: 10.1542/peds.2017-2797
57. Kajbafzadeh A-M, Sharifi-Rad L, Ghahestani SM, Ahmadi H, Kajbafzadeh M, Mahboubi AH. Animated biofeedback: an ideal treatment for children with dysfunctional elimination syndrome. *J Urol.* (2011) 186:2379–84. doi: 10.1016/j.juro.2011.07.118
58. Azevedo RVM de, Oliveira EA, Vasconcelos MM de A, Castro BAC de, Pereira FR, Duarte NFV, et al. Impact of an interdisciplinary approach in children

and adolescents with lower urinary tract dysfunction (LUTD). *Braz J Nephrol.* (2014) 36:451–9. doi: 10.5935/0101-2800.20140065

59. Koppen IJN, Vriesman MH, Saps M, Rajindrajith S, Shi X, van Etten-Jamaludin FS, et al. Prevalence of functional defecation disorders in children: a systematic review and meta- analysis. *J Pediatr.* (2018) 198:121–30.e6. doi: 10.1016/j.jpeds.2018.02.029

8

Developing a Research Mentorship Program: The American Society of Pediatric Nephrology's Experience

Tetyana L. Vasylyeva [1*], *María E. Díaz-González de Ferris* [2], *David S. Hains* [3], *Jacqueline Ho* [4], *Lyndsay A. Harshman* [5], *Kimberly J. Reidy* [6], *Tammy M. Brady* [7], *Daryl M. Okamura* [8], *Dmitry V. Samsonov* [9], *Scott E. Wenderfer* [10] *and Erum A. Hartung* [11]

[1] Department of Pediatrics, Texas Tech University Health Sciences Center, Amarillo, TX, United States, [2] UNC Transition Program, Manning Drive N.C. Children's Hospital, The University of North Carolina, Chapel Hill, NC, United States, [3] Division of Pediatric Nephrology, Indiana University School of Medicine, Indianapolis, IN, United States, [4] UPMC Children's Hospital of Pittsburgh, University of Pittsburgh, Pittsburgh, PA, United States, [5] Division of Pediatric Nephrology, Department of Pediatrics, University of Iowa Stead Family, Iowa City, IA, United States, [6] Department of Pediatrics, Montefiore Medical Center, Albert Einstein College of Medicine, Children's Hospital at Montefiore, Bronx, NY, United States, [7] Division of Pediatric Nephrology, Johns Hopkins University School of Medicine, Baltimore, MD, United States, [8] Center for Developmental Biology and Regenerative Medicine, Seattle Children's Hospital, University of Washington, Seattle, WA, United States, [9] New York Medical College, Valhalla, NY, United States, [10] Renal Section, Baylor College of Medicine, Texas Children's Hospital, Houston, TX, United States, [11] Division of Nephrology, Children's Hospital of Philadelphia, Perelman School of Medicine of the University of Pennsylvania, Philadelphia, PA, United States

***Correspondence:**
Tetyana L. Vasylyeva
tetyana.vasylyeva@ttuhsc.edu

Background: Most pediatric nephrologists work in academia. Mentor-mentee relationships provide support and guidance for successful research career. Mentorship program implementation is valuable in medical fields for providing research opportunities to young faculty.

Methods: The American Society of Pediatric Nephrology (ASPN) established a research mentorship program to (a) assist with matching of appropriate mentor-mentee dyads and (b) establish metrics for desirable mentor-mentee outcomes with two independent components: (1) the grants review workshop, a short-term program providing mentor feedback on grant proposals, and (2) the longitudinal program, establishing long-term mentor-mentee relationships. Regular surveys of both mentors and mentees were reviewed to evaluate and refine the program.

Results: Twelve mentees and 17 mentors participated in the grant review workshop and 19 mentees were matched to mentors in the longitudinal program. A review of NIH RePORTER data indicated that since 2014, 13 NIH grants have been awarded. Mentees in the longitudinal program reported that the program helped most with identifying an outside mentor, improving grant research content, and with general career development. Mentors perceived themselves to be most helpful in assisting with overall career plans. Email communications were preferred over phone or face-to-face communications. Mentees endorsed strong interest in staying in touch with their mentors and 100% of mentors expressed their willingness to serve in the future.

Conclusion: This mentorship program was initiated and supported by a relatively small medical society and has shown early success in cultivating mentoring relationships for a future generation of clinician-scientists.

Keywords: mentorship, research, society, grants, pediatrics

INTRODUCTION

Mentoring is a special partnership between two people based on common goals and expectations, focus, and mutual trust and respect (1). Successful mentoring requires commitment to this process by both mentors and mentees and it serves as an important career advancement mechanism for both (2). Mentors provide guidance and promote a mentee's achievement in any or all of the following: academic pursuits, clinical excellence, life/professional goals and work-life balance. Neely et al. wrote, "Development of an academic career easily follows a clinical course for which there are multiple role models; however, development of an academic research career involves few role models, and rarely do instructional guides reach out to the new faculty" (3). In addition to professional aptitude, two components appear essential for a successful research career: (1) a broad supportive infrastructure, and (2) a person- and time-specific continuous mentor-mentee relationship. Positive mentoring relationships require trust, respect, shared information, resources, and expectations as well as professional, enthusiastic, supportive, and collaborative problem-solving (4).

Although a number of papers and internet resources address mentorship programs (5–8), very few focus on development of an academic research career for physician-scientists (3, 9–12). These resources are mostly institution-based and oriented to students and/or graduate medical trainees (13–15). Two recent papers addressed more sponsorship-type programs instead of structural research mentorships (16, 17). Faculty development programs from medical societies are more oriented toward educational research. For example, the American Society of Hematology developed an educational scholarly project (18) and the American Society of Pediatric Hematology/Oncology supports a mentoring program for early career members (19). The Society for Maternal-Fetal Medicine expressed additional concern about forthcoming training of physician-scientists: uncertainties related to future administration of health care, federal support for research, attrition of physician-scientists, and an inadequate supply of new scholars (20). Furthermore, the Accreditation Council for Graduate Medical Education has increased the scholarly productivity requirements for residency programs, placing even more pressure on faculty to be productive in this realm.

Recognizing the need, the American Society of Nephrology (ASN) recently introduced an extensive set of electronic educational resources, presented in brief animations, podcasts, and other media for internal medicine nephrologists. These resources detail effective communication, identifying the right mentor or mentee, navigating mentorship challenges, and assessing a mentee's understanding of expectations (21). These resources developed by an adult medicine subspecialty professional society addressed universal challenges to academic medicine. Although virtually all ASPN members are also ASN members, gaps remained for those trained in pediatric nephrology.

As with other pediatric subspecialties, many pediatric nephrologists work in small divisions with as few as 1–3 faculty in a group. Thus, the lack of a local, experienced research mentor to guide research development and review early faculty progress is common. Recognizing that many junior investigators could benefit from the addition of established senior investigators to their mentoring team, the ASPN created a research mentorship program in 2014.

The specific goals of the ASPN mentorship program were (1) to provide junior investigators with successful research mentors outside their home institutions who have similar research interests, and (2) to provide mentorship training to more established investigators who are ready to become mentors. This program allowed mentors to support junior faculty career development, academic pursuits, and development of grant funding proposals. In this descriptive paper, we present the unique experiences and early data gathered during the ASPN research mentorship program development and implementation. Our experiences may serve as an example for other medical societies seeking to improve junior faculty research mentoring experiences.

METHODS

Development of the ASPN Mentorship Program

The ASPN Mentorship Program was conceived and developed by the ASPN Research Committee in 2014 to match mentors with self-identified mentees and establish an environment for desirable mentor-mentee research outcomes. The program was designed to be dynamic and open to modifications based on periodic surveys and evaluations by all participants. In 2016, a Quality Improvement (QI) framework was formalized with creation of an American Board of Pediatrics (ABP)-approved Maintenance of Certification (MOC) Part 4 program. The program was administered by the co-chairs of the Research Committee, who typically serve 3-year terms. ASPN senior leadership (Council of the Society) ensures management support and monitors step-by-step progress reports.

The mentoring program had two components: (a) the short-term grant review program, designed to help a mentee with a specific grant submission and (b) the longitudinal program, which facilitates the establishment of long-term mentor-mentee relationships to aid in career development. Mentors and mentees can choose to participate in one or both components. Furthermore, the mentee can participate in the grant review program as often as desired. One of the most important approaches to ensure success of the program is optimal matching of mentors and mentees.

Requirements for Mentors and Mentees

The ASPN Research Committee co-chairs selected potential mentors for each mentee among the existing research committee members, current members of the Society, or established non-Society mentors aligned within the field of pediatric nephrology. The selection process was iterative, with feedback from both mentees and potential mentors to ensure no conflicts of interest or conflicts in commitment. To participate in the program, mentees need only to be ASPN members in good standing. ASPN mentees who entered in the longitudinal program perceived that mentors would help with their career and research development.

Grant Review Program

The grant review program consisted of an annual in-person grant review workshop held in conjunction with a large national meeting. These workshops were held in a "mock study section" format, with 3–4 mentors serving as primary and secondary reviewers for 2–3 grants presented orally by groups of mentees. The structure of these workshops was tailored to the needs of the mentees who were assigned to small groups based on research topic or methodology. Mentors are selected based on proven track record of grantsmanship sufficient for the mentees' stage of training. However, often mid-level and senior investigators were assigned as reviewers for the same career development grants in order to also provide experience for mid-level faculty on grant review. Mentees submitted drafts of their grant applications in advance of the in-person workshop, and the mentors were asked to complete a written review using a standard NIH-style review template. Mentees were required to submit a specific aims page at a minimum and were also encouraged to submit other grant sections (e.g., Research Strategy, Career Development). All participants were asked to keep the review process confidential.

Longitudinal Program

Mentees and mentors in the longitudinal program signed a Mentoring Partnership Agreement on enrollment to formalize the relationship and clarify individual expectations. These expectations included committing to regular meetings (in person at least annually; by phone or virtually at other time points), maintaining confidentiality, reviewing and revising the mentees' goals statements annually, providing each other with honest, direct, and respectful feedback, and providing program feedback to the Research Committee. Mentees were asked to write a goals statement, to be reviewed/updated annually with their mentors. Mentees were also encouraged to contact the mentor regularly via phone or electronic communication to discuss specific needs related to grant review, programmatic development, promotion, and tenure.

Mentors in the program are experienced, independently-funded physician scientists, who are able to work with mentees to develop goals with realistic expectations and individualized career development plans. Mentors who reviewed grants for mentees also participated in the grant review component were often selected to become a longitudinal mentor. It was important for mentors to commit to meeting routinely with the mentees to review progress, give feedback, provide recommendations for improvements, and guide academic career development (e.g., assist with grant proposals, manuscript submissions, and oral presentations). The Program leadership maintains Mentorship Partnership Agreements but does not review goals statements or drafts of grants/manuscripts, which are only shared between mentees and their mentors.

Role of the ASPN in Program Promotion and Support

The role of the ASPN in the mentorship program was to advertise the program, elicit participation, judiciously select and contact mentors for each new mentee in the program, review program feedback and outcome metrics regularly to improve the program organization, and develop education workshops. Research Committee members who participated in the QI project had to attend meetings to review survey data at least twice yearly for 2 years to be eligible to receive ABP MOC Part 4 credit.

Research Mentorship Program Evaluation

Surveys were sent to mentees and mentors using Survey Monkey®. Surveys were designed based on program metrics and questions were left unchanged from year-to-year to allow tracking of program efficacy over time in a standard fashion. Mentees and mentors in the longitudinal program were asked about methods and rates of contact with each other within the context of the program. Mentees and mentors in the grants review workshop were asked about what portions of their grants were specifically reviewed. Metrics selected to rate the quality of the program included expectations, number, and format of meetings between mentors and mentees, type of grants reviewed, number and content of sections of grants reviewed, and perceived helpfulness of mentee-mentor interactions in specific areas (i.e., improving grantsmanship). NIH grants are tracked using the RePORTER database (https://projectreporter.nih.gov/reporter.cfm). Metrics were collated by the ASPN Research Committee co-chairs and reviewed in aggregate at Committee meetings on a quarterly basis. Program improvements were implemented on an ongoing basis.

In response to participants' feedback that the program would benefit from more active oversight from the Research Committee, a mentorship program Oversight Subcommittee was formed in 2017. This Oversight Committee, which consists of former co-chairs of the Research Committee and other senior ASPN members, reaches out to mentees and mentors in the longitudinal program on a regular basis to ensure continued mentor-mentee contact and to provide educational resources.

RESULTS

Outcomes of the ASPN Mentorship Program

Since its inception, 12 mentees and 17 mentors have participated in the grant review program and 19 were matched as mentor-mentee pairs for the longitudinal component. Ten mentees participated in both programs, so there have been 21 unique mentees in the mentoring program. Of these, 16 were women and 5 were men. At the time of enrollment in the mentoring program, 17 mentees were junior faculty and 4 were in pediatric nephrology fellowship. Fellowship mentees were also supported by their local Scholarship Oversight Committees. Of the longitudinal program mentees, 8 have "graduated" from their formal mentoring relationship and were able to submit a grant. Mentees were considered to have "graduated" if they had reached

TABLE 1 | American Society of Pediatric Nephrology longitudinal research mentorship program: Mentees' perceptions on expectations and meetings with mentors over a 2-year period, *n* (%) (Questions were added in 2017, so 2016 data is not available).

Survey year	2017 $n = 7$	2018 $n = 8$
Question 1: What were your expectations going into the program?		
Submit R01	2 (29)	3 (33)
Submit career development grant	4 (57)	5 (56)
Submit institutional or foundation grant	0	0
Formulating a research career	1 (14)	2 (11)
Question 2: Has this program met your expectations?		
Yes	6 (86)	8 (100)
No	1 (14)	0
Question 3: Have you discussed expectations with your mentor?		
Yes	6 (86)	8 (100)
No	1 (14)	0
Question 4: In the past 6 months, how many times did you have contact with your mentor?		
None	2 (29)	1 (12.5)
1	1 (14)	4 (50)
2-3	4 (57)	2 (25)
4 or more	0	1 (12.5)
Question 5: In what manner did you communicate with your mentor?		
Email	2 (29)	3 (44)
Phone	3 (43)	2 (29)
In person	2 (29)	(29)
Video chat	0	0
Question 6: Do you have another meeting scheduled?		
Yes	1 (14)	4 (50)
No	6 (86)	4 (50)

TABLE 2 | American Society of Pediatric Nephrology longitudinal research mentorship program: Mentors' perceptions on expectations and meetings with mentees at the end of the represented year, *n* (%).

Survey year	2016 $n = 5$	2017 $n = 8$	2018 $n = 6$
Question 1: Do you think you were a good fit for your mentee's research focus?			
Yes	5 (100)	8 (100)	8 (100)
No	0	0	0
Question 2: In what manner did you communicate with your mentee?			
Email	5 (100)	8 (100)	6 (100)
Phone	1 (20)	5 (63)	4 (67)
In person	4 (80)	6 (75)	5 (83)
Video chat	1 (20)	0	1 (17)
Question 3: Number of times you met with your mentee?*			
None	–	1 (13)	3 (50)
1	–	3 (38)	2 (33)
2–3	–	3 (38)	0
4 or more	–	1 (13)	1 (17)
Question 4: Would you be willing to serve as a mentor in the future?			
Yes	4 (80)	8 (100)	6 (100)
No	1 (20)	0	0

*Mentors were surveyed after each year of the active program. *Question added to survey in 2017.*

TABLE 3 | American Society of Pediatric Nephrology longitudinal research mentorship program: Mentees' and mentors' reports of which sections of the grant were reviewed [*n* (%) of positive responses].

Grant sections reviewed	Mentees			Mentors		
Years	**2016** $n = 6$	**2017** $n = 7$	**2018** $n = 8$	**2016** $n = 5$	**2017** $n = 8$	**2018** $n = 6$
No comment	2 (33)	1 (14)	2 (25)	0	2 (25)	1 (17)
Concept/plan only	1 (17)	1 (14)	3 (38)	4 (80)	2 (25)	4 (67)
Specific aims	3 (50)	5 (71)	6 (75)	1 (20)	6 (75)	3 (50)
Significance	1 (17)	3 (43)	1 (13)	1 (20)	2 (25)	2 (33)
Innovation	1 (17)	4 (57)	1 (13)	1 (20)	2 (25)	1 (17)
Approach	2 (33)	5 (71)	2 (25)	2 (40)	5 (63)	2 (33)
Career development plan	0	1 (14)	1 (13)	0	1 (13)	0

their goals within the program, which were delineated at the time of program entry, and therefore chose to formally end their participation. From the 21 mentees who have participated in the mentoring program since 2014, review of NIH RePORTER data in October 2018 indicated 13 successful NIH grants following mentorship program participation: 5 R01s, 3 R03s, and 5 K awards. Although non-NIH funding (commercial, private foundations, institutional internal funds, etc.) represents a substantial source of research support this information was more difficult to track. We are planning to collect this information in our upcoming surveys.

Tables 1, 2 detail longitudinal program mentee and mentor responses, respectively, to survey questions regarding expectations, mentee-mentor fit, frequency of communication, future meeting plans. Sections of grant proposals reviewed in the longitudinal program are shown in **Table 3. Figure 1** represents satisfaction with the grant review (A) and longitudinal components (B) of the program in various areas.

In 2018, 100% of mentees in the longitudinal program agreed that the program met their expectations and that expectations were clearly communicated with the mentors. During a 6 month period, 50% of mentees met with their mentors face to face at least once, 25% met 2–3 times, and 12.5% met 4 or more times (**Table 1**). The vast majority of the longitudinal program mentees discussed the *Specific Aims* of their grants but interactions were less focused on their overall career development plan (**Table 3**). For the longitudinal component, email communications were preferred over phone or face-to-face communications.

While every mentor over the initial 3-year-period strongly believed that he/she was a good fit for their mentee, mentors' perceptions of the program differed from mentees' in key aspects. Mentors in both the grants review and longitudinal components

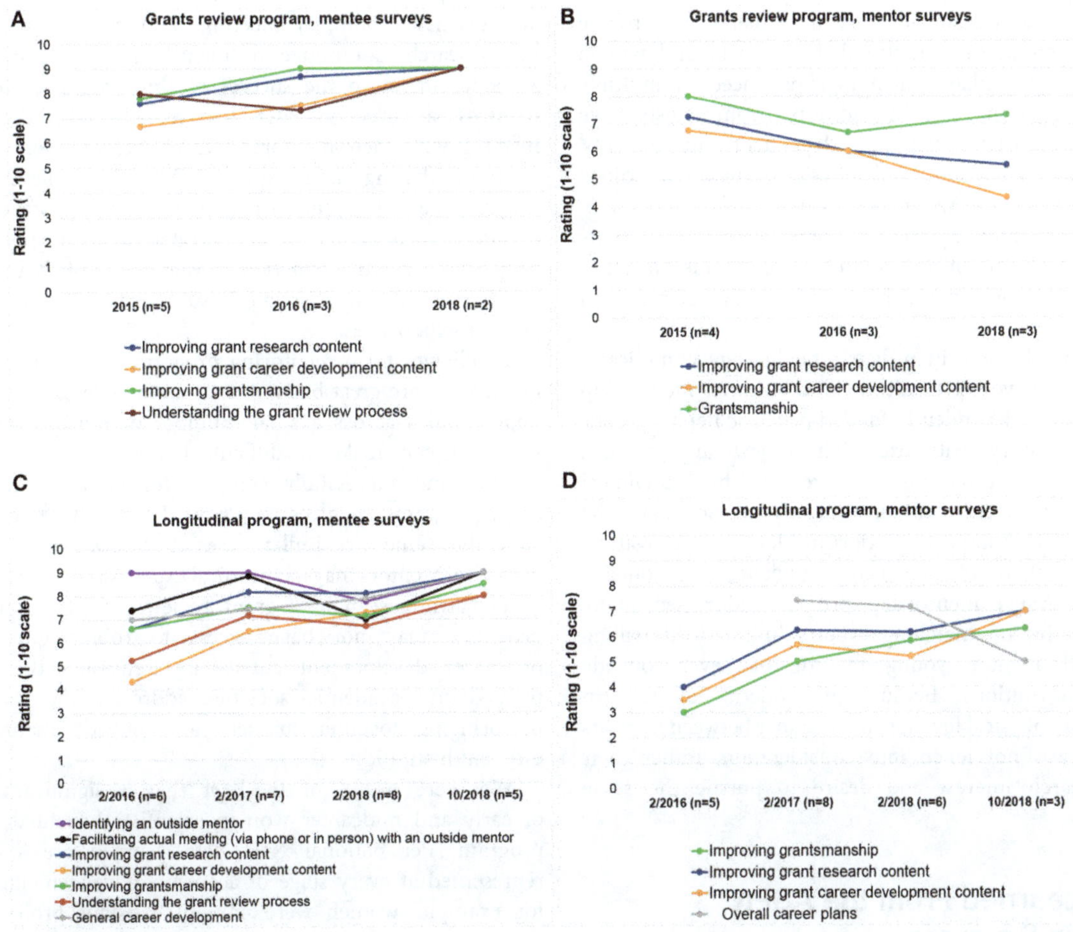

FIGURE 1 | American Society of Pediatric Nephrology research mentorship program: Mentees' ratings of the program's helpfulness in different areas, and mentors' ratings of their own helpfulness to their mentees. **(A)** Grant review mentees, **(B)** Grant review mentors, **(C)** Longitudinal program mentees, and **(D)** Longitudinal program mentors.

of the program perceived their overall helpfulness relatively low on a scale from 1 to 10 (**Figures 1B,D**), despite the mentees rating the program's helpfulness relatively highly (**Figures 1A,C**). Although no more than 14% of longitudinal program mentees reported reviewing long term career development plans with their mentors (**Table 3**), mentees rated the program relatively highly for helpfulness in general career development (score 7.0–7.9 out of 10, **Figure 1B**). Similarly, mentors also reported that they believed they were helpful to their mentees in "overall career plans" (score 7.2–7.4 out of 10, **Figure 1D**). As the program has evolved and improved over the years, 100% of mentors expressed their willingness to serve in the future (**Table 2**). During the course of this program, the longitudinal component demonstrated sustained improvement in satisfaction (**Figures 1C,D**).

DISCUSSION

We described the development and management of a junior faculty oriented research mentorship program within a pediatric medical subspecialty. The ASPN mentorship program experience demonstrates participant satisfaction, mentor-mentee stability, programmatic improvement over time, and notably a high yield of NIH grants during the project implementation period. Development of such a program within a relatively small pediatric society is challenging but essential. This model could serve as an example for other similar medical organizations.

The ASPN mentorship program addresses an important gap identified by academic nephrologists at the start of their careers. While some of the challenges experienced by new faculty in pediatric subspecialties are common with other aspiring physician scientists in other medicine careers, some are unique to those in pediatric medicine and nephrology. New faculty in pediatrics can become overwhelmed with the demands of juggling clinical practice with a research career. Initiating research—from conceptualization, proposal development, grant submission and ultimately to implementation and dissemination—is challenging, but extremely important for academic advancement.

The challenges in pediatric nephrology research are many, including a widespread array of pediatric nephrology divisions throughout the country that are small and with a paucity of locally available mentors experienced in multiple areas of investigation (22). In addition, nephrologists have several specific needs that are dependent on patients' unique psychosocial issues and physiology/pathophysiology of kidney disease (23); these issues are only more complicated in children. Several renal-related conditions are relatively uncommon in children, making identification and recruitment of potential clinical study participants extremely difficult.

The small work force in pediatric nephrology complicates the accessibility of young faculty to find research mentorship from established, independently-funded pediatric nephrologists. Through the country, with exception of few large centers, pediatric nephrology programs are represented by 2–5 clinical faculty (24). Moreover, many institutions do not have the infrastructure to support junior/mid-level investigators, which require networking and career guidance from outside mentors. The ASPN mentorship program addressed many of these obstacles by matching experts in the field willing to teach and mentor young investigators even outside their home institutions. Because of modern advances in communication, physical location and distance between mentors and mentees was not taken into consideration, rather their common research interest and desire to pursue the same scientific goals.

Lessons Learned From the ASPN Mentorship Program

Oversight by the ASPN ensured the success of this program and collection of outcome measurements of the program was critical. Governing the program through the ASPN research committee proved to be a viable option. Customized pairing of mentees with mentors based on academic and research expertise was a high priority for participants. We believe that requesting drafts of mentees' grant applications in advance of the in-person workshop, and requesting that mentors complete a written review, substantially increased the success rate of the program because it ensured that participants were highly motivated.

Mentees highly regarded the ability to receive individualized feedback from established investigators on their research grant proposals. Although not employed by ASPN, similar programs might use an "intelligent match" to achieve the best possible arrangements, using a very specific matching parameters and computerized approach. E-mail was the preferred mode of communication to foster ongoing relationship, with mentors further appreciating the importance of additional face-to-face contact.

We learned that the design and maintenance of a mentoring program should be dynamic with frequent assessments for improvement. An efficient monitoring vehicle was brief periodic online surveys. The frequency of these surveys could depend on the program, but annual surveys were adequate in this experience. In our program response to survey was close to 50% of participants. Results of the surveys were reviewed and discussed both, at meetings and conference calls with the Research Committee to identify process improvements. As a testament to the success of this program, 50% of the mentees surveyed in 2018 had already scheduled another meeting with their mentors, and all mentors were willing to continue sharing their expertise. We also believe that this program helped to enrich a national network of pediatrician scientists with similar research interests. It is possible that people with positive experiences were more likely to complete the survey. As such, some results may be biased toward positive experiences.

Challenges for a mentoring program in academic pediatric nephrology are great but not insurmountable. Limited funding opportunities across a small number of funding agencies in the field can make it difficult for junior investigators to identify and successfully compete for grant funding.Within small programs, mentees may have difficulty finding a mentor with the same or similar research interest or appropriate expertise. Mentors may have topical expertise but lack experience in pediatric research or grant review. Faculty from smaller programs may not have access to robust grant writing or career development curricula. Harnessing the strengths of pediatric academic societies addresses these challenges by bringing together mentees and outside mentors from different institutions.

We were proud of the fact that a significant number of early and midcareer women scientists benefited from the program. Per national NIH data, women are still under-represented at every stage of academic advancement. In 2015, for example, women were 44% of assistant professors, and 35% of professors (25). Our program successfully overcame that disparity.

Our program has some limitations. Due to the relatively small number of participants, we cannot provide detailed characteristics on age, race/ethnicity, and size/resources of their home institution. Although we chose mentors with strong track records of NIH-funded research, we did not collect information about their mentoring activities within their own institutions. In the future we are planning to collect more data about mentee's institutional environment (e.g., size of practice, characteristics of medical centers, local mentoring) as well as data about number of proposals funded by the NIH, industry and foundations.

Suggestions for the Design of Mentoring Programs

It is fundamental that mentors and mentees who entered a mentoring program have a clear understanding of the goals, objectives, and desirable outcomes of the collaboration. Mentors should be willing to commit to working one-on-one with mentees and ideally should have a successful track record of grant awards and research publications. Mentors should help young clinical scientists to plan, develop, grow, and manage their careers. Mentors also have an important role in helping junior faculty members become resilient in times of change, more self-reliant in their careers, and more responsible as self-directed learners. Mentees should clearly understand expectations and should be willing to provide feedback to the program.

Based on our ASPN experience, we identified that the 10 key elements (in no specific order) for successful mentorship programs are to:

1. Provide concrete advice on specific research pursuits and promote interaction between mentors and mentees as well as other content experts with successful research careers;
2. Provide infrastructure that enables pairing of mentors and mentees, completion of goals statements, assurance of confidentiality, and successful program completion;
3. Facilitate planning and management of program assessments, track scheduling, and report documentation;
4. Inform program participants about available specialty focused NIH and non-NIH funding opportunities;
5. Complete thorough and consistent evaluations of the participants' progress;
6. Perform continuous review and evaluation of program assignments and activities throughout the program cycles and make appropriate changes;
7. Employ continuous QI techniques (Plan-Do-Study-Act) to improve programmatic effectiveness;
8. Provide enticements for senior investigators and experienced mentors to stay involved, such as Maintenance of Certification (MOC) Part 4 credits from the American Board of Pediatrics (ABP) for participants;
9. Train a future generation of mentors through role modeling and feedback.
10. Motivate others with dedication, enthusiasm and good will.

In summary, a structured and well-organized research mentorship program with strong medical society leadership, brings professional fulfillment to academic physicians. In addition, providing increased research mentorship helps to increase and sustain the research workforce, which results in more robust research and improved child health.

CONCLUSION

The ASPN Research Mentorship Program, initiated and supported within a relatively small medical society; showed early success in training a future generation of clinician-scientists who will be able to undertake valuable research that we hope will 1 day lead to better patient outcomes.

AUTHOR CONTRIBUTIONS

TV participated in the program and led the writing group, correspondent author. MD-G substantial contribution in Program improvement and correction of manuscript. DH led a mentorship program, participated in writing. JH led mentorship program, participated in writing. LH actively participated in mentorship program and manuscript writing. KR actively participated in mentorship program evaluation and manuscript writing. TB led the program, writing. DO led the program, writing. DS manuscript revision, suggestions, writing. SW led the program, participated in survey, data analysis and writing. EH led the program, survey, data analysis, graphs for paper, writing and revisions.

ACKNOWLEDGMENTS

The recommendations in this paper are the work of authors representing the American Society of Pediatric Nephrology (ASPN) and are endorsed by the ASPN Council, but are not necessarily representative of the opinions of each individual member of the ASPN.

REFERENCES

1. Mentoring Program. Guidance and Program Plan. U.S. *Department of Energy. Office of Learning and Workforce Development.* Prepared by: June Robinson, Learning & Development Programs Division (HC-22), Office of Learning & Workforce Development. (2014). Available online at: https://www.energy.gov/sites/prod/files/2014/11/f19/DOE_Mentoring%20Guidance%20%20Pgrm%20Plan2_0.pdf/ (accessed October 30, 2018).
2. Frei E, Stamm M, Buddeberg-Fischer B. Mentoring programs for medical students - a review of the PubMed literature 2000 – 2008. *BMC Med Educ.* (2010) 10:32. doi: 10.1186/1472-6920-10-32
3. Gail Neely J, Smith RJ, Graboyes EM, Paniello RC, Gubbels SP, Guide to academic research career development. *Laryngoscope Invest Otolaryngol.* (2016) 1:19–24. doi: 10.1002/lio2.5
4. Hudson P. Forming the mentor-mentee relationship. *J Mentoring Tutoring.* (2016) 24:30–43. doi: 10.1080/13611267.2016.1163637
5. Chronus. *How to Start a High-Impact Mentoring Program.* A Five-Step Guide to Launching a Mentoring Program. Available online at: https://chronus.com/how-to-start-a-mentoring-program/ (accessed October 30, 2018).
6. MonsteR. *9 Companies With Solid Mentorship Programs.* Available online at: https://www.monster.com/career-advice/article/9-companies-with-solid-mentorship-programs-0816/ (accessed October 30, 2018).
7. Mentor. *Start a Program.* Available online at: https://www.mentoring.org/program-resources/start-a-program/ (accessed October 30, 2018).
8. Henry-Noel N, Bishop M, Gwede CK, Petkova E, Szumacher E. Mentorship in medicine and other health professions. *J Cancer Educ.* (2018) 1–9. doi: 10.1007/s13187-018-1360-6. [Epub ahead of print].
9. Spence JP, Buddenbaum JL, Bice PJ, Welch JL, Carroll AE. Independent investigator incubator (I3): a comprehensive mentorship program to jumpstart productive research careers for junior faculty. *BMC Med Educ.* (2018) 18:186. doi: 10.1186/s12909-018-1290-3
10. Alvira CM, Steinhorn RH, Balistreri WF, Fineman JR, Oishi PE, Padbury JF, et al. Enhancing the development and retention of physician-scientists in academic pediatrics: strategies for success. *J Pediatr.* (2018) 200:277–84. doi: 10.1016/j.jpeds.2018.06.019
11. Lalani N, Griffith KA, Jones RD, Spratt DE, Croke J, Jagsi R. Mentorship experiences of early-career academic radiation oncologists in North America. *Int J Radiat Oncol Biol Phys.* (2018) 101:732–40. doi: 10.1016/j.ijrobp.2018.03.035
12. Walensky RP, Kim Y, Chang Y, Porneala BC, Bristol MN, Armstrong K, et al. The impact of active mentorship: results from a survey of faculty in the department of medicine at massachusetts general hospital. *BMC Med Educ.* (2018) 18:108.doi: 10.1186/s12909-018-1191-5
13. Jordan J, Hwang M, Kaji AH, Coates WC. Scholarly tracks in emergency medicine residency programs are associated with increased choice of academic career. *West J Emerg Med.* (2018) 19:593–9. doi: 10.5811/westjem.2018.1.36753

14. Amonoo HL, Barreto EA, Stern TA, Donelan K. Residents' experiences with mentorship in academic medicine. *Acad Psychiatry.* (2018) 43:71–5. doi: 10.1007/s40596-018-0924-4
15. Moye J, Molinari VA, Karel MJ, Naik AD, Sakai E, Carpenter BD. Come, join, lead: attracting students to careers in aging and promoting involvement in gerontological societies. *Gerontol Geriatr Educ.* (2017) 27:1–11. doi: 10.1080/02701960.2017.1287075
16. Ayyala MS, Skarupski K, Bodurtha JN, González-Fernández M, Ishii LE, Fivush B, et al. Mentorship is not enough: exploring sponsorship and its role in career advancement in academic medicine. *Acad Med.* (2018) 94:94–100.doi: 10.1097/ACM.0000000000002398
17. Gottlieb AS, Travis EL. Rationale and models for career advancement sponsorship in academic medicine: the time is here; the time is now. *Acad Med.* (2018) 93:1620–3. doi: 10.1097/ACM.0000000000002342
18. Kesselheim JC, Clayton CP, Fritz J, Smith RE, Gitlin SD, Reid E, et al. The American society of hematology (ASH) medical educators institute: a pilot faculty development project for hematology educators. *J Cancer Educ.* (2018) doi: 10.1007/s13187-018-1363-3. [Epub ahead of print].
19. Badawy SM, Black V, Meier ER, Myers KC, Pinkney K, Hastings C, et al. Early career mentoring through the American society of pediatric hematology/oncology: lessons learned from a pilot program. *Pediatr Blood Cancer.* (2017) 64:e26252. doi: 10.1002/pbc.26252
20. Sadovsky Y, Caughey AB, DiVito M, D'Alton ME, Murtha AP. SMFM research committee. research to knowledge: promoting the training of physician-scientists in the biology of pregnancy. societyfor maternal-fetal medicine (SMFM). *Am J Obstet Gynecol.* (2018) 218:B9–13. doi: 10.1016/j.ajog.2017.09.024
21. American Society of Nephrology. *Mentoring Resources.* Available online at: https://www.asn-online.org/education/training/mentors/ (accessed October 30, 2018).
22. Primack WA, Meyers KE, Kirkwood SJ, Ruch-Ross HS, Radabaugh CL, Greenbaum LA. The US pediatric nephrology workforce: a report commissioned by the American academy of pediatrics. *Am J Kidney Dis.* (2015) 66:33–9. doi: 10.1053/j.ajkd.2015.03.022
23. Ibrahim T. Academic internal medicine in the United States: current trends, future implications for academic nephrology. *Clin J Am Soc Nephrol.* (2008) 3:1887–94. doi: 10.2215/CJN.02110508
24. Glenn D, Ocegueda S, Nazareth M, Zhong Y, Weinstein A, Primack W, et al. The global pediatric nephrology workforce: a survey of the international pediatric nephrology association. *BMC Nephrol.* (2016) 15:17–83. doi: 10.1186/s12882-016-0299-2
25. National Institute of Health. *Funding Longevity by Gender Among NIH-Supported Investigators.* Available online at: https://nexus.od.nih.gov/all/2018/09/07/funding-longevity-by-gender-among-nih-supported-investigators/ (accessed October 30, 2018).

9

Mycophenolate Mofetil in the Treatment of Steroid-Dependent or Frequently Relapsing Nephrotic Syndrome in Children

Xin Xiang [1,2], Shi-Yuan Qiu [1,2] and Mo Wang [1,2]*

[1] Ministry of Education Key Laboratory of Child Development and Disorders, Department of Nephrology, National Clinical Research Center for Child Health and Disorders, China International Science and Technology Cooperation Base of Child development and Critical Disorders, Children's Hospital of Chongqing Medical University, Chongqing, China, [2] Chongqing Key Laboratory of Pediatrics, Chongqing, China

***Correspondence:**
Mo Wang
wangmo_cqmu@163.com

Objectives: This meta-analysis aims to evaluate the efficacy and safety of the mycophenolate mofetil (MMF) in the treatment of steroid-dependent nephrotic syndrome (SDNS) or frequently relapsing nephrotic syndrome (FRNS) in children.

Methods: We searched for the studies especially the randomized controlled trials in PubMed, Cochrane Library, Embase, China National Knowledge Infrastructure, and Wan Fang database. The data were analyzed by Review Manager 5.3 software. We used the GRADE pro-Guideline Development Tool online software to evaluate the quality of evidence.

Results: Finally, we identified 620 studies, of which we included five randomized controlled trials and one prospective cohort study with 447 children. The results showed the following: (1) the relapse-free survival rate within 1 year—the MMF group was superior to the levamisole group [ratio difference (RD) = 0.13, 95% CI (0.02, 0.24), $P = 0.02$] but not to the calcineurin inhibitors (CNIs) group [RD = −0.27, 95%CI (−0.40, −0.14), $P < 0.0001$]; (2) the number of relapses within 1 year—the MMF group was less than that in the CNIs and levamisole group [mean difference (MD) = −0.26, 95%CI (−0.45, −0.08), $P = 0.005$]; (3) the cumulative prednisone dosage—the MMF group was lower than that in the control group [standardized mean difference (SMD) = −0.32, 95%CI (−0.53, −0.11), $P = 0.003$]; (4) incidence of adverse reactions—there was no significant difference between the MMF group and the control group [RD = 0.02, 95%CI (−0.04, 0.09), $P = 0.46$].

Conclusion: The therapy of mycophenolate mofetil in the treatment of SDNS or FRNS in children has a certain advantage in reducing the number of relapses and cumulative prednisone dosage within 1 year when compared with the CNIs and levamisole. However, due to the limited quantity and quality of the included studies, the conclusions above need to be confirmed by more high-quality randomized controlled trials.

Keywords: mycophenolate mofetil, frequently relapsing nephrotic syndrome, steroid-dependent nephrotic syndrome, children, meta-analysis

INTRODUCTION

Nephrotic syndrome (NS) is a common glomerular disease in childhood characterized by proteinuria, hypoproteinemia, hyperlipidemia, and edema. The pathogenesis of the disease has not been fully elucidated. At present, it is mainly related to immune imbalance (1), systemic circulatory factors (2), and abnormal podocyte genetic mutations (3). Ninety percent of cases of nephrotic syndrome presenting in childhood are idiopathic (4), and glucocorticoid therapy has been considered a first-line treatment for PNS in children since the 1950s. According to the response to steroid treatment, PNS can be classified as steroid-sensitive nephrotic syndrome (SSNS), steroid-resistant nephrotic syndrome (SRNS), and steroid-dependent nephrotic syndrome (SDNS). SDNS and FRNS are refractory patterns of steroid responsiveness in nephrotic syndrome that account for about 40% of PNS in children whose goal is to choose appropriate second-line immunosuppressants, to induce a response as soon as possible, and to maintain a long-term response. The Kidney Disease: Improving Global Outcomes (KDIGO) guidelines (5) recommend a variety of immunosuppressants for the treatment of SDNS or FRNS in children, including mycophenolate mofetil (MMF), cyclophosphamide, cyclosporine A (CsA), tacrolimus (TAC), rituximab, and the immunomodulator levamisole. However, due to the responsiveness of different patients to different drugs and adverse reactions, making the best plan of pharmacotherapy is still a great challenge for most pediatric nephrologists.

MMF, as a novel immunosuppressant, is a 2-ethyl ester derivative of mycophenolic acid, which is taken off the esterification *in vivo* to form a metabolite with immunosuppressive activity. Mycophenolic acid can selectively act on T and B lymphocytes and the first or second signal in the process of activation to achieve the purpose of immunosuppression. In addition, the inhibitory effect of MMF on other cytokines *in vivo* can also play a role in delaying the progression of the disease. In 1998 (6), American doctors used MMF for the first time in the treatment of adult RNS and achieved good results. Subsequently, the role of MMF in the treatment of kidney disease has received widespread attention. Previous studies have confirmed its positive effect on the treatment of SDNS or FRNS in children. However, most of these studies are based on retrospective analysis, and only a few randomized controlled trials (RCTs) have focused on its efficacy and safety. Therefore, in this study, a meta-analysis was conducted to evaluate the efficacy and safety of MMF in the treatment of SDNS or FRNS in children to provide higher-strength evidence for the usage of MMF.

METHODS

Study Design

In accordance with the principle of "PICOS," it was defined as following: (1) P: the children with SDNS or FRNS; (2) I: treated with MMF or other immunosuppressants (TAC, CsA, and levamisole; (3) C: MMF vs. other immunosuppressants (TAC, CsA, and levamisole); (4) O: relapse-free survival rate within 1 year, the number of relapses within 1 year, cumulative prednisone dosage, and incidence of adverse reactions; (5) S: a meta-analysis of RCTs and a prospective cohort study.

Abbreviations: SDNS, steroid-dependent nephrotic syndrome; FRNS, frequently relapsing nephrotic syndrome; SRNS, steroid-resistant nephrotic syndrome; RNS, refractory nephrotic syndrome; SSNS, steroid-sensitive nephrotic syndrome; PNS, primary nephrotic syndrome.

Literature Search

Chinese Literature

We searched the China National Knowledge Infrastructure (CNKI) and Wan Fang database with the keywords including "nephrotic syndrome," "mycophenolate mofetil," and "children."

English Literature

We used the combination of subject words and free words to search PubMed, Embase, and The Cochrane Library. For example, the free words of "nephrotic syndrome" include "nephrotic syndromes," "syndrome, nephrotic," "syndromes, nephrotic," and "nephrotic."

Search Time

Unlimited–December 2020.

Study Selection and Data Extraction

Inclusion criteria

Inclusion criteria were as follows: (1) the prospective studies, especially RCTs, of MMF in the treatment of SDNS or FRNS in children aged from 3 months to 18 years old; (2) the follow-up period of at least 1 year; and (3) the diagnostic criteria refers to the 2012 KDIGO guidelines (7, 8): (a) SDNS, two consecutive relapses during corticosteroid therapy or within 14 days of ceasing therapy; (b) FRNS, >2 relapses within 6 months of initial relapse, or ≥ 4 relapses in any 12 months. Among them, steroid sensitivity showed that urinary protein turned negative after 4 weeks of treatment with a sufficient amount of prednisone [2 mg/(kg·day) or 60 mg/(m^2·day)].

Exclusion criteria

Exclusion criteria were as follows: (1) all kinds of secondary nephrotic syndrome, such as nephrotic syndrome caused by lupus, hepatitis B virus infection, and antineutrophil-associated glomerulonephritis; (2) retrospective studies, review, meeting, and literature that is not consistent with the purpose of evaluation.

Data Extraction

Based on the inclusion and exclusion criteria, independent duplicate data extraction was performed by two reviewers (Xin Xiang and Shi-Yuan Qiu) using a predesigned data collection form, and the results were reviewed by a third investigator (Mo Wang). In this study, a small number of data in the original literature are expressed by the quartile method, which needs to be converted into mean and standard deviation by using Luo (9) and other methods.

Types of Outcome Measures

Primary Outcomes

Relapse-free survival rate within 1 year, the number of relapses within 1 year, and cumulative prednisone dosage.

Relapse

Twenty-four-hour urine protein ≥50 mg/kg for 3 consecutive days, urinary protein/creatinine (mg/mg) ≥2.0 in morning urine or morning urine protein changed from negative to positive or (+ + +)–(+ + ++).

Secondary Outcome

Incidence of adverse reactions (mainly considering serious adverse reactions, such as severe infection, agranulocytosis, etc.).

Statistical Methods

Statistical analysis of the data was carried out by RevMan5.3 software provided by The Cochrane collaboration network. Heterogeneity analysis was carried out in selected trials. When $P > 0.05$ and $I^2 < 50\%$, the homogeneity of the study was not significant. A fixed-effect model was used. On the contrary, the random effect model was adopted. Ratio difference (RD) and its 95% confidence interval (95%CI) were used for count data. Mean difference (MD) or standardized mean difference (SMD) and its 95% CI were used for measurement data. If there was obvious heterogeneity in the study, its sensitivity was analyzed and postprocessed. Only descriptive analysis was carried out if it cannot be determined.

Evidence Quality Assessment

We used the GRADE pro-Guideline Development Tool online software (GRADEpro GDT, Evidence Prime, Hamilton, ON) to evaluate the quality of evidence.

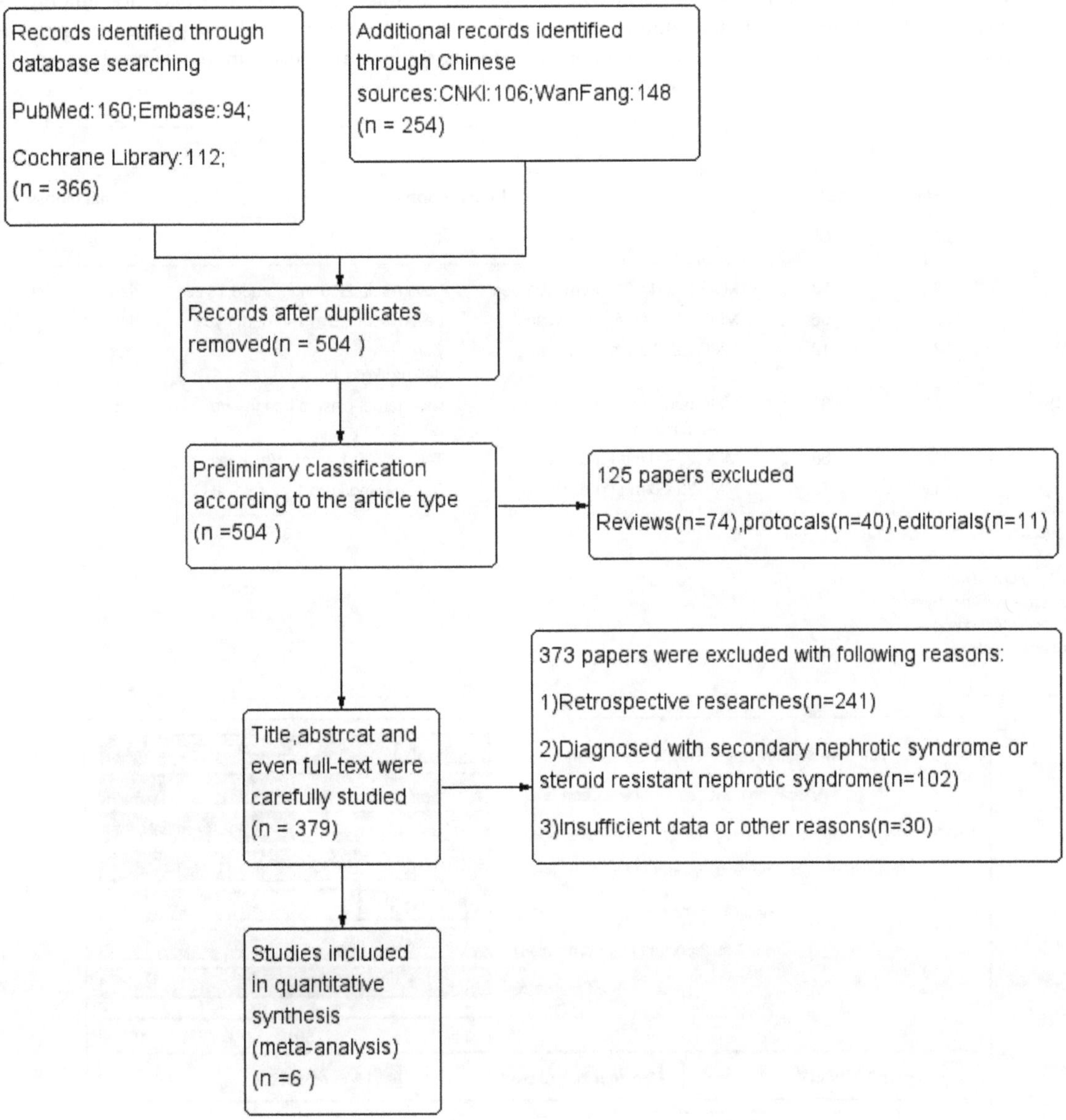

FIGURE 1 | Flow diagram of the study identification.

RESULTS

Literature Retrieval Results

Six hundred twenty articles were retrieved according to the above method. We excluded the repetitions, reviews, retrospective studies, nonclinical studies, and the studies inconsistent with the purpose of evaluation by reading titles, abstracts, and some of the specific contents of the literature. Finally, a total of six articles were included: one Chinese literature (10) and five English articles (11–15). The total number of subjects analyzed was 447 children. **Figure 1** shows the process of literature retrieval. **Table 1** shows the characteristics of the included studies.

Risk of Bias

The Cochrane Collaboration (16) was used for assessing the risk of bias. Of the six articles, one was randomly generated by a computer, one was stratified by randomized numbers in Excel table, one was randomized by central computer minimization, and the other two were randomly grouped, whose random allocation method was not indicated. Two of them were hidden in design allocation but without indicating the specific hiding method. One article adopted the blind method, but others did not mention whether to use blind methods. Follow-up after publication was not mentioned in almost all literature. All the studies clearly explained that there was no significant statistical difference in the baseline data between the experimental group and the control group, which means that they were balanced and comparable. **Figure 2** shows the authors' judgment about each risk bias item presented as percentages across all included studies.

1-Year Relapse-Free Survival Rate

The definition of relapse of SDNS or FRNS in children is as mentioned above. All of the six articles included in this study reported the relapse-free survival rate within 1 year. When analyzing all the data extracted from the literature, we found that there was significant heterogeneity among the studies. Thus, we conducted the subgroups according to the types of immunosuppressants used in the control group. The results

TABLE 1 | Characteristics of the included study.

Trial	Patient number		Intervention		Renal biopsy	Outcome
	E[a]	C[b]	E	C		
Sinha (14)	76	73	MMF 750–1,000 $mg/m^2/d$, 1 year	Levamisole 22.5 mg/kg/qod,1 year	No	1[c] 2[d] 3[e] 4[f]
Basu (15)	56	56	MMF 1,200 $mg/m^2/d$,1 year	Levamisole 2.5 mg/kg/qod,1 year	No	1 2 3 4
Dorresteijn (13)	12	12	MMF 1,200 $mg/m^2/d$,1 year	CsA 4–5 mg/kg/d,1 year	Yes	1 2 3 4
Gellermann (11)	28	30	MMF, target plasma trough level 1.5–2.5 mg/ml	CsA, target plasma trough level 80–100 ng/ml	Yes	1 4
Wang (12)	34	38	MMF 20–30 mg/kg/d, 1 year	TAC 0.05–0.15 mg/kg/d, 1 year	Yes	1 3 4
Geng (10)	14	18	MMF 20–30 mg/kg/d, 1 year	CsA 3–5 mg/kg/d,1 year	Yes	1 2 4

[a] *Experiment group.*
[b] *Control group.*
[c] *1-year relapse-free survival rate.*
[d] *The number of relapses within 1 year.*
[e] *Cumulative glucocorticoid dosage.*
[f] *Incidence of adverse reactions.*

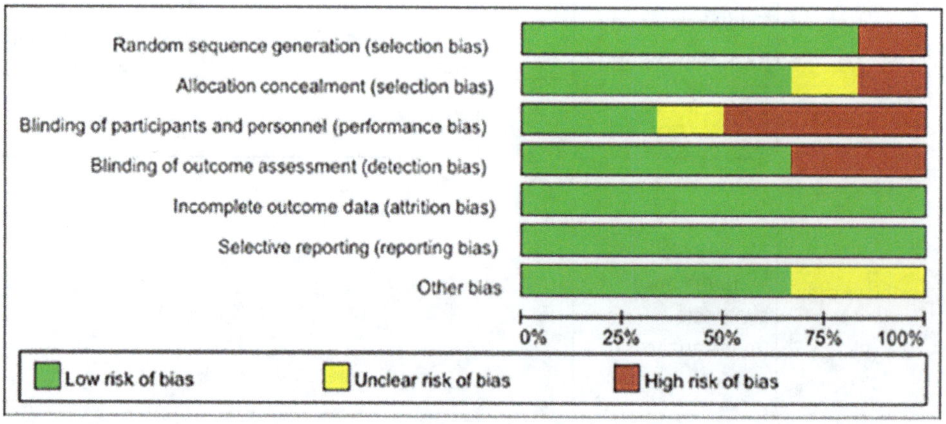

FIGURE 2 | Inclusion bias.

Study or Subgroup	MMF Events	MMF Total	Control group Events	Control group Total	Weight	Risk Difference M-H, Fixed, 95% CI
1.9.1 MMF Vs Levamisole						
Aditi Sinha 2018	31	76	25	73	57.1%	0.07 [-0.09, 0.22]
Biswanath Basu 2015	21	56	9	56	42.9%	0.21 [0.06, 0.37]
Subtotal (95% CI)		**132**		**129**	**100.0%**	**0.13 [0.02, 0.24]**
Total events	52		34			
Heterogeneity: Chi² = 1.75, df = 1 (P = 0.19); I² = 43%						
Test for overall effect: Z = 2.27 (P = 0.02)						
1.9.2 MMF Vs CNIs						
Eiske 2008	7	12	11	12	13.0%	-0.33 [-0.65, -0.01]
Geng 2018	2	14	8	18	17.0%	-0.30 [-0.60, -0.01]
Jutta Gellermann 2013	9	28	21	30	31.3%	-0.38 [-0.62, -0.14]
WANG 2016	13	34	20	38	38.8%	-0.14 [-0.37, 0.08]
Subtotal (95% CI)		**88**		**98**	**100.0%**	**-0.27 [-0.40, -0.14]**
Total events	31		60			
Heterogeneity: Chi² = 2.17, df = 3 (P = 0.54); I² = 0%						
Test for overall effect: Z = 3.97 (P < 0.0001)						

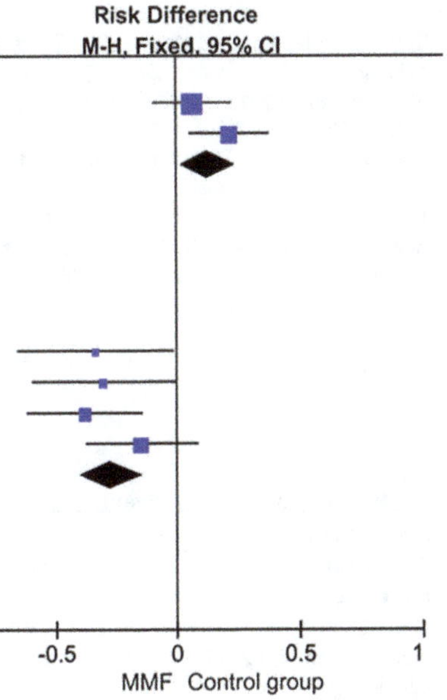

FIGURE 3 | Forest plot showing ratio difference (RD) of the 1-year relapse-free survival rate between the groups.

Study or Subgroup	MMF Mean	MMF SD	MMF Total	Control group Mean	Control group SD	Control group Total	Weight	Mean Difference IV, Fixed, 95% CI
Aditi Sinha 2018	1.11	0.6	76	1.36	0.63	73	87.8%	-0.25 [-0.45, -0.05]
Biswanath Basu 2015	1.1	1.2	30	1.7	1.5	30	7.3%	-0.60 [-1.29, 0.09]
Geng 2018	1	1.48	14	1	0.67	18	4.9%	0.00 [-0.83, 0.83]
Total (95% CI)			**120**			**121**	**100.0%**	**-0.26 [-0.45, -0.08]**
Heterogeneity: Chi² = 1.32, df = 2 (P = 0.52); I² = 0%								
Test for overall effect: Z = 2.78 (P = 0.005)								

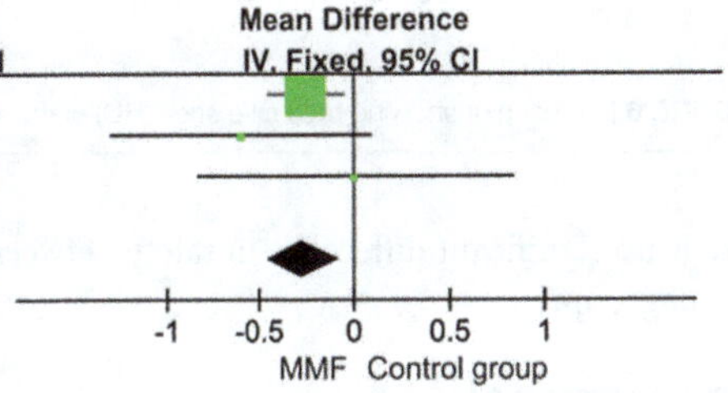

FIGURE 4 | Forest plot showing mean difference (MD) of the number of relapses within 1 year between the groups.

shown in **Figure 3** indicate that MMF was superior to levamisole but not to calcineurin inhibitors (CNIs), and the differences were statistically significant.

The Number of Relapses Within 1 Year

Four articles reported the number of relapses within 1 year. The total number of patients after treatment was analyzed. The results showed that there was heterogeneity among the studies. We have to find the source of heterogeneity by eliminating one by one. After removing the literature of Eiske2008, the heterogeneity was significantly reduced. Re-reading the literature, we found that the renal biopsy results of the subjects included in this study were minimal change diseases (MCDs). We thought it to be the source of heterogeneity, so the literature was deleted. The remaining three articles were analyzed by the fixed-effect model, and the specific results of the meta-analysis were as follows in **Figure 4** [MD $= -0.26$, 95%CI (-0.45, -0.08), $P = 0.005$]. The number of relapses within 1 year was statistically significant between the two groups. Thus, it was considered that the MMF group was superior to the control group in reducing the number of relapses within 1 year.

Cumulative Prednisone Dosage

Four articles reported the data of cumulative prednisone dosage. There was no obvious heterogeneity among the studies, so the fixed effect model was used for analysis. The specific meta-analysis results are shown in **Figure 5**. The difference in cumulative hormone usage between children with SDNS or FRNS treated with MMF and the control group was statistically significant [SMD $= -0.32$, 95%CI (-0.53, -0.11), $P = 0.003$], indicating that MMF is more effective in reducing cumulative prednisone dosage than the CNIs and levamisole.

Incidence of Adverse Reactions

Heterogeneity analysis was conducted on six articles reporting the incidence of adverse reactions. Then, the fixed-effect model was used for analysis. The results of meta-analysis are shown in **Figure 6**. There was no significant difference in the incidence of adverse reactions between the MMF group and the control group [RD $= 0.02$, 95%CI (-0.04, 0.09), $P = 0.46$]. We believe that

Study or Subgroup	MMF Mean	MMF SD	MMF Total	Control group Mean	Control group SD	Control group Total	Weight	Std. Mean Difference IV, Fixed, 95% CI
Aditi Sinha 2018	0.24	0.2	76	0.3	0.2	73	42.0%	-0.30 [-0.62, 0.02]
Biswanath Basu 2015	0.12	0.09	56	0.18	0.16	56	31.1%	-0.46 [-0.83, -0.08]
Eiske 2008	0.13	0.16	12	0.08	0.12	12	6.7%	0.34 [-0.47, 1.15]
WANG 2016	0.16	0.02	34	0.17	0.03	38	20.1%	-0.38 [-0.85, 0.08]
Total (95% CI)			**178**			**179**	**100.0%**	**-0.32 [-0.53, -0.11]**

Heterogeneity: Chi² = 3.19, df = 3 (P = 0.36); I² = 6%
Test for overall effect: Z = 3.02 (P = 0.003)

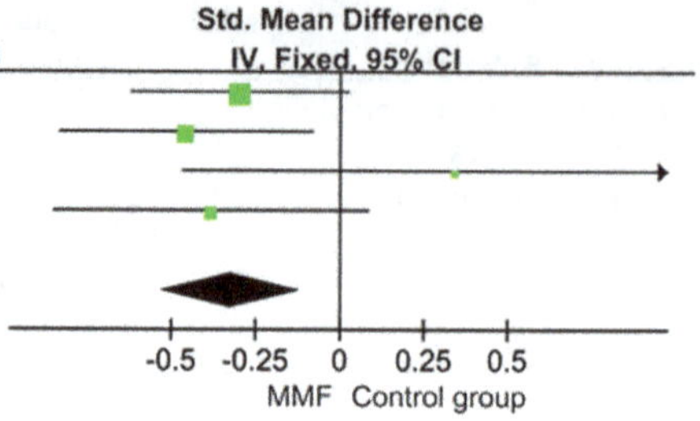

FIGURE 5 | Forest plot showing standardized mean difference (SMD) of the cumulative prednisone dosage between the groups.

Study or Subgroup	MMF Events	MMF Total	Control group Events	Control group Total	Weight	Risk Difference M-H, Fixed, 95% CI
Aditi Sinha 2018	3	76	3	73	28.0%	-0.00 [-0.06, 0.06]
Biswanath Basu 2015	10	56	7	56	21.1%	0.05 [-0.08, 0.19]
Eiske 2008	2	12	0	12	4.5%	0.17 [-0.07, 0.41]
Geng 2018	5	28	6	34	11.5%	0.00 [-0.19, 0.19]
Jutta Gellermann 2013	20	54	21	60	21.4%	0.02 [-0.16, 0.20]
WANG 2016	10	34	11	38	13.5%	0.00 [-0.21, 0.21]
Total (95% CI)		**260**		**273**	**100.0%**	**0.02 [-0.04, 0.09]**
Total events	50		48			

Heterogeneity: Chi² = 2.27, df = 5 (P = 0.81); I² = 0%
Test for overall effect: Z = 0.74 (P = 0.46)

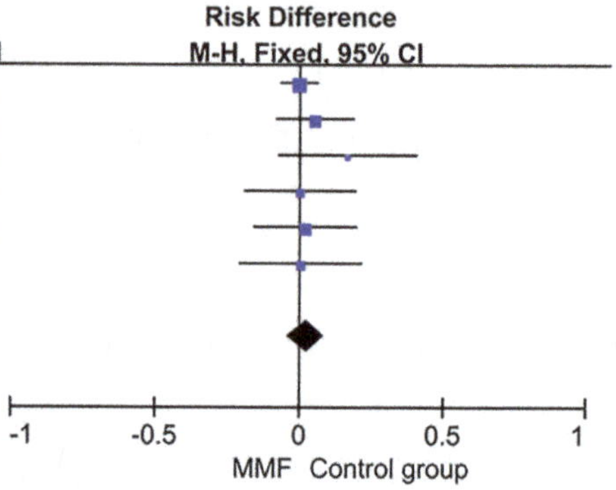

FIGURE 6 | Forest plot showing ratio difference (RD) of the incidence of adverse reactions between the groups.

there is no significant difference in safety between MMF and the control group.

DISCUSSION

The objective of this study was to evaluate the efficacy and safety of mycophenolate mofetil in the treatment of SDNS or FRNS in children by meta-analysis. Six prospective studies were included, with a total number of 447 children. The results show that when compared with other immunosuppressants (including tacrolimus, cyclosporine A, and levamisole), MMF has some advantages in reducing the number of relapses and cumulative prednisone dosage within 1 year. As for the relapse-free survival, MMF was superior to levamisole but not to CNIs. At the same time, the incidence of adverse reactions did not decrease, which was not consistent with previous research and clinical experience (17, 18). In addition, in order to explore the optimal dose of MMF, we conducted a subgroup analysis of different doses of MMF according to the RCTs included in the study. However, we did not find that the effects of different subgroups on the main outcomes were statistically significant.

We also used GRADE pro-GDT to evaluate the quality of the primary outcomes and secondary outcomes (**Table 2**). The results suggested that the quality of the evidence in the 1-year relapse-free survival rate was high, while the quality of the evidence for the cumulative prednisone dosage and the incidence of adverse reactions were moderate. However, the certainty of the number of relapses within 1 year was low.

One of the main outcomes of this study is the incidence of adverse reactions, which are mainly concerned with serious adverse reactions, such as severe infection and agranulocytosis. However, the mild adverse reactions such as rash and medicated fever may be ignored. Almost all kinds of immunosuppressants have varying degrees of side effects. This also has become one of the reasons why it is difficult for us to choose appropriate treatment plans in clinical work. It was reported that the side effects of MMF are cytopenia and diarrhea. Levamisole has an immunomodulatory function that is usually well-tolerated. Its main side effect is elevated liver enzymes. Calcineurin inhibitors have long been used in SDNS or FRNS. Their major side effects are hirsutism, gum hypertrophy, and nephrotoxicity, leading to interstitial kidney fibrosis and chronic kidney disease. Cyclophosphamide is an efficient treatment, but its gonadal toxicity is a major drawback to its use. More recent drugs such as rituximab are very effective but induce an increased risk of opportunistic infection, prolonged neutropenia, and anaphylaxis.

MMF can be used not only in the treatment of PNS but also in other kidney diseases in children. By comparing the different efficacy of MMF combined with steroid and steroid alone in the treatment of 76 children with Henoch–Schoenlein purpura nephritis (HSPN), Lu et al. (19) found that the

TABLE 2 | Evaluation of GRADE pro GDT of MMF or others for the treatment of SDNS or FRNS in children.

Certainty assessment							№ of patients		Effect		Certainty	Importance
Outcomes (No of studies)	**Study design**	**Risk of bias**	**Inconsistency**	**Indirectness**	**Imprecision**	**Other considerations**	**MMF**	**Others**	**Relative (95% CI)**	**Absolute (95% CI)**		
1-year relapse-free survival rate (6)	Random-ized trials (5/6)	Not serio-us	Not serious	Not serious	Not serious	None	80/220 (37.9%)	94/227 (41.4%)	RD−0.02 (-0.12 to 0.05)	-	⊕⊕⊕⊕ **HIGH**	IMPORTANT
The number of relapses within 1 year (3)	Randomized trials	Not serious	Not serious	Serious[a]	Serious[b]	None	120	121	-	MD 0.26 lower (0.45 lower to 0.08 lower)	⊕⊕◯◯ **LOW**	CRITICAL
Cumulative prednisone dosage (4)	Randomized trials (3/4)	Not serio-us	Not serious	Not serious	Serious[b]	None	178	179	-	SMD 0.32 lower (0.53 lower to 0.11 lower)	⊕⊕⊕◯ **MODERATE**	CRITICAL
Incidence of adverse reactions (6)	Randomized trials (5/6)	Not serious	Serious[c]	Not serious	Not serious	None	50/260 (19.2%)	48/273 (17.6%)	RD 0.02 (−0.04 to 0.09)	-	⊕⊕⊕◯ **MODERATE**	IMPORTANT

[a] *The mean and standard deviation of the article with largest weight are converted from the quartile notation by Luo's methods.*
[b] *Limited sample size.*
[c] *Different articles have different definitions of severe and mild adverse reactions.*
⊕, Evidence quality symbol; ◯, Downgraded one level.

combination of MMF and steroid was superior to steroid alone in relieving proteinuria. In the treatment of antineutrophil cytoplasmic antibody (ANCA)-associated vasculitis (AAV). Hu et al. (20) found that MMF effectively ameliorates disease activity and considerably improves renal function in patients. Similarly, MMF also plays a significant role in renal transplant patients (21).

Due to the limited number of clinical researches in pediatric population and short application history of MMF, the data included in this study were insufficient. By consulting the Chinese Clinical Trail Registry (ChiCTR) and International Clinical Trails Registry Platform (WHO ICTRP), we found that some clinical projects in line with the theme of our research, including IRCT20130812014333n113, NCT04048161, CTRI/2019/04/018517, and JPRN-jRCTs051180081. We hope that our conclusions will be further confirmed after the successful completion of the above studies. In addition, some of the literature reports included in this study have shortcomings in the quality of methodology, such as unknown methods of randomization, unclear hidden distribution, and not using a blinded study design, as examples. In addition, this study has some incompleteness in obtaining literature data. For example, there are reports on the number of relapses within 1 year in the literature of Gellermann (11), but there are only the mean value and no standard deviation, without response through searching the original text or contacting the author. Thus, the study has to be excluded from the analysis of the outcome index. The authenticity of the research results may be affected. It is also suggested that when we carry out RCTs in the future, we should strictly abide by the above methodological requirements and report accordingly. In short, the treatment of mycophenolate mofetil in children with SDNS or FRNS still needs to be verified by more well-designed, large-sample, multicenter, long-term, and close follow-up RCTs.

AUTHOR CONTRIBUTIONS

XX was responsible for the concept, design, definition of intellectual content, literature search, data acquisition, and statistical analysis. S-YQ was responsible for the manuscript preparation and editing. MW took responsibility for the manuscript review and integrity of the work as a whole from inception to published article. All authors contributed to the article and approved the submitted version.

and technology innovation project demonstration category—application of total exon detection in the management with steroid-resistant nephrotic syndrome. The role of the fund is to provide financial support and technical advice.

ACKNOWLEDGMENTS

The authors appreciate the medical statisticians from the Pediatric College of Chongqing Medical University, China, for their consultations of statistical methods.

REFERENCES

1. Zhang L, Yan J, Yang B, Zhang G, Wang M, Dong S, et al. IL-23 activated gammadelta T cells affect Th17 cells and regulatory T cells by secreting IL-21 in children with primary nephrotic syndrome. *Scand J Immunol.* (2018) 87:36–45. doi: 10.1111/sji.12629
2. Tulpar S, Gunduz Z, Sahin U, Hakan Poyrazoglu M, Dursun I, Dusunsel R, et al. Trace elements in children suffering from idiopathic nephrotic syndrome. *The Eurasian J Med.* (2014) 46:187–91. doi: 10.5152/eajm.2014.36
3. Ogawa-Akiyama A, Sugiyama H, Kitagawa M, Tanaka K, Kano Y, Mise K, et al. Podocyte autophagy is associated with foot process effacement and proteinuria in patients with minimal change nephrotic syndrome. *PLoS ONE.* (2020) 15:e0228337. doi: 10.1371/journal.pone.0228337
4. Banh TH, Hussain-Shamsy N, Patel V, Vasilevska-Ristovska J, Borges K, Sibbald C, et al. Ethnic differences in incidence and outcomes of childhood nephrotic syndrome. *Clin J Am Soc Nephrol.* (2016) 11:1760–8. doi: 10.2215/CJN.00380116
5. Lombel RM, Gipson DS, Hodson EM. Treatment of steroid-sensitive nephrotic syndrome: new guidelines from KDIGO. *Pediatr Nephrol.* (2013) 28:415–26. doi: 10.1007/s00467-012-2310-x
6. Briggs WA, Choi MJ, Scheel PJ, Jr. Successful mycophenolate mofetil treatment of glomerular disease. *Am J Kidney Dis.* (1998) 31:213–7. doi: 10.1053/ajkd.1998.v31.pm9469489
7. Floege J, Barbour SJ, Cattran DC, Hogan JJ, Nachman PH, Tang SCW, et al. Management and treatment of glomerular diseases (part 1): conclusions from a kidney disease: improving global outcomes (KDIGO) controversies conference. *Kidney Int.* (2019) 95:268–80. doi: 10.1016/j.kint.2018.10.018
8. Rovin BH, Caster DJ, Cattran DC, Gibson KL, Hogan JJ, Moeller MJ, et al. Management and treatment of glomerular diseases (part 2): conclusions from a kidney disease: improving global outcomes (KDIGO) controversies conference. *Kidney Int.* (2019) 95:281–95. doi: 10.1016/j.kint.2018.11.008
9. Luo D, Wan X, Liu J, Tong T. Optimally estimating the sample mean from the sample size, median, mid-range, and/or mid-quartile range. *Stat Methods Med Res.* (2018) 27:1785–805. doi: 10.1177/0962280216669183
10. Geng HY, Ji LN, Chen CY, Tu J, Li HR, Bao R, et al. Mycophenolate mofetil versus cyclosporine A in children with primary refractory nephrotic syndrome. *Zhonghua er ke za zhi = Chin JPediatr.* (2018) 56:651–6. doi: 10.3760/cma.j.issn.0578-1310.2018.09.004
11. Gellermann J, Weber L, Pape L, Tönshoff B, Hoyer P, Querfeld U. Mycophenolate mofetil versus cyclosporin a in children with frequently relapsing nephrotic syndrome. *J AmSoci Nephrol.* (2013) 24:1689–97. doi: 10.1681/ASN.2012121200
12. Wang J, Mao J, Chen J, Fu H, Shen H, Zhu X, et al. Evaluation of mycophenolate mofetil or tacrolimus in children with steroid sensitive but frequently relapsing or steroid-dependent nephrotic syndrome. *Nephrology.* (2016) 21:21–7. doi: 10.1111/nep.12537
13. Dorresteijn EM, Holthe JEK-v, Levtchenko EN, Nauta J, Hop WCJ, Heijden AJ. Mycophenolate mofetil versus cyclosporine for remission maintenance in nephrotic syndrome. *Pediatr Nephrol.* (2008) 23:2013–20. doi: 10.1007/s00467-008-0899-6
14. Sinha A, Puraswani M, Kalaivani M, Goyal P, Hari P, Bagga A. Efficacy and safety of mycophenolate mofetil versus levamisole in frequently relapsing nephrotic syndrome: an open-label randomized controlled trial. *Kidney Int.* (2019) 95:210–8. doi: 10.1016/j.kint.2018.08.039
15. Basu B, Pandey R, Mondal N, Schaefer F. Efficacy and safety of mycophenolate-mofetil vs. Levamisole in children with idiopathic nephrotic syndrome: results of a randomized clinical trial. *Nephrol Dial Transplant.* (2014) 29:iii7. doi: 10.1053/j.ajkd.2015.04.048
16. Cumpston M, Li T, Page MJ, Chandler J, Welch VA, Higgins JP, et al. Updated guidance for trusted systematic reviews: a new edition of the cochrane handbook for systematic reviews of interventions. *Cochrane Database Syst Rev.* (2019) 10:Ed000142. doi: 10.1002/14651858.ED000142
17. Ogarek I, Szczesny-Choruz E, Wierzchowska-Slowiaczek E, Kwinta-Rybicka J, Stec Z, Moczulska A, et al. [Mycophenolate mofetil (MMF) as the first choice immunosuppressive drug in treatment of steroid-dependent nephrotic syndrome in children]. *Polski merkuriusz lekarski: organ Polskiego Towarzystwa Lekarskiego.* (2018) 44:192–5.
18. Hackl A, Cseprekal O, Gessner M, Liebau MC, Habbig S, Ehren R, et al. Mycophenolate mofetil therapy in children with idiopathic nephrotic syndrome: does therapeutic drug monitoring make a difference? *Ther Drug Monit.* (2016) 38:274–9. doi: 10.1097/FTD.0000000000000258
19. Lu Z, Song J, Mao J, Xia Y, Wang C. Evaluation of mycophenolate mofetil and low-dose steroid combined therapy in moderately severe henoch-schonlein purpura nephritis. *Med Sci Monit.* (2017) 23:2333–9. doi: 10.12659/MSM.904206
20. Hu W, Liu C, Xie H, Chen H, Liu Z, Li L. Mycophenolate mofetil versus cyclophosphamide for inducing remission of ANCA vasculitis with moderate renal involvement. *Nephrol Dial Transplant.* (2008) 23:1307–12. doi: 10.1093/ndt/gfm780
21. Zhang J, Luo Y, Zhu Z, Feng G, Sun Z, Zhang X. Pharmacokinetic comparison of two mycophenolate mofetil formulations in kidney transplant recipients. *Ther Drug Monit.* (2018) 40:649–54. doi: 10.1097/FTD.0000000000000545

10

Febrile Proteinuria in Hospitalized Children: Characterization of Urinary Proteins

Evgenia Gurevich[1,2], Eytan Israel[1,2], Yael Segev[3] and Daniel Landau[3,4]*

[1] Soroka University Medical Center, Ben-Gurion University of the Negev, Beersheba, Israel, [2] Division of Pediatrics, Ben-Gurion University of the Negev, Beersheba, Israel, [3] Department of Microbiology and Immunology, Ben-Gurion University of the Negev, Beersheba, Israel, [4] Department of Pediatrics B, Schneider Children's Medical Center, Sackler School of Medicine, Tel Aviv University, Tel Aviv, Israel

***Correspondence:**
Daniel Landau
danny_l@clalit.org.il

Background: Transient proteinuria during febrile illness is a common phenomenon. Recent studies have re-examined the pathophysiology of proteinuria and new urinary markers to characterize it, including B7-1 (CD80), which is expressed also in glomerular podocytes and influences the glomerular barrier.

Aim: To investigate the pattern of proteinuria in febrile non-renal diseases, including B7-1.

Methods: We prospectively analyzed urine samples of 44 febrile children and 28 afebrile controls for different protein components: albumin (glomerular marker), β2-microglobulin (tubular marker), uromodulin (Tamm Horsfall protein-THP, a renal endogenous protein) and B7-1. Febrile illness was characterized as focal bacterial vs. viral. Exclusion criteria were underlying renal disease, steroid treatment or urinary tract infection.

Results: Elevated urine albumin (64.5 ± 10.3 vs. 17.8 ± 4 mg/g, mean ± S.E.M., $p = 0.0009$) and β2-microglobulin (1.44 ± 0.34 vs. 0.182 ± 0.03 mg/g, mean ± S.E.M., $p = 0.005$] and decreased uromodulin (10.5 ± 1 vs. 26.7 ± 2.2 Arbitrary units, mean ± S.E.M., $p = 0.0001$) excretion were found during febrile illness vs. controls. Urine B7-1 was also increased in the febrile group (0.27 ± 0.05 vs. 0.07 ± 0.01 ng/ml, mean ± S.E.M., $p = 0.001$), and was the only marker which was significantly higher in bacterial vs. viral disease.

Conclusions: Febrile proteinuria is not generalized: while proteins of both glomerular and tubular origin increase, uromodulin decreases. Urine B7-1 is increased during fever, more significantly in bacterial infections. Thus, urinary B7-1 may be used as an additional marker to differentiate between febrile states of bacterial vs. viral origin.

Keywords: β2-microglobulin, uromodulin, CD80 (B7-1) protein, albuminuria, proteinuria, fever

INTRODUCTION

Normal glomerular barrier prevents the filtration of high molecular weight proteins into the Bowman's capsule. Subsequently, proximal tubular reabsorption retrieves proteins of lower molecular weight that escaped glomerular barrier, leading to a minimal amount of protein of circulation origin in urine. In addition, uromodulin, or Tamm Horsfall protein is synthesized and partly secreted by the distal tubule and found in urine in normal states (1, 2). Transient proteinuria is a common finding in several illness states. It has been described during fever, sepsis, trauma and anaphylaxis, without relation to renal disease (3). Several studies in the past have described transient proteinuria during febrile illness and whether its origin was glomerular or tubular (4, 5). However, no studies have been performed on the role of urinary uromodulin in this process. Recent studies have reported new evidence on the pathophysiology of infection related proteinuria, including the role of B7-1(CD80) protein, expressed on both circulating leucocytes as well as on glomerular epithelial cells (podocytes). This protein was shown to modulate the podocyte cytoskeleton and influence on glomerular filtration barrier in different proteinuric states (6, 7). No studies have been performed to simultaneously examine the involvement of markers of different renal compartments (glomerular, tubular, and endogenously synthesized), including B7-1, in this common phenomenon. We hypothesized that glomerular B7-1 may be upregulated also in transient febrile proteinuria. Therefore, in this study we characterized the type of urinary proteins (albumin, β2-microglobulin, uromodulin, and B7-1) in children with febrile proteinuria.

PATIENTS AND METHODS

The research protocol of the study has been approved by the local Helsinki committee. Study consent was signed by patients' parents. In this prospective study, children with febrile illness (temperature above 38°C) of infectious origin, hospitalized in pediatric wards were enrolled. The exclusion criteria were underlying renal disease, signs of urinary tract infection, or corticosteroid treatment. Children without fever who were hospitalized for elective surgical procedures served as controls. Clinical, laboratory and imaging data were recorded for each patient and the child was finally diagnosed as having a viral [no specific focus of infection, normal peripheral blood leucocyte (WBC) count] or a specific bacterial disease.

TABLE 1 | Demographic characteristics.

	Febrile	Afebrile	P value
Number	44	28	
Age (mean ± S.E.M.)	6.6 ± 0.79	4.9 ± 0.72	0.12
Male (%)	27 (60%)	21 (75%)	NS
Background illness	17 (39%)	3 (11%)	0.02
Previous hospitalization	18 (41%)	8 (29%)	NS
Temperature on admission (°C), (mean ± S.E.M)	38.6 ± 0.9		
Maximal temperature (°C), (mean ± S.E.M)	39 ± 0.74		
Hours of fever prior to admission (mean ± S.E.M)	31 ± 4		
Suspected bacterial disease (%)	23 (52%)		

Urine samples in both study and control groups were collected at the time of admission. Urine samples were checked with Multistix® urinalysis strips for white blood cells, nitrites, protein, blood and specific gravity. Then urine samples were biochemically tested for total protein, albumin (as glomerular injury marker), β2-microglobulin (tubular marker), uromodulin (Tamm Horsfall protein-THP, a renal endogenous protein), and B7-1 (CD-80) protein. Urine protein response on the sticks was determined using a semi quantitative determination (+1 to +4) method by photometric color test. Urine creatinine was determined using kinetic color test (Jaffé method). Urine albumin was determined by immune turbidometric test. All these tests were performed using an Olympus Life &[[Inline Image]]Material Science system. Urinary β2-microglobulin was determined using Microparticle Enzyme Immunoassay (MEIA)(Abbott Ax SYM, Germany). Tamm Horsfall protein (THP)/uromodulin concentration was analyzed by Western blot analysis using rabbit anti THP antibody (Santa Cruz). Protein expression was quantified densitometrically using *Image J* software and expressed as arbitrary units (AU). Urine B7-1 (CD80) protein concentration was analyzed using an enzyme-linked immunosorbent assay kit (Human sCD80 Instant Elisa Kit, eBioscience, Affymetrix, North America), according to the test protocol. Briefly, after a 3 h incubation of 50 μl urine samples at room temperature, the microwell strips were washed 3 times with approximately 400 μl wash buffer per well. Then 100 μl of TMB substrate solution was pipetted to all wells and the microwell strips were incubated again at room temperature for 10 min. The substrate reaction was stopped by quickly pipetting 100 μl of Stop Solution, and then immediately read for absorbance at 450 nm using a spectro-photometer (SpectraMax Paradigm Multi-Mode Microplate Reader, SoftMax Pro Software, 2014). A standard curve was created by plotting the mean absorbance for each standard concentration on the ordinate against the measured sCD80 concentration on the abscissa.

Group comparison was performed using standard statistical tests: *t*-test for continuous variables, chi square for categorical values and ANOVA test for comparison of more than 2 continuous variables. Analyzing receiver operating characteristic (ROC curves) was assessed using *pROC*, an open-source package (8).

RESULTS

Fifty-six febrile children admitted to the hospital were approached for consent. 12 patients were excluded, 11 because of insufficient amount of urine and one patient because of positive urine culture. Finally 44 febrile children age 2 months–17.7 years, (6.6 ± 0.79 years, mean ± S.E.M.) were enrolled and compared with 28 controls age 3 months–16.5 years (4.9 ± 0.72 years, mean ± S.E.M., $p = 0.12$). There were 27 (60%) males in febrile group vs. 21 (75%) ones in the control group. Seventeen patients (39%) in febrile group vs. 3 patients (11%) in the control group had some background illness, 18 (41%) in febrile group vs. 8 (29%) in the control group were previously hospitalized (**Table 1**). Temperature on admission in febrile group was 38.6 ± 0.9°C, maximal temperature was 39 ± 0.74°C, the fever duration prior to admission was similar for both bacterial and viral groups and averaged 31 ± 4 h (mean ± S.E.M). In the study group febrile disease was of bacterial origin in 52% of cases and of viral origin in 48%. Bacterial diagnoses included: pneumonia (9), rickettsiosis (2), dysentery (4), cellulitis with abscess (1), mastoiditis (1), acute otitis media (1), and occult bacteremia (1). The diagnosis of pneumonia was based on positive findings on chest X-Ray examinations (lobar infiltrate). In one patient blood serologic test was positive for Mycoplasma Pneumonia. Blood cultures were negative in all the patients with pneumonia except one which was positive for Pneumococcus Pneumonia. All patients with pneumonia except two had elevated leucocyte count (24 ± 2.6*10^3/ul, mean ± S.E.M.). In the patient with rickettsiosis, the diagnosis was based on clinical and laboratory findings and confirmed serologically. Mastoiditis was diagnosed based on clinical findings and leukocytosis (17*10^3/μl). In the patient with dysentery, stool cultures were positive for shigella (2), salmonella (1), and campylobacter (1). In the patient with an abscess and cellulitis, positive culture for Staph aureus was obtained from the pus. Otitis media was diagnosed clinically, but this patient was also diagnosed with pneumonia, confirmed by a chest X-ray. The diagnosis of occult bacteremia was made based on fever and leukocytosis (20*10^3/μl). Febrile patients without specific focus of infection and normal peripheral blood leucocyte count were diagnosed as having viral infections.

Urine samples were obtained 31 ± 4.1 h (mean ± S.E.M.) from the beginning of fever. The assessment of different urinary proteins is summarized in **Table 2**. Multistix® urinalysis strips were positive for protein (in those samples with specific gravity of more than 1010) in 13 out of 43 febrile patients (30%) and only in 1 patient from the control group (3.7%) (two-tailed $\chi^2 = 0.005$). In the febrile group urine protein/creatinine ratio was above normal (200 mg/g) in 32 cases (72.2%) vs. 5 cases (18%) in the control group ($\chi^2 = 0.001$). In the febrile group 27 patients (60%) had a urine albumin\creatinine ratio above 30 mg/g (upper limit of norm) vs. 3 patients in the control group ($\chi^2 < 0.005$). Urinary albumin\creatinine ratio in the febrile group was 64.5 ± 10.3 mg/g, mean ± S.E.M. Of note, the albumin fraction in urine was less than half of the total protein. There was a wide distribution in urine β2-microglobulin excretion in the study group: 1.44 ± 0.34 mg\g, mean ± S.E.M. In the control group, urine β2-microglobulin was significantly lower (0.182 ± 0.03 mg/g, mean ± S.E.M, $p = 0.01$) (**Table 2**). Tamm-Horsfall Protein (THP) excretion in urine was significantly decreased in febrile children vs. control (10.5 ± 1 vs. 26.7 ± 2.2 arbitrary units, mean ± S.E.M, $p = 0.0001$).

The study group comparison was further subdivided into three groups: afebrile children, patients having febrile disease of bacterial origin (according to above mentioned criteria) vs. non-bacterial origin. As mentioned, total protein excretion was higher in febrile children vs. controls. However, there was no difference between bacterial and nonbacterial febrile groups. Albumin excretion was also elevated in febrile children vs. control without a clear difference between nonbacterial and bacterial groups (**Table 2**). There was no significant difference in urine

TABLE 2 | Characteristics of proteinuria.

Urine values (mean ± S.E.M)	Normal value	Afebrile (*n* = 28)	Febrile		*P*-value AF vs. F	*P*-value Bacterial vs. Viral
Protein/creatinine (mg/g)	<200	150 ± 17	Total (*n* = 44)	430 ± 54.5	0.0001	
			Bacterial (*n* = 23)	480 ± 83.3		NS
			Viral (*n* = 21)	380 ± 65.3		
Albumin/creatinine (mg/g)	<30	17.8 ± 4	Total (*n* = 44)	64.5 ± 10.3	0.0009	
			Bacterial (*n* = 23)	44.7 ± 8.85		NS
			Viral (*n* = 21)	117.9 ± 33.2		
β2mgl/creatinine (mg/g)	≤0.132	0.182 ± 0.03	Total (*n* = 44)	1.44 ± 0.34	0.005	
			Bacterial (*n* = 23)	1.218 ± 0.35		NS
			Viral (*n* = 21)	1.693 ± 0.58		
B7-1 (ng/ml)	NA	0.07 ± 0.01	Total (*n* = 25)	0.27 ± 0.05	0.001	
			Bacterial (*n* = 11)	0.4 ± 0.07		0.002
			Viral (*n* = 14)	0.14 ± 0.04		
Tamm-Horsfall protein (AU)	NA	26.7 ± 2.2	Total (*n* = 44)	10.5 ± 1	0.0001	
			Bacterial (*n* = 23)	7 ± 1		0.14
			Viral (*n* = 21)	9.5 ± 1.3		

AF-afebrile, F-febrile, NA-not available, NS-not significant, AU-arbitrary units. AF-afebrile, AU-arbitrary units, β2mgl-beta-2 microglobulin, F-febrile, NA-not available, NS-not significant.

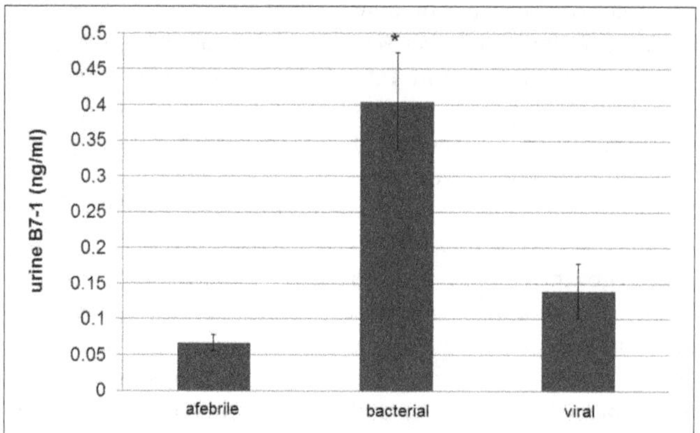

FIGURE 1 | Urine B7-1 excretion in febrile disease of bacterial vs. viral origin and vs. control afebrile group: urine B7-1 concentration was significantly higher in cases of bacterial disease vs. viral and in comparison with the control group *$p < 0.0001$.

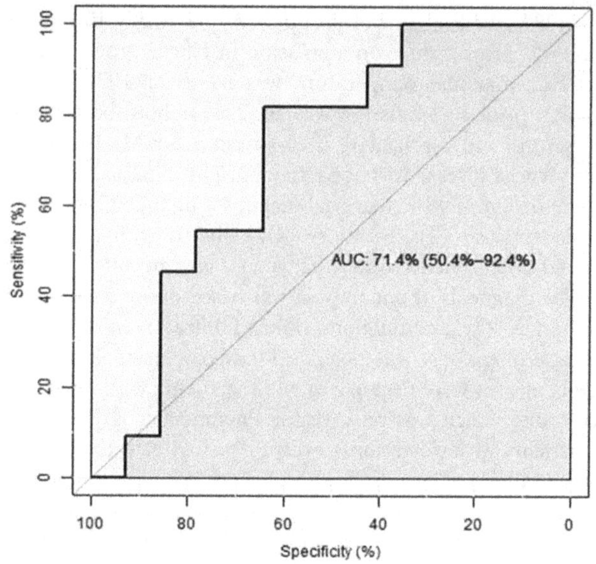

FIGURE 2 | ROC curve assessing the predictive value of urine B7-1 for bacterial infection in febrile children (8).

β2-microglobulin excretion between bacterial and nonbacterial groups but its excretion was significantly elevated in each of these groups vs. control ($p < 0.05$). Uromodulin (THP) excretion was lower in the bacterial vs. nonbacterial group, but this difference was not significant ($p = 0.14$).There was a significantly higher excretion of B7-1 in urine in the febrile group vs. afebrile controls (0.27 ± 0.05 vs. 0.07 ± 0.01 ng/ml, mean ± S.E.M., $p = 0.0001$). Urine B7-1 concentration was also significantly higher in cases of bacterial disease vs. nonbacterial (0.4 ± 0.07 vs. 0.14 ± 0.04 ng/ml, mean ± S.E.M., $p < 0.002$) (**Table 2**) (**Figure 1**). An ROC curve that tests the performance of urine B7-1 to differentiate between viral and bacterial infections yielded an AUC value (±S.E.M) of 0.85 ± 0.08 (95% CI: 0.71–0.99, $p = 0.003$) (**Figure 2**). The optimal mathematical point along the curve is a urine B7-1 value of 0.132, providing a sensitivity of 91.7% and a specificity of 61.5%. Thus, there was no significant difference in urine excretion of any of the checked proteins in the cases of bacterial vs. viral infection except for urine B7-1 that was significantly higher in the cases of bacterial infections.

DISCUSSION

In this study we first characterized the type of urinary proteins in children with febrile proteinuria. Elevated urinary total protein (in the mild-non-nephrotic range), urine albumin and β2-microglobulin excretion were found in febrile children. Urine B7-1 excretion also was higher in the cases of febrile states. Not all urinary proteins showed a pattern of transient elevation during febrile illness. For example, uromodulin (Tamm-Horsfall protein), that is excreted in urine in normal states, was actually significantly decreased during fever. This protein is secreted by the kidney and is thought to play role in water\electrolyte balance and kidney innate immunity. Studies in *Umod* knockout mice showed that uromodulin has a defensive role against urinary tract infection (UTI) (10, 11), since this protein binds to pathogens of the urinary tract, such as type 1-fimbriated *E. coli*, and interferes with their binding to uroplakins on the urothelium (12). Several *in vitro* studies showed that THP is able to bind to immunity-related molecules, such as immunoglobulin G, complement 1q, and tumor necrosis factor-α (9, 13, 14). Uromodulin also acts as a chemoattractant (15) and as a proinflammatory molecule. It interacts with monocytes, neutrophils and myeloid dendritic cells leading to activation of components of the immune system via toll-like receptor 4 (16). The physiological role of this process is still unclear. Saemann et al. hypothesize that uromodulin is released into kidney parenchyma in cases of tubular damage and serves as a signal to activate local immune response to prevent bacterial invasion (16). This unexpected decreased urinary THP excretion during fever can be explained by its excessive excretion into blood, as Prajcer et al. showed that inflammatory damage in thick ascending limb leads to decreased urinary and increased blood uromodulin level (17). Medullary cystic kidney disease type 2 (MIM 603860) and familial juvenile hyperuricemic nephropathy (MIM 162000) are autosomal dominant tubulointerstitial kidney diseases that are due to UMOD gene mutations and are collectively called uromodulin-associated kidney disease (UAKD). Decreased urine uromodulin excretion in these diseases leads to nephropathy, interstitial nephritis, hyperuricemia, renal stone formation and renal insufficiency. In this study, in spite of elevated albumin and β2-microglobulin urine excretion during febrile disease, most of urine protein was neither albumin nor β2-microglobulin. The increase in urinary albumin excretion suggests that additional high molecular weight proteins may also be excreted, most probably due to a transient disturbance in glomerular barrier. Recent studies have reported new evidences on the pathophysiology of proteinuria of glomerular origin, including the role of B7-1. This protein is expressed in glomerular epithelial cells (podocytes) and influences glomerular anatomical barrier in different proteinuric states. B7-1 influences the actin cytoskeleton of podocytes and slit diaphragm organization leading to proteinuria. Both genetic aberrations (e.g., deletion of α3 integrin or nephrin), toxic stimuli (such as PAN induced reactive oxygen species), or direct stimulation of the TLR-4/CD14 receptor on the podocyte can cause B7-1 induction. B7-1 then induces the podocyte's foot process effacement and disruption of the slit diaphragm complex, leading to proteinuria. Reiser et al. (6) also showed rapid upregulation of B7-1 in podocytes and nephrotic-range proteinuria by *in vivo* exposure to low-dose LPS in wild type and SCID mice. B7-1 knockout mice were protected from this LPS induced nephrotic range proteinuria, suggesting a role of podocyte (and not white blood cell) B7-1 expression in the pathogenesis of proteinuria. Podocyte's B7-1 is upregulated in patients with certain glomerular diseases. Positive B7-1 immunostaining was observed in biopsy specimen from patients with recurrent focal segmental glomerulosclerosis (FSGS) a disease associated with severe proteinuria. Yu et al. showed the resolution of nephrotic range proteinuria after B7-1 inhibition with Abatacept (CTLA-4–Ig) treatment in patients with rituximab-resistant recurrent FSGS and in patients with glucocorticoid-resistant primary FSGS (18), suggesting that B7-1 can be a target for the treatment of proteinuria. However, these findings have recently been challenged by Baye et al. (19). These new observations led us to explore the possible role of B7-1 in febrile children. As mentioned, B7-1 was found to be the only urine biomarker that was not just significantly higher in febrile disease vs. controls, but also higher in febrile cases of bacterial disease vs. viral origin.

Activation of toll-like receptors (TLRs) is basic in the initiation of innate immunologic response (20, 21). For example, exposure to lipopolysaccharide (LPS) induces B7-1 expression via TLR-4 in podocytes, leading to reorganization of its cytoskeleton, foot process effacement and proteinuria. B7-1 acts as a costimulatory molecule in this process, as previously mentioned (6). We suppose that in the cases of bacterial infections toxins or other bacterial components lead to proteinuria via similar mechanism and B7-1 acts as a co-stimulatory molecule in this process, being upregulated and eventually found in urine.

LIMITATIONS OF THE STUDY

The study was performed on a relatively small sample of patients, due to budget limitations. Thus, the negative statistically significant differences found between the bacterial and viral groups may become significant in larger study groups. In addition, only a limited number of urinary excreted proteins were analyzed in this study, and the correlation between blood level of these proteins and their excretion was not assessed.

In summary, in this first study we have shown that febrile proteinuria is not a generalized nonspecific phenomenon: while proteins of both glomerular and tubular origin increase, uromodulin decreases. Urine B7-1, a possible marker of increased glomerular permselectivity is increased during fever, more significantly in bacterial infections. Thus, if verified by larger studies, urinary B7-1 may be used as an additional marker to differentiate between febrile states of bacterial and viral origin.

ETHICS STATEMENT

The research protocol of the study has been approved by the Soroka University Medical Center local Helsinki committee. Study consent was signed by patients' parents.

AUTHOR CONTRIBUTIONS

EG and EI recruited the patients. EI wrote a preliminary report. EG wrote the manuscript's first draft. YS performed the laboratory analyses and reviewed the manuscript. DL conceived the study design and finalized the manuscript's last version.

ACKNOWLEDGMENTS

The study was supported by an unconditioned research grant of the Israeli Society of Clinical Pediatrics. No honorarium, grant, or other form of payment was given to anyone to produce the manuscript.

REFERENCES

1. Devuyst O, Dahan K, Pirson Y. Tamm-Horsfall protein or uromodulin: new ideas about an old molecule. *Nephrol Dial Transplant.* (2005) 20:1290–4. doi: 10.1093/ndt/gfh851
2. Rampoldi L, Scolari F, Amoroso A, Ghiggeri G, Devuyst O.The rediscovery ofuromodulin (Tamm-Horsfall protein): from tubulointerstitial nephropathy to chronic kidney disease. *Kidney Int.* (2011) 80:338–47. doi: 10.1038/ki.2011.134
3. Jensen H, Henriksen K. Proteinuria in non-renal infectious diseases. *Acta MedScand.* (1974) 196:75–82. doi: 10.1111/j.0954-6820.1974.tb00971.x
4. Marks MI, McLaine PN, Drummond KN. Proteinuria in children with febrile illnesses. *Arch Dis Child.* (1970) 45:250–3. doi: 10.1136/adc.45.240.250
5. Hemmingsen L, Skaarup P. Urinary excretion of ten plasma proteins in patients with febrile diseases. *Acta Med Scand.* (1977) 201:359–64. doi: 10.1111/j.0954-6820.1977.tb15712.x
6. Reiser J, von Gersdorff G, Loos M, Oh J, Asanuma K, Giardino L, et al. Induction of B7-1 in podocytes is associated with nephrotic syndrome. *J Clin Invest.* (2004) 113:1390–7. doi: 10.1172/JCI20402
7. Garin EH, Mu W, Arthur JM, Rivard CJ, Araya CE, Shimada M, et al. Urinary CD80 is elevated in minimal change disease but not in focal segmental glomerulosclerosis. *Kidney Int.* (2010) 78:296–302. doi: 10.1038/ki.2010.143
8. Robin X, Turck N, Hainard A, Tiberti N, Lisacek F, Sanchez JC, et al. pROC: an open-source package for R and S+ to analyze and compare ROC curves. *BMC Bioinformatics* (2011) 12:77. doi: 10.1186/1471-2105-12-77
9. Hession C, Decker JM, Sherblom AP, Kumar S, Yue CC, Mattaliano RJ, et al. Uromodulin (Tamm-Horsfall glycoprotein): a renal ligand for lymphokines. *Science* (1987) 237:1479–84. doi: 10.1126/science.3498215
10. Bates JM, Raffi HM, Prasadan K, Mascarenhas R, Laszik Z, Maeda N, et al. Tamm-Horsfall protein knockout mice are more prone to urinary tract infection: rapid communication. *Kidney Int.* (2004) 65:791–7. doi: 10.1111/j.1523-1755.2004.00452.x
11. Mo L, Zhu XH, Huang HY, Shapiro E, Hasty DL, Wu XR. Ablation of the Tamm-Horsfall protein gene increases susceptibility of mice to bladder colonization by type1-fimbriated *Escherichia coli*. *Am J Physiol Renal Physiol.* (2004) 286:F795–802. doi: 10.1152/ajprenal.00357.2003
12. Pak J, Pu Y, Zhang ZT, Hasty DL, Wu XR. Tamm-Horsfall protein binds to type1 fimbriated *Escherichia coli* and prevents *E. coli* from binding to uroplakin Ia and Ib receptors. *J Biol Chem.* (2001) 276:9924–30. doi: 10.1074/jbc.M008610200
13. Rhodes DC, Hinsman EJ, Rhodes JA. Tamm-Horsfall glycoprotein binds IgG with high affinity. *Kidney Int.* (1993) 44:1014–21. doi: 10.1038/ki.1993.343

14. Rhodes DC. Binding of Tamm-Horsfall protein to complement 1q measured by ELISA and resonant mirror biosensor techniques under various ionic-strength conditions. *Immunol Cell Biol.* (2001) 78:474–82. doi: 10.1111/j.1440-1711.2000.t01-3-.x
15. Schmid M, Prajczer S, Gruber LN, Bertocchi C, Gandini R, Pfaller W, et al. Uromodulin facilitates neutrophil migration across renal epithelial monolayers. *Cell Physiol Biochem.* (2010) 26:311–8. doi: 10.1159/000320554
16. Saemann MD, Weichhart T, Zeyda M, Staffler G, Schunn M, Stuhlmeier KM, et al. Tamm-Horsfall glycoprotein links innate immune cell activation with adaptive immunity via a Toll like receptor-4-dependent mechanism. *J Clin Invest.* (2005) 115:468–75. doi: 10.1172/JCI200522720
17. Prajczer S, Heidenreich U, Pfaller W, Kotanko P, Lhotta K, Jennings P. Evidence for a role of uromodulin in chronic kidney disease progression. *Nephrol Dial Transplant.* (2010) 25:1896–903. doi: 10.1093/ndt/gfp748
18. Yu CC, Fornoni A, Weins A, Hakroush S, Maiguel D, Sageshima J, et al. Abatacept in B7-1-positive proteinuric kidney disease. *N Engl J Med.* (2013) 369:2416–23. doi: 10.1056/NEJMoa1304572
19. Baye E, Gallazzini M, Delville M, Legendre C, Terzi F, Canaud G. The co-stimulatory receptor B7-1 is not induced in injured podocytes. *Kidney Int.* (2016) 90:1037–44. doi: 10.1016/j.kint.2016.06.022
20. Takeda K, Kaisho T, Akira S. Toll-like receptors. *Annu Rev Immunol.* (2003) 21:335–76. doi: 10.1146/annurev.immunol.21.120601.141126
21. Beutler B, Rietschel ET. Innate immune sensing and its roots: the story of endotoxin. *Nat Rev Immunol.* (2003) 3:169–76. doi: 10.1038/nri1004

11

Childhood Idiopathic Nephrotic Syndrome: Does the Initial Steroid Treatment Modify the Outcome? A Multicentre, Prospective Cohort Study

Andrea Pasini [1], Cristina Bertulli [1], Luca Casadio [2], Ciro Corrado [3], Alberto Edefonti [4], GianMarco Ghiggeri [5], Luciana Ghio [4], Mario Giordano [6], Claudio La Scola [1], Cristina Malaventura [7], Silvio Maringhini [3], Antonio P. Mastrangelo [4], Marco Materassi [8], Francesca Mencarelli [1], Giovanni Messina [6], Elena Monti [9], William Morello [4], Giuseppe Puccio [10], Paola Romagnani [8], Giovanni Montini [4,11] and the NefroKid Study Group*

[1] Nephrology and Dialysis Unit, Department of Pediatrics, IRCCS Azienda Ospedaliero-Universitaria di Bologna, Bologna, Italy, [2] Unità Operativa Complessa of Paediatrics and Neonatology, Local Health Authority of Romagna, Ravenna, Italy, [3] Pediatric Nephrology Unit, Children's Hospital "G. Di Cristina", A.R.N.A.S. "Civico", Palermo, Italy, [4] Pediatric Nephrology, Dialysis and Transplant Unit, Fondazione Ca' Granda Istituto di Ricovero e Cura a Carattere Scientifico Ospedale Maggiore Policlinico, Milan, Italy, [5] Division of Nephrology, Dialysis, Transplantation, Laboratory on Pathophysiology of Uremia, Istituto G. Gaslini, Genoa, Italy, [6] Nephrology Unit, Giovanni XXIII Children's Hospital, Bari, Italy, [7] Section of Pediatrics, Department of Medical Sciences, University of Ferrara, Ferrara, Italy, [8] Nephrology and Dialysis Unit, Meyer Children's Hospital, Florence, Italy, [9] Specialty School of Paediatrics - Alma Mater Studiorum, Università di Bologna, Bologna, Italy, [10] Retired, Palermo, Italy, [11] Giuliana and Bernardo Caprotti Chair of Pediatrics, Department of Clinical Sciences and Community Health, University of Milano, Milan, Italy

***Correspondence:**
Andrea Pasini
andrea.pasini@aosp.bo.it

Background: A great majority of children with idiopathic nephrotic syndrome will relapse after successful treatment of the initial episode. The possibility that different steroid dosing regimens at onset, adjusted for risk factors, can reduce the rate of relapse represents an interesting option to investigate.

Objectives: To evaluate the effect of the initial steroid regimen, adjusted for time to remission (TTR), on the frequency of relapses and steroid dependence, and to verify the influence of prognostic factors on disease course.

Methods: A multicentre, prospective, cohort study. Children with nephrotic syndrome, with TTR $\leq$10 days (Group A), were given a 20-week prednisone regimen (2,828 mg/m^2) and those with a TTR >10 days, a 22-week regimen (3,668 mg/m^2) (Group B). Previously published retrospective data from the same centers were also evaluated. Main outcomes were: relapse rate, number of frequent relapsers + steroid dependent children and total prednisone dose after induction.

Results: 143 children were enrolled. Rate of relapsed subjects (77 vs. 79%) and frequent relapsers + steroid dependent subjects (40 vs. 53%) did not differ between Groups A and B, or between the retrospective and prospective cohorts. The cumulative prednisone dose taken after the induction treatment was similar in both groups and in the retrospective and prospective cohorts. TTR was not associated with relapse risk. Age at onset and total serum protein were significantly lower in relapsing patients. At ROC analysis, the best cut-off was 5.3 years for age at onset and 4.2 g/dL for total serum protein. According to these cut-offs, older children with higher total serum protein had a higher relapse free survival rate (58%) than younger children with lower total serum protein (17%).

Conclusions: TTR was not found to be a prognostic factor of relapse; because of this, different steroid regimens, adjusted for TTR, did not modify the relapse rate in any relevant measure. Conversely, younger age and low total serum protein were independent predictors of relapse risk, however this outcome was not modified by higher prednisone regimens.

Clinical Trial Registration: https://www.ClinicalTrials.gov/, identifier: NCT01386957 (www.nefrokid.it).

Keywords: childhood idiopathic nephrotic syndrome, steroid treatment, frequent relapsers, steroid dependency, prognostic factors, age at onset, total serum protein

INTRODUCTION

Steroid therapy is the first-line treatment for idiopathic nephrotic syndrome (INS), inducing remission in 80–90% of children (1–3). However, 75–80% of responders will relapse, and 40–50% will show frequent relapses or steroid dependence (4-9). No consensus exists regarding optimal dosing or treatment duration (10–16). In 2000, a Cochrane meta-analysis showed that 3 months of steroid treatment resulted in a lower relapse rate at 12 and 24 months, with an increased benefit being demonstrated for up to 7 months of treatment (17). While new trials focused on modifying the clinical evolution of INS, many study groups began looking for prognostic factors of relapse and steroid dependence [early age at onset (18–21), male gender (21), intrauterine growth retardation (22), and time to remission (23-25)]. Vivarelli et al. identified time to remission (TTR) >14 days as a main prognostic factor for relapse, with all subjects relapsing within 3 months, while 20% of subjects with a TTR ≤7 days were still in remission at 18 months.

On these bases, we designed an epidemiological, observational, prospective, multicenter study to evaluate the role of the initial steroid regimen as regards relapse occurrence and steroid dependence, and to verify the influence of potential prognostic factors on disease course (23–25).

Moreover, we took the clinical decision to differentiate the steroid regimen on the basis of TTR (≤10 or >10 days), with the aim of protecting later responders from the higher risk of relapse, as reported by some authors (23–25).

METHODS

This is an epidemiological, multicenter, prospective cohort study involving 49 Italian pediatric units, performed between 2011 and 2016 (ClinicalTrials.gov Id: NCT01386957). An additional cohort, compiled using retrospective data from children treated at the same centers, was used for further analyses (13). Ethics Committee approval from the participating hospitals and written informed consent were obtained.

Diagnosis

All children with a first episode of INS, defined as proteinuria >40 mg/m^2/h or urine protein/creatinine ratio (uPr/uCr) >2 mg/mg and albuminemia <2.5 g/dL, were enrolled. Inclusion criteria were age at onset >6 months and <18 years and a diagnosis of INS. Exclusion criteria were congenital and secondary forms of nephrotic syndrome and steroid resistance. During the treatment protocol, dipstick urinalysis was performed daily, in order to identify TTR (first day of negative/trace dipstick).Relapse was defined as 3 days of dipstick ≥2+, confirmed by uPr/uCr >2 mg/mg. Time to relapse was defined as the time elapsed since the start of treatment to the first relapse. At the end of the 24-month follow-up period, patients were classified as non-relapser (NR), infrequent relapser (IR), frequent relapser (FR), or steroid-dependent (SD) according to standard definitions (26). Non-relapsers and infrequent relapsers (NR + IR) and frequent relapsers and steroid-dependent (FR + SD) subjects were grouped and compared.

Therapy Protocol

Subjects with a TTR ≤10 days (Group A) received prednisone 60 mg/m^2/day for 4 weeks, those with a TTR >10 days (Group B) for 6 weeks. Patients not achieving remission within 6 weeks received 3 alternate-day pulses of iv methylprednisolone (1 g/1.73 m^2, max 1g), followed by alternate-day prednisone at 40 mg/m^2. Those who had not achieved remission after a further 2 weeks were classified as steroid-resistant (SR). Steroid tapering was identical for all patients: 4 weeks of alternate-day prednisone (40 mg/m^2), followed by 14 weeks of tapering. The first episode cumulative prednisone dose was 2,828 mg/m^2 (20 weeks) in Group A, and 3,668 mg/m^2 (22 weeks) in Group B. First relapses were treated with prednisone 60 mg/m^2/day, until proteinuria was negative for 5 consecutive days, then a single alternate-day 40 mg/m^2 dose (4 weeks). Subsequent relapses were treated according to each individual center's relapse protocol.

Abbreviations: INS, idiopathic nephrotic syndrome; TTR, time to remission; uPr/uCr, urine protein/creatinine; NR, non-relapser; IR, infrequent relapse; FR, frequent relapser; SD, steroid-dependent; SR, steroid-resistant; SDS, systolic and diastolic blood pressure; SS, steroid-sensitive.

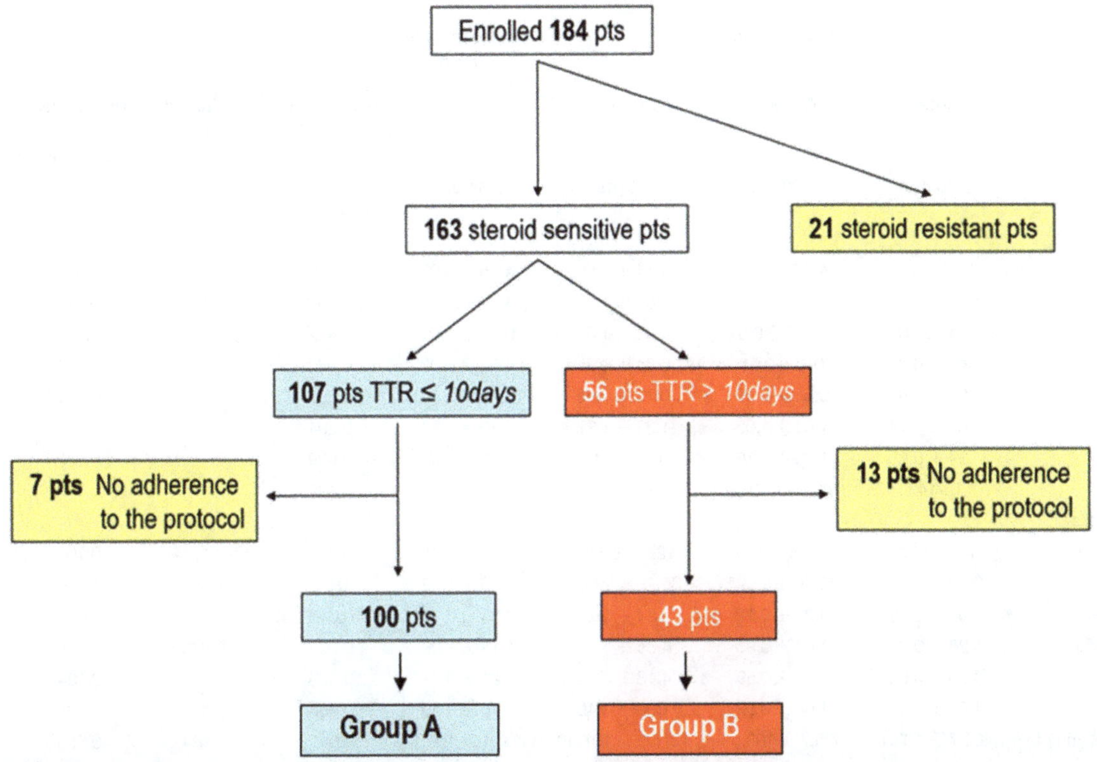

FIGURE 1 | Study flow chart.

Clinical and Laboratory Data

Height, weight, body mass index, systolic and diastolic blood pressure (SDS), complete blood count, urea, creatinine, uricemia, serum protein electrophoresis, albumin, total cholesterol, triglycerides, electrolytes, urinalysis, 24-h proteinuria, or uPr/uCr were recorded in an online database (www.nefrokid.it) at diagnosis, 12 and 24 months. Total number of relapses, time to relapse, total steroid dose at 12 and 24 months, and the use of other immunosuppressors were also recorded.

Additional Retrospective Cohort

We acknowledged that the original design of the prospective study was somewhat flawed. Therefore, we decided to get a wider perspective in order to draw more reliable conclusions (see Discussion). To that purpose, a previously published retrospective study of 144 INS children diagnosed between January 2007 and December 2009 and followed up for 24 months was used as an additional cohort for further analyses (13). Inclusion criteria were identical, while steroid treatment was not standardized. Steroid induction dose was 2,013 ± 617 mg/m^2, with a 5 (2.5–8) week duration. The first episode mean cumulative prednisone dose was 3,582 ± 881 mg/m^2, ranging from 1,904 to 6,035 mg/m^2, with a 21 (9–48) week duration.

Study Aims

(a) To evaluate and compare the clinical course of patients (Group A vs. Group B and prospective vs. retrospective cohort) at 24 months.

(b) To evaluate the prognostic relevance of the following factors: age and laboratory data at onset, TTR in continuous form, total prednisone induction dose (4 weeks of daily prednisone vs. 6 weeks).

Outcomes

(a) Relapse free survival, percentage of patients with at least one relapse at 24 months, number of relapses per patient and time to first relapse.

(b) Steroid sensitivity (prevalence of FR + SD subjects) at 24 months.

(c) Cumulative post-induction prednisone dose (cumulative prednisone dose administered from induction to 24 months).

Statistical Analysis

Statistical analysis was performed using the open source software R (27). The Chi-Square test of independence was used to analyze the association between categorical variables. Non-parametric tests (Wilcoxon, Kruskal-Wallis) were used to compare the distribution of a continuous variable in two or more different groups.

Linear regression models were used to analyse the association between continuous variables and the Kaplan Meier estimator to build relapse free survival curves. Cox hazard ratio models were used to evaluate significance of

TABLE 1 | Comparison of clinical and laboratory data at onset: Group A vs. Group B and prospective vs. retrospective cohort.

	Prospective cohort			Restrospective cohort	*p*-value			
	Total (143 pts)	Group A (100 pts)	Group B (43 pts)	Total (144 pts)	Group A vs. Group B	Adjusted (Holm's method)	Prospective vs. retrospective	Adjusted (Holm's method)
Clinical data								
Age (years)	4.55 ± 2.7	4.73 ± 2.53	4.14 ± 3.06	4.75 ± 3.06	0.01	0,21	0.885	1
Sex (Male)	93 (65.0%)	65 (65.0%)	28 (65.1%)	96 (66.7%)	0.989	1	0.771	1
Height (SDS)	−0.04 ± 0.87	−0.08 ± 0.81	0.05 ± 1.01	0.02 ± 1.00	0.412	1	0.481	1
Weight (SDS)	0.46 ± 0.89	0.4 ± 0.91	0.64 ± 0.84	0.55 ± 1.03	0.082	1	0.171	1
BMI (SDS)	0.65 ± 0.93	0.60 ± 0.92	0.79 ± 0.95	0.72 ± 0.89	0.207	1	0.541	1
sBP (SDS)	1.07 ± 1.12	1.01 ± 1.05	1.23 ± 1.27	0.86 ± 1.14	0.294	1	0.083	1
dBP (SDS)	1.34 ± 0.88	1.28 ± 0.76	1.5 ± 1.12	1.13 ± 0.91	0.529	1	0.150	1
SGA	16/143	10/100 (10%)	6/43 (13.8%)		0.491	1		
Laboratory data								
Hemoglobin (g/dL)	13.0 ± 1.2	13.08 ± 1.09	12.97 ± 1.34	13.3 ± 1.2	0.323	1	0.104	1
Urea (mg/dL)	29.3 ± 16.5	26.66 ± 13.25	35.26 ± 21.07	28.6 ± 13.2	0.01	0,21	0.936	1
Creatinine (mg/dl)	0.30 ± 0.15	0.29 ± 0.12	0.34 ± 0.21	0.35 ± 0.15	0.653	1	0.001	0.022
Uricemia (mg/dL)	4.23 ± 0.99	4.04 ± 0.93	4.65 ± 1.01	4.13 ± 1.09	0.004	0,088	0.546	1
Total proteins (g/dL)	4.23 ± 0.58	4.26 ± 0.59	4.18 ± 0.58	4.21 ± 0.67	0.323	1	0.734	1
Albumin (g/dL)	1.63 ± 0.50	1.64 ± 0.52	1.60 ± 0.46	1.40 ± 0.40	0.955	1	0.001	0.022
Tot. cholesterol (mg/dL)	403.7 ± 108.1	395.7 ± 108.05	421.09 ± 107.49	400.1 ± 102.1	0.049	0,784	0.665	1
Triglycerides (mg/dL)	197.20 ± 110.2	184.2 ± 92.12	225.86 ± 139.03	217.62 ± 138.5	0.074	1	0.331	1
Na (mmol/L)	136.8 ± 3.5	137.25 ± 3.54	135.84 ± 3.11	136.2 ± 3.4	0.03	0,522	0.240	1
K (mmol/L)	4.47 ± 0.50	4.42 ± 0.43	4.61 ± 0.52	4.51 ± 0.56	0.02	0,38	0.921	1
Ca (mg/dL)	8.18 ± 0.55	8.15 ± 0.61	8.24 ± 0.42	8.18 ± 0.70	0.439	1	0.652	1
P (mg/dL)	4.93 ± 0.82	4.84 ± 0.81	5.12 ± 0.82	5.08 ± 1.09	0.029	0,522	0.287	1
uPr/uCr (mg/mg)	13.39 ± 10.7	11.74 ± 9.41	17.44 ± 12.6	10.32 ± 7.22	0.002	0.046	0.056	1
Proteinuria (g/L)	9.32 ± 9.13	8.29 ± 8.27	11.91 ± 10.71	8.05 ± 8.17	0.088	1	0.230	1
Microhematuria	58 (40.6%)	37 (37.0%)	22 (51.2%)	59 (41.0%)	0.114	1	0.943	1
Steroid response								
TTR (days)	10.3 ± 7.8			14.8 ± 12.4			0.00025	0.00575

Mean ± SD for numerical variables, number (%) for categorical variables. BMI, body mass index; sBP, systolic blood pressure; dBP, dyastolic blood pressure; SGA, small for gestational age. The red color values represent the significant values.

prognostic factors in relation to survival curves and for multivariate analysis.

RESULTS

Clinical Course

Prospective Cohort

One hundered and eighty-four children (median age at diagnosis: 3.9, range 0.6–17 years; Male:Female 1.9:1) with INS were enrolled. One hundred and sixty-three (89%) were steroid-sensitive (SS), 21 (11%) were SR and were excluded alongside an additional 20 patients due to non-compliance. The final cohort comprised 143 subjects. Among them, 100 (70%) had a TTR ≤10 days and were administered the 4-week induction regimen (Group A), whilst the 43 with a later TTR were given the 6-week induction regimen (Group B) (**Figure 1**).

Retrospective Cohort

One hundred forty-four steroid sensitive patients from a retrospective study (13), followed-up for 24 months, were evaluated. Steroid induction dose was 2,013 ± 617 mg/m^2, with a 5 (2.5–8) week duration.

Data at Onset

Clinical characteristics and laboratory data are shown in **Table 1**. The two cohorts were similar, except for higher serum creatinine and lower serum albumin values in the retrospective cohort. Groups A and B were also similar, except for age at onset, which was significantly lower in Group B, while urea, uricemia, total cholesterol, Na, K, P, and PrU/CrU were significantly higher in Group B.

The median TTR was 8 (1–47) days in the prospective cohort, with 156 (96%) patients achieving remission within 4 weeks, and

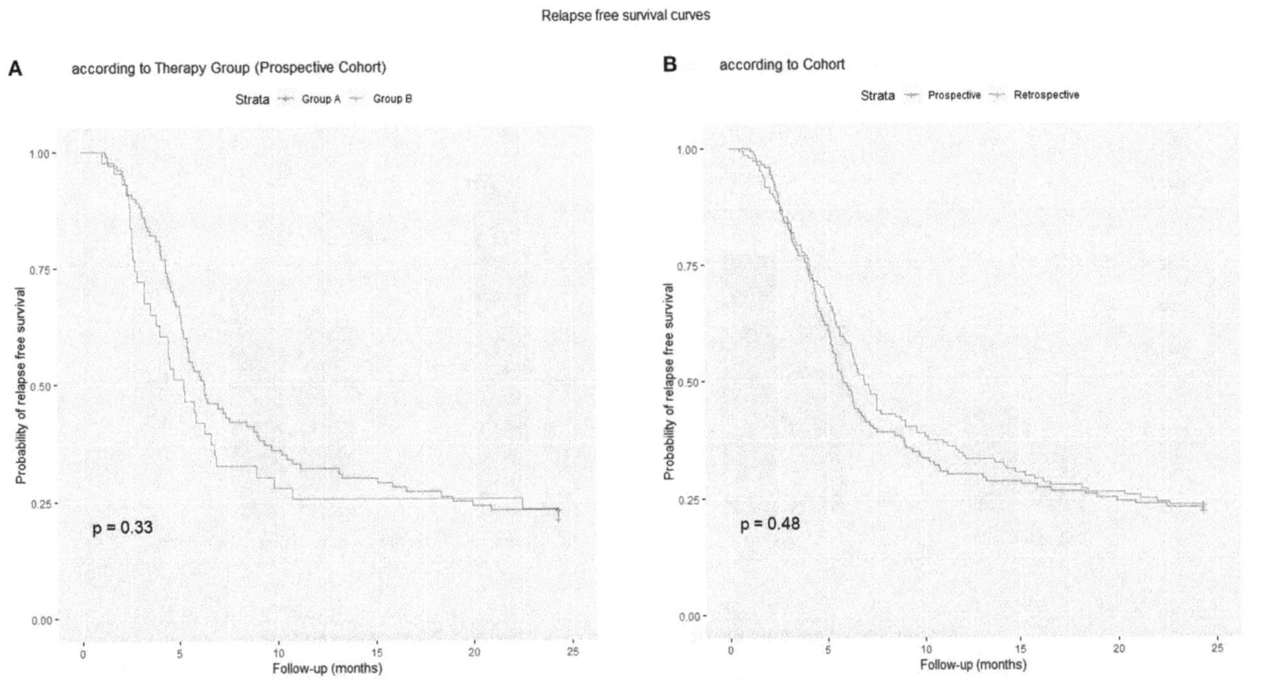

FIGURE 2 | Relapse-free survival curves: **(A)** Group A vs. Group B; **(B)** Prospective vs. Retrospective Cohort.

7 (4%) in more than 4 weeks (3 after iv methylprednisolone boluses). The median TTR was significantly longer (11; range 3–77 days) in the retrospective cohort. The mean total induction prednisone dose was 1,685 ± 107 mg/m^2 in Group A, 2,648 ± 426 in Group B, and 2,013 ± 617 in the retrospective cohort.

Relapses

In the prospective cohort, 111 (78%) subjects relapsed after a mean time of 188 ± 140 days from the start of treatment. At 12 months, 100 subjects (70%) had relapsed. There were a total of 268 relapses (182 in Group A, 86 in Group B), ranging from 1 (42 patients) to 7 (1 patient) per patient. The mean number of relapses per patient (1.8 vs. 2; $p = 0.43$), and the percentage of patients who had relapsed at 12 (68 vs. 74%; $p = 0.44$) and 24 months (77 vs. 79%; $p = 0.78$) did not differ between Groups A and B. The relapse rate in the retrospective vs. the prospective cohort (77 vs. 78% at 24 months, $p = 0.91$) and the number of relapses per patient (2.1 vs. 1.9, $p = 0.44$) did not differ. The time to first relapse was longer in Group A vs. Group B (mean = 205.6 vs. 166.8 days; $p = 0.05$). The relapse-free survival curve up to the end of follow-up did not differ between Groups A and B (p=0.30), or between the two cohorts ($p = 0.50$; **Figures 2A,B**).

Steroid Sensitivity

In the prospective cohort, 32 children (22%) were NR, 48 (34%) IR, 5 (3%) FR, 58 (41%) SD. The prevalence of FR + SD subjects was similar in Groups A and B (40 vs. 53%, $p = 0.14$) and in the two cohorts (43 vs. 44%, $p = 0.8$).

Cumulative Post-induction Prednisone Doses

The Group A induction dose was lower per protocol (4 vs. 6 weeks) and the cumulative dose remained significantly lower at 12 and 24 months ($p = 0.002$ and $p = 0.018$, respectively), compared to Group B. Therefore, the cumulative post-induction prednisone dose did not differ significantly ($p = 0.28$; **Figure 3A**). Steroid sparing agents were utilized more frequently in Group B than in Group A (42 vs. 25%, $p = 0.04$). When comparing the retrospective and prospective cohorts, the mean total induction prednisone dose (2013 vs. 1977, $p = 0.49$), the mean cumulative prednisone dose at 12 (5,656 vs. 5,355, $p = 0.3$) and 24 months (7,668 vs. 7,203, $p = 0.5$) and the mean cumulative prednisone dose administered from induction to 24 months (5,682 vs. 5,245, $p = 0.6$) did not differ (**Figure 3B**).

Prognostic Factors

The significance of prognostic factors for the whole population (prospective + retrospective cohort) is shown in **Table 2**, and separately for the prospective and retrospective cohorts in **Supplementary Tables 1, 2**, respectively.

Age at Onset

Age at onset was significantly associated with all outcomes in the whole population (**Table 2**) and in the prospective cohort. In the retrospective cohort, only time to relapse and prednisone dose were not significantly associated with age.

TTR

In the whole population, TTR in continuous form was only significantly associated with a higher prevalence of FR-SD

A

B

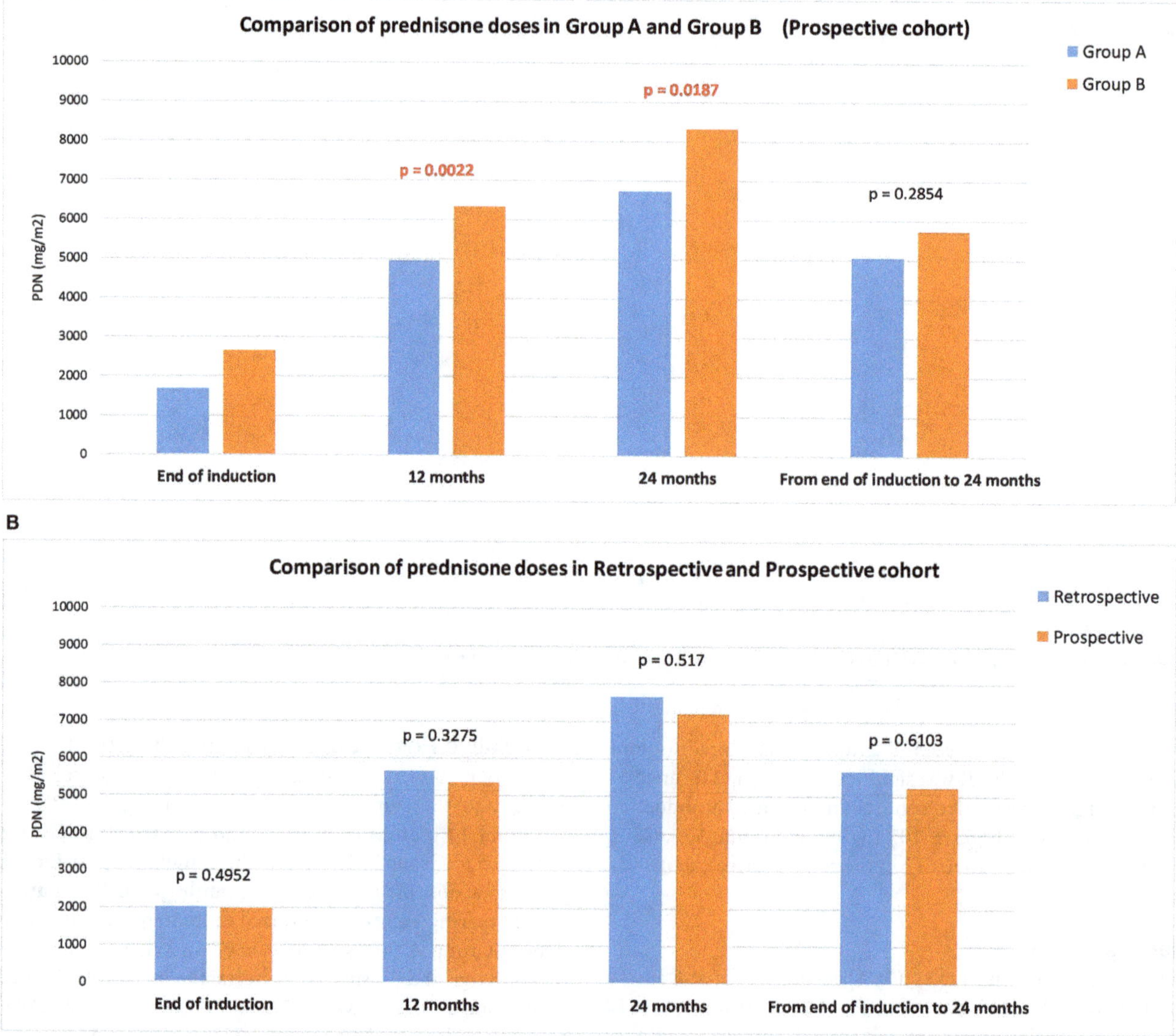

C

Total prednisone doses (mg/m2)				
	Induction	12 months	24 months	From end of induction to 24 months
Group A	1685±107	4953 ± 2152	6736 ± 3521	5048 ± 3242
Group B	2648±426	6316 ± 2287	8320 ± 3568	5717 ± 795
Retrospective	2013 ± 617	5656 ± 2355	7668 ± 4000	5682 ± 4011
Prospective	1977 ± 509	5355 ± 2270	7203 ± 3411	5245 ± 3348

FIGURE 3 | Cumulative prednisone doses. Total daily PRED dose, cumulative PRED dose at 12, 24 months and from the end of induction to the end of follow-up: Group A vs. B **(A)**, prospective vs. retrospective cohort **(B)**. All values are means ± SD (mg/m^2) **(C)**.

patients (**Table 2**). This association held true in the retrospective cohort, where a weak association with a higher relapse rate was also seen ($p = 0.02$). No associations were observed in the prospective cohort (**Supplementary Tables 1, 2**).

In order to exclude the confounding factor of a different induction therapy in the evaluation of TTR, we decided to perform a separate sub-analysis for Group A (induction prednisone dose 1,685 ± 107) and Group B (induction prednisone dose 2,648 ± 426) (**Figure 4**), categorizing patients as "lower TTR" and "higher TTR" in each group. In both groups, there was no detectable effect of TTR as a negative prognostic factor. When patients from the retrospective cohort were categorized for TTR in the same way as the prospective cohort, data did not show a significant prognostic role for TTR.

TABLE 2 | Prognostic factors evaluated in the whole population according to the different outcomes.

	Relapse	Time to relapse	N. of relapses	Prevalence of FR-SD	PDN after remission	Relapse-free survival	Relapse-free survival adjusted (Holm's method)
Whole population							
Age at onset (years)	0.00002	0.0006	0.0009	0.00005	0.046	0.0000001	0.000002
TTR (days)	0.088	NS	NS	0.003	NS	NS	NS
Prednisone dose in induction (mg/m2)	NS	NS	NS	NS	NS	NS	NS
Hemoglobin (g/dL)	NS	NS	NS	NS	NS	NS	NS
Urea (mg/dL)	NS	NS	NS	NS	0.005	NS	NS
Creatinine (mg/dl)	0.016	NS	0.012	0.042	0.017	0.0037	0.056
Uricemia (mg/dL)	NS	NS	NS	0.07	NS	0.096	NS
Total proteins (g/dL)	0.0003	0.009	0.005	0.019	0.00002	0.00001	0.00019
Albumin (g/dL)	0.058	0.004	NS	0.086	0.025	0.0009	0.0162
Alpha 2 globulins (g/L)	NS	NS	NS	NS	NS	NS	NS
Gamma globulins (g/L)	NS	NS	NS	NS	NS	0.068	NS
Tot. cholesterol (mg/dL)	0.049	NS	NS	NS	0.09	NS	NS
Triglycerides (mg/dL)	0.08	NS	NS	0.056	NS	0.059	NS
Na (mmol/L)	0.06	0.02	NS	NS	0.06	0.039	NS
K (mmol/L)	NS	NS	NS	NS	NS	NS	NS
Ca (mg/dL)	NS	NS	NS	NS	0.014	NS	NS
P (mg/dL)	NS	NS	NS	NS	NS	NS	NS
uPr/uCr (mg/mg)	0.039	0.016	NS	0.00016	0.026	0.001	0.017
Proteinuria (g/L)	NS	0.007	0.046	0.002	0.0006	0.001	0.017
Microhematuria	NS	NS	NS	NS	NS	NS	NS

p-values are in red if <0.05, in green if ≥0.05, and <0.10. All p > 0.10 are labeled as NS (not significant).

All total prednisone doses (taken by Group A, Group B, prospective and retrospective cohort) expressed as means ± SD (mg/m^2), are shown in **Figure 3C**.

Total Induction Prednisone Dose

In the whole population, induction dose was not associated with any of the outcomes (**Table 2**). The same was seen when the two cohorts were analyzed separately.

Laboratory Values at Onset (Table 2)

Total protein values were significantly associated with all outcomes in the entire population. Albumin behaved similarly for three outcomes. A lower total protein or albumin value was associated with higher relapse rate. The behavior was similar in the two cohorts (**Supplementary Tables 1, 2**). Among other values, only creatinine, proteinuria, and the PrU/CrU ratio showed a consistent association with most outcomes (**Table 2**). Creatinine showed a paradoxical association: higher values were associated with a better prognosis. As creatinine showed a strong collinearity with age, this association was not analyzed further. The other laboratory values were not consistently associated with the outcomes.

Relapse Free Survival Analysis

The last two columns in **Table 2** report the results of bivariate analysis for each prognostic factor using relapse free survival as outcome. Both raw *p*-values and adjusted *p*-values are shown. Time to first relapse was always computed from start of therapy, and follow-up was 24 months from start of therapy for all patients.

We chose to use relapse-free survival as outcome for our final multivariate analysis, because it includes information about both relapse rate and time to relapse.

Multivariate analysis was performed using a Cox proportional hazards model, including all the variables with a $p < 0.1$ in the bivariate analysis performed on the whole population. The following variables were excluded because of strong collinearity: albumin with total serum protein, creatinine with age, and PrU/CrU with proteinuria and age. In the final model, age at onset (coefficient $= -0.128$; $p = 0.000004$) and total serum protein (coefficient $= -0.488$; $p = 0.00002$) were the only significant independent predictors of relapse free survival (total likelihood ratio = 1.774e-10). Younger patients with lower total serum protein values at onset had a higher risk of earlier and more frequent relapses. None of the other risk factors were independent prognostic factors.

A ROC analysis showed that the best cut-offs (Youden's index) for age at onset (AUC = 0.681) and serum protein (AUC = 0.653) were 5.3 years and 4.2 g/dL, respectively. Using these cut-offs, children were categorized as follows: Group 1: not at risk for either total protein or age (n = 41, 15%), Group 2: at risk for total protein only (n = 34, 12%), Group 3: at risk

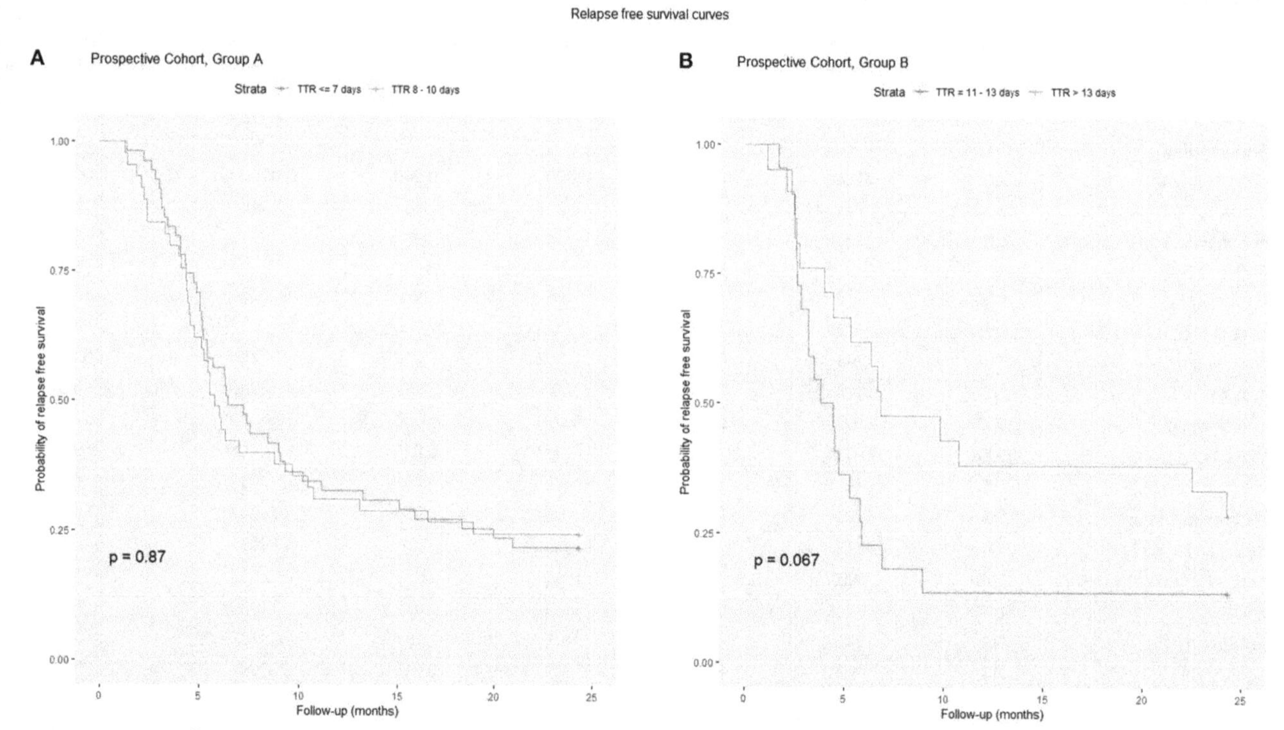

FIGURE 4 | A sub-analysis of TTR and relapse risk was performed on Group A and B. On the left **(A)** for Group A, the relapse-free survival curve did not differ between the two subgroups. On the right **(B)** for Group B patients with higher TTR have a better curve, but the difference is not significant.

for age only (n = 78, 29%) and Group 4: at risk for both total protein and age (n = 120, 44%).This categorization significantly predicted relapse free survival (**Figure 5A**). **Figure 5B** shows instead that total induction prednisone dose (threshold 2,000 mg/m^2) was not significant (p = 0.70). Even when analyzing induction prednisone dose in each of the abovementioned risk groups separately, no significant effect on relapse free survival was observed (**Figures 6A–D**).

These 4 groups were also good predictors of FR-SD prevalence (p = 0.007). In Group 1, 24% of patients were FR-SD vs. 54% in Group 4. Groups 2 and 3 showed similar behavior, with 38 and 41% of FR-SD patients, respectively.

DISCUSSION

This is the first published prospective study to use a steroid regimen adjusted for a prognostic factor. When this study was conceived, the Cochrane review (28) recommended prolonging the total prednisone dose and steroid protocol duration. In accordance with this, we prolonged and diversified our steroid regimen on the basis of TTR $\leq$10 or >10 days. The rationale was to administer a higher daily prednisone dose to children at risk of more frequent relapses or steroid dependence (23–25).

However, we do acknowledge that the original design of the prospective study was not really appropriate, for two important reasons:

1) It was based on the assumption that TTR is a strong negative prognostic factor for relapse. That assumption was based on rather limited evidence from the literature, and was not confirmed in successive studies. Moreover, our same results did not seem to support our initial assumption.
2) The lack of randomization and the association of TTR with different steroid therapy make it very difficult to distinguish between the possible effects of the two variables in our prospective data.

In particular, our results showed that a higher-dose and longer initial steroid therapy for childhood INS, diversified according to TTR, was not associated with a significantly different clinical course. At first glance, this result may appear to mean that treating the patients at higher risk of relapse with higher prednisone doses was successful, having reduced their relapse rate. Unfortunately, that conclusion holds only if the assumption of a strong negative prognostic role of TTR is confirmed.

To draw more reliable conclusions, we decided to expand our data by adding data from a previous retrospective cohort of patients, as described in Methods. At the same time, we performed specific sub analyses of our data aimed at differentiating, as much as possible, between the effect of TTR and the effect of therapy.

As a result of a more in-depth evaluation of our prospective data and a re-evaluation of all the prognostic factors in the whole population of our patients (prospective + retrospective), we found no evidence the TTR can be considered a major prognostic factor of relapse (**Figure 4**, **Supplementary Figures 1, 2**). Similarly, no detectable effect of different steroid doses (in the range of those tested) was found.

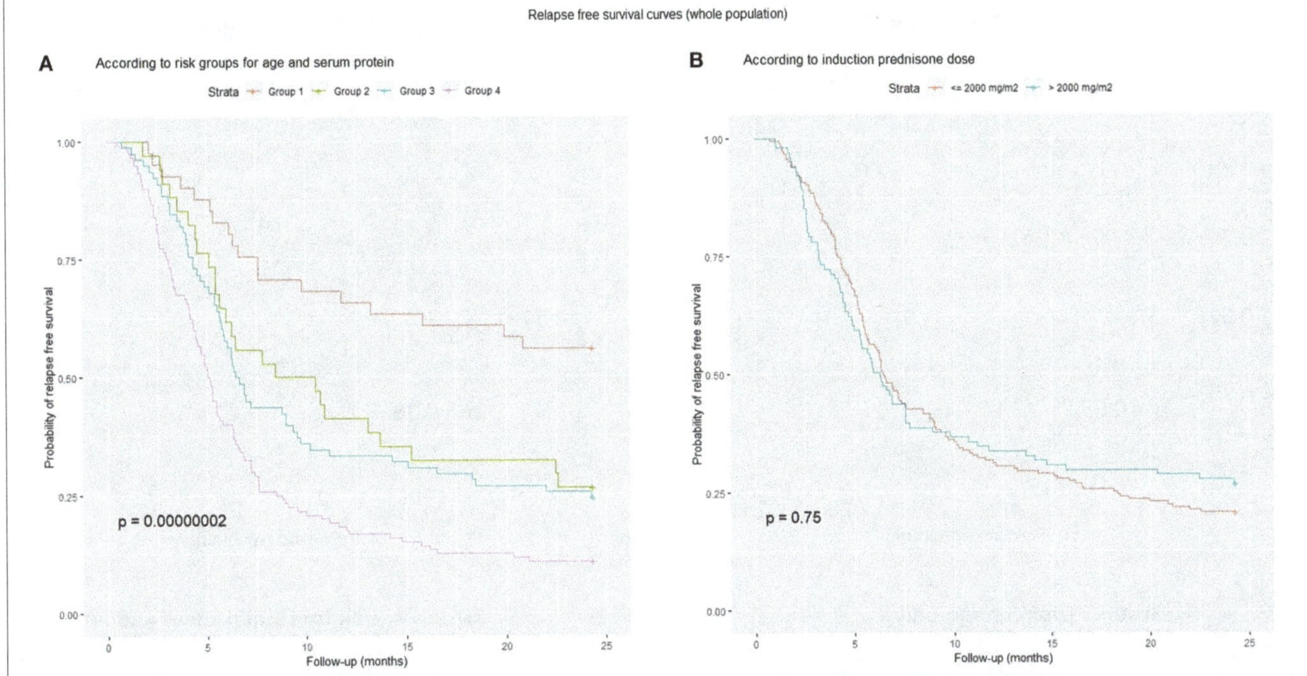

FIGURE 5 | Relapse-free survival curves: **(A)** combined risk groups according to age (cut-off 5.3 years) and serum protein (cut-off 4.2 g/dl): Group 1, low-risk for both; Group 2, high-risk for total proteins only; Group 3, high-risk for age only; Group 4, high-risk for both; **(B)** induction prednisone dose in binary form (threshold 2,000 mg/m^2).

Relapse Rate

Relapse rate at 24 months, time to relapse, the number of relapses per patient and the percentage of FR+SD subjects did not differ significantly either between Groups A and B, or between the prospective and retrospective cohorts, where no TTR-based categorization was applied.

Our data confirm the results of three RCTs, published when our study was ongoing, which showed that relapse rate was not modified by initial steroid regimen. In 2013, Teeninga demonstrated that extending initial prednisone treatment without increasing cumulative dose did not benefit clinical outcome (29). In 2015, Sinha et al. (30) and Yoshikawa et al. (31), comparing a 3-month (2,792 ± 287 mg/m^2) vs. a 6-month regimen (3,530 ± 399 mg/m^2), and a 2- vs. a 6-month regimen (2,240 vs. 3,885 mg/m^2), respectively, found no differences in relapse rate or the number of FR subjects (32). These findings were confirmed both by the authors of the 2015 Cochrane review (33) and the results of a recent RCT (34).

In particular, in our study, considering the total induction dose in binary form in the whole population, low-dose (<2,000 mg/m^2) was as effective as high-dose (>2,000 mg/m^2) in terms of relapse free survival (**Figure 5B**), and the same was true considering each risk group (based on age and total protein) separately (**Figures 6A–D**). Sinha obtained similar results in his RCT (30), comparing 3- vs. 6-month regimens.

As TTR was apparently associated with some differences in laboratory data at diagnosis, we suggest that it could be perhaps considered as a consequence of delayed diagnosis and more serious renal involvement at onset, rather than as a prognostic factor for a subsequent higher relapse rate.

On the contrary, both age and total serum protein concentrations at onset (but also proteinuria and uPr/uCr) were shown to be consistent predictors of relapse, independently of TTR and steroid induction doses.

Indeed, a more immature immunological status in younger patients could be related to a higher frequency of relapses and steroid dependency, as reported by many studies (18–21). Concurrently, a massive proteinuria causing a greater reduction of total serum protein concentrations, could be, at onset, a clinical prognostic sign of subsequent frequent relapses.

Cumulative Prednisone Doses

Another aspect we wanted to investigate in our study was the possible role of higher steroid dose at onset in reducing the need for steroids after remission. Our data definitely do not support that hypothesis, as shown by the evaluation of the mean cumulative doses taken from the end of the induction to 24 months (**Figure 3A**). This result cannot be attributed to a different use of steroid sparing agents.

Prognostic Factors

As previously discussed, our data did not confirm a major prognostic role for TTR, contrary to published studies (20, 22, 35–39).

Conversely, age at onset and total serum protein were significant and strong prognostic factors, associated with all the outcomes. A correlation between age at onset and risk of relapse

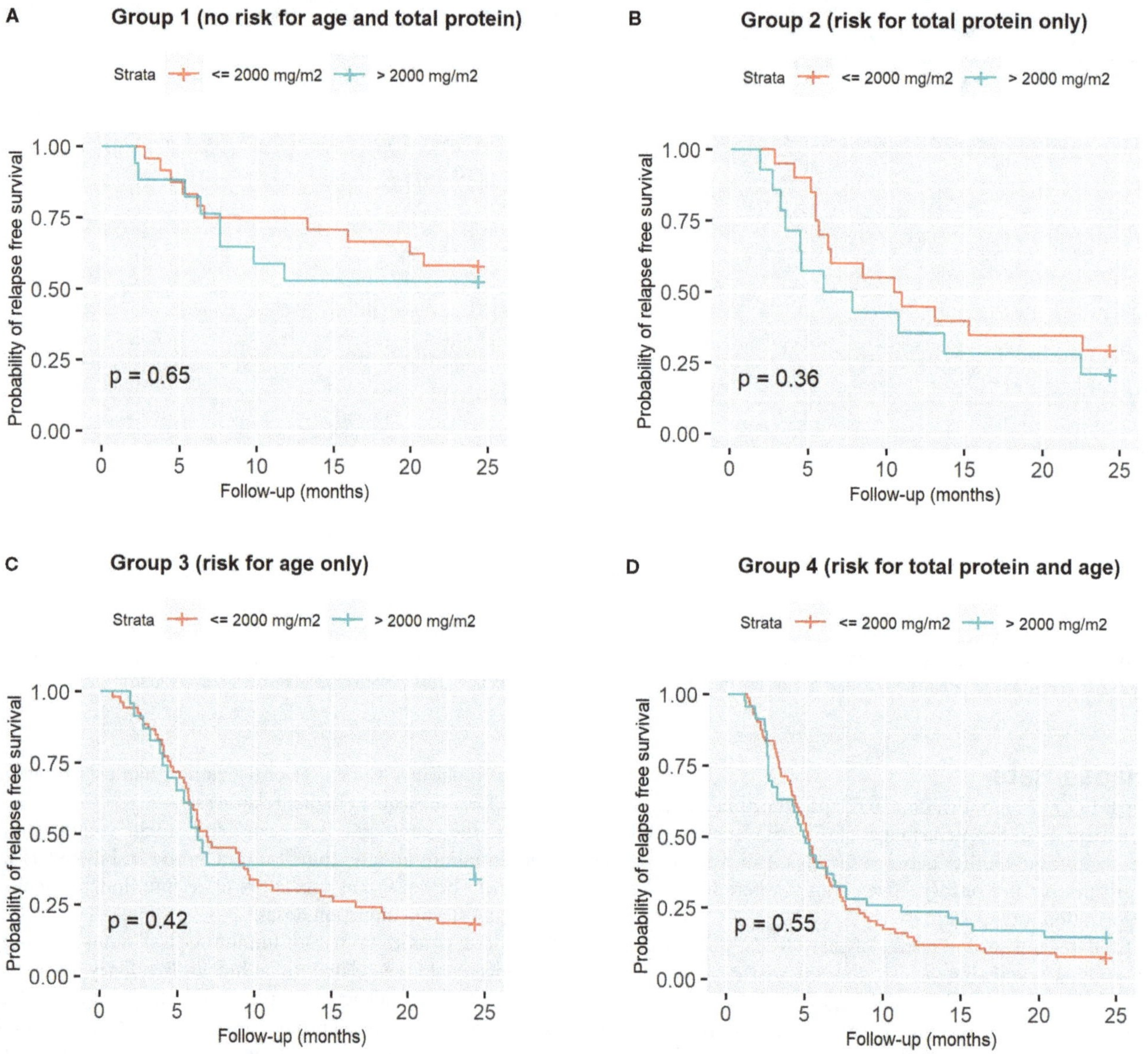

FIGURE 6 | Relapse-free survival curves according to induction prednisone dose in binary form (threshold 2,000 mg/m^2), analyzed in each of the 4 combined risk groups based on age (cut-off 5.3 years) and serum protein (cut-off 4.2 g/dl): **(A)** Group 1, low-risk for both; **(B)** Group 2, high-risk for total proteins only; **(C)** Group 3, high-risk for age only; **(D)** Group 4, high-risk for both.

has been shown by many authors (15, 16, 18, 30, 40, 41), but not by others (37). In 2003, an RCT comparing long vs. short-course prednisolone regimens (42) showed that younger children were more susceptible to relapse and benefitted from the long alternate-day regimen. In 2015, Sinha's *post-hoc* analysis (30) showed that age ≤3 years was associated with an increased relapse risk, but the number of FR children was not reduced by prolonged steroid therapy. The relapse rate and number of FR + SD subjects was not lower in younger children treated with higher prednisone doses.

In a multivariate analysis performed for relapse free survival in our whole population, total serum protein and age at onset were confirmed as the only independent prognostic factors. Based on the ROC analysis cut-offs (5.3 years and 4.2 g/dL), it was possible to categorize children into groups with different relapse risks (**Figure 5A**).

Nevertheless, a small percentage of younger subjects with lower serum protein never relapsed. Other factors are probably involved. Recent research has focused on the impact of genetic polymorphisms on glucocorticoid response (43–45).

Limitations

The non-optimal design of the original prospective study motivated us to add a retrospective cohort of patients to perform a more reliable analysis. Of course, that can be in itself a cause of bias and of difficulties in interpretation of the results. However, we believe that that procedure allowed us to comprehensively analyse a large population of patients, especially for prognostic factor analysis. Our analysis shows that data from the two cohorts are comparable enough, and that our main conclusions are reliable and consistent across the two individual cohorts.

The choice of 10 days as a cut-off value for TTR was based on our retrospective study. In the prospective study, the distribution of TTR was shifted toward the left, with a median of 8 days, resulting in an unbalanced number of patients (100 vs. 43). Moreover, we did not confirm TTR as a significant predictive factor, as also suggested by recent studies.

Further limitations include the number of dropouts (20) for non-adherence.

CONCLUSIONS

Steroid doses, adjusted for TTR, did not modify either the relapse rate or the number of FR + SD children at 24 months. However, a more refined analysis of our data showed that TTR cannot be considered a major prognostic factor of relapse, differently from what was reported by some other authors.

Conversely, younger age and low total serum protein values at onset were reliable prognostic factors for relapse and steroid dependence, with no apparent effects of higher prednisone regimens at onset. According to our data, a 4-week steroid induction regimen does not require higher cumulative doses throughout 24 months of follow-up, and thus represents a valid option for pediatric INS. However, a deeper understanding of the pathogenetic mechanisms involved in INS will help us detect subjects at higher risk of relapse and choose new therapeutic options (46–50).

ETHICS STATEMENT

The studies involving human participants were reviewed and approved by Comitato Etico Indipendente di Area Vasta Emilia Centro (CE-AVEC) della Regione Emilia-Romagna IRCCS Azienda Ospedaliero-Universitaria di Bologna, Policlinico S.Orsola-Malpighi. Written informed consent to participate in this study was provided by the participants' legal guardian/next of kin.

AUTHOR CONTRIBUTIONS

AP, AE, GMo conceptualized and designed the study, coordinated and supervised data collection, drafted the initial manuscript, reviewed, and revised the manuscript. GP carried out the initial analyses, drafted the initial manuscript, reviewed, and revised the manuscript. CB, LC, CC, GG, LG, MG, CL, CM, SM, AM, MM, FM, GMe, EM, WM, and PR collected data and reviewed and revised the manuscript. All authors approved the final manuscript as submitted and agree to be accountable for all aspects of the work.

ACKNOWLEDGMENTS

We thank all the members of Nefrokid Study Group, whose collaboration was essential to performing the study. We would also thank the non-profit association Il Sogno di Stefano and The Nando Peretti Foundation for their generous financial support. The authors thank Alexandra Teff for her linguistic assistance.

MEMBERS OF THE NEFROKID STUDY GROUP (ITALY)

Andrea Pasini, Francesca Mencarelli, Chiara De Mutiis, Claudio La Scola, Cristina Bertulli: Nephrology and Dialysis Unit, Department of Pediatrics, IRCCS Azienda Ospedaliero-Universitaria di Bologna; Elena Monti: Specialty School of Paediatrics - Alma Mater Studiorum, Università di Bologna, Italy; Gabriella Aceto, Giovanni Messina, Laura Spagnoletta, Mario Giordano, Tommaso De Palo: Nephrology Division, Giovanni XXIII Children's Hospital, Bari; Giovanni Montini, Alberto Edefonti, Luciana Ghio, Gianluigi Ardissino, Antonio Mastrangelo, William Morello, Elena Groppali, Marta Lepore: Pediatric Nephrology and Dialysis Unit, Fondazione Ca' Granda IRCCS Ospedale Maggiore Policlinico, Milan; Silvio Maringhini, Vitalba Azzolina, Ciro Corrado: Pediatric Nephrology Unit, Children's Hospital G. Di Cristina, A.R.N.A.S. Civico, Palermo; Carmelo Fede, Roberto Chimenz, Giovanni Conti: Pediatric Nephrology and Dialysis, AOU G.Martino, Messina; Paola Romagnani, Marco Materassi, Fiammetta Ravaglia: Nephrology and Dialysis Unit, Meyer Children's Hospital, Florence; Maria D'Agostino: Pediatric Unit, S.Giovanni XXIII Hospital, Bergam; Sante Cantatore: Department of Pediatrics, Azienda Ospedaliera - University of Modena, Modena; Anita Ammenti, Claudio Ruberto: Department of Pediatrics, University of Parma, Parma; Chiara Gualeni: Pediatric Unit, Children's Hospital, Brescia; Elena Cama: Department of Pediatrics and Neonatology, Desenzano del Garda; Mariotti Paola: Pediatric Unit, San Jacopo Hospital, Pistoia; Amata Negri: Pediatric Unit, Filippo Del Ponte Hospital, Varese; Alberto Bettinelli: Pediatric Unit, San Leopoldo Mandic Hospital, Merate; Gianluca Vergine, Elisa Ravaioli, Alessandra Lavacchini: Pediatric Unit, Ospedale degli Infermi, Rimini; Alessandra Dozza: Pediatric Unit, Ospedale Maggiore, Bologna; Angela Simoni: Pediatric Unit, Ramazzini Hospital, Carpi; Marina Piepoli: Pediatric Unit, Guglielmo da Saliceto Hospital, Piacenza; Felice Sica: Pediatric Unit, AOU Ospedali Riuniti, Foggia; Gabriele Ripanti: Pediatric Unit, San Salvatore Hospital, Pesaro; Marina Milani: Pediatric Unit, Fondazione MBBM, S. Gerardo Hospital, Monza; Paola Tommasi: Pediatric Unit, Vittore Buzzi Hospital, Milan; Carla Romanello: Pediatric Unit, S. Maria della Misericordia Hospital, Udine; Manuela Pasini: Pediatric Unit, Maurizio Bufalini Hospital, Cesena; Paola Mastinu: Pediatric Unit, S.Chiara Hospital, Trento; Laura Luti: Pediatric Unit, AOU Pisa; Antonella Amendolea: Pediatric Unit, Cecina; Silvia Manfredi: Pediatric Unit, Massa Carrara; Fabrizio Pugliese: Pediatric Emergency Department, Salesi Children's Hospital, University of Marche; Emanuela Lanfranchi: Pediatric

Unit, Fermo; Maria Principi: Pediatric Unit, Macerata; Agrippino Reciputo: Pediatric Unit, Cinisello Balsamo; Marialuisa Casciana: Pediatric Unit, C. Poma Hospital, Mantova; Antonio Pellegatta: Pediatric Unit, Busto Arsizio; Fiorella Russo: Pediatric Unit, Desio; Nicola Altamura: Pediatric Unit, Sesto San Giovanni; Lorena Ruzza: Pediatric Unit, San Carlo Hospital, Milan; Stefano Sardini: Pediatric Unit, Asola; Ines L'Erario: Pediatric Unit, Burlo Garofalo Hospital, Trieste; Antonella Crisafi: Pediatric Unit, Santa Maria Nuova Hospital, Reggio Emilia; Andrea Zucchini: Pediatric Unit, Faenza; Laura Serra: Pediatric Unit, Santa Maria della Scaletta Hospital, Imola; Peter Bertamini: Pediatric Unit, Santa Maria del Carmine Hospital, Rovereto; Rita Bini: Pediatric Unit, Grosseto; Patrizia Cortesi: Pediatric Unit, Pescia; Caterina Balducci: Pediatric Unit, Prato; Francesca Simoni: Pediatric Unit, Pianadi Lucca Hospital, Lucca; Patrizia Fonduli, Franca Paola Zurrida: Pediatric Unit, Brotzu Hospital, Cagliari; Laura De Petris: Pediatric Unit, Mazzoni Hospital, Ascoli Piceno; Vinicio Goj: Pediatric Unit, Fatebenefratelli Hospital, Milan; Gian Luigi Marsiglia: Pediatric Unit, IRCCS Policlinico S Matteo, Pavia; Patrizia Caruso: Pediatric Unit, Cremona; Filippo Salvini: Pediatric Unit, S. Paolo Hospital, Milan; Paola Perotti: Pediatric Unit, Voghera; Anna Bussolini: Pediatric Unit, Tradate; Stefano Poli, Barbara Balduzzi: Pediatric Unit, Esine; Barbara Roman: Pediatric Unit, Vimercate; Sergio Mariani, Laura Cafarelli: Pediatric Unit, Saronno; Vittorio Venturoli: Pediatric Unit, Morgagni-Pierantoni Hospital, Forlì; Andrea Corsini Pediatric Unit, Bentivoglio; Luca Casadio: Pediatric Unit, Ravenna.

REFERENCES

1. A Report of the International Study of Kidney Disease in Children. Nephrotic syndrome in children: Prediction of histopathology from clinical and laboratory characteristics at time of diagnosis. *Kidney Int.* (1978) 13:159–65. doi: 10.1038/ki.1978.23
2. Arneil GC. The nephrotic syndrome. *Pediatr Clin North Am.* (1971) 18:547–59. doi: 10.1016/S0031-3955(16)32565-2
3. Koskimies O, Vilska J, Rapola J, Hallman N. Long-term outcome of primary nephrotic syndrome. *Arch Dis Child.* (1982) 57:544–8. doi: 10.1136/adc.57.7.544
4. Anonymous. Early identification of frequent relapsers among children with minimal change nephrotic syndrome. A report of the international study of kidney disease in children. *J Pediatr.* (1982) 101:514–8. doi: 10.1016/S0022-3476(82) 80692-6
5. Arbeitsgemeinschaft für Pädiatrische Nephrologie. Short versus standard prednisone therapy for initial treatment of idiopathic nephrotic syndrome in children. *Lancet.* (1988) 1:380–3. doi: 10.1016/S0140-6736(88)91182-8
6. Lande MB, Leonard MB. Variability among pediatric nephrologists in the initial therapy of nephrotic syndrome. *Pediatr Nephrol.* (2000) 14:766–9. doi: 10.1007/PL00013433
7. Eddy AA, Symons JM. Nephrotic syndrome in childhood. *Lancet.* (2003) 362:629–39. doi: 10.1016/S0140-6736(03)14184-0
8. Hogg R, Portman RJ, Milliner D, Lemley KV, Eddy A, Ingelfinger J. Evaluation and management of proteinuria and nephrotic syndrome in children: recommendations from a pediatric nephrology panel established at the national kidney foundation conference on proteinuria, albuminuria, risk, assessment, detection and elimination (PARADE). *Pediatrics.* (2000) 106:1242–9. doi: 10.1542/peds.105.6.1242
9. Bagga A, Hari P, Srivastava RN. Prolonged versus standard prednisolone therapy for initial episode of nephrotic syndrome. *Pediatr Nephrol.* (1999) 13:824–7. doi: 10.1007/s004670050708
10. Schulman SL, Kaiser BA, Polinsky MS, Srinivasan R, Baluarte HJ. Predicting the response to cytotoxic therapy for childhood nephrotic syndrome: superiority of response to corticosteroid therapy over histopathologic patterns. *J Pediatr.* (1988) 113:996–1001. doi: 10.1016/S0022-3476(88)80570-5
11. MacHardy N, Miles PV, Massengill SF, Smoyer WE, Mahan JD, Greenbaum L, et al. Management patterns of childhood-onset nephrotic syndrome. *Pediatr Nephrol.* (2009) 24:2193–201. doi: 10.1007/s00467-009-1282-y
12. Fujinaga S, Endo A, Ohtomo Y, Ohtsuka Y, Shimizu T. Uncertainty in management of childhood-onset idiopathic nephrotic syndrome: is the long-term prognosis really favorable? *Pediatr Nephrol.* (2013) 28:2235–8. doi: 10.1007/s00467-013-2553-1
13. Pasini A, Aceto G, Ammenti A, Ardissino G, Azzolina V, Bettinelli A, et al. Best practice guidelines for idiopathic nephrotic syndrome: recommendations versus reality. *Pediatr Nephrol.* (2015) 30:91–101. doi: 10.1007/s00467-014-2903-7
14. Ehrich JH, Brodehl J. Long versus standard prednisone therapy for initial treatment of idiopathic nephrotic syndrome in children. Arbeitsgemeinschaft fur padiatrische nephrologie. *Eur J Pediatr.* (1993) 152:357–61. doi: 10.1007/BF01956754
15. Ksiazek J, Wyszynska T. Short versus long initial prednisone treatment in steroid-sensitive nephrotic syndrome in children. *Acta Paediatr.* (1995) 84:889–93. doi: 10.1111/j.1651-2227.1995.tb13787.x
16. Ueda N, Chihara M, Kawaguchi S, Niinomi Y, Nonoda T, Matsumoto J, et al. Intermittent vs. long-term tapering prednisolone for initial therapy in children with idiopathic nephritic syndrome. *J Pediatr.* (1998) 112:122–6. doi: 10.1016/S0022-3476(88)80136-7
17. Hodson EM, Willis NS, Craig JC. Corticosteroid therapy for nephrotic syndrome in children. *Cochrane Datab Syst Rev.* (2007) CD001533. doi: 10.1002/14651858.CD001533.pub3
18. Takeda A, Matsutani H, Niimura F, Ohgushi H. Risk factors for relapse in childhood nephrotic syndrome. *Pediatr Nephrol.* (1996) 10:740–1. doi: 10.1007/s004670050205
19. Kabuki N, Okugawa T, Hayakawa H, Tomizawa S, Kasahara T, Uchiyama M. Influence of age at onset on the outcome of steroid-sensitive nephrotic syndrome. *Pediatr Nephrol.* (1998) 12:467–70. doi: 10.1007/s004670050489
20. Hiraoka M, Tsukahara H, Haruki S, Hayashi S, Takeda N, Miyagawa K, et al. The West Japan cooperative study of kidney disease in children: older boys benefit from higher initial prednisolone therapy for nephrotic syndrome. *Kidney Int.* (2000) 58:1247–52. doi: 10.1046/j.1523-1755.2000.00279.x
21. Andersen RF, Thrane N, Noergaard K, Rytter L, Jespersen B, Rittig S. Early age at debut is a predictor of steroid-dependent and frequent relapsing nephrotic syndrome. *Pediatr Nephrol.* (2010) 25:1299–304. doi: 10.1007/s00467-010-1537-7
22. Zidar N, Avgustin Cavic M, Kenda RB, Ferluga D. Unfavorable course of minimal change nephrotic syndrome in children with intrauterine growth retardation. *Kidney Int.* (1998) 54:1320–3. doi: 10.1046/j.1523-1755.1998.00121.x
23. Yap HK, Han EJ, Heng CK, Gong WK. Risk factors for steroid dependency in children with idiopathic nephrotic syndrome. *Pediatr Nephrol.* (2001) 16:1049–52. doi: 10.1007/s004670100024
24. Letavernier B, Letavernier E, Leroy S, Baudet-Bonneville V, Bensman A, Ulinski T. Prediction of high-degree steroid dependency in pediatric idiopathic nephrotic syndrome. *Pediatr Nephrol.* (2008) 23:2221–6. doi: 10.1007/s00467-008-0914-y
25. Vivarelli M, Moscaritolo E, Tsalkidis A, Massella L, Emma F. Time for initial response to steroids is a major prognostic factor in idiopathic nephrotic syndrome. *J Pediatr.* (2010) 156:965–71. doi: 10.1016/j.jpeds.2009.12.020
26. Kidney Disease: Improving Global Outcomes (KDIGO) Glomerulonephritis Work Group. KDIGO clinical practice guideline for glomerulonephritis. *Kidney Int Suppl.* (2012) 2:156–62. doi: 10.1038/kisup.2012.15
27. R Core Team. *R: A Language and Environment for Statistical Computing.* Vienna: R Foundation for Statistical Computing (2019). Available online at: https://www.R-project.org/.

28. Hodson EM, Willis NS, Craig JC. Corticosteroid therapy for nephrotic syndrome in children. *Cochrane Database Syst Rev.* (2007) 4:CD001533. doi: 10.1002/14651858.CD001533.pub4
29. Teeninga N, Kist-van Holthe JE, van Rijswijk N, de Mos NI, Hop WC, Wetzels JF, et al. Extending prednisolone treatment does not reduce relapses in childhood nephrotic syndrome. *J Am Soc Nephrol.* (2013) 24:149–59. doi: 10.1681/ASN.2012070646
30. Sinha A, Saha A, Kumar M, Sharma S, Afzal K, Mehta A, et al. Extending initial prednisolone treatment in a randomized control trial from 3 to 6 months did not significantly influence the course of illness in children with steroid-sensitive nephrotic syndrome. *Kidney Int.* (2015) 87:217–24. doi: 10.1038/ki.2014.240
31. Yoshikawa N, Nakanishi K, Sako M, Oba MS, Mori R, Ota E, et al. A multicenter randomized trial indicates initial prednisolone treatment for childhood nephrotic syndrome for two months is not inferior to six-month treatment. *Kidney Int.* (2015) 87:225–32. doi: 10.1038/ki.2014.260
32. Hoyer PF. New lessons from randomized trials in steroid-sensitive nephrotic syndrome: clear evidence against long steroid therapy. *Kidney Int.* (2015) 87:17–9. doi: 10.1038/ki.2014.354
33. Hahn D, Hodson EM, Willis NS, Craig JC. Corticosteroid therapy for nephrotic syndrome in children. *Cochrane Database Syst Rev.* (2015) 2015:CD001533. doi: 10.1002/14651858.CD001533.pub5
34. Webb NJA, Woolley RL, Lambe T, Frew E, Brettell EA, Barsoum EN, et al. Long termtaperingversusstandardprednisolonetreatment for firstepisode of childhoodnephroticsyndrome: phaseIIIrandomisedcontrolledtrial and economicevaluation. *BMJ.* (2019) 365:l1800. doi: 10.1136/bmj.l1800
35. Constantinescu AR, Shah HB, Foote EF, Weiss LS. Predicting first-year relapses in children with nephrotic syndrome. *Pediatrics.* (2000) 105:492–5. doi: 10.1542/peds.105.3.492
36. Fujinaga S, Hirano D, Nishizaki N. Early identification of steroid dependency in Japanese children with steroid sensitive nephrotic syndrome undergoing short-term initial steroid therapy. *Pediatr Nephro.* (2011) 26:485–6. doi: 10.1007/s00467-010-1642-7
37. Nakanishi K, Iijima K, Ishikura K,Hataya H, Nakazato H, Sasaki S, et al. Two-Year outcome of the ISKDC regimen and frequent-relapsing risk in children with idiopathic nephrotic syndrome. *Clin J Am Soc Nephrol.* (2013) 8:756–62. doi: 10.2215/CJN.09010912
38. Harambat J, Godron A, Ernould S, Rigothier C, Llanas B, Leroy S. Prediction of steroid-sparing agent use in childhood idiopathic nephrotic syndrome. *Pediatr Nephrol.* (2013) 28:631–8. doi: 10.1007/s00467-012-2365-8
39. Sureshkumar P, Hodson EM, Willis NS, Barzi F, Craig JC. Predictors of remission and relapse in idiopathic nephrotic syndrome: a prospective cohort study. *Pediatr Nephrol.* (2014) 29:1039–46. doi: 10.1007/s00467-013-2736-9
40. Situmorang D, Sekarwana N, Fadlyana E. Risk factor of frequent relapse in pediatric nephrotic syndrome. *Am J Med Biol Res.* (2016) 4:10–2. doi: 10.12691/ajmbr-4-1-3
41. Sinha A, Hari P, Sharma PK, Gulati A, Kalaivani M, Mantan M, et al. Disease course in steroid sensitive nephrotic syndrome. *Indian Pediatr.* (2012) 49:881–7. doi: 10.1007/s13312-012-0220-4
42. Hiraoka M, Tsukahara H, Matsubara K, Tsurusawa M, Takeda N, Haruki S, et al. West Japan Cooperative Study Group of Kidney Disease in Children. A randomized study of two long-course prednisolone regimens for nephrotic syndrome in children. *Am J Kidney Dis.* 2003 41:1155–62. doi: 10.1016/s0272-6386(03)00346-9
43. Cuzzoni E, De Iudicibus S, Stocco G, Favretto D, Pelin M, Messina G, et al. *In vitro* sensitivity to methyl-prednisolone is associated with clinical response in pediatric idiopathic nephrotic syndrome. *Clin Pharmacol Ther.* (2016) 100:268–74. doi: 10.1002/cpt.372
44. Teeninga N, Kist-van Holthe JE, van den Akker EL, Kersten MC, Boersma E, Krabbe HG, et al. Genetic and *in vivo* determinants of glucocorticoid sensitivity in relation to clinical outcome of childhood nephrotic syndrome. *Kidney Int.* (2014) 85:1444–53. doi: 10.1038/ki.2013.531
45. Turolo S, Edefonti A, Lepore M, Ghio L, Cuzzoni E, Decorti G, et al. SXR rs3842689: a prognostic factor for steroid sensitivity or resistance in pediatric idiopathic nephrotic syndrome. *Pharmacogenomics.* (2016) 17:1227–33. doi: 10.2217/pgs-2016-0029
46. Schijvens AM, Ter Heine R, de Wildt SN, Schreuder MF. Pharmacology and pharmacogenetics of prednisone and prednisolone in patients with nephrotic syndrome. *Pediatr Nephrol.* (2019) 34:389–403. doi: 10.1007/s00467-018-3929-z
47. Cuzzoni E, Franca R, De Iudicibus S, Marcuzzi A, Lucafò M, Pelin M, et al. MIF plasma level as a possible tool to predict steroid responsiveness in children with idiopathic nephrotic syndrome. *Eur J Clin Pharmacol.* (2019) 75:1675–83. doi: 10.1007/s00228-019-02749-3
48. Sibley M, Roshan A, Alshami A, Catapang M, Jöbsis JJ, Kwok T, et al. Induction prednisone dosing for childhood nephrotic syndrome: how low should we go? *Pediatr Nephrol.* (2018) 33:1539–45. doi: 10.1007/s00467-018-3975-6
49. Musah S, Mammoto A, Ferrante TC, Jeanty SSF, Hirano-Kobayashi M, Mammoto T, et al. Mature induced-pluripotent-stem-cell-derived human podocytes reconstitute kidney glomerular-capillary-wall function on a chip. *Nat Biomed Eng.* (2017) 1:0069. doi: 10.1038/s41551-017-0069
50. Veissi S, Smeets B, van den Heuvel LP, Jansen J, Schreuder MF. Nephrotic syndrome in a dish: recent developments in modeling *in vitro*. *Pediatr Nephrol.* (2019) 35:1363–72. doi: 10.1007/s00467-019-4203-8

12

Rituximab for Children With Difficult-to-Treat Nephrotic Syndrome: Its Effects on Disease Progression and Growth

Rezan Topaloğlu[1], Bora Gülhan[1], Kübra Çelegen[1], Mihriban İnözü[1], Mutlu Hayran[2], Ali Düzova[1] and Fatih Ozaltin[1,3,4]*

[1] Division of Pediatric Nephrology, Department of Pediatrics, School of Medicine, Hacettepe University, Ankara, Turkey, [2] Department of Preventive Oncology, School of Medicine, Hacettepe University, Ankara, Turkey, [3] Nephrogenetics Laboratory, School of Medicine, Hacettepe University, Ankara, Turkey, [4] Center for Biobanking and Genomics, School of Medicine, Hacettepe University, Ankara, Turkey

***Correspondence:**
Rezan Topaloğlu
rezantopaloglu@hacettepe.edu.tr

Background: Since the early 2000s rituximab (RTX) has been thought of as an alternative treatment for steroid-sensitive nephrotic syndrome (SSNS) and steroid-resistant nephrotic syndrome (SRNS).

Objective: This study aimed to determine the effects of RTX treatment on disease outcome and growth in pediatric SSNS and SRNS patients.

Materials and Methods: The medical records of pediatric SSNS and SRNS patients that began RTX treatment at the mean age of 10.8 ± 5.1 years between 2009 and 2017 were retrospectively reviewed. Additionally, the effect of RTX on growth was evaluated based on patient height, weight, and BMI z scores.

Results: The study included 41 children, of which 21 had SSNS and 20 had SRNS. Mean age at diagnosis of NS was 5.8 ± 4.7 years. Mean duration of post-RTX treatment follow-up was 2.3 ± 1.6 years. Among the SSNS patients, 6 and 11 patients were steroid free and calcineurin inhibitor free at the last follow-up visit, respectively. The 1-year cumulative steroid and calcineurin inhibitor doses both decreased after RTX treatment, as compared to before RTX ($P = 0.001$ and $P = 0.015$, respectively). The median height *z*-score at the time of RTX initiation was −1.2 and the median height *z*-score at the last follow-up visit was −0.6 ($P = 0.044$). The median BMI *z*-score decreased from 1.6 (IQR; 0.9–3.0) at the time RTX was initiated to 1.1 IQR; [(−0.7)−2.5] at the last follow-up visit ($P = 0.007$). At the last follow-up visit 4 SRNS patients had complete remission and 4 had partial remission. The 1-year cumulative steroid dosage in the SRNS patients decreased significantly after RTX, as compared to before RTX ($P = 0.001$). The median height *z*-score at the time of RTX initiation was −0.8 and the median height *z*-score at the last follow-up visit was −0.7 ($P = 0.81$). The median BMI *z*-score decreased from 0.3 at the time RTX was initiated to −0.1 at the last follow-up visit ($P = 0.11$).

Conclusion: RTX has a more positive effect on disease outcome and growth in SSNS patients than in those with SRNS.

Keywords: rituximab, nephrotic syndrome, steroid, cyclosporine, growth

INTRODUCTION

Idiopathic nephrotic syndrome (NS) is a major challenge in pediatric nephrology. The mainstay of NS treatment is steroid therapy. Nearly 80–90% of NS patients respond to steroid therapy and are considered to have steroid-sensitive NS (SSNS) (1). Approximately 60% of SSNS patients develop frequently relapsing NS (FRNS) or steroid-dependent NS (SDNS). In contrast, 10–20% of NS patients have steroid-resistant NS (SRNS) and do not respond to steroid therapy (2). Some SRNS patients can achieve partial or complete remission with calcineurin inhibitor (CNI) treatment (3). How best to treat NS patients that do not respond to steroids or CNIs remains a challenge. Moreover, patients with both FRNS/SDNS and SRNS usually require long-term steroid therapy, which is associated with the risk of serious side effects, including obesity, growth retardation, osteoporosis, glaucoma, cataracts, and hypertension (2).

Due to the problems associated with treating NS with steroids and CNIs, rituximab (RTX) has recently become an important alternative treatment option. RTX is an immunoglobulin IgG1-kappa type, mouse-human chimeric monoclonal antibody, with murine anti-CD20 variable sequence regions and human constant sequence regions. RTX binds specifically to the CD20 antigen, which is expressed on pre B-cells, and immature, mature, and memory B-cells, but not on plasma cells (4). Benz et al. (5) were the first to report the use of RTX in NS patients. Subsequently, additional case reports provided additional observational evidence of the positive effect of RTX on NS (6). Large series on the use of RTX reported that other immunosuppressive drugs could be withdrawn. However, the relapse rate is high when the CD19 and CD20 counts returned to normal (7). Reports of the efficacy of RTX for treating both SSNS and SRNS have been encouraging (8, 9).

The first RTX protocols for NS were based on lymphoma, with a once-weekly dose of 375 mg/m^2 for 4 weeks. This protocol was modified in many institutions as 2 weekly doses of 750 mg/m^2 plus maintenance dosing at regular intervals (4). In addition, some RTX researchers focused on RTX's effect on height and weight in children (2). Accordingly, the present study aimed to determine the long-term effects of RTX treatment on disease progression in children with SSNS and SRNS, and to analyze its effect on height and weight.

MATERIALS AND METHODS

Patients and Definitions

Medical records of Caucasian SSNS and SRNS patients aged 1–20 years that were treated with RTX between 2009 and 2017 were retrospectively reviewed. Patients that were included in the study met the following criteria: 1. Onset of idiopathic NS at age >1 year; 2. Initiation of RTX treatment at age <19 years. Standard definitions were used for NS, remission, relapse, and steroid resistance (10, 11). Frequently relapsing NS was defined as ≥2 relapses within 6 months of achieving initial remission or ≥4 relapses in any 12-month period. SDNS was defined as 2 consecutive relapses while tapering the prednisolone dose or within 15 d of prednisolone discontinuation. SRNS was defined as lack of remission despite prednisolone 2 mg/kg/d (maximum: 60 mg/d) for 4 weeks, followed by 3 methylprednisolone pulses (12). Complete remission was defined as a urinary protein/creatinine ratio (Up/Uc) <0.2 mg/mg and partial remission was defined as a Up/Uc of 0.2–2 mg/mg and serum albumin >2.5 g/dL. All SRNS patients were screened for genetic mutations that cause steroid resistance.

The study protocol was approved by the Hacettepe University Ethics Committee (GO18/1136) and written informed consent was provided by the patients' parents and patients who were >10 years of age. The study was conducted in accordance with the World Medical Association Declaration of Helsinki.

Immunosuppressive Therapies

Steroid therapy was initiated as 2 mg/kg/d (maximum: 60 mg/d) and continued for 4 weeks, followed by tapering as 1.5 mg/kg/d (maximum: 60 mg/d) q.o.d. for 4 weeks, 1 mg/kg/d q.o.d. for 4 weeks, 0.5 mg/kg/d q.o.d. for 4 weeks, and then 0.25 mg/kg/d on q.o.d. for 6–12 months (13). Relapse was treated with prednisolone 2 mg/kg/d (maximum: 60 mg/d) until remission (zero or trace proteinuria for 3 consecutive d), followed by prednisolone 2 mg/kg/d q.o.d. for 2 weeks, and then tapering (1 mg/kg/d q.o.d. for 2 weeks, 0.5 mg/kg/d q.o.d. for 2 weeks, and 0.25 mg/kg/d q.o.d. for 2 weeks and continued for 12 months). Cyclosporine 1–4 mg/kg/d b.i.d. was administered to maintain a through level of 50–100 ng/mL. Cumulative steroid and CNI dosages before and after RTX were also calculated. After obtaining parental/patient consent, patients were administered 2–4 weekly doses of RTX (375 mg/m^2/dose).

Each patient's attending physician decided on the number of RTX doses for induction and maintenance. Premedication consisted of diphenhydramine, acetaminophen, and methylprednisolone (1 mg/kg, max. 60 mg) 30 min before RTX infusion. The standard methylprednisolone dose was also included in the calculation of cumulative steroid doses. Maintenance RTX treatment was given to some patients every 6–12 months, according to the clinical assessment made by their physician. Following RTX treatment, prophylactic trimethoprim-sulfamethoxazole t.i.w. was routinely administered. In order to prevent relapse, maintenance immunosuppressive therapy was continued, which could be stopped in some of the patients. CD19 and CD20 counts were not performed in all the patients on a regular basis.

Growth Parameters

Height, weight, and BMI z-scores were assessed at the time RTX was initiated and at the last follow-up visit. Standard height, weight, and BMI scores were based on Turkish children growth curves. BMI was calculated as kg/height (m)^2.

Statistical Analysis

Descriptive statistical analysis was used to evaluate demographic and clinical data. Mean ± SD, median, and IQR (interquartile range) were calculated for numeric variables. Frequency tables were used to describe categorical data. The Mann-Whitney U-test or the independent t-test was used to compare 2 independent samples. Survival analysis was performed using Kaplan-Meier analysis with overall log-rank testing. All data were analyzed using IBM SPSS Statistics for Windows v.21 (IBM Corp., Armonk, NY).

RESULTS

Among the 41 pediatric NS patients included in the study, 21 (51.2%) had SSNS (20 SDNS and 1 FRNS) and 20 (48.8%) had SRNS. Mean duration of follow-up after RTX treatment was 2.3 ± 1.6 years. Additional patient clinical characteristics are given in the **Table 1**.

SSNS Patients

In all, 21 (51.2%) of the NS patients had SSNS. All of these patients used steroid and CNI before RTX. Additional clinical features are given in the **Table 1**. The mean time from diagnosis of NS to the first RTX infusion was 6.4 ± 3.8 years. As induction treatment, RTX was given as 2, 3, and 4 doses in 4, 10, and 7 patients, respectively. Regular maintenance RTX treatment (every 6–12 months) was given to 10 patients (47.6%). Median number of cumulative RTX infusions was 4 (IQR; 3–6). Following RTX treatment, as maintenance treatment cyclosporine A was given to 10 of the patients and mycophenolate mofetil (MMF) was given to 2.

The median number of relapses during the first 2 years after RTX was 0 (IQR; 0–2), as compared to 4 (IQR; 2.5–6) during the 2 years before RTX ($P = 0.001$). In total, 8 (38%) of the SSNS patients relapsed after RTX. Among the relapsed patients, the mean time from RTX discontinuation to first relapse was 14.6 ± 11.7 months. In addition, among the relapsed patients RTX induction treatment was administered as 2 doses in 2 patients, 3 doses in 2 patients, and 4 doses in 4 patients. Kaplan-Meier analysis showed that age at diagnosis of NS, time from diagnosis of NS to RTX, age at initiation of RTX, renal histological diagnosis before RTX, and the number of RTX doses for both induction and maintenance were not associated with the first relapse after RTX treatment. The post-RTX relapse-free period did not differ significantly between the patients that received RTX induction treatment as 2, 3, and 4 doses ($p = 0.48$).

At the last follow-up visit 2 (9.5%) of the SSNS patients were in relapse, 3 (14.3%) in partial remission, and 16 (76.2%) in complete remission. At the last follow-up visit 6 of the patients were steroid free, 11 were still receiving steroid treatment of ≤0.5 mg/kg/d, and 4 were receiving steroid treatment at 0.5–1.1 mg/kg/d. At last follow-up visit, 11 of the SSNS patients were CNI free, 10 were still receiving CNI 2.4 ± 1.0 mg/kg/d, and 4 were both CNI free and steroid free.

Median cumulative steroid dose was 117.8 mg/kg (IQR; 75.6–152 mg/kg) for 0–12 months before RTX and 69.6 mg/kg (IQR; 51.4–133 mg/kg) for 12–24 months before RTX. At 0–12 months post RTX treatment the median cumulative steroid dose decreased to 34 mg/kg (IQR; 20–48 mg/kg; $P = 0.001$) and 24.5 mg/kg (7.5–74.8 mg/kg) 12–24 months post RTX ($P = 0.013$). The median cumulative cyclosporine dose was 811.5 mg/kg (IQR; 594.8–937.5 mg/kg) 0–12 months before RTX and 782.5 mg/kg (IQR; 519–1057.3 mg/kg) 12–24 months before RTX. At 0–12 months post RTX the median cumulative cyclosporine dose decreased to 583.5 mg/kg (IQR; 305.8–903 mg/kg) mg/kg ($P = 0.015$) and 725 mg/kg (IQR; 81.5–798 mg/kg) 12–24 months post RTX ($P = 0.028$; **Figures 1A,B**). Mean GFR at initiation of RTX and at the last follow-up visit was 202.1 ± 55.8 mL/min/1.73 m^2 and 176.9 ± 50.1 mL/min/1.73 m^2, respectively ($P = 0.14$).

At the initiation of RTX 18 (85.7%) of the SSNS patients had a height z-score <0 and their mean time from NS diagnosis to initiation of RTX was 6.6 ± 4.1 years. Among the SSNS patients, 3 (14.3%) had a height z-score >0 at initiation of RTX and their median time from NS diagnosis to initiation of RTX was 5.5 ± 1.4 years ($P = 0.60$). Steroid treatment duration of the patients with a height z-score <0 (6.8 ± 4.0 years) and >0 (4.0 ± 1.4 years) at the time of RTX was not statistically different ($P = 0.35$). Similarly, mean duration of cyclosporine treatment did not differ significantly according to height z-score (z-score <0: 3.7 ± 2.8 years; z-score >0: 2.0 ± 2.0 years; $P = 0.51$). In total, the height z-score in 11 (52.3%) SSNS patients improved after RTX treatment; the median height z-score at initiation of RTX was −1.2 [IQR; (−2.5)–(−0.3)], vs. −0.6 [IQR; (−1.9)–(−0.1)] at the last follow-up visit ($P = 0.044$). At the last follow-up visit the BMI z-score in 15 (71.4%) SSNS patients was lower than at initiation of RTX; the median BMI z-score decreased from 1.6 (IQR; 0.9–3.0) at the time of initiation of RTX treatment to 1.1 (IQR; [(−0.7)–2.5] at the last follow-up visit ($P = 0.007$).

SRNS Patients

In total, 20 of the NS patients (48.8%) had SRNS, all of which were also resistant to CNIs. Mean duration of follow-up after RTX was 2.0 ± 1.4 years. Additional clinical features are given in the **Table 1**. RTX induction treatment was administered as 2 doses in 2 patients, 3 doses in 4 patients, and 4 doses in 14 patients. Among the SRNS patients, 14 (70%) received maintenance RTX every 6–12 months. Median number of cumulative RTX infusions was 6 (IQR; 4–7). Rituximab treatment was discontinued in 5 SRNS patients that progressed to chronic renal failure (<90 ml/min/1.73 m^2).

At the last follow-up visit 4 (20%) of the SRNS patients had complete remission and 4 (20%) had partial remission, whereas 6 patients still had active disease with normal GFR (≥90 ml/min/1.73 m^2) and 6 others had a GFR <90 mL/min/1.73 m^2. Steroids were discontinued in 2 SRNS patients with complete remission and partial remission, and cyclosporine was withdrawn in 4 patients with partial remission. The 1-year cumulative steroid dose decreased significantly after RTX, as compared to before RTX (0–12 months). In contrast, the 1-year cumulative cyclosporine dose before and after RTX did not differ significantly (**Figures 1C,D**).

The median cumulative steroid dose 0–12 months before RTX was 77 mg/kg (IQR; 46.7–240.5 mg/kg), and 166 mg/kg (IQR: 56.3–572.3 mg/kg) for 12–24 months before RTX. The median cumulative steroid dose 0–12 months post RTX decreased to 56.2 mg/kg (IQR; 21.8–95.5 mg/kg; $P = 0.01$) and 56.5 mg/kg (IQR: 9.4–83.5 mg/kg) 12–24 months post RTX ($P = 0.063$). The median cumulative cyclosporine dose was 927 mg/kg (IQR; 496–1187.5 mg/kg) 0–12 months before

TABLE 1 | Demographic and clinical characteristics of the SSNS and SRNS patients.

Parameters	Total	SSNS	SRNS	P**
Boys (n) (%)/Girls (n) (%)	22(53.7)/19 (46.3)	10 (47.6)/11 (52.4)	8 (40)/12 (60)	0.43
Age of diagnosis of NS* (mean ± SD) (years)	5.8 ± 4.7	4.4 ± 3.6	7.3 ± 5.2	0.17
Age of first RTX* treatment (mean ± SD) (years)	10.8 ± 5.1	10.8 ± 4.3	10.9 ± 5.6	0.62
Duration of follow-up after RTX* treatment (mean ± SD) (years)	2.3 ± 1.6	2.5 ± 1.8	2.0 ± 1.4	0.44
Age at last visit (mean ± SD) (years)	13.0 ± 5.5	13.1 ± 5.6	12.9 ± 5.5	0.95
Number of the patients with renal biopsy before RTX* (FSGS/MCD/MGN/C1qN*) (n = 36)	19/14/2/1	5/10/1/0	14/4/1/1	0.64
Duration of steroid treatment before RTX* treatment (for SSNS; mean ± SD, for total and SRNS; median, IQR) (years)	4.3 (2.0–8.4)	6.4 ± 3.8	2.2 (1–5.8)	**0.028**
Duration of cyclosporine treatment before RTX* treatment (for SSNS; mean ± SD, for total and SRNS; median, IQR) (years)	1.5 (0.8–6)	3.5 ± 2.7	0.8 (0.5–2.8)	**0.018**
Serum albumin level at the time of RTX* (mean ± SD) (g/dl)	3.1 ± 0.9	3.7 ± 0.7	2.5 ± 0.8	**<0.001**
Urinary protein/creatinine ratio at the time of RTX* (median) (IQR) (mg/mg)	5.6 (0.14–7.9)	0.14 (0.1–1.3)	6.8 (1.4–15.4)	**<0.001**
Steroid dosage before RTX* (0–12 months) (median) (IQR) (mg/kg)	112.5 (57.6–176)	117.8 (75.6–152)	77 (46.7–240.5)	0.98
Steroid dosage after RTX* (0–12 months) (median) (IQR) (mg/kg)	36.3 (21–62)	34 (20–48)	56.2 (21.8–95.5)	0.15
Steroid dosage before RTX* (12–24 months) (median) (IQR) (mg/kg)	87.5 (53.5–220.5)	69.6 (51.4–133)	166 (56.3–572.3)	0.19
Steroid dosage after RTX* (12–24 months) (median) (IQR) (mg/kg)	28.7 (7.5–74.8)	24.5 (7.5–74.8)	56.5 (9.4–83.5)	0.68
Cyclosporine dosage before RTX* (0–12 months) (median) (IQR) (mg/kg)	831 (596.5–1057)	811.5 (594.8–937.5)	927 (496–1187.5)	0.34
Cyclosporine dosage after RTX* (0–12 months) (median) (IQR) (mg/kg)	743 (316.8–909)	583.5 (305.8–903)	770.5 (336.8–925.4)	0.63
Cyclosporine dosage before RTX* (12–24 months) (median) (IQR) (mg/kg)	750 (446–934.5)	782.5 (519–1057.3)	630 (397–929.5)	0.49
Cyclosporine dosage after RTX* (12–24 months) (median) (IQR) (mg/kg)	436 (0–735)	725 (81.5–798)	405.5 (0–555.5)	0.32

FSGS, focal segmental glomerulosclerosis; GN, glomerulonephritis; IQR, inter-quartile range; MCD, minimal change disease; MGN, membranous glomerulonephritis; NS, nephrotic syndrome; RTX, rituximab; SD, standard deviation. P is for comparison of related values of SSNS and SRNS.*
Bold values indicate the statistically significant (<0.05) parameters.

RTX, and 630 mg/kg (IQR; 397–929.5 mg/kg) 12–24 months before RTX. The median cumulative cyclosporine dose 0–12 months post RTX decreased to 770.5 mg/kg (IQR; 336.8–925.4 mg/kg; $P = 0.51$), as compared to 405.5 mg/kg (IQR; 0–555.5 mg/kg) 12–24 months post RTX ($P = 0.80$; **Table 1**). Mean GFR at initiation of RTX and at the last follow-up visit was 214.6±181.6 mL/min/1.73 m^2 and 128.5±63.2 mL/min/1.73 m^2, respectively ($P = 0.28$).

At the initiation of RTX 15 of the SRNS patients had a height z-score <0 and their median time from NS diagnosis to RTX initiation was 3.9 ± 3.9 years. Five patients had a height z-score >0 and their median time from NS diagnosis to RTX initiation was 2.8 ± 2.5 years ($P = 0.80$). The duration of steroid treatment did not differ significantly between the SRNS patients with a height z-score <0 (7.2 ± 10.4 years) and >0 zero (2.0 ± 1.5 years) at RTX initiation ($P = 0.23$). Similarly, the duration of cyclosporine treatment in the patients with a height z-score <0 (2.4 ± 3.7 years) and >0 (1.7 ± 1.3 years) at initiation of RTX did not differ significantly ($P = 0.74$). The height z-score improved in 8 of the SRNS patients after RTX treatment; the median height z-score at initiation of RTX was −0.8 [IQR; (−2.2)-(0.03)], vs. −0.7 [IQR; (−2.1)−0.4] at the last follow-up visit ($p = 0.81$). At the last follow-up visit the BMI z-score in 13 (65%) SRNS patients was lower than at initiation of RTX; the median BMI z-score decreased from 0.3 [IQR; (−0.8)−1.0] at initiation of RTX to −0.1 [IQR;(−1.0)−0.8] at the last follow-up visit ($p = 0.11$).

Adverse Effects

Only 1 SSNS patient and 2 SRNS patients had mild RTX infusion-related adverse reactions (tingling of the throat). In all patients, the rate of RTX infusion was decreased and these adverse effects did not persist. Additionally, they did not re-occur in following RTX doses. All patients continued RTX doses. None of the patients had serious infections, such as peritonitis, cellulitis, and thrombosis, or other adverse events.

DISCUSSION

The present study aimed to determine the effects of RTX on disease outcome and growth parameters in pediatric SSNS and SRNS patients. Fornoni et al. (14) observed that RTX can bind directly to the sphingomyelin phosphodiesterase

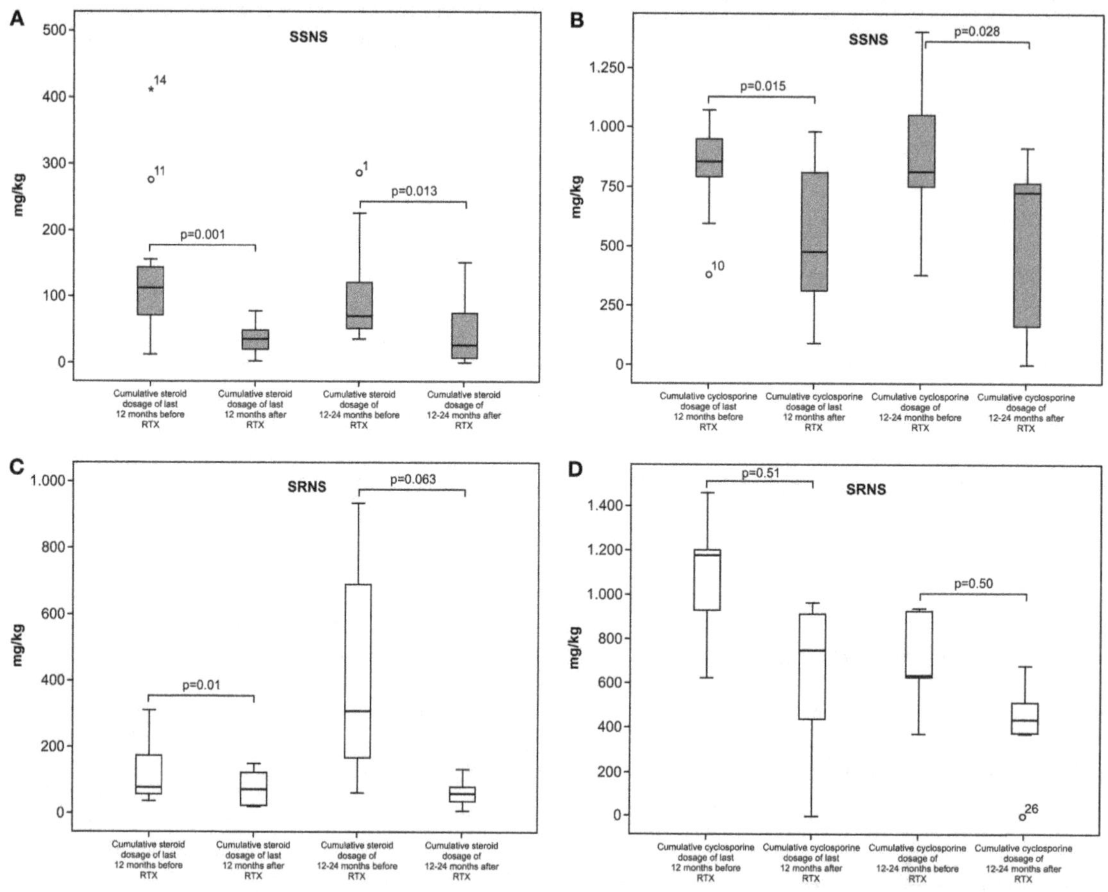

FIGURE 1 | (A,B) cumulative steroid and cyclosporine doses in the SSNS patients 12 months before and 12 months after RTX treatment. **(C,D)** cumulative steroid and cyclosporine doses in the SRNS patients 12 months before and 12 months after RTX treatment.

acid-like 3b protein (SMPDL3b), which is a component of phospholipid membranes that prevents SMPDL3b down-regulation in podocytes. RTX's relevance to NS was first reported in 2004 (5); subsequently, numerous studies on RTX and NS were performed: however, there remains a lack of consensus regarding the use of RTX for treating NS, including the optimal regimen for initial treatment (dose and number of doses). Kamei et al. (15) reported that Japanese patients with a single dose of RTX had a higher rate (75%) of relapse than those given multiple doses. The researchers concluded that the ability of a single RTX dose to prevent relapses was transient and that most relapses occur in association with recovery of B-cells. Kemper et al. (7) studied 37 SDNS patients and reported that among the 21 that received 1 dose of RTX, 64.8% relapsed. The researchers also noted that the time to first relapse was shorter in the patients that received 1 or 2 doses of RTX, as compared to those that received 3 or 4 doses. Lastly, they reported that the number of RTX induction doses did not affect long-term prognosis.

Fujinaga et al. (16) studied the predictors of relapse and long-term outcome in 43 SDNS patients given a single dose of RTX as induction treatment. In all, 91% of their patients relapsed. In addition, the relapse-free survival rate in the patients aged <12.5 years at the time of initial RTX treatment was shorter than in those aged ≥12.5 years. Furthermore, age at RTX initiation and the duration of relapse-free periods was positively correlated. The researchers also noted that the early relapse rate after RTX was significantly higher in the patients with shorter CD19 depletion. Tellier et al. (17) studied the long-term outcome in 18 SDNS patients with a median duration of follow-up of 3.2 years. They observed a relapse rate of 56% during a 2-year period following RTX treatment. In addition, 44.5% of the patients were free of therapy at the last follow-up visit. In the present study 38% of the SSNS patients relapsed following RTX treatment, but age and the number of RTX doses administered for both induction and maintenance were not associated with the first post-RTX relapse. Furthermore, in the present study 20% of SSNS patients were free of oral drug therapy.

Findings regarding the efficacy of maintenance immunosuppressive drug treatment following RTX are inconsistent. Ito et al. (18) reported that maintenance therapy with MMF is effective in SDNS patients, whereas Fujinaga et al. (19) compared MMF and cyclosporine after 1 dose of RTX in SDNS patients, reporting that treatment failure occurred more frequently in those given MMF and that the sustained remission rate was higher in the cyclosporine group. In the present study most of the NS patients received cyclosporine as maintenance therapy and the type of maintenance therapy did not affect the time to first relapse after RTX treatment.

Sinha et al. (8) published one of the largest studies on RTX in NS (SSNS and SRNS) patients. They included 101 SDNS patients, of which 82 received 2 doses of RTX initially. The authors found that both cumulative steroid dosage and number of relapses were lower at in time periods 6 and 12 months after RTX compared to 6 and 12 months prior RTX. Similarly, in the present study the cumulative steroid dose 12 months after RTX was lower than 12 months before RTX. Moreover, the present study also calculated the cyclosporine dose before and after RTX, observing that the cumulative cyclosporine dose was lower after RTX than before RTX. More recently, Ravani et al. (20) performed a multicenter, open label, non-inferiority trial with pediatric SDNS patients that had developed SDNS during the previous the 6–12 months and were maintained in remission with high-dose prednisone. Their patients were divided into 2 groups: prednisone (control) and single-dose RTX (intervention). They concluded that RTX was not inferior to steroids for the treatment of SDNS.

The rate of response to RTX in SRNS patients is lower than in SSNS patients, even when SSNS patients receive RTX during periods of relapse. The first report of RTX treatment in SRNS patients included 5 Indian children treated with RTX, of which 3 achieved complete remission and 2 achieved partial remission (21). Prytula et al. (22) studied 27 SRNS patients with different RTX regimes. In this cohort, 17 patients received two doses of 750 mg/m^2 every 14 days and 6 patients received single dose of RTX (375 mg/m^2). The rest of the patients received other treatment regimes of RTX. After these RTX doses, 6 patients (22%) achieved full remission and 6 patients (22%) had proteinuria with serum albumin >30 g/L. Sinha et al. (8) reported a series of 58 NS patients that were steroid and calcineurin resistant. Most of the patients ($n = 39$) received 4 doses of RTX, and complete remission and partial remission were observed in 12.1 and 17.2% of the patients, respectively. Fujinaga et al. (23) studied the long-term outcome of early RTX treatment in 6 NS patients that were both cyclosporine and steroid resistant. Following RTX treatment, and then intravenous pulse methylprednisolone and/or high-dose prednisolone, all patients achieved complete remission.

The findings above, in whole, show that the response to RTX varies geographically. The present study's findings fall between those of the 2 geographic regions described above. Complete or partial remission was observed in 40% of the present study's patients, respectively. Some of the SSNS and SRNS patients in the present study received periodic RTX dose, as reported earlier (24). Based on the present findings, we think that such dosing regimens might have a positive effect on remission.

The effect of RTX on growth in children is another contentious issue. Kamei et al. (25) measured the height of 21 SSNS patients aged ≤10 years at initiation of RTX and at the last follow-up visit, reporting that the height z-score did not differ significantly between the 2 time points. Sato et al. (2) investigated the effect of RTX on height and weight in 13 SDNS patients, and observed that the height z-score for all 13 patients was higher at the last follow-up visit and the height z-score of 10 of the 13 patients increased significantly following RTX treatment. Lastly, they noted that the obesity index in 12 of the 13 patients improved significantly following RTX treatment. More recently, Basu et al. (26) compared the efficacy of RTX and tacrolimus in SDNS patients in a randomized clinical trial. They reported a higher 12-month absolute change in the height z-score in the RTX arm, as compared to the tacrolimus arm. In the present study the height z-score in 50% of the patients improved following RTX treatment and the median height z-score at the last follow-up visit was higher than at the time of initiation of RTX treatment. RTX had a similarly positive effect on BMI in the present study's SSNS and SRNS patients. These positive effects of RTX on growth were less prominent in SRNS patients than in the SSNS patients; only 40% of the SRNS had an improved height z-score after RTX treatment, and the median height z-score among the SRNS patients at the last follow-up visit and at the time of initiation of RTX did not differ significantly. These findings might have been due to the shorter duration of steroid treatment before RTX in SRNS patients than in the SSNS patients.

In conclusion, the positive effects of RTX on disease progression and growth (height and BMI) are more prominent in SSNS patients than in SRNS patients. RTX causes decreased number of relapses, cumulative steroid, and calcineurin dosages.

AUTHOR CONTRIBUTIONS

RT, BG, FO, and AD: research formulation and study design. KÇ, Mİ, and BG: data acquisition. RT, BG, and MH: data analysis/interpretation. MH and BG: statistical analysis. RT: supervision/mentorship. Each of the authors contributed important intellectual content during manuscript drafting and/or revision, and approved the final version. Furthermore, they all accept responsibility for the overall work, including the accuracy and integrity of all portions of the work.

REFERENCES

1. Iijima K, Sako M, Kamei K, Nozu K. Rituximab in steroid-sensitive nephrotic syndrome: lessons from clinical trials. *Pediatr Nephrol.* (2018) 33:1449–55. doi: 10.1007/s00467-017-3746-9
2. Sato M, Ito S, Ogura M, Kamei K. Impact of rituximab on height and weight in children with refractory steroid-dependent nephrotic syndrome. *Pediatr Nephrol*. (2014) 29:1373–9. doi: 10.1007/s00467-014-2792-9
3. Tullus K, Webb H, Bagga A. Management of steroid-resistant nephrotic syndrome in children and adolescents. *Lancet Child Adolesc Health.* (2018) 2:880–90. doi: 10.1016/S2352-4642(18)30283-9
4. Tullus K, Marks SD. Indications for use and safety of rituximab in childhood renal diseases. *Pediatr Nephrol.* (2013) 28:1001–9. doi: 10.1007/s00467-012-2260-3
5. Benz K, Dotsch J, Rascher W, Stachel D. Change of the course of steroid-dependent nephrotic syndrome after rituximab therapy. *Pediatr Nephrol.* (2004) 19:794–7. doi: 10.1007/s00467-004-1434-z

6. Iijima K, Sako M, Nozu K. Rituximab for nephrotic syndrome in children. *Clin Exp Nephrol.* (2017) 21:193–202. doi: 10.1007/s10157-016-1313-5
7. Kemper M, Gellermann J, Habbig S, Krmar RT, Dittrich K, Jungraithmayr T, et al. Long-term follow-up after rituximab for steroid-dependent idiopathic nephrotic syndrome. *Nephrol Dial Transplant.* (2012) 27:1910–5. doi: 10.1093/ndt/gfr548
8. Sinha A, Bhatia D, Gulati A, Rawat M, Dinda AK, Hari P, et al. Efficacy and safety of rituximab in children with difficult-to treat nephrotic syndrome. *Nephrol Dial Transplant.* (2015) 30:96–106. doi: 10.1093/ndt/gfu267
9. Basu B, Mahapatra TK, Mondal N. Mycophenolate mofetil following rituximab in children with steroid-resistant nephrotic syndrome. *Pediatrics.* (2015) 136:e132–9. doi: 10.1542/peds.2015-0486
10. Kidney Disease Improving Global Outcomes (KDIGO). Steroid-sensitive nephrotic syndrome in children. *Kidney Int.* (2012) 2(Suppl 2):163–71. doi: 10.1038/kisup.2012.16
11. Indian Pediatric Nephrology Group. Management of steroid sensitive nephrotic syndrome. revised guidelines. *Indian Pediatr.* (2008) 45:203–14.
12. Niaudet P, Gagnadoux MF, Broyer M. Treatment of childhood steroid-resistant idiopathic nephrotic syndrome. *Adv Nephrol Necker Hosp.* (1998) 28:43–61.
13. Saatçi Ü, Beşbaş N. *Primer Nefrotik Sendromda Tedavi Yaklaşımları.* Ankara: Çocuk Nefroloji Derneği Yayınları (1990).
14. Fornoni A, Sageshima J, Wei C, Merscher-Gomez S, Aguillon-Prada R, Jauregui AN, et al. Rituximab targets podocytes in recurrent focal segmental glomerulosclerosis. *Sci Transl Med.* (2011) 3:85ra46. doi: 10.1126/scitranslmed.3002231
15. Kamei K, Ito S, Nozu K, Fujinaga S, Nakayama M, Sako M, et al. Single dose of rituximab for refractory steroid-dependent nephrotic syndrome in children. *Pediatr Nephrol.* (2009) 24:1321–8. doi: 10.1007/s00467-009-1191-0
16. Fujinaga S, Hirano D, Mizutani A, Sakuraya K, Yamada A, Sakurai S, et al. Predictors of relapse and long-term outcome in children with steroid-dependent nephrotic syndrome after rituximab treatment. *Clin Exp Nephrol.* (2017) 21:671–6. doi: 10.1007/s10157-016-1328-y
17. Tellier S, Brochard K, Garnier A, Bandin F, Llanas B, Guigonis V, et al. Long-term outcome of children treated with rituximab for idiopathic nephrotic syndrome. *Pediatr Nephrol.* (2013) 28:911–8. doi: 10.1007/s00467-012-2406-3
18. Ito S, Kamei K, Ogura M, Sato M, Fujimaru T, Ishikawa T, et al. Maintenance therapy with mycophenolatemofetil after rituximab in pediatric patients with steroid-dependent nephrotic syndrome. *Pediatr Nephrol.* (2011) 26:1823–8. doi: 10.1007/s00467-011-1886-x
19. Fujinaga S, Someya T, Watanabe T, Ito A, Ohtomo Y, Shimizu T, et al. Cyclosporine versus mycophenolate mofetil for maintenance of remission of steroid-dependent nephrotic syndrome after a single infusion of rituximab. *Eur J Pediatr.* (2013) 172:513–8. doi: 10.1007/s00431-012-1913-3
20. Ravani P, Rossi R, Bonanni A, Quinn RR, Sica F, Bodria M, et al. Rituximab in children with steroid-dependent nephrotic syndrome: a multicenter, open-label, noninferiority, randomized controlled trial. *J Am Soc Nephrol.* (2015) 26:2259–66. doi: 10.1681/ASN.2014080799
21. Bagga A, Sinha A, Moudgil A. Rituximab in patients with the steroid-resistant nephrotic syndrome. *N Engl J Med.* (2007) 356:2751–2. doi: 10.1056/NEJMc063706
22. Prytula A, İijima K, Kamei K, Geary D, Gottlich E, Majeed A, et al. Rituximab in refractory nephrotic syndrome. *Pediatr Nephrol.* (2010) 25:461–8. doi: 10.1007/s00467-009-1376-6
23. Fujinaga S, Nishino T, Umeda C, Tomii Y, Watanabe Y, Sakuraya K. Long-term outcomes after early treatment with rituximab for Japanese children with cyclosporine- and steroid-resistant nephrotic syndrome. *Pediatr Nephrol.* (2019) 34:353–7. doi: 10.1007/s00467-018-4145-6
24. Takahashi T, Okamoto T, Sato Y, Yamazaki T, Hayashi A, Aoyagi H, et al. Periodically repeated rituximab administrations in children with refractory nephrotic syndrome: 2-year multicentre observational study. *Pediatr Nephrol.* (2019) 34:87–96. doi: 10.1007/s00467-018-4063-7
25. Kamei K, Ishikura K, Sako M, Aya K, Tanaka R, Nozu K, et al. Long-term outcome of childhood-onset complicated nephrotic syndrome after a multicenter, double-blind, randomized, placebo-controlled trial of rituximab. *Pediatr Nephrol.* (2017) 32:2071–8. doi: 10.1007/s00467-017-3718-0
26. Basu B, Sander A, Roy B, Preussler S, Barua S, Mahapatra TKS, et al. Efficacy of rituximab vs tacrolimus in pediatric corticosteroid-dependent nephrotic syndrome: a randomized clinical trial. *JAMA Pediatr.* (2018) 172:757–64. doi: 10.1001/jamapediatrics.2018.1323

13

Adrenal Insufficiency in Children With Nephrotic Syndrome on Corticosteroid Treatment

Karmila Abu Bakar[1,2], Khairunnisa Khalil[2,3], Yam Ngo Lim[2], Yok Chin Yap[2], Mirunalini Appadurai[2], Sangeet Sidhu[2], Chee Sing Lai[2], Azriyanti Anuar Zaini[1], Nurshadia Samingan[1] and Muhammad Yazid Jalaludin[1]*

[1] *Pediatric Unit, Faculty of Medicine, University of Malaya, Kuala Lumpur, Malaysia,* [2] *Pediatric Institute of the Hospital, Kuala Lumpur, Malaysia,* [3] *Paediatric Nephrology Unit, Institute of Paediatrics, Kuala Lumpur, Malaysia*

***Correspondence:**
Muhammad Yazid Jalaludin
yazidj@ummc.edu.my

Background: Adrenal insufficiency can result from impaired functions at all levels of hypothalamic-pituitary-adrenal (HPA) axis. We here studied risk factors associated with adrenal insufficiency in children receiving prolonged exogenous steroid treatment for nephrotic syndrome.

Method: We performed low-dose Synacthen tests (LDSTs, 0.5 μg/m²) in children with steroid-sensitive nephrotic syndrome 4–6 weeks after discontinuation of the corticosteroid therapy. We measured early morning serum cortisol levels at baseline and at intervals of 10, 20, 30, and 60 min following the stimulation test. We defined normal HPA axis stimulation responses as those with peak cortisol cut-off values >550 nmol/L.

Result: We enrolled 37 children for this study research. All children enrolled had normal early morning cortisol levels. However, 13 (35.1%) demonstrated HPA axis suppression (by LDST) 4–+6 weeks after discontinuation of oral prednisolone. Nephrotic syndrome diagnosed before 5 years of age (OR, 0.75; 95% CI, 0.57–0.99; $p = 0.043$), and steroid-dependence [OR, 5.58; 95% confidence interval (CI), 1.06–29.34; $p = 0.042$] were associated with increased risk of developing adrenal suppression after steroid discontinuation.

Conclusion: HPA axis suppression, may go unnoticed without proper screening. A normal early morning cortisol level (275–555 nmol/L) does not exclude adrenal insufficiency in children with steroid-sensitive nephrotic syndrome. Further screening with LDSTs, particularly in children younger than 5 years at diagnosis, may be warranted.

Keywords: adrenal insufficiency, steroid withdrawal, nephrotic syndrome, HPA axis, cortisol, low-dose Synacthen test, adrenal suppression

INTRODUCTION

The most common glomerular disease in childhood is idiopathic nephrotic syndrome (NS), for which corticosteroids are the first line of treatment. Almost 80% of children with NS demonstrate steroid responsiveness, achieving complete remission within 4 weeks. However, ~40–50% of these children are steroid dependent and require a long course of steroids, leaving them vulnerable to the adverse effects of chronic steroid usage, such as stunted growth, hypertension, obesity, secondary diabetes, vitamin D deficiency and secondary osteoporosis, cardiomyopathy, and hypothalamic-pituitary-adrenal (HPA) axis suppression. Most of these conditions are well known, but HPA axis suppression has to date been understudied and under-reported.

The recommended treatment regimen for NS at diagnosis, according to the KDIGO guidelines (1), is with induction of prednisolone at 60 mg/m^2/day, or 2 mg/kg/day, (maximum 60 mg/day) for 4–6 weeks. This will be followed by alternate-day prednisolone given in single doses at 40 mg/m^2 or 1.5 mg/kg (maximum 40 mg on alternate days), for 2–5 months with tapering of the dose. This is a longer duration of steroid therapy compared to the original ISKDC guideline (2) which consisted of 4 weeks induction and 4 weeks of 40 mg/m^2 3 days a week. Recently, PREDNOS trial (3) compared the pattern of disease relapse in patients receiving 8 weeks vs. extended 16 weeks of corticosteroids. There was no significant difference in time to first relapse in these two groups. They found that extended corticosteroid treatment reduced the healthcare resource use and only made a small improvement in quality of life. Treatment of relapse is different from initial presentation. Alternate day dosing of 0.1–1 mg/kg for at least 3 months is recommended in frequently relapsing and steroid dependent NS. The steroid weaning regimen may vary based on the individual patient's previous experiences with relapses, steroid dependency, frequency of relapses, steroid toxicity and the use of steroid sparing agent. Close monitoring is imperative to detect complications associated with prolonged use of high-dose corticosteroids.

The physiological secretory rate of endogenous steroids in the intact HPA axis was ~6 mg/m^2/day. Exogenous steroid doses were adjusted above this secretory rate (8–10 mg/m^2/day) as their bioavailability is reduced by gastric acids and first-pass metabolism in the liver. High-dose steroids are defined as supraphysiological steroid levels. HPA axis suppression is dependent on the total duration, total cumulative dose, and potency of the steroid used (4).

Adrenal insufficiency can be primary, secondary, or tertiary. Primary adrenal insufficiency results from intrinsic adrenal cortex diseases. Secondary and tertiary adrenal insufficiencies are caused by impaired production or action of corticotrophin, and are collectively known as central adrenal insufficiency. Overall, the prevalence of secondary adrenal insufficiency is 150–280 per million inhabitants in a population (5) and the condition can occur in children on high-dose and prolonged steroid prescriptions (4).

Various stimuli may activate the HPA axis to maintain normal body homeostasis and to combat stress, such as that induced by infections and endotoxins (6),absence or reduced glucocorticoid negative feedback (7), and hypoglycemia. Suppression of this critical mechanism via endogenous or exogenous pathways may alter the body's adaptive processes, triggering a pathogenic cascade. Adrenal insufficiency is associated with significant morbidity and mortality when inadequately treated during periods of intercurrent illness (8).

Different methods of assessing the HPA axis function exist. The insulin tolerance test and the Standard Short Synacthen test (SSST) were frequently used, but their limited reliability, tediousness, and associated adverse events led to the low-dose Synacthen test (LDST) being the preferred test nowadays. Moreover, LDST can detect mild degrees of adrenal insufficiency missed by SSST (9).

MATERIALS AND METHODS

Study Population

We identified 119 patients from the admissions list of the Pediatrics Institute of the Hospital Kuala Lumpur (Malaysia) between January 2017 and January 2018. We identified 119 patients as having steroid-sensitive NS, and enrolled 37 patients who fit the study inclusion criteria. Eligible patients had: (i) steroid-sensitive idiopathic NS; (ii) achieved remission; and (iii) been off steroids for 4–6 weeks. We excluded patients with: (i) steroid-resistant NS; or (ii) secondary NS. **Figure 1** summarizes the selection process (**Table 1**).

Data Collection

We used a pre-defined standardized data collection sheet for extracting data that contained information on patients' socio-demographic information (gender, age, ethnicity), anthropometric measurements, age at diagnosis, total number of relapses, and total duration of steroid use before LDST.

We collected blood samples for morning serum cortisol and ACTH levels, and for the LDST after steroid discontinuation during a planned visit. We then examined the patients every 3 months for a year to monitor their disease progress, their growth parameters, and to detect relapses or steroid toxicity.

LDST

Synacthen was given intravenously (0.5 μg/m^2) and serum cortisol levels were measured before and after the administration. The peak cortisol response at any time within 60 min should exceed 550 nmol/L (10). We used a lower Synacthen dose 0.5 μg/m^2 than the conventional 250 μg/m^2 dose based on the observation that the low-dose ACTH stimulation test using 1 μg of tetracosactrin can be used to detect mild secondary adrenal insufficiency (9). A cortisol increment at 30 min above the basal level is a measure of adrenal reserve and a low absolute level indicates adrenal insufficiency.

We educated parents about hydrocortisone replacement at times of illness or stress during transient adrenal insufficiency periods (11, 12). We informed parents to give oral hydrocortisone at three times the physiological replacement dose (30 mg/m^2/day) divided into three equal doses) during moderate illnesses such as fever and minor injury (this is called hydrocortisone "stress dosing"). During severe illnesses such as serious injury or trauma, or for anesthesia for surgery, we prescribed intravenous hydrocortisone at 10 times the physiological replacement dose (100 mg/m^2/day divided into four equal doses) (11).

For study subjects who relapsed during the study period, treatment was instituted as per International Study of Kidney Disease in Children (ISKDC) guideline. Patients who developed an intercurrent illness during the study period were treated as per other children with NS. Assessment of the volume status, the need for antibiotics and steroid replacement therapy was on the discretion of the treating physician.

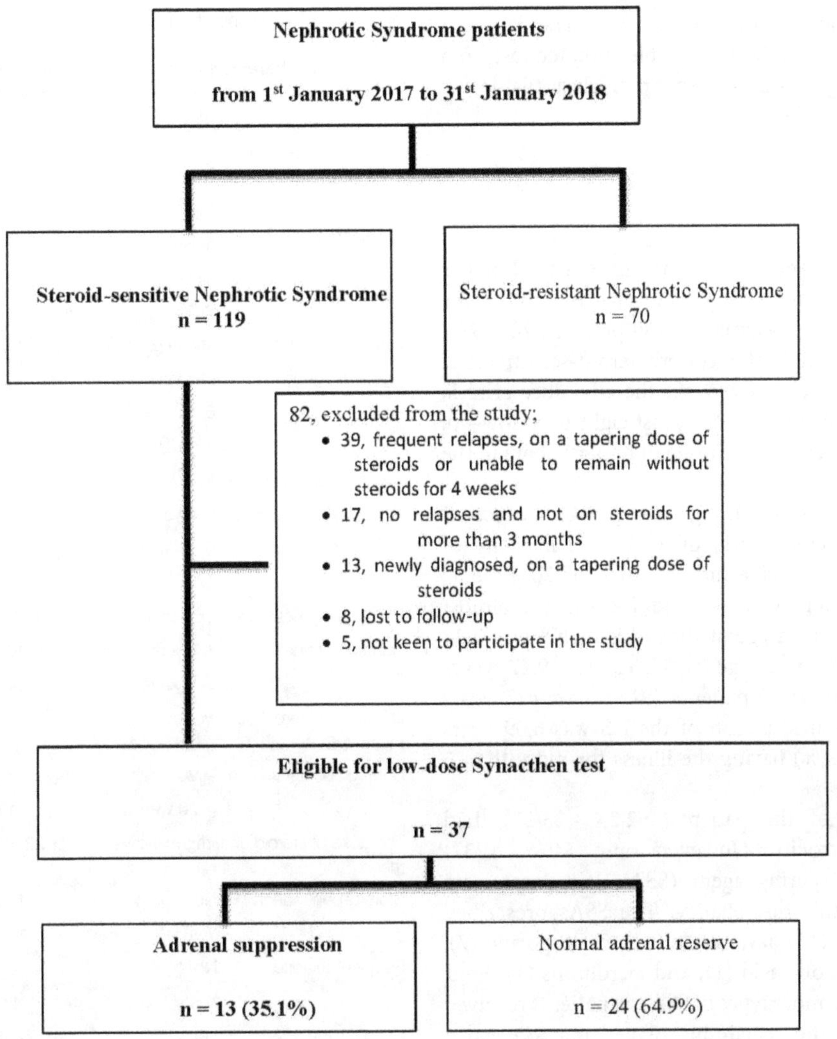

FIGURE 1 | Overview of the study flow.

TABLE 1 | Common definitions in nephrotic syndrome.

Remission	Urine albumin nil or trace for three consecutive days
Relapse	Urine albumin 3+ or more for three consecutive days
Frequent relapses	Two or more relapses in the initial 6-month period or more than three relapses in any 12 months
Steroid dependence	Two consecutive relapses when on alternate day steroid therapy or within 14 days of its discontinuation
Steroid resistance	Absence of remission despite therapy with daily prednisolone at a dose of 60 mg/m^2/day

Ethical Considerations

We registered this study with the National Medical Research Register (NMRR) under the identification number NMRR-16-1427-30586 (IIR). The Medical Research Ethics Committee (MREC), the University Malaya Medical Centre (UMMC) approved the study under the registration number MREC UMMC ID: 2016816-4142. This study was supported by a grant from the University Malaya Research Fund Assistance (BKP034-2015). We obtained written informed consent from all parents or guardians of the patients prior to starting the study. All children enrolled were also required to sign an assent form or to agree verbally. We performed all tests in accordance with approved guidelines.

Statistical Analysis

We used descriptive statistics to compare baseline characteristics between children with adrenal suppression and those with normal adrenal function. We expressed numerical data as means and standard deviations, and tabulated categorical variables as predicted numbers and percentages. We first used simple logistic regression analyses to determine unadjusted associations of factors of interest, and then applied multivariate analyses using the logistic regression model to identify predictors of HPA insufficiency. We performed data analyses using the Statistical Package for Social Science software version 23.0. The data that support the findings of this study are available upon request from the corresponding author. The data are not publicly available due to privacy or ethical restrictions.

RESULTS

Between 1st January 2017 and 31st January 2018, a total of 189 patients received treatment for NS in the Pediatric Institute of the Hospital Kuala Lumpur in Malaysia. Of 189 patients, 70 (37%) were steroid-resistant and 119 patients were steroid-sensitive, but only 31% of the patients (37 of 119) fit the eligibility criteria for enrolment; we excluded 69 patients, lost eight to follow-up, and encountered five patients who chose not to participate in the study (**Figure 1**).

Our study population showed a greater preponderance of males, with a male to female ratio of 3.6:1. The majority of patients were of Malay ethnicity and consisted of 26 patients (70.3%) and the rest were Chinese and Indians (in almost equal proportion). The mean age at diagnosis of NS was 3.38 years (±2.28), and the mean age at LDST was 9.47 years (±3.73). Thirty-four out of 37 patients (91.9%) were 5 years old or younger. The mean duration of the NS was 6.09 years (±3.44), with 21/37 (43.2%) having the illness for more than 5 years (**Table 2**).

Almost two thirds of the patients, 62.2% (23/37), had evidence of steroid toxicity. However, only 54% (20/37) had received a steroid-sparing agent (SSA). We possess no data that can explain this discrepancy. The SSAs prescribed were cyclophosphamide (13), levamisole (12), cyclosporine (7), rituximab (3), mycophenolic acid (1), and tacrolimus (1). Four patients received three or more types of SSA, six patients received two types of SSA, and the remaining 10 patients received a single agent. We categorized the steroid toxicities according to the affected system: immunosuppression; cardiovascular (hypertension); eye involvement (cataract, glaucoma); and musculoskeletal (short stature, cushingoid features, and skin striae). Eight out of 37 patients (21.6%) had frequent relapses and 20 (54.1%) patients were steroid dependent.

Thirteen out of 37 patients (35.1%) had HPA axis suppression. All of them were younger than 5 years of age and 76.9% were boys ($n = 10/13$). The mean durations of steroid usage were 66 (±121.25) weeks in those who developed HPA axis suppression and 30 (±35.31) weeks in those who did not. Ten of those patients with HPA axis suppression (76.9%) were steroid dependent.

We found that children with a younger age (mean age at diagnosis of 2.54 years) were more likely to develop HPA axis suppression than older children (95% CI, 0.567–0.990). Steroid-dependent patients were six times more likely to develop HPA axis suppression than to maintain normal HPA axis function (95% CI, 1.06–29.34) (**Table 3**).

The mean basal plasma cortisol concentration was significantly higher by 40% in patients with a normal adrenal response than in patients with a suppressed adrenal response [303.92 (±133.99) vs. 215.69 (±102.61) nmol/L, $p = 0.012$]. After the injection of 0.5 μg/m² Synacthen, both groups of patients demonstrated serum cortisol peaks at 20 min. The mean 20-min peak serum cortisol concentration was lower in the children with suppressed responses than in those with

TABLE 2 | Demographic and clinical characteristics of patients with normal HPA axis and HPA axis suppression.

Characteristics		Normal HPA axis (*n* = 24) (64.9%)	HPA axis suppression (*n* = 13) (35.1%)
Gender	Male	19 (79.2)	10 (76.9)
	Female	5 (20.8)	3 (23.1)
Race	Malay	16 (66.7)	10 (76.9)
	Chinese	5 (20.8)	1 (7.7)
	Indian	3 (12.5)	2 (15.4)
Age at diagnosis, years, mean ± SD*		3.83 ± 2.69	2.54 ± 0.80
Age at diagnosis	0–5 years	21 (87.5)	13 (100)
	6–11 years	2 (8.3)	0 (0.0)
	12–18 years	1 (4.2)	0 (0.0)
Age at LDST, years, mean ± SD*		10.44 ± 4.25	7.67 ± 1.32
Age at LDST	0–5 years	5 (20.8)	2 (15.4)
	6–11 years	10 (41.7)	11 (84.6)
	12–18 years	9 (37.5)	0 (0.0)
Duration of illness, years, mean ± SD*		6.61 ± 3.99	5.13 ± 1.86
Duration of illness	≤ 5 years	10 (41.7)	6 (46.2)
	> 5 years	14 (58.3)	7 (53.8)
Duration of steroid use, weeks, mean ± SD*		30.54 ± 35.31	66.05 ± 121.25
Duration of steroid use	< 20 weeks	13 (54.2)	7 (53.8)
	≥ 20 weeks	11 (45.8)	6 (46.2)
The dose of steroid use, mg/m²/days, mean (SD)*		22.37 ± 8.30	25.63 ± 11.36
Steroid-dependent	No	14 (58.3)	3 (23.1)
	Yes	10 (41.7)	10 (76.9)
Frequent relapse	No	20 (83.3)	9 (69.2)
	Yes	4 (16.7)	4 (30.8)
Steroid toxic	No	8 (33.3)	6 (46.2)
	Yes	16 (66.7)	7 (53.8)
Use of steroid-sparing agent (SSA)	No	9 (37.5)	8 (61.5)
	Yes	15 (62.5)	5 (38.5)
Immuno-suppression prior to LDST	Prednisolone alone	19 (79.2)	11 (84.6)
	Combination with SSA	5 (20.8)	2 (15.4)
Comorbid diseases	No	17 (70.8)	11 (84.6)
	Yes	7 (29.2)	2 (15.4)
ACTH, pmol/L, mean ± SD		20.52 ± 14.20	40.92 ± 85.14
ACTH Result	Normal	22 (91.7)	10 (76.9)
	Abnormal	2 (8.3)	3 (23.1)

**SD, standard deviation.*

normal responses; this difference, however, was not statistically significant [467.54 (±69.16) and 630.33 (±97.86), respectively, $p = 0.869$] (**Figure 2**).

DISCUSSION

We analyzed cortisol levels in patients with steroid-sensitive NS using LDST and confirmed that 13 of them (35.1%) had HPA axis suppression. Multivariate analyses showed that younger age at diagnosis and steroid dependency were the two significant factors associated with HPA axis suppression. We defined HPA axis suppression as cortisol levels <550 nmol/L despite stimulation. This definition may help to anticipate adverse outcomes associated with inappropriate cortisol responses during "stress periods" in children on steroid therapy.

The duration of steroid usage in children with NS varies with the frequency of relapses, steroid dependency, presence of steroid toxicity, and different medical practices. In our center, we administer steroids as per the ISKDC guideline. Case-to-case evaluations are frequent as some patients maintain remission states and avoid relapses when given prolonged steroid courses.

The HPA axis functions as a complex neuroendocrine feedback mechanism crucial during stress adaptation (14); it is influenced by circadian and ultradian rhythms (15). Animal studies have shown that the HPA axis regulates the secretion of glucocorticoids, which have dominant effects in regulating cardiovascular, metabolic, cognitive, and immunological states (13, 16, 17). The paraventricular nuclei (PVN) of the hypothalamus initiate axis activation (18, 19). Exposure to stressors stimulates the secretion of corticotrophin-releasing hormone (CRH), and this hormone eventually stimulates the pituitary gland to secrete adrenocorticotropic hormone (ACTH). ACTH in turn binds to its receptors on the adrenal gland and induces cortisol secretion (20, 21), which inhibits ACTH and CRH production (negative feedback mechanism), in a manner similar to that in children with excess exogenous glucocorticoids (22).

Children with NS receive supraphysiologic doses of steroids that may potentially inhibit cortisol production. When this inhibition lasts longer than the duration of the corticosteroid exposure, it is called adrenal suppression. Although the effect may be transient, it can result in significant morbidity during periods of physiologic stress (23). In children receiving high-dose steroids, adrenal suppression is not apparent and clinicians need to be aware that abrupt withdrawal may trigger adrenal crises (4, 22).

The suppression of the HPA axis can occur after a single dose of steroid, but it typically recovers quickly. However, the long-term use of systemic corticosteroids may take a long time to recover (24). Studies have looked at the effects of corticosteroid use on the HPA axis and at the corresponding recovery times. The recovery time depends on the glucocorticoid potency and its types, the duration of therapy, and the weaning protocols; therefore, estimations are difficult, and comparisons between studies are complex also because of the different diagnostic tests used to assess the adrenal function.

In our study, the local prevalence of adrenal suppression in children with NS 4–6 weeks after steroid discontinuation was 35.1%. This figure is lower than that reported in a study by Abeyagunawardena et al. (25), which showed that 20 of 32 (62.5%) children on alternate-day prednisolone for

TABLE 3 | Multivariate analysis for children with nephrotic syndrome on corticosteroid treatment.

Variables		ß*	Df**	*p*-value	Adjusted +OR (95% ++CI)
Age at diagnosis		−0.288	1	0.043	0.749 (0.567–0.990)
Steroid-dependent	No	1.719	1	0.042	5.58 (1.06–29.34)
	Yes				

*ß, beta; **Df, degrees of freedom; +OR, odd ratio; ++CI, confidence interval; LDST, low-dose Synacthe n test.*

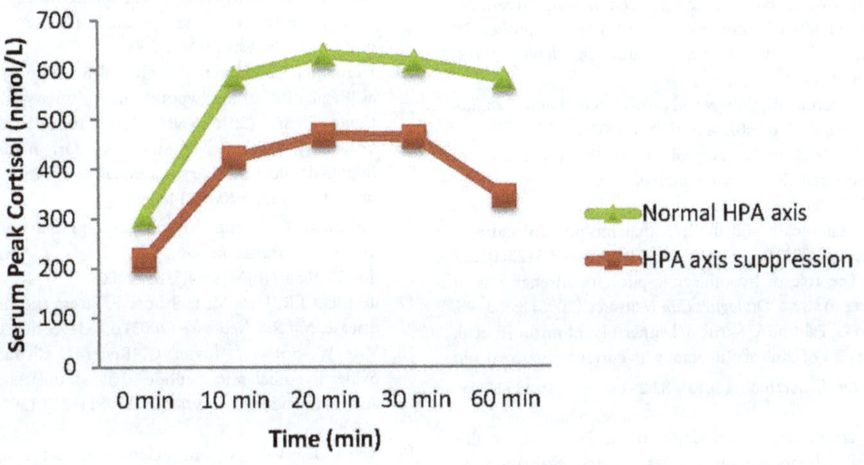

FIGURE 2 | Serum peak cortisol concentrations (means) from baseline (time 0) following stimulation with 0.5 μg/m² Synacthen (10, 20, 30, and 60 timepoints).

steroid-dependent NS had HPA axis suppression. Furthermore, their cut-off cortisol level to diagnose adrenal suppression was found to be <500 nmol/L. Mantan et al. (26) also studied children on low dose steroids and 28 of 70 children had adrenal suppression. Diagnosis is based on a single early morning dose of serum cortisol. Those at a risk of acquiring adrenal suppression in his study were mainly frequent relapsers and steroid resistant NS.

The variety of investigations used and different cut-off values to examine the HPA axis are potential caveats concerning the validity of the assessment results. Recently, Mongioi et al. (27) studied the accuracy of LDST in 103 adults. All of them had primary AI or hypothalamic-pituitary diseases. Those receiving steroids were excluded. The receiver operating characteristic curve showed 100% sensitivity and 67.3% specificity when 500 nmol/L was used as the serum cortisol cut-off value. Our study, however, is based on the study done by Tordjman et al. (9), which used 550 nmol/L of serum cortisol as the cut-off value in LDST, resulting in 100% sensitivity and 89% specificity.

We found steroid toxicity in 62.2% of our cohort, suggesting that predicting which patients are at risk of developing adrenal crisis is impossible based on steroid toxicity alone. In a resource limited setting, conducting screening tests for HPA axis suppression in every patient on corticosteroid treatment is additionally unfeasible. Therefore, predicting patients who warrant screening for adrenal suppression is important. Based on our study findings, patients younger than 5 years, and who are steroid-dependent, should be screened for adrenal suppression by measuring both a morning serum cortisol level and an LDST. Identifying children at risk for adrenal suppression early would reduce the burden of illness in terms of morbidity, mortality, and cost of care.

We acknowledge the limitations of our study. We had no data on the frequency of hospital admissions, severity of intercurrent illnesses, or recovery rates to compare between patients with HPA axis suppression and those without HPA axis suppression. We also failed to examine the recovery periods in children with HPA axis suppression.

In conclusion, a life-threatening HPA axis suppression may go unnoticed without proper screening. A normal early morning cortisol level (275–555 nmol/L) does not rule out adrenal insufficiency in children with steroid-sensitive NS. Further screening with LDSTs may be warranted, particularly in children younger than 5 years of age at diagnosis.

ETHICS STATEMENT

The studies involving human participants were reviewed and approved by NMRR. Written informed consent to participate in this study was provided by the participants' legal guardian/next of kin. Written informed consent was obtained from the individual(s), and minor(s)' legal guardian/next of kin, for the publication of any potentially identifiable images or data included in this article.

AUTHOR CONTRIBUTIONS

All authors worked together in designing the study, getting ethics approval, recruiting patients, performing the low-dose synacthen test, analyzing the data, and writing up the paper.

REFERENCES

1. Kidney Disease Improving Global Outcome. *Treatment of the Initial Episode of Steroid Sensitive Nephrotic Syndrome (KDIGO Guideline No. 3.1)* (2012). Retrieved from: https://kdigo.org
2. Tarshish P, Tobin JN, Bernstein J Edelmann CM. Prognostic significance of the early course of minimal change nephrotic syndrome: report of the International Study of Kidney Disease in Children. *JASN.* (1997) 8:769–76.
3. Webb NJA, Woolley RL, Lambe T, Frew E, Brettell EA, Barsoum EN, et al. Long term tapering versus standard prednisolone treatment for first episode of childhood nephrotic syndrome : phase III randomised controlled trial and economic evaluation. *BMJ.* (2019) 365:l1800. doi: 10.1136/bmj.l1800
4. Gupta P, Bhatia V. Corticosteroid physiology and principles of therapy. *Indian J Pediatr.* (2008) 75:1039–44. doi: 10.1007/s12098-008-0208-1
5. Laureti S, Vecchi L, Santeusanio F, Falorni A. Is the prevalence of Addison's disease underestimated? *J Clin Endocrinol Metab.* (1999) 84:1762 doi: 10.1210/jcem.84.5.5677-7
6. Beishuizen A, Thijs LG. Endotoxin and the hypothalamo-pituitary-adrenal (HPA) axis. *J Endotoxin Res.* (2003) 9:3–24 doi: 10.1179/096805103125001298
7. Smith SM, Vale WW. The role of hypothalamic-pituitary-adrenal axis in neuroendocrine responses to stress. *Dialogues Clin Neurosci.* (2006) 8:383–95.
8. Quinkler M, Johannsson G, Falorni A, Skrtic S, Lennern H, Monson JP, et al. Adrenal insufficiency : review of clinical outcomes with current glucocorticoid replacement therapy. *Clin Endocrinol.* (2015) 82:2-11. doi: 10.1111/cen.12603
9. Tordjman K, Jaffe A, Grazas N, Apter C, Stern N. The role of the low dose (1 microgram) adrenocorticotropin test in the evaluation of patients with pituitary diseases. *J Clin Endocrinol Metab.* (1995) 80:1301–5. doi: 10.1210/jcem.80.4.7714104
10. Gonc EN, Kandemir N, Kinik ST. Significance of low-dose and standard-dose ACTH tests compared to overnight metyrapone test in the diagnosis of adrenal insufficiency in childhood. *Horm Res.* (2003) 60:191–7 doi: 10.1159/000073232
11. Shulman DI, Palmert MR, Kemp SF. Adrenal insufficiency: still a cause of morbidity and death in childhood. *Pediatrics.* (2007) 119:e484–94. doi: 10.1542/peds.2006-1612
12. Merke DP, Bornstein SR. Congenital adrenal hyperplasia. *Lancet.* (2005) 365:2125–36. doi: 10.1016/S0140-6736(05)66736-0
13. McEwen BS. Physiology and neurobiology of stress and adaptation: central role of the brain. *Physiol Rev.* (2007) 87:873–904. doi: 10.1152/physrev.00041.2006
14. Herman JP, Mcklveen JM, Ghosal S, Kopp B, Wulsin A, Makinson R, et al. Regulation of the hypothalamic-pituitary-adrenocortical stress response. *Compr Physiol.* (2016) 6:603–21. doi: 10.1002/cphy.c150015
15. Walker JJ, Terry JR, Lightman SL. Origin of ultradian pulsatility in the hypothalamic - pituitary - adrenal axis. *Proc Biol Sci.* (2010) 277:1627–33. doi: 10.1098/rspb.2009.2148
16. Chrousos GP. The hypothalamic-pituitary-adrenal axis and immune-mediated inflammation. *N Engl J Med.* (1995) 332:1351–62. doi: 10.1056/NEJM199505183322008
17. de Kloet ER, Joels M, Holsboer F. Stress and the brain: from adaptation to disease. *Nat Rev Neurosci.* (2005) 6:463–75. doi: 10.1038/nrn1683
18. Vale W, Spiess J, Rivier C, Rivier J. Characterization of a 41-residue ovine hypothalamic peptide that stimulates secretion of corticotropin and beta-endorphin. *Science.* (1981) 213:1394–7. doi: 10.1126/science.6267699
19. Rivier C, Vale W. Modulation of stress-induced ACTH release by corticotropin-releasing factor, catecholamines and vasopressin. *Nature.* (1983) 305:325–7. doi: 10.1038/305325a0

20. Mountjoy KG, Robbins LS, Mortrud MT, Cone RD. The cloning of a family of genes that encode the melanocortin receptors. *Science.* (1992) 257:1248–51. doi: 10.1126/science.1325670
21. Cone RD, Lu D, Koppula S, Vage DI, Klungland H, Boston B, et al. The melanocortin receptors: agonists, antagonists, and the hormonal control of pigmentation. *Recent Prog Horm Res.* (1996) 51:287–317.
22. Paragliola RM, Papi G, Pontecorvi A, Corsello SM. Treatment with synthetic glucocorticoids and the hypothalamus-pituitary-adrenal axis. *Int J Mol Sci.* (2017) 18:2201. doi: 10.3390/ijms18102201
23. Ahmet A, Brienza V, Tran A, Lemieux J, Aglipay M, Barrowman N, et al. Frequency and duration of adrenal suppression following glucocorticoid therapy in children with rheumatic diseases. *Arthritis Care Res.* (2017) 69:1224–30. doi: 10.1002/acr.23123
24. Sperling MA. *Pediatric Endocrinology E-Book.* Elsevier Health Sciences (2014).
25. Abeyagunawardena AS, Hindmarsh P, Trompeter RS. Adrenocortical suppression increases the risk of relapse in nephrotic syndrome. *Arch Dis Child.* (2007) 92:585–8. doi: 10.1136/adc.2006.108985
26. Mantan M, Grover R, Kaushik S, Yadav S. Adrenocortical suppression in children with nephrotic syndrome treated with low-dose alternate day corticosteroids. *Indian J Nephrol.* (2018) 28:203–8. doi: 10.4103/ijn.IJN_80_17
27. Mongioì LM, Condorelli RA, Barbagallo F, Cannarella R, La Vignera S, Calogero AE. Accuracy of the low-dose ACTH stimulation test for adrenal insufficiency diagnosis: a re-assessment of the cut-off value. *J Clin Med.* (2019) 8:806. doi: 10.3390/jcm8060806

14

Risk Factors for Poor Prognosis of Severe Infection in Children With Idiopathic Nephrotic Syndrome: A Double-Center, Retrospective Study

Hengci Zhang[1,2†], Shiyuan Qiu[1,3†], Cheng Zhong[1,2], Lin Shi[1,2], Jiacheng Li[1,2], Tao Zhang[2,4], Xiaoping Zhu[2,4] and Mo Wang[1,2*]*

[1] Department of Nephrology, Children's Hospital of Chongqing Medical University, Ministry of Education Key Laboratory of Child Development and Disorders, National Clinical Research Center for Child Health and Disorders, China International Science and Technology Cooperation Base of Child Development and Critical Disorders, Chongqing Key Laboratory of Pediatrics, Chongqing, China, [2] Western Pediatric Development Union, Chongqing, China, [3] Pediatric Internal Medicine Department, Chongqing You You Baobei Women's and Children's Hospital, Chongqing, China, [4] Department of Pediatrics, The Affiliated Hospital of Guizhou Medical University, Guiyang, China

***Correspondence:**
Xiaoping Zhu
zxp_1963819@163.com
Mo Wang
wangmo_cqmu@163.com

These authors have contributed equally to this work and share first authorship

Background: Infection is the most common complication of Idiopathic Nephrotic Syndrome (INS) and the main cause of INS recurrence, severe infection and even leading to mortality. The purpose of this study was to investigate the risk factors of severe infection in INS children and the clinical parameters influencing prognosis.

Methods: Totally 147 children with INS and concomitant infections were enrolled and classified into the severe infection group (SIG) and Non-severe infection group (Non-SIG). The clinical characteristics and auxiliary examination results were compared between the two groups, and the early-warning parameters for severe infection and risk factors for poor prognosis were evaluated.

Results: There were 49 patients in the SIG, 98 patients in the Non-SIG. In the SIG, the most common severe infections disease included severe pneumonia (63.6%), severe sepsis (30.6%), septic shock (4.1%). In SIG, Gram-positive bacteria (GPB) were more common, as was respiratory syncytial virus (RSV), and the three most common strains were Pseudomonas aeruginosa, Staphylococcus aureus (SA) and Staphylococcus epidermidis. There were more steroid-resistant nephrotic syndrome and combination of steroids and immunosuppressants in SIG, compared with the Non-SIG ($P = 0.000$). Patients in the SIG has lower complement 3 (C3, $\leq$0.55 g/L,) and absolute lymphocyte count (ALC, $\leq 1.5 \times 10^9$/L) ($P = 0.004$). Logistic regression analysis revealed that the independent risk factors for severe infections were the combined use of immunosuppressants [95% confidence interval (CI):1.569–463.541, $P = 0.023$], steroid resistance (95% CI: 4.845–2,071.880, $P = 0.003$), C-reactive protein (CRP) $\geq$8 mg/L (95% CI: 43.581–959, 935.668, $P = 0.001$), and infections caused by GPB (95% CI: 27.126–2,118, 452.938, $P = 0.002$), influenza (95% CI: 2.494–1, 932.221, $P = 0.012$) and RSV (95% CI: 5.011–24 963.819, $P = 0.007$). The patients in the SIG were classified into the survival group ($N = 39$) and the mortality group ($N = 5$). Logistic regression analysis showed that white blood cell count (WBC) $> 15 \times 10^9$/L (95% CI: 1.046–2.844, $P = 0.033$) was an independent risk factor of poor prognosis for these patients.

Conclusions: Resistance to steroids, combined with steroids and IS agents, and GPB infections (especially SA) are high-risk factors for severe infection in children with INS. We should monitor CRP $\geq$ 8 mg/L, C3 $\leq$ 0.55 g/L and ALC $\leq$ 1.5 $\times$ 10^9/L to avoid developing severe infection. Accompanied by an increase in ANC, WBC significantly increased, suggesting a fatal infection.

Keywords: idiopathic nephrotic syndrome, severe infection, risk factor, prognosis, children

INTRODUCTION

Idiopathic nephrotic syndrome (INS) is one of the most common kidney diseases in children. It is characterized by heavy proteinuria, pitting edema, hypoalbuminemia, and hyperlipidemia. INS occurs in 1.15–16.9 per 100,000 children, and its incidence varies by ethnicity and region (1). Infection is the most common complication of INS; it hampers the treatment of the underlying kidney disease, leads to INS relapse, increases rates of unplanned hospitalizations, and even leads to increased mortality. Several recent reports have evaluated the clinical characteristics and risk factors in children with INS and infections (2, 3). However, few studies have assessed the risk factors for serious infections associated with INS and the risk factors for poor prognosis of infections. The purpose of this study was to investigate the risk factors of severe infections in children with INS and the clinical parameters leading to poor prognosis.

MATERIALS AND METHODS

Study Population

This study enrolled children aged 0–18 years with INS and concomitant infections who were hospitalized in the Children's Hospital of Chongqing Medical University and the Affiliated Hospital of Guizhou Medical University, from January 2013 to October 2019. Written informed consent was obtained from parents or legal guardians, and this study complied with the ethical principles of the Helsinki Declaration of the World Medical Association. All the patients met the following criteria: (1) An onset age from birth to 18 years. (2) The definition of nephrotic syndrome (NS) included: ① nephrotic- range proteinuria: urine protein/creatinine ratio (UPCR) $\geq$ 200.0 (mg/mmol) in spot morning urine or 24 h urine quantification $\geq$50 mg/kg/day ② hypoproteinaemia: serum albumin < 25 g/L, ③ hyperlipidemia: serum cholesterol higher than 5.7 mmol/L and ④ varied degrees of edema. ① and ② are necessary for diagnosis. Children were excluded from congenital nephrotic syndrome, any other secondary NS, such as Henoch–Schoenlein purpura nephritis, lupus nephritis.

Clinical Data

The retrieved clinical data of children with INS who met the inclusion criteria were as follows: (1) Baseline characteristics, including sex, age, duration, usage, duration of steroid and immunosuppressive (IS) therapy. IS agents included cyclosporine, tacrolimus, mycophenolate, cyclophosphamide; (2) Laboratory data were collected, including complete blood count, urinalysis, alanine aminotransferase (ALT), aspartate aminotransferase (AST), alkaline phosphatase (ALP), serum urea nitrogen, serum creatinine, uric acid, serum albumin, serum potassium, serum sodium, serum chlorine, serum calcium, C-reactive protein (CRP), procalcitonin (PCT), total cholesterol (Tch), triglycerides, high-density lipoprotein (HDL), low-density lipoprotein (LDL), prothrombin time (PT), activated partial thromboplastin time (APTT), fibrinogen (Fib), D-dimer, immunoglobulin G (IgG), immunoglobulin A (IgA), immunoglobulin M (IgM), immunoglobulin E (IgE), complement 3 (C3), complement 4 (C4), and pathogens isolated by specimen culture (e.g., blood, urine, sputum, cerebrospinal fluid, and bronchoalveolar lavage fluid), antigen testing from blood, or histological material from a definite site of infection. Because complement detection helped to rule out nephropathy caused by autoimmune diseases (4), and children with INS were often accompanied by IgG deficiency, resulting in an increased risk of infection (5), almost all of the subjects in this study were tested for complement and immunoglobulin.

Definitions

The Standard definitions of the outcome of INS were in **Table 1** (6). Infection was defined as a suspected or proven infection caused by any pathogen or a clinical syndrome associated with a high probability of infection. Evidence of infection includes positive findings on clinical exam, imaging, or laboratory tests. We referred to the clinical manifestations, biochemical indicators, the definitions of severe infections in adults with INS (7, 8) and related diseases that cause INS infection in children (9–12). Finally, based on the International Guidelines for Management of Severe Sepsis and Septic Shock (2012) (13), the principle of severe infection was when children with INS have signs and symptoms of inflammation with following conditions occur: variations in general signs (at least two), variations in indicators of inflammation (at least one) and at least one of the variations in organ function, tissue perfusion or hemodynamic variations, as detailed in **Table 2.** The prognosis was determined based on the post-treatment conditions of the children, who were classified into good prognosis (survival group) and poor prognosis (mortality group) groups. The good prognosis was defined as symptoms and signs of inflammation are restored, without the manifestations of infection. The poor prognosis was defined as mortality.

Statistical Analysis

Statistical analysis was conducted using the SPSS 22.0 statistical software (IBM Corporation, NY, United States). In the

TABLE 1 | Relevant definitions in nephrotic syndrome.

	Definition
Term	
Relapse	Urine albumin 3+ or 4+ or proteinuria >40 mg/m ^{2} per h or urinary protein: creatinine ratio >2.0 (mg/mg) for 3 consecutive days
SSNS	Complete remission within 4 weeks of prednisone or prednisolone (PDN) at the standard dose (60 mg/m^2/day or 2 mg/kg/day, maximum 60 mg/day)
SRNS	Persistent proteinuria despite 60 mg/m^2 or 2 mg/kg for 8 weeks, after ensuring no infection or non-adherence to medication
SDNS	2 consecutive relapses occurring while weaning to alternate-day steroids or within 2 weeks of steroid discontinuation

SSNS, steroid-sensitive nephrotic syndrome; SRNS, steroid-resistant nephrotic syndrome; SDNS, steroid-dependent nephrotic syndrome.

TABLE 2 | General variables and definitions of severe infection.

General signs
Fever (>38.5°C)
Hypothermia (<35°C)
Heart rate more than two SD above the normal value for age
Tachypnea (Respiratory rate higher than WHO classification for age)
Altered mental status
Inflammatory variables
Leukocytosis (WBC count > 12,000 μL^{-1} or higher than the normal value for age)
Leukopenia (WBC count <4,000 μL^{-1} or below the normal value for age)
Plasma C-reactive protein more than two SD above the normal value
Plasma procalcitonin more than two SD above the normal value
Hemodynamic variables
Arterial hypotension (SBP less than two SD below normal value for age)
Organ dysfunction variables
Arterial hypoxemia (PaO_2/FiO_2 < 300)
Acute oliguria (urine output <0.5 mL kg^{-1} h^{-1} for at least 2 h despite adequate fluid resuscitation)
Coagulation abnormalities
Ileus (absent bowel sounds)
Tissue perfusion variables
Hyperlactatemia (Lactate above upper limits laboratory normal)
Decreased capillary refill or mottling

SD, standard deviation; WBC, white blood cell; SBP, systolic blood pressure; WHO, World Health Organization.

assessment of differences in clinical parameters, categorical data were evaluated using contingency tables and the chi-square test. Quantitative data with a normal distribution were analyzed using an independent sample *t*-test. On the contrary, quantitative data that did not follow a normal distribution were analyzed using the rank-sum test. Normality testing was performed using the one-sample Kolmogorov-Smirnov test. In the binary logistic regression analysis, parameters were entered following the "forward Wald" method. The sensitivity and specificity of each parameter were compared using a univariate receiver operating characteristic (ROC) curve. For significance criteria, values of $P < 0.05$ were considered statistically significant, and values of $P < 0.01$ were considered highly statistically significant.

Study Design

Patients who met the criteria and were complicated by infections and admitted to the Children's Hospital of Chongqing Medical University and the Affiliated Hospital of Guizhou Medical University, from January 2013 to October 2019 were into our research. According to the severity of the infections, the patients were divided into severe infection group (SIG) or Non-severe infection group (Non-SIG) (who didn't match the criteria of severe infection) and matched according to the ratio of 1:2. We retrospectively reviewed the medical data, including baseline characteristics, laboratory testing, pathogens. The flowchart of this study is shown in **Figure 1**.

RESULTS

Baseline Characteristics

In total, 147 children, including 111 (63.8%) boys and 36 (36.2%) girls, suffering from INS with concomitant infections were enrolled in this study. The youngest child was 6 months old, and the oldest was 16.4 years old. The median age was 5.25 years old, and there was no statistically significant difference between the two groups ($P > 0.05$) (**Table 3**). Among the children, the shortest and longest disease durations were 0.03 and 106.13 months, respectively, and the median was 0.67 months. There were 49 children in the SIG and 98 in the Non-SIG. The SIG primarily developed severe pneumonia ($n = 31$, 63.3%), severe sepsis ($n = 15$, 30.6%), septic shock ($n = 2$, 4.1%), and severe chickenpox ($n = 1$, 2.0%); whereas, the Non-SIG primarily developed pneumonia ($n = 81$, 82.7%), urinary tract infection (UTI) ($n = 12$, 12.2%), and upper respiratory tract infection (URTI) ($n = 5$, 5.1%).

Clinical Data Analysis

Through statistical analysis of clinical data, we found that there were many differences between SIG and Non-SIG. The percentage of relapsed cases and SRNS in SIG were higher than those Non- SIG (63.3 vs. 30.6%, 51.0 vs. 10.2%, respectively). The number of steroids (≥0.5 mg/kg) users and immunosuppressant users in SIG was significantly higher than that in the Non-SIG (46.9 vs. 16.3%, 36.7 vs. 4.1%). There were 18 cases using immunosuppressive agents, including 12 cases using tacrolimus, of which 2 cases were combined with mycophenolate mofetil and 1 case was combined with cyclophosphamide. The remaining 4 cases used mycophenolate mofetil alone and 2 cases used cyclophosphamide alone. Steroids and immunosuppressants for SIG were used longer than for Non -SIG. In the auxiliary examination, we also found that there were significant differences between the two groups. The ANC, PCT, PT, and APTT in

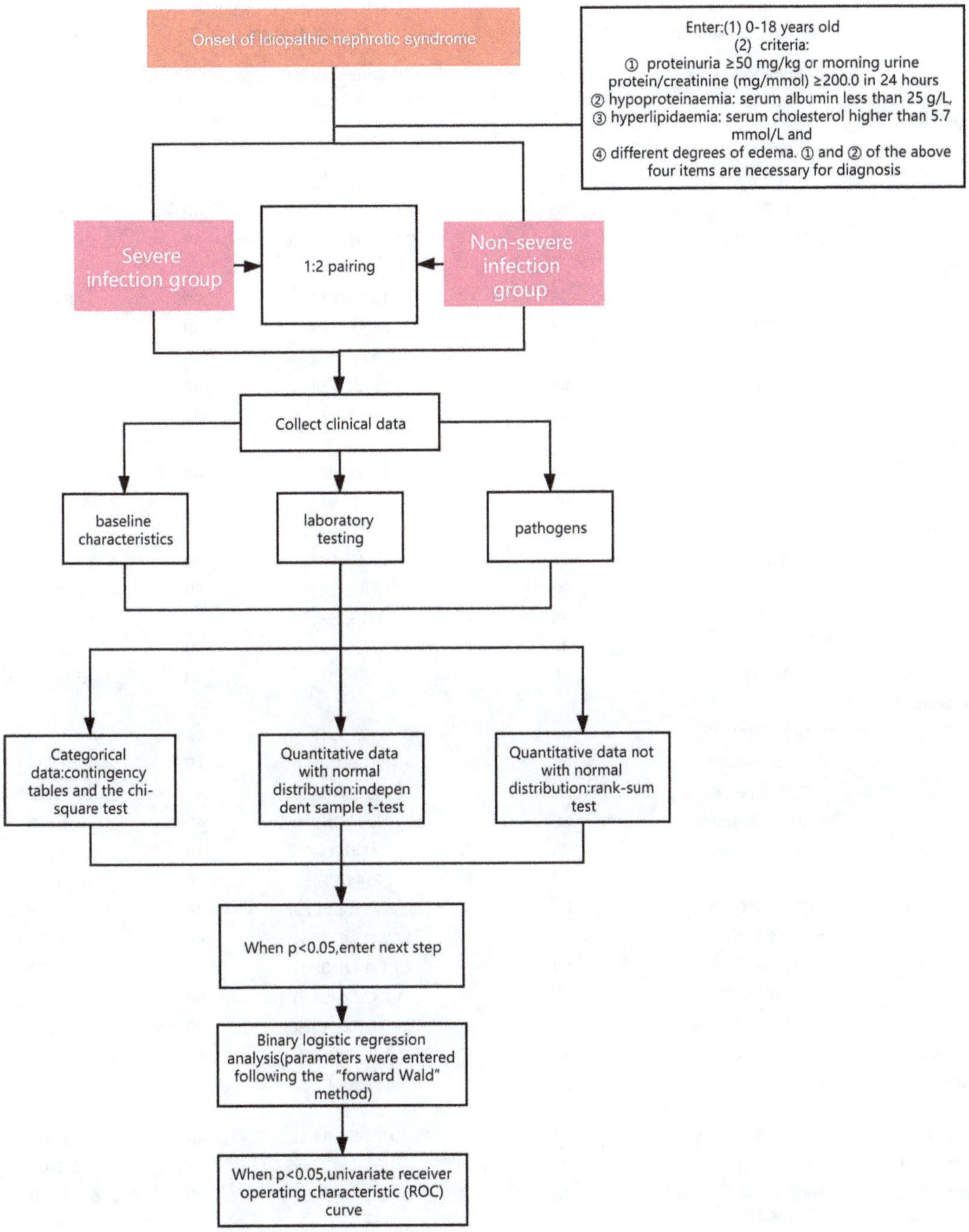

FIGURE 1 | Experimental design process.

the SIG were significantly higher than those in the Non-SIG, while ALC, Tch, LDL, and C3 were significantly lower than those in the Non-SIG. Other indicators were also significantly different, such as WBC, CRP, uric acid, urea nitrogen, and other indicators SIG are higher than Non-SIG. The SIG group's Fib, serum potassium, sodium, etc. were lower than the Non-SIG group (**Table 3**).

Analysis of Pathogens and Drug Resistance in the Non-SIG and SIG

Based on the data from blood, sputum, and urine cultures obtained from 147 children with INS and infections during hospitalization, 30 of them were detected and 46 strains were isolated. The three most common types in the SIG were Pseudomonas aeruginosa (three strains), Staphylococcus aureus

TABLE 3 | Demographic characteristics, laboratory data of children with INS in the severe and non-severe infection group.

	Non-SIG (N = 98)		SIG (N = 49)		X^2 value	p-value
	Summary	***N***	**Summary**	***N***		
Baseline characteristics						
Male	73 (74.5%)	98	38 (77.6%)	49	0.166	0.684
Female	25 (25.5%)	98	11 (22.4%)	49		
Duration (months)	0.37 (0.23, 1.78)	98	3.00 (0.67, 12.00)	49	$Z = -3.846$	0.000**
Age (years)	5.17 (2.52, 9.38)	98	6.00 (2.67, 10.00)	49	$Z = -0.321$	0.749
Disease conditions						
Initial episode	68 (69.4%)	98	18 (36.7%)	49	14.347	0.000**
Relapse	30 (30.6%)	98	31 (63.3%)	49		
SSNS	82 (83.7%)	98	19 (38.8%)	49	32.434	0.000**
SRNS	10 (10.2%)	98	25 (51.0%)	49		
SDNS	6 (6.1%)	98	5 (10.2%)	49		
Treatments before infection						
Duration of steroid (days)	0 (0, 0)	98	63 (0.362)	49	$Z = -5.135$	0.000**
MP pulse	1 (1.0%)	98	4 (8.2%)	49	3.132	0.077
Steroid dosage per day						
<0.5 mg/kg	82 (83.7%)	98	26 (53.1%)	49		
0.5–1.5 mg/kg	10 (10.2%)	98	15 (30.6%)	49	15.146	0.001**
>1.5 mg/kg	6 (6.1%)	98	8 (16.3%)	49		
IS therapy (n)	4 (4.1%)	98	18 (36.7%)	49	27.369	0.000**
Duration of IS (days)	0 (0, 0)	98	0 (0, 11)	49	−5.141	0.000**
Auxiliary examinations						
WBC ($\times 10^9$/L)	10.18 (8.25, 12.13)	98	13.25 (9.79, 17.34)	49	$Z = -3.850$	0.000**
ALC ($\times 10^9$/L)	3.27 (2.23, 4.71)	98	2.46 (1.56, 3.74)	49	$Z = -2.889$	0.004**
ANC ($\times 10^9$/L)	5.46 (3.92, 8.58)	98	9.99 (6.33, 12.33)	49	$Z = -4.442$	0.000**
PLT ($\times 10^9$/L)	390.0 (313.5, 459.5)	98	345.0 (244.0, 484.5)	49	$Z = -1.448$	0.147
Hb (g/L)	137 (125, 149)	98	122 (96, 144)	49	$Z = -3.276$	0.001**
CRP $\geq$ 8 mg/L (n)	1 (1.0%)	98	22 (44.9%)	49	47.651	0.000**
PCT (ng/ml)	0.05 (0.05, 0.10)	85	0.65 (0.10, 11.29)	46	$Z = -5.812$	0.000**
Serum albumin (g/L)	16.7 (14.7, 19.3)	98	17.2 (13.4, 22.7)	49	$Z = -0.072$	0.943
ALT (U/L)	16.0 (10.4, 23.8)	98	25.1 (14.8, 32.1)	49	$Z = -3.493$	0.000**
AST (U/L)	33.3 (24.7, 43.2)	98	31.2 (22.4, 51.3)	49	$Z = -0.557$	0.578
ALP (U/L)	163.6 (122.8, 199.3)	98	101.6 (77.3, 139.3)	49	$Z = -5.519$	0.000**
Serum uric acid (μmol/L)	326.5 (258.5, 374.0)	98	360.0 (234.0, 506.2)	49	$Z = -2.624$	0.009**
Serum urea nitrogen (mmol/L)	4.90 (3.78, 6.93)	98	7.64 (4.21, 12.32)	49	$Z = -2.750$	0.006**
Serum creatinine (μmol/L)	33.50 (25.68, 50.50)	98	45.90 (29.35, 116.25)	49	$Z = -1.354$	0.176
Serum potassium (mmol/L)	4.50 ± 0.71	98	4.04 ± 0.72	49	$t = 3.670$	0.000**
Serum sodium (mmol/L)	136.30 (132.55, 138.75)	98	132.20 (128.95, 137.10)	49	$Z = -3.048$	0.002**
Serum chlorine (mmol/L)	103.85 (100.20, 106.83)	98	101.50 (96.50, 105.05)	49	$Z = -2.554$	0.011*
Serum calcium (mmol/L)	1.94 (1.82, 2.05)	98	1.87 (1.73, 2.09)	49	$Z = -1.459$	0.145
Tch (mmol/L)	10.76 ± 3.10	98	8.86 ± 3.53	49	$t = 3.337$	0.001**
Triglyceride (mmol/L)	2.98 (2.01, 4.36)	98	3.14 (2.43, 4.17)	49	$Z = -0.489$	0.625
LDL (mmol/L)	7.86 ± 2.96	98	5.66 ± 3.23	49	$t = 4.112$	0.000**
HDL (mmol/L)	1.71 (1.23, 2.21)	98	1.50 (0.81, 2.16)	49	$Z = -1.724$	0.085
IgG (g/L)	2.24 (1.36, 3.02)	97	1.88 (0.83, 4.29)	48	$Z = -0.534$	0.594
IgA (g/L)	0.85 (0.63, 1.35)	97	0.89 (0.62, 1.30)	48	$Z = -0.089$	0.929
IgM (g/L)	1.76 (1.31, 2.40)	97	1.49 (1.09, 2.22)	48	$Z = -1.589$	0.112
IgE (g/L)	176.0 (46.2, 458.5)	97	76.3 (23.8, 372.0)	48	$Z = -1.790$	0.073

(Continued)

TABLE 3 | Continued

	Non-SIG ($N = 98$)		SIG ($N = 49$)		X^2 value	p-value
	Summary	N	Summary	N		
C3 (g/L)	0.99 ± 0.21	97	0.85 ± 0.30	48	$t = 2.947$	0.004**
C4 (g/L)	0.24 (0.19, 0.30)	97	0.23 (0.17, 0.27)	48	$Z = -0.854$	0.393
PT (s)	10.4 (9.7, 11.1)	87	11.2 (10.2, 13.3)	48	$Z = -3.151$	0.002**
APTT (s)	31.00 (26.90, 35.70)	87	36.75 (28.15, 53.23)	48	$Z = -2.882$	0.004**
Fib (g/L)	5.97 ± 1.70	87	5.31 ± 2.02	48	$t = 2.023$	0.045*
D-dimer	1.26 (0.58, 2.31)	87	1.83 (0.69, 5.80)	48	$Z = -1.836$	0.066

*$p < 0.05$, **$p < 0.01$. Continuous parameters were expressed as ($\bar{X} \pm s$) or P50 (P25, P75), and discrete parameters were expressed as a percentage (%). SIG, severe infection group; MP, methylprednisolone; IS, immunosuppressive; WBC, white blood cells; ALC, absolute lymphocyte count; ANC, absolute neutrophil count; PLT, platelets count; Hb, hemoglobin; CRP, C-reactive protein; PCT, procalcitonin; ALT, alanine aminotransferase; AST, aspartate aminotransferase; ALP, alkaline phosphatase; Tch, total cholesterol; LDL, low-density lipoprotein; HDL, high-density lipoprotein; PT, prothrombin time; APTT, activated partial thromboplastin time; Fib, fibrinogen.

(SA) (three strains), and Staphylococcus epidermidis (three strains). On the contrary, the three most common types in the Non-SIG were Haemophilus influenzae (three strains), Streptococcus pneumonia (SP) (three strains), and Enterococcus faecium (three strains). The detection rate of Gram-positive bacteria (GPB) was higher in the SIG than in the Non-SIG (**Table 4**). The pathogen profiles indicated that the SIG was more likely to be infected with GPB, respiratory syncytial virus (RSV) and influenza viruses (FLu), and fungi than the Non-SIG ($P < 0.05$). In total, 10 drug-resistant strains were detected in the two groups. The incidence of Methicillin-resistant strains was significantly higher in the SIG ($n = 4$) than in the Non-SIG ($n = 0$) ($P = 0.000$).

Risk Factor Analysis for Severe Infections in INS

To identify the risk factors of severe infections in children with INS, the aforementioned clinical parameters that were statistically different between the two groups were entered into the binary logistic regression analysis model. The results obtained using the "forward Wald" method were shown in **Table 5**. Binary logistic regression analysis showed that the combined use of immunosuppressants (OR: 26.969, 95% CI: 1.569–463.541), CRP ≥8 mg/L (OR: 6,468.029, 95% CI: 43.581–959,935.668), steroid resistance (OR: 100.191, 95% CI: 4.845–2,071.880), infection with gram-positive cocci (OR: 7,580.545, 95% CI: 27.126–2,118,452.938), infection with influenza virus (OR: 69.426, 95% CI: 2.494–1,932.221), and infection with respiratory syncytial virus (OR: 353.681, 95% CI: 5.011–24,963.819) were independent risk factors for severe infections in children with INS. ALC (increase > 1.5×10^9/L) (OR: 0.356, 95% CI: 0.188–0.675) and complement C3 (increase > 0.55 g/L) (OR: 0.000, 95% CI: 0.000–0.276) were protective factors.

Through the ROC curve model analysis, it was found that when children with nephropathy were co-infected, the risk of infection progression often needed to consider the combined effect of multiple influencing factors at the same time. The sensitivity and specificity reflected by the area under the ROC curve (AUC) showed that when infection occurred in children with INS, when one or more factors including steroid resistance, IS treatment and increased CRP were combined, a more severe infection was very likely to occur (**Figures 2A,B**).

Analysis of Prognosis of INS Patients With Concomitant Severe Infections

In the SIG, 39 patients survived, five died, and five gave up treatment. Five patients who gave up treatment were excluded because of incomplete data and unclear prognosis. The causes of death included multiple organ failure syndromes (2 cases), brain herniation (1 case), and circulatory failure (2 cases). The patients were classified into the survival group ($N = 39$) and the mortality group ($N = 5$). The statistically significant parameters between two groups by univariate analysis entered into the binary logistic regression analysis model. There was no significant difference in baseline characteristics, treatment, and disease condition between the two groups. However, in the auxiliary examination, WBC, Serum chlorine, and ANC in the mortality group were significantly higher than those in the survival group, and ALT, AST, serum calcium, IgG, IgA, and C3 were significantly lower than those in the survival group (**Table 6**). Binary logistic regression analysis showed that WBC (increased > 15×10^9/L) (OR: 1.725, 95% CI: 1.046–2.844) is an independent risk factor for the poor prognosis of INS children with severe infections, often accompanied by an increase in the ANC(> 10×10^9/L), whereas serum calcium level (increase > 1.30 mmol/L) (OR: 0.000, 95% CI: 0.000–0.698) was a protective factor. The area under the ROC curve shows that serum calcium and WBC are highly specific and sensitive in predicting the risk of poor prognosis (**Figures 2C,D**).

DISCUSSION

Infection is one of the main complications of childhood idiopathic nephrotic syndrome, which can lead to frequent relapses of INS, treatment failures, and even death (14). Children with INS are more likely to have a poor prognosis after infection due to the primary disease and therapeutic drugs. At present, most studies on children's INS focus on the analysis of risk factors for infection, and there is a lack of large-scale reports on the risk factors and outcome factors

TABLE 4 | Pathogen spectrum and the analysis in the severe and non-severe infection group.

Pathogens	Non-severe infection group	Severe infection group	Total (*N*, %)	X^2 value	*p*-value
Gram-negative bacteria	12	14	26 (56.52)	2.577	0.108
Morganella	1	2	3 (6.52)		
Escherichia coli	3	1	4 (8.70)		
Acinetobacter baumannii	1	2	3 (6.52)		
Enterobacter cloacae	0	1	1 (2.17)		
Klebsiella pneumonia	0	2	2 (4.35)		
Pseudomonas aeruginosa	1	3	4 (8.70)		
Haemophilus influenzae	3	2	5 (10.87)		
Haemophilus parainfluenzae	2	0	2 (4.35)		
Elizabethkingia	0	1	1 (2.17)		
Pantoea agglomerans	1	0	1 (2.17)		
Gram-positive bacteria	7	13	20 (43.48)	10.256	0.001
Staphylococcus aureus	1	3	4 (8.70)		
Staphylococcus epidermidis	0	3	3 (6.52)		
Staphylococcus hominis	0	2	2 (4.35)		
Staphylococcus haemolyticus	0	1	1 (2.17)		
Streptococcus pneumoniae	3	2	5 (10.87)		
Enterococcus faecium	3	2	5 (10.87)		
Fungus	0	4	4	5.429	0.020
Virus	18	25	43		
Cytomegalovirus	8	5	13 (30.23)	0.011	0.918
Epstein-Barr virus	2	2	4 (9.30)	0.032	0.858
Adenovirus	1	0	1 (2.33)	0.000	1.000
Influenza virus	3	7	10 (23.26)	4.842	0.028
Parainfluenza virus	3	3	6 (13.95)	0.195	0.658
Respiratory syncytial virus	1	8	9 (20.93)	10.785	0.001
Mycoplasma pneumoniae	7	1	8	0.8100	0.368

TABLE 5 | Binary logistic regression analysis of risk factors of severe infections in children with INS.

	Coefficient (B)	Wald value	*p*	OR	95% Confidence interval for EXP (B)	
					Lower limit	Upper limit
Steroid Combined with IS	3.295	5.155	0.023	26.969	1.569	463.541
SSNS		9.375	0.009			
SRNS	4.607	8.886	0.003	100.191	4.845	2,071.880
SDNS	1.979	1.208	0.272	7.233	0.212	246.345
Increased ALC	−1.033	10.025	0.002	0.356	0.188	0.675
CRP ≥ 8 mg/L	8.775	11.831	0.001	6,468.029	43.581	959,935.668
Increased C3	−8.205	5.405	0.020	0.000	0.000	0.276
Infection with gram-positive bacteria	8.933	9.662	0.002	7,580.545	27.126	2,118,452.938
Infection with influenza virus	4.240	6.243	0.012	69.426	2.494	1,932.221
Infection with RSV	5.868	7.301	0.007	353.681	5.011	24,963.819
Constant	3.318	1.269	0.260	27.612		

IS, Immunosuppressant; ALC, absolute lymphocyte count; RSV, respiratory syncytial virus.

for severe infection. Referring to the definition of severe infection in adult INS and the indicators of severe infection in children (7, 8), we defined the manifestations of severe infection in children with INS and analyzed the relevant risk factors.

In this study, it was observed that pneumonia and urinary tract infection were dominant in Non-severely infective INS children, while severe pneumonia, sepsis was dominant in severely infective INS children. In Taiwan (15), pneumonia is the main type of infection in children with INS, which is consistent

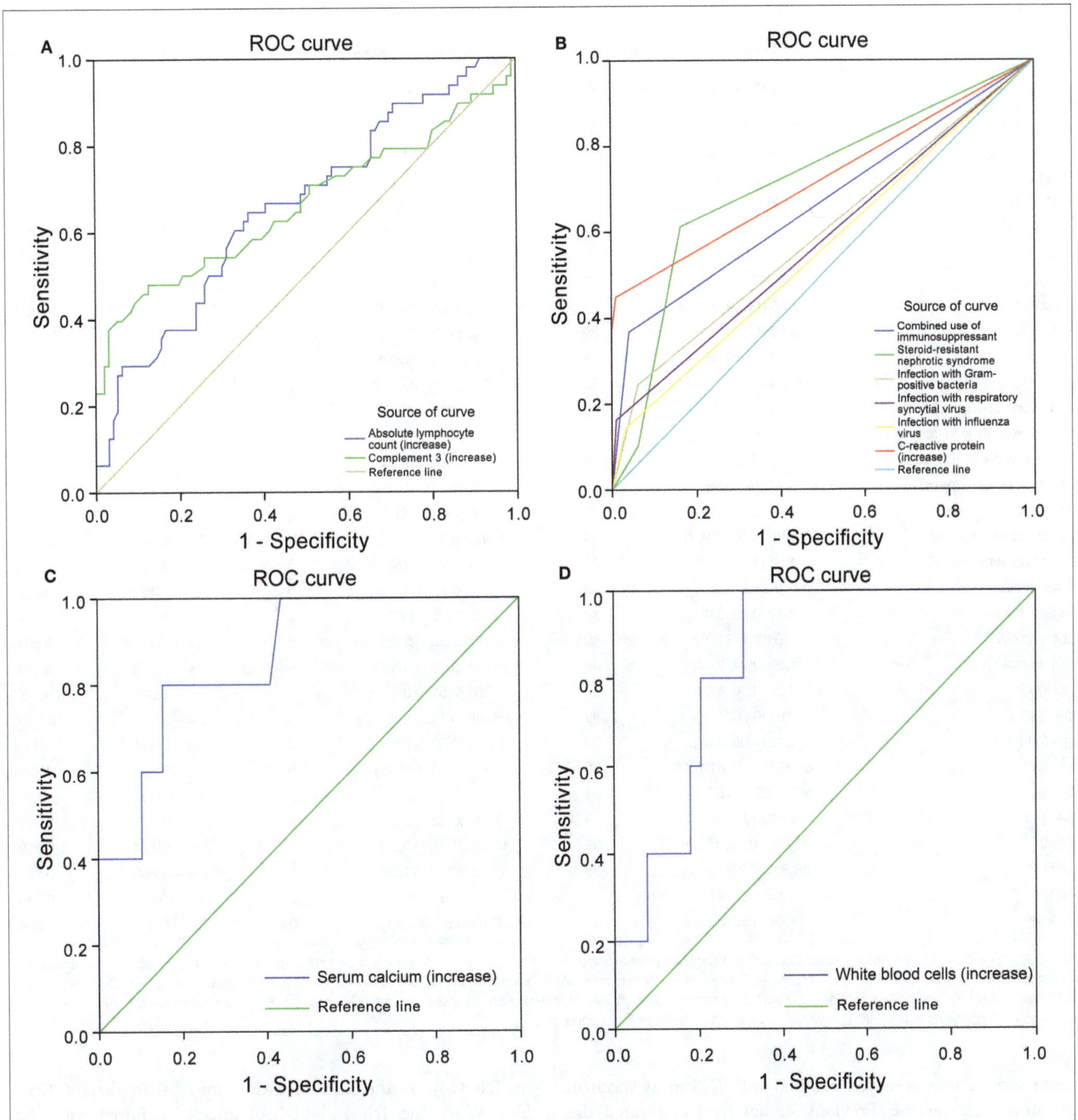

FIGURE 2 | Receiver operating characteristics (ROC) curve. Protective factors of severe infection **(A)**. Risk factors of severe infection **(B)**. Protective factors for poor prognosis of severe infection **(C)**. Risk factors for poor prognosis of severe infection **(D)**.

with the Non-SIG in our study, while in India, Saudi Arabia, and other regions (2, 16, 17), the upper respiratory tract infection is the main type, but these studies did not grade the infection. Although in Israel (18), the infections were mainly pneumonia and bacteremia/sepsis, but they defined the infection as a serious bacterial infection, which has limitations. From our research, it is found that both severe and Non-severe infections are mainly respiratory infections. Therefore, our treatment should be more active when pneumonia is complicated. We found that the pathogen spectrum of the two groups is significantly different, and GPB are an independent risk factor for severe infections. In SIG, the respiratory pathogens are mainly SA, while Non-SIG is mainly composed of SP and Haemophilus influenzae, and it is more common for SIG strains to have drug resistance. Therefore, when patients are infected with methicillin-resistant SA or other methicillin-resistant GPB, they are more likely to

TABLE 6 | Univariate analysis of risk factors for poor prognosis of SIG in children with INS.

	Survival group (*N* = 39)		Mortality group (*N* = 5)		X^2 value	*p*-value
	Summary	***N***	**Summary**	***N***		
WBC (×10⁹/L)	12.75 (8.98, 15.99)	39	21.20 (15.78, 30.96)	5	$Z = -2.496$	0.013*
PLT (×10⁹/L)	366 (298, 499)	39	155 (91, 461)	5	$Z = -1.498$	0.134
Hb (g/L)	126 (106, 145)	39	80 (68, 125)	5	$Z = -1.998$	0.046
ALC (×10⁹/L)	2.36 (1.57, 3.43)	39	2.47 (1.38, 4.43)	5	$Z = -0.296$	0.767
ANC (×10⁹/L)	9.27 (5.18, 11.39)	39	12.21 (10.84, 20.15)	5	$Z = -2.034$	0.042 *
CRP ≥ 8 mg/L (*n*)	17 (43.6%)	39	4 (80.0%)	5		0.176$^{\Delta}$
PCT (ng/ml)	0.43 (0.10, 8.65)	39	5.52 (0.62, 45.64)	5	$Z = -1.423$	0.155
Serum albumin (g/L)	17.06 (14.30, 23.80)	39	12.60 (10.20, 15.35)	5	$Z = -1.029$	0.303
ALT (U/L)	25.10 (15.10, 28.50)	39	13.40 (9.75, 67.75)	5	$Z = -2.663$	0.008**
AST (U/L)	31.20 (25.40, 46.50)	39	22.10 (18.65, 242.05)	5	$Z = -2.422$	0.015*
ALP (U/L)	102.60 (81.20, 137.50)	39	78.00 (63.05, 164.50)	5	$Z = -1.091$	0.275
Serum uric acid (μmol/L)	346 (224, 485)	39	360 (271, 449)	5	$Z = -0.185$	0.853
Serum urea nitrogen (mmol/L)	6.33 (3.70, 11.70)	39	8.20 (5.67, 28.08)	5	$Z = -1.183$	0.237
Serum creatinine (μmol/L)	40.60 (27.00, 74.50)	39	82.00 (37.00, 284.75)	5	$Z = -1.738$	0.082
Serum potassium (mmol/L)	4.11 ± 0.68	39	3.61 ± 1.04	5	$t = 1.440$	0.157
Serum sodium (mmol/L)	131.5 (129.2, 136.7)	39	132.4 (122.0, 141.0)	5	$Z = -0.129$	0.897
Serum chlorine (mmol/L)	101.9 (96.0, 104.1)	39	109.6 (101.1, 114.6)	5	$Z = -2.238$	0.025 *
Serum calcium (mmol/L)	1.91 (1.75, 2.09)	39	1.67 (1.29, 1.78)	5	$Z = -2.626$	0.009**
Tch (mmol/L)	9.24 ± 3.62	39	8.36 ± 2.69	5	$t = 0.519$	0.607
Triglyceride (mmol/L)	3.10 (2.38, 3.86)	39	3.73 (3.05, 10.27)	5	$Z = -1.110$	0.267
LDL (mmol/L)	5.89 ± 3.30	39	5.05 ± 3.10	5	$t = 0.541$	0.591
HDL (mmol/L)	1.53 (0.94, 2.04)	39	0.81 (0.56, 1.33)	5	$Z = -1.923$	0.054
IgG (g/L)	2.06 (0.96, 4.02)	39	0.66 (0.51, 0.86)	5	$Z = -2.644$	0.008**
IgA (g/L)	0.91 (0.66, 1.31)	39	0.48 (0.40, 0.62)	5	$Z = -2.570$	0.010*
IgM (g/L)	1.48 (1.08, 2.51)	39	1.74 (0.82, 1.85)	5	$Z = -0.481$	0.631
IgE (g/L)	81.30 (21.30, 410.00)	39	32.20 (27.66, 187.95)	5	$Z = -0.795$	0.427
C3 (g/L)	0.88 ± 0.30	39	0.63 ± 0.09	5	$t = 3.940$	0.001**
C4 (g/L)	0.22 (0.16, 0.27)	39	0.25 (0.23, 0.26)	5	$Z = -0.981$	0.326
PT (s)	11.05 (10.18, 12.83)	39	11.20 (10.00, 13.20)	5	$Z = -0.114$	0.909
APTT (s)	36.30 (26.78, 53.83)	39	37.50 (32.40, 44.20)	5	$Z = -0.265$	0.791
Fib (g/L)	5.56 ± 1.97	39	5.22 ± 1.99	5	$t = 0.369$	0.714
D-dimer	1.44 (0.55, 3.20)	39	3.10 (0.86, 32.25)	5	$Z = -1.137$	0.256

*$p < 0.05$, **$p < 0.01$. $^{\Delta}$Fisher exact method. Continuous parameters were expressed as ($\bar{X} \pm s$) or P50 (P25, P75), and discrete parameters were expressed as a percentage (%). SIG, severe infection group; WBC, white blood cells; ALC, absolute lymphocyte count; ANC, absolute neutrophil count; Hb, hemoglobin; PLT, platelets count; CRP, C-reactive protein; PCT, procalcitonin; ALT, alanine aminotransferase; AST, aspartate aminotransferase; ALP, alkaline phosphatase; Tch, total cholesterol; LDL, low-density lipoprotein; HDL, high-density lipoprotein; PT, prothrombin time; APTT, activated partial thromboplastin time; Fib, fibrinogen.

cause serious infections. So, children with INS must vaccinate pneumococcal vaccine. Previous studies have confirmed that the use of high cumulative doses of steroids and IS agents (8, 17, 19–23) all increase the risk of INS infection. Besides, we found that children with SRNS or relapse are more susceptible to severe infection, and the risk of severe infection is higher when treated with steroids combined with immunosuppressive agents such as tacrolimus or mycophenolate mofetil. From the auxiliary inspection point of view, SIG has higher CRP and PCT, but their Tch and LDL are lower. The Tch and LDL of the two groups were higher than the normal range, but studies have shown that inflammation can cause a decrease in Tch (24), so the LDL of SIG is lower than that of Non-SIG. When the Tch and LDL of infected children with INS decrease, we need to be vigilant. SIG's PT and APTT are also higher, suggesting that when there is a problem with the coagulation function of Non-SIG, we need to be alert to the progress of the infection, and even cause diffuse intravascular coagulation. C3 (<0.55 g/L) and ALC (<1.5 × 10^9/L) are predictors of severe infections, which had not been previously reported. We believe that this is because the use of high-dose steroids and IS agents and INS itself will cause ALC and C3 to decrease. Co-infection will further reduce the ALC and C3 (25–27). Therefore, When C3 ≤ 0.55 g/L or ALC ≤ 1.5 ×

10^9/L, the infection should be timely and controlled to avoid further aggravation.

Regarding prognosis, we found that children in the mortality group had lower immunity. The serum calcium of the mortality group was significantly reduced, which is one of the factors of poor prognosis. In INS, hypoalbuminemia is often accompanied by a decrease in serum calcium. The cause of hypocalcemia may not only be caused by INS itself, but also infection. Serum calcium lower than 1.30 mmol/L may cause death. WBC ($>15 \times 10^9$/L) was the only independent risk factor for poor prognosis, no similar results have been reported in children with INS, whereas reports involving adults with INS have shown that hypotension and decreased platelet count were risk factors for a poor prognosis (14). Although decreased ALC is a risk factor for severe infection, however, due to an increase in ANC, the resulting increase in white blood cells became an early warning indicator of fatal severe infection, especially the increase in WBC increased ($>15 \times 10^9$/L).

Several limitations of this study should be mentioned. First, although we have found some risk factors of severe infection in children with INS, as a retrospective study, it might lead to the bias in data collection and uniform availability of information from the medical records. Second, the age span of children in this study was large, and the results could not well-reflect the clinical characteristics of children with INS complicated with severe infection in each age period. We tried to divide the children into infant, childhood and adolescence group based on tanner staging. However, due to the relatively small sample size, it was hard to perform statistical analysis. In the future, we will expand the sample size and design a prospective study based on the results of this study, so as to avoid poor prognosis of children with INS caused by severe infection, and to find more risk factors of severe infection in children with INS in different age period.

In summary, our double-center retrospective study showed that resistance to steroids, combined use of steroids and IS agents, and GPB infections (especially SA) are high risk factors for severe infection. We should monitor CRP $\geq$ 8 mg/L, C3 $\leq$ 0.55 g/L and ALC $\leq 1.5 \times 10^9$/L to avoid developing severe infection.

The WBC of severely infected patients increases significantly, especially when ANC increases, which can lead to fatal infections.

ETHICS STATEMENT

The studies involving human participants were reviewed and approved by Ethics Committee of the Children's Hospital of Chongqing Medical University (reference number 2020-12, 2020-03-24). Written informed consent to participate in this study was provided by the participants' legal guardian/next of kin.

AUTHOR CONTRIBUTIONS

MW and XZ designed this study. HZ and SQ wrote the draft. CZ, LS, and TZ has participated in data collection and case follow-up. JL designed the statistical analysis of the study. All authors contributed to the article and approved the submitted version.

ACKNOWLEDGMENTS

First, we would like to thank Western Pediatric Development Union of China for setting up a platform for academic exchange. Besides, we would thank all of the medical staff at the department of nephrology, Children's Hospital of Chongqing Medical University, and the department of pediatrics, the Affiliated Hospital of Guizhou Medical University for their support in this research. At last, we would like to thank Haiping Yang, Gaofu Zhang, Qin Yang, Daoqi Wu for their help in data collection.

REFERENCES

1. Noone DG, Iijima K, Parekh R. Idiopathic nephrotic syndrome in children. *Lancet.* (2018) 392:61–74. doi: 10.1016/S0140-6736(18)30536-1
2. Ajayan P, Krishnamurthy S, Biswal N, Mandal J. Clinical spectrum and predictive risk factors of major infections in hospitalized children with nephrotic syndrome. *Indian Pediatr.* (2013) 50:779–81. doi: 10.1007/s13312-013-0214-x
3. Gulati A, Sinha A, Sreenivas V, Math A, Hari P, Bagga A. Daily corticosteroids reduce infection-associated relapses in frequently relapsing nephrotic syndrome: a randomized controlled trial. *Clin J Am Soc Nephrol.* (2011) 6:63–9. doi: 10.2215/CJN.01850310
4. International Study of Kidney Disease in Children. Nephrotic syndrome in children: prediction of histopathology from clinical and laboratory characteristics at time of diagnosis. A report of the International Study of Kidney Disease in Children. *Kidney Int.* (1978) 13:159–65. doi: 10.1038/ki.1978.23
5. Giangiacomo J, Cleary TG, Cole BR, Hoffsten P, Robson AM. Serum immunoglobulins in the nephrotic syndrome. A possible cause of minimal-change nephrotic syndrome. *New Engl J Med.* (1975) 293:8–12. doi: 10.1056/NEJM197507032930103
6. Kidney Disease: Improving Global Outcomes (KDIGO) Glomerulonephritis Work Group. KDIGO clinical practice guideline for glomerulonephritis. *Kidney Int.* (2012) 2(Suppl.):139–274. doi: 10.1038/kisup.2012.9
7. Lebo CH, Jianhua DO, Shutian XU. Clinical characteristics and risk factors of severe infections in hospitalized adult patients with primary nephrotic syndrome. *Chin J Nephrol Dial Transplant.* (2018) 1:18–23. doi: 10.3969/cndt.j.issn.1006-298X.2018.01.004
8. Li J, Zhang Q, Su B. Clinical characteristics and risk factors of severe infections in hospitalized adult patients with idiopathic nephrotic syndrome. *J Int Med Res.* (2017) 45:2139–45. doi: 10.1177/0300060517715339
9. UNICEF, WHO. *Pneumonia: The Forgotten Killer of Children.* New York, NY: United Nations Children's Fund (2006).
10. Bradley JS, Byington CL, Shah SS, Alverson B, Carter ER, Harrison C, et al. Executive summary: the management of community-acquired pneumonia in infants and children older than 3 months of age: clinical practice guidelines by the Pediatric Infectious Diseases Society and the Infectious Diseases Society of America. *Clin Infect Dis.* (2011) 53:617–30. doi: 10.1093/cid/cir625
11. Pediatric Acute Lung Injury Consensus Conference Group. Pediatric acute respiratory distress syndrome: consensus recommendations from the Pediatric Acute Lung Injury Consensus Conference. *Pediatr Crit Care Med.* (2015) 16:428–39. doi: 10.1097/PCC.0000000000000350
12. Cameron JC, Allan G, Johnston F, Finn A, Heath PT, Booy R. Severe complications of chickenpox in hospitalised children in the UK and Ireland. *Arch Dis Childhood.* (2007) 92:1062–6. doi: 10.1136/adc.2007.123232

13. Dellinger RP, Levy MM, Rhodes A, Annane D, Gerlach H, Opal SM. Surviving Sepsis Campaign: international guidelines for management of severe sepsis and septic shock. *Intens Care Med.* (2012) 39:165–228. doi: 10.1007/s00134-012-2769-8
14. Latta K, von Schnakenburg C, Ehrich JH. A meta-analysis of cytotoxic treatment for frequently relapsing nephrotic syndrome in children. *Pediatr Nephrol.* (2001) 16:271–82. doi: 10.1007/s004670000523
15. Wei CC, Yu IW, Lin HW, Tsai AC. Occurrence of infection among children with nephrotic syndrome during hospitalizations. *Nephrology.* (2012) 17:681–8. doi: 10.1111/j.1440-1797.2012.01650.x
16. Narain U, Gupta A. Urinary tract infection in children with nephrotic syndrome. *Pediatr Infect Dis J.* (2018) 37:144–6. doi: 10.1097/INF.0000000000001747
17. Alfakeekh K, Azar M, Sowailmi BA, Alsulaiman S, Makdob SA, Omair A, et al. Immunosuppressive burden and risk factors of infection in primary childhood nephrotic syndrome. *J Infect Public Health.* (2019) 12:90–4. doi: 10.1016/j.jiph.2018.09.006
18. Lebel A, Kropach N, Ashkenazi-Hoffnung L, Huber-Yaron A, Davidovits M. Infections in children with nephrotic syndrome: twenty years of experience. *Clin Pediatr.* (2020) 59:692–8. doi: 10.1177/0009922820908583
19. Abeyagunawardena A, Brogan PA, Trompeter RS, Dillon MJ. Immunosuppressive therapy of childhood idiopathic nephrotic syndrome. *Exp Opin Pharmacother.* (2002) 3:513–9. doi: 10.1517/14656566.3.5.513
20. Youssef J, Novosad SA, Winthrop KL. Infection risk and safety of corticosteroid use. *Rheumat Dis Clin N Am.* (2016) 42:157. doi: 10.1016/j.rdc.2015.08.004
21. Lionakis MS, Kontoyiannis DP. Glucocorticoids and invasive fungal infections. *Lancet.* (2003) 362:1828–38. doi: 10.1016/S0140-6736(03)14904-5
22. Orlicka K, Barnes E, Culver EL. Prevention of infection caused by immunosuppressive drugs in gastroenterology. *Ther Adv Chronic Dis.* (2013) 4:167–85. doi: 10.1177/2040622313485275
23. Alwadhi RK, Mathew JL, Rath B. Clinical profile of children with nephrotic syndrome not on glucorticoid therapy, but presenting with infection. *J Paediatr Child Health.* (2004) 40:28–32. doi: 10.1111/j.1440-1754.2004.00285.x
24. Liu Y, Coresh J, Eustace JA, Longenecker JC, Jaar B, Fink NE, et al. Association between cholesterol level and mortality in dialysis patients: role of inflammation and malnutrition. *JAMA.* (2004) 291:451–9. doi: 10.1001/jama.291.4.451
25. Li W, Li H, Song W, Hu Y, Liu Y, Da R, et al. Differential diagnosis of systemic lupus erythematosus and rheumatoid arthritis with complements C3 and C4 and C-reactive protein. *Exp Ther Med.* (2013) 6:1271–6. doi: 10.3892/etm.2013.1304
26. Wesche DE, Lomas-Neira JL, Perl M, Chung CS, Ayala A. Leukocyte apoptosis and its significance in sepsis and shock. *J Leukoc Biol.* (2005) 78:325–37. doi: 10.1189/jlb.0105017
27. Felmet KA, Hall MW, Clark RS, Jaffe R, Carcillo JA. Prolonged lymphopenia, lymphoid depletion, and hypoprolactinemia in children with nosocomial sepsis and multiple organ failure. *J Immunol.* (2005) 174:3765–72. doi: 10.4049/jimmunol.174.6.3765

15

Psychosocial Assessment of Candidates for Transplantation (PACT) Score Identifies High Risk Patients in Pediatric Renal Transplantation

*Kyle W. Freischlag[1], Vivian Chen[2], Shashi K. Nagaraj[2], Annabelle N. Chua[2], Dongfeng Chen[3], Delbert R. Wigfall[2], John W. Foreman[2], Rasheed Gbadegesin[2], Deepak Vikraman[4] and Eileen T. Chambers[2]**

[1] School of Medicine, Duke University, Durham, NC, United States, [2] Department of Pediatrics, Duke University, Durham, NC, United States, [3] Department of Pathology, Duke University, Durham, NC, United States, [4] Department of Surgery, Duke University, Durham, NC, United States

***Correspondence:**
Eileen T. Chambers
eileen.chambers@duke.edu

Background: Currently, there is no standardized approach for determining psychosocial readiness in pediatric transplantation. We examined the utility of the Psychosocial Assessment of Candidates for Transplantation (PACT) to identify pediatric kidney transplant recipients at risk for adverse clinical outcomes.

Methods: Kidney transplant patients <21-years-old transplanted at Duke University Medical Center between 2005 and 2015 underwent psychosocial assessment by a social worker with either PACT or unstructured interview, which were used to determine transplant candidacy. PACT assessed candidates on a scale of 0 (poor candidate) to 4 (excellent candidate) in areas of social support, psychological health, lifestyle factors, and understanding. Demographics and clinical outcomes were analyzed by presence or absence of PACT and further characterized by high (≥3) and low (≤2) scores.

Results: Of 54 pediatric patients, 25 (46.3%) patients underwent pre-transplant evaluation utilizing PACT, while 29 (53.7%) were not evaluated with PACT. Patients assessed with PACT had a significantly lower percentage of acute rejection (16.0 vs. 55.2%, $p = 0.007$). After adjusting for HLA mismatch, a pre-transplant PACT score was persistently associated with lower odds of acute rejection (Odds Ratio 0.119, 95% Confidence Interval 0.027–0.52, $p = 0.005$). In PACT subsection analysis, the lack of family availability (OR 0.08, 95% CI 0.01–0.97, $p = 0.047$) and risk for psychopathology (OR 0.34, 95% CI 0.13–0.87, $p = 0.025$) were associated with a low PACT score and post-transplant non-adherence.

Conclusions: Our study highlights the importance of standardized psychosocial assessments and the potential use of PACT in risk stratifying pre-transplant candidates.

Keywords: renal transplantation, pediatrics, kidney, adherence, psychosocial factors

INTRODUCTION

Renal transplantation is the treatment of choice for end-stage renal disease in children and adolescents. Identification of psychosocial factors that can negatively impact post-transplant care is important to ensure successful clinical outcomes, which include adherence to medications, freedom from rejection and long-term patient and allograft survival. For children with end-stage renal disease, psychosocial stressors associated with increased morbidity and mortality include lower socioeconomic status and limited parental support (1, 2). Currently, there is no standardized approach to determine psychosocial readiness in pediatric kidney transplantation.

Multiple pre-transplant assessment tools have been developed for adults with scant data in pediatrics. These include the Stanford Integrated Psychosocial Assessment for Transplant (SIPAT), the Structured Interview for Renal Transplantation (SIRT), and the Transplant Evaluation Rating Scale (TERS) (3–5). The Pediatric Transplant Rating Instrument (P-TRI) attempted to address this gap in pediatric transplantation; however, follow-up studies have shown inconsistency with poor inter-rater reliability (6, 7). Other studies have simply used clinical judgement without a tool to risk-stratify patients (8).

The most widely used tool, the Psychosocial Assessment of Candidates for Transplantation (PACT), was developed in the 1980s as a standardized pre-transplant psychosocial evaluation tool (9). Since its development, PACT has shown good inter-rater reliability, improved clinical ease of use, and is a uniform framework for pre-transplant evaluation across all organ systems (9–11). As PACT has shown clinical utility and reliability in adult solid organ transplantation (12–15), we hypothesized that PACT could identify high risk pediatric transplant recipients and potentially improve transplant outcomes. In this pilot study, we aimed to assess the effect of implementing a standardized assessment such as PACT on clinical outcomes.

MATERIALS AND METHODS

Study Design

In this retrospective analysis, eligible patients for inclusion were <21 years of age at time of transplantation, had continued post-transplant follow-up, and underwent renal transplantation for end-stage renal disease from January 1, 2005 to December 31, 2015 at Duke University Medical Center. Patients were excluded for missing transplant data or not receiving their primary transplantation or follow-up at our institution. The Duke University Institutional Review Board (IRB Protocol #0078991) approved this study.

Study Outcomes

The primary endpoint of our study was biopsy proven acute rejection graded by Banff criteria within 3 years post-transplantation (16). Secondary endpoints included post-transplant dialysis, length of hospital stay, 30-day readmission, missed post-transplant appointments per year, non-adherence, renal allograft survival, and patient death. Non-adherence was determined by patient self-report, undetectable drug levels, or missed appointments (17, 18).

Pact Score and Psychosocial Analysis

The PACT assessed candidates on 4 domains including social support, psychological health, lifestyle factors, and understanding of transplant and follow-up. PACT contained 8 subsection items: family support, family availability, personality factors, risk for psychopathology, ability to sustain change, drug and alcohol abuse, medical adherence, and relevant knowledge. The social support domain included evaluation of family support and family availability with an emphasis on relationships. The psychological health domain incorporated assessment of personality factors/psychiatric disorders and risk for psychopathology, which focused on coping mechanisms and family history of psychiatric disorders. The lifestyle factors domain evaluated dietary/exercise habits and the ability to change unhealthy behaviors, drug and alcohol use, and compliance with medications/medical advice. Finally, the understanding of transplant and follow-up domain encompassed relevant transplant knowledge and receptiveness to education. (19). Each category was assessed by scale of mild, moderate, or severe (9, 20). An overall final transplant candidacy score from 0 (contraindication to transplant) to 4 (excellent candidate) was assigned by the social worker. A low PACT score was defined as a score ≤2 and a high PACT score was defined as ≥3 (21). The psychosocial assessment was incorporated into the decision to transplant and patients with low PACT score were monitored more closely after transplant.

The psychosocial assessment was one of the initial steps for assessing transplant candidacy and was completed 1–2 months prior to listing for transplant. Trained licensed hospital social workers who specialize in pre-transplant evaluations performed our psychosocial assessments using language suitable for a 5th grade reading level. All psychosocial assessments were incorporated into multidisciplinary meetings to help evaluate the readiness of potential candidates alongside other concerns such as medical comorbidities. Preceding the PACT, all patients received a pre-transplant psychosocial analysis by a licensed social worker from 2005 to 2010. However, the pre-transplant psychosocial rating before the implementation of the PACT was not standardized, subject to variability in content (home life, finances, transportation, school, and adherence) depending on the evaluator and differed in the criteria for candidate suitability. The PACT was implemented to standardize pediatric renal pre-transplant assessments in 2010. All pre-transplants assessments were completed using PACT from 2010 to 2015. Final subsection scores represented the abilities and risk factors present in the primary caregivers and the child, starting at the developmental age of 12. Patients were listed regardless of PACT score. Increased pre-transplant visits with social worker intervention were initiated for patients with a low PACT score and transplanted only for score of >1. Patients with psychiatric illnesses were referred to outpatient psychiatry for titration of medications and counseling pre-transplant and not transplanted until issues controlled. Patients with low PACT scores defined as <2, were monitored more closely post-transplantation by medical team,

TABLE 1 | Demographic characteristics between recipients with and without a PACT assessment.

	PACT assessment	No PACT assessment	*p*
n	25	29	
Age at transplant (median [IQR])	14.80 [8.51, 17.08]	13.39 [4.12, 15.30]	0.249
Female (%)	9 (36.0)	8 (27.6)	0.711
Race (%)			0.766
African American	10 (40.0)	11 (37.9)	
Caucasian	10 (40.0)	14 (48.3)	
Other	5 (20.0)	4 (13.8)	
BMI at transplant (median [IQR])	22.00 [12.00, 35.00]	25.00 [12.00, 37.00]	0.952
HLA Mismatch [mean (sd)]	1.00 (1.55)	2.52 (1.70)	0.001
Class I PRA > 20% (%)	1 (4.0)	1 (3.4)	0.999
Class II PRA > 20% (%)	2 (8.0)	4 (13.8)	0.809
Pre-transplant dialysis (%)	19 (76.0)	17 (58.6)	0.289
Induction (%)			0.443
Anti-thymocyte Globulin	8 (33.3)	6 (21.4)	
IL-2 inhibitor	11 (45.8)	18 (64.3)	
None	4 (16.7)	2 (7.1)	
Other	1 (4.2)	2 (7.1)	
MAINTENANCE IMMUNOSUPPRESSION			
Calcineurin inhibitors	25 (100.0)	26 (89.7)	0.29
Steroids	25 (100.0)	26 (89.7)	0.29
Anti-metabolites	25 (100.0)	26 (89.7)	0.809
EBV immune	11 (44.0)	11 (37.9)	0.861
CMV immune	7 (28.0)	10 (34.5)	0.828
Diagnosis (%)			0.449
Dysplasia	5 (20.0)	12 (41.4)	
FSGS	8 (32.0)	8 (27.6)	
Glomerulonephritis	3 (12.0)	1 (3.4)	
Obstructive Uropathy	3 (12.0)	3 (10.3)	
Other	6 (24.0)	5 (17.2)	
Re-transplant (%)	1 (4.0)	2 (6.9)	0.999
Living donor (%)	6 (24.0)	16 (55.2)	0.041
Total ischemia (hours, median [IQR])	11.75 [2.18, 15.23]	1.50 [1.00, 16.00]	0.339
Follow-up time [years, mean (sd)]	2.87 (2.30)	8.34 (4.12)	<0.001

social workers, and when appropriate by psychiatrist and/or psychologists. In cases with multiple psychosocial assessments over time, the PACT score closest to the time of transplant was used.

Statistical Analysis

Patients were stratified based on presence or absence of a PACT assessment. Of those with a PACT assessment, sub-analysis by low vs. high PACT score was performed. Baseline characteristics and unadjusted outcomes were compared using the Kruskal-Wallis test for continuous variables and Pearson χ^2 test for categorical variables. For acute rejection, a multivariable linear model was used adjusting for HLA mismatch. A model examining probability of freedom from acute rejection was generated using the Kaplan-Meier method.

A *p*-value of less than 0.05 was deemed statistically significant. Statistical analysis was performed using R version 3.3.1 (R Foundation for Statistical Computing, Vienna, Austria).

TABLE 2 | Clinical outcomes in recipients with a PACT assessment and with no PACT assessment.

	PACT assessment	No PACT assessment	*p*
n	25	29	
Post-transplant dialysis (%)	9 (36.0)	12 (42.9)	0.819
Patient death [mean (sd)]	1.00 (0.00)	1.07 (0.26)	0.188
Missed appointments per year [mean (sd)]	0.44 (0.78)	0.17 (0.30)	0.108
Non-adherence (%)	7 (28.0)	16 (55.2)	0.082
Graft failure (%)	0 (0.0)	3 (10.3)	0.29
30-day readmission (%)	5 (20.0)	3 (10.3)	0.541
Hospital stay (days, median [IQR])	7.00 [5.00, 9.50]	7.00 [6.00, 10.00]	0.506
Acute rejection [mean (sd)]	4 (16.0)	16 (55.2)	0.007
Delayed graft function (%)	6 (25.0)	3 (10.3)	0.295

RESULTS

Demographics

A total of 54 pediatric patients who underwent renal transplantation at Duke University from 2005 to 2015 met the inclusion criteria. Of these, 25 (46.3%) patients had a PACT assessment while 29 (53.7%) patients had no PACT assessment. Demographics and clinical characteristics between the two groups are shown in **Table 1**. Recipients with a PACT assessment were better matched (HLA mismatch 1.00, 2.52 $p = 0.001$), received a lower percentage of their allografts from living donors (24 vs. 55.2%, $p = 0.04$), and had less follow-up time (2.87 vs. 8.34 years, $p < 0.001$) when compared to their no PACT assessment counter parts. In PACT assessment recipients, the median PACT score was 3 (IQR 3.00–4.00). Additionally, 4 patients met the definition of a low PACT score (≤ 2) while 21 patients had a high PACT score ($\geq$3) (21). Otherwise, there were no significant differences in gender, race, BMI, PRA, pre-transplant dialysis, PRA, immunosuppression regimen, viral serology status, diagnosis, re-transplant, or cold ischemia time between the two groups (**Table 1**).

Clinical Outcomes

Unadjusted clinical outcomes between PACT assessment and no PACT assessment patients are displayed in **Table 2.** Patients with PACT assessment had a significantly lower percentage of acute rejection within the first 3 years post-transplant (16.0 vs. 55.2%, $p = 0.007$) and a lower percentage of non-adherence (28.0 vs. 55.2%, $p = 0.08$). After adjustment for HLA mismatch, lower odds of acute rejection remained associated with having a

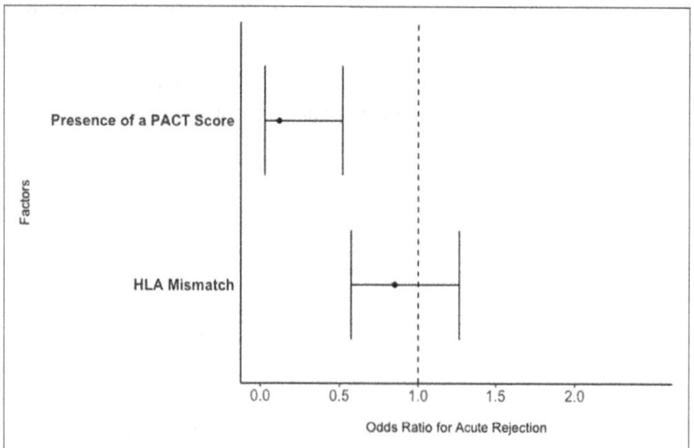

Variables	Odds ratio	*p*-value
Presence of a PACT score	0.119 (95% Confidence Interval 0.027–0.52)	0.005
HLA mismatch	0.851 (95% CI 0.576–1.259)	0.42

FIGURE 1 | The effect of PACT score and HLA mismatch on the odds of acute rejection in pediatric kidney transplantation. The presence of a PACT score remained significantly associated with lower odds of rejection within 3-years post-transplant even after adjusting for HLA mismatch.

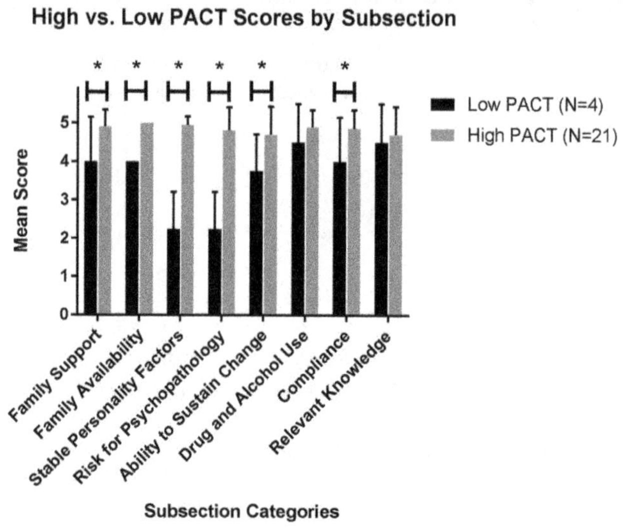

FIGURE 2 | Differences in PACT subcategories between candidates with high vs. low PACT scores. Patients with a low PACT score ≤2 had less family support, family availability, stable personality factors, ability to change and compliance and increased risk for psychopathology than those with high PACT score ≥3. *denotes significance ($p < 0.05$).

TABLE 3 | Clinical outcomes between high PACT (≥3) and low PACT scores (≤2) in recipients with a PACT assessment.

	Low PACT	High PACT	*p*
Post-transplant dialysis (%)	3 (75.0)	6 (28.6)	0.228
Patient death [mean (sd)]	0 (0.0)	0 (0.0)	
Missed appointments per year [mean (sd)]	1.22 (0.68)	0.32 (0.74)	0.062
Non-adherence (%)	3 (75.0)	4 (19.0)	0.094
Graft Failure	0 (0.0)	0 (0.0)	
30-day readmission (%)	0 (0.0)	5 (23.8)	0.682
Hospital stay (days, median [IQR])	14.00 [5.50, 22.25]	7.00 [5.00, 9.00]	0.64
Acute rejection in 3 years of transplant [mean (sd)]	0 (0.0)	4 (19.0)	0.835
Delayed graft function (%)	1 (25.0)	5 (25.0)	0.999

TABLE 4 | Odds of non-adherence by PACT subsection in recipients with a PACT assessment.

Variable	Odds ratio	95% confidence interval	*p*-value
Family support	0.38	0.11–1.41	0.15
Family availability	0.08	0.01–0.97	0.047
Personality factors	0.37	0.13–1.03	0.056
Risk for psychopathology	0.34	0.13–0.87	0.025
Ability to sustain change	1.03	0.34–3.06	0.97
Drug and alcohol abuse	4314	0.00–Inf	0.99
Medical adherence	0.44	0.13–1.53	0.2
Relevant knowledge	1.1	0.32–3.74	0.88

PACT score (Odds Ratio 0.119, 95% Confidence Interval 0.027–0.52, $p = 0.005$) but not HLA mismatch (OR 0.851, 95% CI 0.576–1.259) (**Figure 1**).

When comparing High PACT (≥ 3) vs. Low PACT Scores (≤ 2), the high PACT mean was 3.52 (SD 0.51) while the low PACT group mean was 1.75 (SD 0.50). The low PACT group had a higher percentage of non-adherence and increased rate of missed appointments per year than the high PACT group (**Table 3**). Compared to the high PACT group, patients with lower PACT scores had less family support ($p = 0.01$) and family availability ($p < 0.0010$), more unstable personality factors ($p < 0.001$), increased risk for psychopathology ($p < 0.001$), less ability to sustain change ($p = 0.03$), and less medical adherence ($p = 0.02$) (**Figure 2**). Overall, non-adherence in the low PACT group was associated with less family availability (Odds Ratio 0.08, 95% Confidence Interval 0.01–0.97, $p = 0.047$) and increased risk for psychopathology (OR 0.34, 95% CI 0.13–0.87, $p = 0.025$; **Table 4**).

DISCUSSION

Our study was the first to examine the clinical utility of PACT in a pediatric renal transplantation. Our overall goals were to understand the impact of introducing a standardized psychosocial assessment such as PACT and to elucidate any differences in the clinical outcomes between patients with low and high PACT scores. Similar to adult transplant studies in BMT, lung, and liver recipients, our pilot investigation demonstrated that assessment with PACT was associated with modest improvement in clinical outcomes. Previous studies have shown PACT to be associated with lower in-hospital mortality, shorter length of stay and readmission duration (10, 12, 13, 22, 23). Similar to prior studies, we demonstrated an association between using a standardized assessment, such as PACT, and lower post-transplant morbidity, specifically less acute rejection and non-adherence. Compared to a non-standardized assessment, incorporating PACT into the pre-transplant approach was helpful to identify high risk patients that required more frequent post-transplant monitoring by the medical team including monthly labs, social worker visits, and psychiatry/psychology appointments when appropriate.

The need for pre-transplant psychosocial evaluation has been known for decades, however, standardization of tools or criteria remain insufficient in modern solid organ transplantation (20). Adult measures such as The Stanford Integrated Psychosocial Assessment for Transplant (SIPAT), the Structured Interview for Renal Transplantation (SIRT), and the Transplant Evaluation Rating Scale (TERS) (3–5) have not been studied in pediatrics. PACT has been shown to correlate with outcomes and is among the most studied in adult transplantation. In order to provide one unifying pre-transplant assessment for both pediatric and adults, we evaluated PACT in transplanted children. Our study bridges a gap in the PACT literature and provides important information regarding its potential utility in pediatric renal transplantation to identify those at risk for rejection and non-adherence. Pediatric measures such as the Pediatric Transplant Rating Instrument (P-TRI) and the Psychosocial Assessment Tool (PAT) (24), adapted for pediatric kidney transplantation, suffer from inter-rater variability and did not correlate with clinical outcomes (6, 7, 25).

While outcomes by overall PACT score have been examined, few studies have examined differences in subscales. In bone marrow transplantation (BMT), several subscales were correlated with better outcomes. Foster et al found that adherence was associated with lower in-hospital mortality, shorter length of stay and readmission duration, and faster engraftment. Additionally, higher scores on family availability and on relevant knowledge/receptiveness to education were associated with decreased mortality (12). While our pilot study was not powered for mortality analysis, our results showed that the difference between a high and low PACT score in this pediatric population was driven by family support, innate personality factors, and adherence, similar to what was reported for the BMT population. Additionally, a low PACT score was found in patients with missed appointments and non-adherence. Of those with a PACT score, non-adherence was more likely found in candidates with a higher risk of psychopathology and lack of family support.

Although our pilot study highlights the potential utility of PACT in children, there are limitations. Retrospective analyses are affected by selection and indication biases. By adjusting for HLA mismatch in our analysis, we attempted to minimize significant differences between recipients with no PACT assessment and a PACT assessment. Despite the known association of *de novo* donor specific antibodies (DSA) and non-adherence, baseline DSA and *de novo* DSA were not routinely screened in all patients at our institution until recently (17, 26, 27). Thus, it could not be included as a clinical outcome. Additionally, patients in the two cohorts were transplanted during two different time periods. Patients transplanted between 2005 and 2010 were not assessed with PACT, while those transplanted between 2010 and 2015 were evaluated utilizing PACT. Potential differences in pre- and post-transplant care between these time periods may have impacted our results. One notable difference due to time of transplant was percentage of living related donors in the PACT negative group, most likely due to these recipients undergoing transplant prior to the Share 35 kidney allocation policy. After this policy, which gave pediatrics priority for the best deceased donor allografts, the rate of deceased donor transplantation increased for children (28). We were unable to account for this difference in our final model, but a higher percentage of living donors would be predicted to decrease rates of acute rejection and not increase (29, 30). Lastly, patients without the PACT assessment had longer follow-up time and thus more time to develop poor clinical outcomes. To eliminate this bias, we only evaluated acute rejection episodes within the first 3 years post-transplantation. Although our sample size is small, and our study was not designed to be powered for mortality or graft failure analyses, we found significant findings that warrant further investigation.

In conclusion, renal transplantation requires significant attention to psychosocial factors for successful clinical outcomes. Currently, a standard psychosocial evaluation for transplant candidates across all centers is lacking. Our study highlights that implementation of a standardized measure, such as the PACT, can identify pediatric kidney transplant candidates at risk for poor outcomes, which can align with pre-transplant measures utilized in the adult setting. Thus, future prospective studies may be indicated prior to widespread use.

AUTHOR CONTRIBUTIONS

KF significantly contributed to the acquisition of data, analysis and interpretation of data for the work. He drafted the manuscript. VC contributed to the acquisition of data and interpretation of data. SN, AC, DW, JF, RG, and DV all contributed to the interpretation of data and critical revisions of the manuscript that significantly added to the scientific content. DC contributed to the analysis and interpretation of data that added to the content of the manuscript. EC contributed to the design of the study, interpretation of data, and drafting of the manuscript. All authors agree to be accountable for all aspects of the work in ensuring that questions related to the accuracy or integrity of any part of the work are appropriately investigated and resolved.

ACKNOWLEDGMENTS

We would like to acknowledge Dr. Chamber's funding from the Duke Health Scholars Award. We would also like to acknowledge the Lunch Pail Defense Fund and the Willie Stargell Foundation for their support.

REFERENCES

1. Fielding D, Brownbridge G. Factors related to psychosocial adjustment in children with end-stage renal failure. *Pediatr Nephrol.* (1999) 13:766–70. doi: 10.1007/s004670050695
2. Shonkoff JP, Garner AS, Committee on Psychosocial Aspects of Child and Family Health, Committee on Early Childhood, Adoption, and Dependent Care, Section on Developmental and Behavioral Pediatrics. The lifelong effects of early childhood adversity and toxic stress. *Pediatrics.* (2012) 129:e232–46. doi: 10.1542/peds.2011-2663
3. Twillman RK, Manetto C, Wellisch DK, Wolcott DL. The Transplant Evaluation Rating Scale. A revision of the psychosocial levels system for evaluating organ transplant candidates. *Psychosomatics.* (1993) 34:144–53. doi: 10.1016/S0033-3182(93)71905-2
4. Maldonado JR, Dubois HC, David EE, Sher Y, Lolak S, Dyal J, et al. The Stanford integrated psychosocial assessment for transplantation (SIPAT): a new tool for the psychosocial evaluation of pre-transplant candidates. *Psychosomatics.* (2012) 53:123–32. doi: 10.1016/j.psym.2011.12.012
5. Mori DL, Gallagher P, Milne J. The structured interview for renal transplantation—SIRT. *Psychosomatics.* (2000) 41:393–406. doi: 10.1176/appi.psy.41.5.393
6. Fisher M, Storfer-Isser A, Shaw RJ, Bernard RS, Drury S, Ularntinon S, et al. Inter-rater reliability of the pediatric transplant rating instrument (P-TRI): challenges to reliably identifying adherence risk factors during pediatric pre-transplant evaluations. *Pediatr Transplant.* (2011) 15:142–7. doi: 10.1111/j.1399-3046.2010.01428.x
7. Fung E, Shaw RJ, Pediatric transplant rating instrument-a scale for the pretransplant psychiatric evaluation of pediatric organ transplant recipients. *Pediatr Transplant.* (2008) 12:57–66. doi: 10.1111/j.1399-3046.2007.00785.x
8. Stone D, Banerjee M, Dupuis J, Leleszi J, Allasio D, Singh TP, et al. Association of parental pretransplant psychosocial assessment with post-transplant morbidity in pediatric heart transplant recipients. *Pediatr Transplant.* (2006) 10:602–7. doi: 10.1111/j.1399-3046.2006.00543.x
9. Mary Ellen Olbrisch JLL, Robert Hamer. The PACT: A rating scale for the study of clinical decision-making in psychosocial screening of organ transplant candidates. *Clin Transplant.* (1989) 3:164–9.
10. Hitschfeld MJ, Schneekloth TD, Kennedy CC, Rummans TA, Niazi SK, Vasquez AR, et al. The psychosocial assessment of candidates for transplantation: a cohort study of its association with survival among lung transplant recipients. *Psychosomatics.* (2016) 57:489–97. doi: 10.1016/j.psym.2016.05.003
11. Presberg BA, Levenson JL, Olbrisch ME, Best AM. Rating scales for the psychosocial evaluation of organ transplant candidates. Comparison of the PACT and TERS with bone marrow transplant patients. *Psychosomatics.* (1995) 36:458–61. doi: 10.1016/S0033-3182(95)71626-7
12. Foster LW, McLellan L, Rybicki L, Dabney J, Visnosky M, Bolwell B, et al. Utility of the psychosocial assessment of candidates for transplantation (PACT) scale in allogeneic BMT. *Bone Marrow Transplant.* (2009) 44:375–80. doi: 10.1038/bmt.2009.37
13. Telles-Correia D, Barbosa A, Mega I, Monteiro E. Adherence correlates in liver transplant candidates. *Transplant Proc.* (2009) 41:1731–4. doi: 10.1016/j.transproceed.2009.02.067
14. Woodman CL, Geist LJ, Vance S, Laxson C, Jones K, Kline JN. Psychiatric disorders and survival after lung transplantation. *Psychosomatics.* (1999) 40:293–7. doi: 10.1016/S0033-3182(99)71221-1
15. Dew MA, Switzer GE, DiMartini AF, Matukaitis J, Fitzgerald MG, Kormos RL, et al. Psychosocial assessments and outcomes in organ transplantation. *Prog Transplant.* (2000) 10:239–59, quiz 260–1. doi: 10.1177/152692480001000408
16. Haas M, Loupy A, Lefaucheur C, Roufosse C, Glotz D, Seron D, et al. The Banff 2017 kidney meeting report: revised diagnostic criteria for chronic active T cell-mediated rejection, antibody-mediated rejection, and prospects for integrative endpoints for next-generation clinical trials. *Am J Transplant.* (2018) 18:293–307. doi: 10.1111/ajt.14625
17. Pizzo HP, Ettenger RB, Gjertson DW, Ettenger RB, Gjertson DW, Reed EF, et al. Sirolimus and tacrolimus coefficient of variation is associated with rejection, donor-specific antibodies, and nonadherence. *Pediatr Nephrol.* (2016) 31:2345–52. doi: 10.1007/s00467-016-3422-5
18. Pearl MH, Zhang Q, Palma Diaz MF, Grotts J, Rossetti M, Elashoff D, et al. Angiotensin II Type 1 receptor antibodies are associated with inflammatory cytokines and poor clinical outcomes in pediatric kidney transplantation. *Kidney Int.* (2018) 93:260–9. doi: 10.1016/j.kint.2017.06.034
19. Olbrisch ME JLL, Hamer R. The PACT: a rating scale for the study of clinical decision making in psychosocial screening of organ transplant candidates. *Clin Transplant.* (1989) 3:164–9.
20. Annunziato RA, Fisher MK, Jerson B, Bochkanova A, Shaw RJ. Psychosocial assessment prior to pediatric transplantation: a review and summary of key considerations. *Pediatr Transplant.* (2010) 14:565–74. doi: 10.1111/j.1399-3046.2010.01353.x
21. Maltby MC, Flattery MP, Burns B, Salyer J, Weinland S, Shah KB. Psychosocial assessment of candidates and risk classification of patients considered for durable mechanical circulatory support. *J Heart Lung Transplant.* (2014) 33:836–41. doi: 10.1016/j.healun.2014.04.007
22. Grover S, Sarkar S. Liver transplant-psychiatric and psychosocial aspects. *J Clin Exp Hepatol.* (2012) 2:382–92. doi: 10.1016/j.jceh.2012.08.003
23. Singal AK, Chaha KS, Rasheed K, Anand BS. Liver transplantation in alcoholic liver disease current status and controversies. *World J Gastroenterol.* (2013) 19:5953–63. doi: 10.3748/wjg.v19.i36.5953
24. Pai AL, Patino-Fernandez AM, McSherry M, Beele D, Alderfer MA, Reilly AT, et al. The Psychosocial Assessment Tool (PAT2.0): psychometric properties of a screener for psychosocial distress in families of children newly diagnosed with cancer. *J Pediatr Psychol.* (2008) 33:50–62. doi: 10.1093/jpepsy/jsm053
25. Pai AL, Tackett A, Ittenbach RF, Goebel J. Psychosocial Assessment Tool 2.0_General: validity of a psychosocial risk screener in a pediatric kidney transplant sample. *Pediatr Transplant.* (2012) 16:92–8. doi: 10.1111/j.1399-3046.2011.01620.x
26. Lionaki S, Panagiotellis K, Iniotaki A, Boletis JN. Incidence and clinical significance of de novo donor specific antibodies after kidney transplantation. *Clin Dev Immunol.* (2013) 2013: 849835. doi: 10.1155/2013/849835
27. Kuhne L, Jung B, Poth H, Schuster A, Wurm S, Ruemmele P, et al. Renal allograft rejection, lymphocyte infiltration, and de novo donor-specific antibodies in a novel model of non-adherence to immunosuppressive therapy. *BMC Immunol.* (2017) 18:52. doi: 10.1186/s12865-017-0236-6
28. Hart A, Gustafson SK, Skeans MA, Stock P, Stewart D, Kasiske BL, et al. OPTN/SRTR 2015 Annual Data Report: Early effects of the new kidney allocation system. *Am J Transplant.* (2017) 17(Suppl. 1):543–64. doi: 10.1111/ajt.14132
29. Andre M, Huang E, Everly M, Bunnapradist S. The UNOS renal transplant registry: review of the last decade. *Clin Transpl.* (2014) 1–12.
30. Van Arendonk KJ, Boyarsky BJ, Orandi BJ, James NT, Smith JM, Colombani PM, et al. National trends over 25 years in pediatric kidney transplant outcomes. *Pediatrics.* (2014) 133:594–601. doi: 10.1542/peds.2013-2775

16

The Incidence of Paediatric Acute Kidney Injury Identified Using an AKI E-Alert Algorithm in Six English Hospitals

Sheetal Bhojani[1], Jelena Stojanovic[2], Nabil Melhem[2], Heather Maxwell[1], Peter Houtman[3], Angela Hall[3], Cheentan Singh[4], Wesley Hayes[5], Rachel Lennon[6], Manish D. Sinha[2,7], David V. Milford[8] and the British Association for Paediatric Nephrology*

[1] Royal Hospital for Children, Glasgow, United Kingdom, [2] Evelina London Children's Hospital, London, United Kingdom, [3] Leicester Royal Infirmary, Leicester, United Kingdom, [4] North Middlesex University Hospital NHS Trust, London, United Kingdom, [5] Bristol Royal Hospital for Children, Bristol, United Kingdom, [6] Royal Manchester Children's Hospital, Manchester, United Kingdom, [7] Kings College London, London, United Kingdom, [8] Birmingham Women's and Children's Hospital, Birmingham, United Kingdom

***Correspondence:**
Manish D. Sinha
manish.sinha@nhs.net

Objective: Acute kidney injury (AKI) is a significant cause of morbidity and mortality among hospitalised patients. The objectives in this study were (i) to investigate the incidence of AKI using the National Health Services (NHS) AKI e-alert algorithm as a means of identifying AKI; and (ii) in a randomly selected sub-group of children with AKI identified using the algorithm, to evaluate the recognition and management of AKI.

Patients and Methods: Retrospective cross-sectional study with initial electronic retrieval of creatinine measurements at six hospitals in England over a six-month period. Results were evaluated using the NHS AKI e-alert algorithm with recognition and management of AKI stages 1, 2 and 3 reviewed in a sub-set of randomly selected patient case notes. Patients aged 29 to 17 years were included. AKI stage 1 was defined as a rise of 1.5 – ≤2x baseline creatinine level; AKI stage 2 a rise of ≤ 2.0 and < 3.0; AKI stage 3 a rise of ≥ 3.0. Urine output was not considered for AKI staging.

Results: 57,278 creatinine measurements were analysed. 5,325 (10.8%) AKI alerts were noted in 1,112 patients with AKI 1 (62%), AKI 2 (16%) and AKI 3 (22%). There were 222 (20%) <1y, 432 (39%) 1 ≤ 6y, 192 (17%) 6 ≤ 11y, 207 (19%) 11 ≤ 16y, and 59 (5%) 16–17y. Case notes of 123 of 1,112 [11.1%] children with AKI alerts were reviewed. Confirmed AKI was recognised with a documented management plan following its identification in $n = 32$ [26%] patients only.

Conclusions: In this first multicentre study of the incidence of AKI in children admitted to selected hospitals across England, the incidence of AKI was 10.8% with most patients under the age of 6 years and with AKI stage 1. Recognition and management of AKI was seen in just over 25% children. These data highlight the need to improve recognition of AKI in hospitalised children in the UK.

Keywords: acute kidney injury, hospital, epidemiology, alerts, algorithm

INTRODUCTION

Acute kidney injury (AKI) is characterised by a reversible loss of normal kidney function and is recognised by a reduction in urine output and/or an increase in serum creatinine, indicative of a reduction in glomerular filtration rate (GFR). It is also usually accompanied by an inability of the kidneys to maintain water, acid-base and electrolyte balance (1, 2). The definition of AKI has undergone several iterations (3) and to define and stratify the severity of AKI several classification systems have been proposed and include the RIFLE, AKIN, and KDIGO criteria (4). These consensus definitions are to be welcomed as they help to standardise the diagnosis of AKI, stratify AKI severity and allow the development of predictors of outcomes based on the AKI staging. In children AKI is staged using broadly similar criteria to adults modified as pRIFLE (1).

In adults, AKI is commonly seen in hospitalised patients and associated with increased morbidity and mortality, with worse outcomes in the sickest patients and those with co-morbidities (5–8). Over the past decade several studies have described AKI in hospitalised children and although the incidence is lower, children also have increased morbidity and mortality associated with AKI (9). Recently, Sutherland et al., described rates of AKI in hospitalised children across North America and observed 3.9 episodes of AKI per 1,000 admissions (10). Similar data have been reported from other parts of the world (11, 12).

In those admitted to paediatric ICU, recent data from the AWARE study highlights that AKI is common and is associated with poor outcome including increased mortality (13). Early detection of AKI and implementation of strategies to minimise progression is therefore essential for acute management, but is also likely to improve long term outcomes, particularly in those with the most severe illness (e.g., those admitted to PICU, those undergoing cardiac surgery or those with prematurity), although further data are awaited to prove this (14, 15).

In England, a national algorithm, standardising the definition of AKI was agreed and provides the ability to ensure that a timely and consistent approach to the detection and diagnosis of patients with AKI across the National Health Service (NHS) (16), termed the "NHS AKI e-alert algorithm" in the manuscript [online **Supplement**]. Following integration of the algorithm into the Laboratory Information Management Systems the algorithm will identify potential cases of AKI from laboratory data in real time and produce a test result. The laboratory system will then send the test result, using existing IT connections to patient management systems in use in hospitals in England. Full implementation across all NHS England sites was intended by 9th March 2015 but has taken longer and this is often due to individual local hospital issues. Nonetheless, studies in adults have shown the implementation of AKI alerts and using an AKI care bundle improved recognition and management of acute kidney injury in hospitalised patients (17, 18).

The objectives of this study were (i) to investigate the incidence of AKI using the NHS AKI e-alert algorithm as a means of identifying AKI; and (ii) in a randomly selected sub-group of children identified using the algorithm, to evaluate the recognition and management of AKI.

METHODS

This project was a retrospective cross-sectional study including six centres across England including three district general hospitals [Leicester Royal Infirmary hospital (Centre #1–centre sees both secondary and tertiary care patients), North Middlesex Hospital (Centre #2) and Worcestershire Acute Hospitals (Centre #3)] and three tertiary children's hospitals [Bristol Royal Hospital for Children (Centre #4), Evelina London Children's Hospital (Centre #5) and Royal Manchester Children's Hospital (Centre #6)]. The participating hospitals in this study are centres geographically placed across England. They are also representative for level of care, including both secondary and tertiary level hospital-based acute services for children in England. The tertiary level participating centres provide specialist paediatric nephrology services including management of children with chronic kidney disease, dialysis, and transplantation [Centres #4, #5, and #6]. This multi-centre project was supported by the membership of the British Association for Paediatric Nephrology and its Acute Kidney Injury Interest Group.

The study was designed in two parts; in the first part of the study, all plasma creatinine measurements performed over a 6 month study period between 01/07/2012 to 31/12/2012 were electronically retrieved and compared to any creatinine measurements that may have been performed over the previous year, allowing staging of AKI using the NHS AKI e-alert algorithm (16). Patients aged 29 days to 16 years 364 days were included in the study. Plasma creatinine was measured using the enzymatic method.

AKI stage 1 was defined as a rise of 1.5 – < 2x baseline creatinine level; AKI stage 2 a rise of $\geq$ 2.0 and < 3.0; AKI stage 3 a rise of $\geq$ 3.0. The baseline creatinine was defined as the lowest creatinine value in the previous 12 months (if available) or the upper limit of the reference value for the age (19).

The lead centre (Centre #5) requested electronic retrieval of all creatinine measurements performed at participating centres during the study period. In addition to the plasma creatinine measurements a brief dataset associated with each measurement was included: age, gender, date and time of creatinine measurement, stage of AKI and number of AKI alerts. All centres sent data electronically to the lead centre and data analysed by investigators.

In the second part of the study, a subset of children identified to have AKI were randomly selected for case note review from 5 of 6 centres. Study investigators visited participating centres to collect data from paper and electronic case notes. Notes from Centre #2 were unavailable for review.

Data collected included patient demographics, documented evidence of AKI recognition by the clinical team, the stage of AKI, if appropriate investigations and management were carried out, and if a specialist nephrology opinion was sought and outpatient follow up arranged. This was a retrospective analysis evaluating the incidence of AKI from results of clinically indicated investigations and therefore no consent from patients and ethical approval was required. There was no direct patient or public involvement in this study.

STATISTICAL ANALYSES

Summary statistics are presented as means for continuous data and median and inter-quartile range (IQR) for non-normally distributed data. Comparisons between the two groups in this study were tested as appropriate using the independent samples t-test for continuous data, Mann–Whitney U-test for non-normally distributed data and the Chi-squared test for categorical data. Statistical analyses were performed using SPSS version 22 (SPSS Inc., Chicago, Illinois). All tests were two-tailed and a $p < 0.05$ was taken to represent a statistically significant result.

TABLE 1 | Number of creatinine measurements per centre analysed over a 6 month period across six participating centres*, including $n = 57,278$ measurements.

Centre	Number of measurements
#1	14,029 (24.5%)
#2	1,775 (3.1%)
#3	965 (1.7%)
#4	7,900 (13.8%)
#5	12,095 (21.1%)
#6	20,514 (35.8%)

Centre #1, Leicester Royal Infirmary hospital; Centre #2, North Middlesex Hospital; Centre #3, Worcestershire Acute Hospitals; Centre #4, Bristol Royal Hospital for Children; Centre #5, Evelina London Children's Hospital; Centre #6, Royal Manchester Children's Hospital.

RESULTS

57278 creatinine measurements over a 6 month period were retrieved from the six centres; measurements from individual centres are shown in **Table 1**. Of these 75.2% measurements [$n = 43,080$] had a baseline creatinine measurement over the previous year to compare with and 24.8% [$n = 14,198$] creatinine measurements had no previous baseline measurements. There were 5,325 [10.8%] creatinine values resulting an AKI alert in 1,112 patients using the NHS AKI e-alert algorithm. The incidence of AKI was higher when restricted to those in whom a previous creatinine measurement 12.4% [5325/43080] was available. Of these AKI alerts, 33,24 (62%) were AKI stage 1, 843 (16%) were AKI stage 2 and 1,158 (22%) were AKI stage 3 alerts. In those with no previous baseline measurement, 7.7% [1088/14198] had creatinine measurement above the upper limit of the reference value for their age and this was significantly lower than those in whom a baseline creatinine was available and who had an AKI alert [$p < 0.0001$]. The age distribution of children with AKI alerts was 222 (20%) <1 year, 432 (39%) 1 $\leq$ 6 years, 192 (17%) 6 $\leq$ 11 years, 207 (19%) 11 $\leq$ 16 years, and 59 (5%) 16–17 years. Their distribution by percentage in each age band by worst stage of AKI is shown in **Figure 1**. AKI stage 1 was the largest group across all ages and 59% of all AKI alerts occurred in those aged <6 years. In those patients with AKI, there were 176, 20, 11, 251, 294, and 360 children with AKI in Centres #1, #2, #3, #4, #5, and #6, respectively, and a statistically significant difference in the incidence of AKI between the centres [$p < 0.0001$]. The incidence of AKI in 1,112 patients shown by percentage of children in each centre by worst stage of AKI is shown in **Figure 2**.

In the second part of the study, 123 of 1,112 (11.1%) patients with AKI alerts were randomly selected for case notes review across 5 of the 6 centres (**Table 2**). There were 68 males (55.2%).

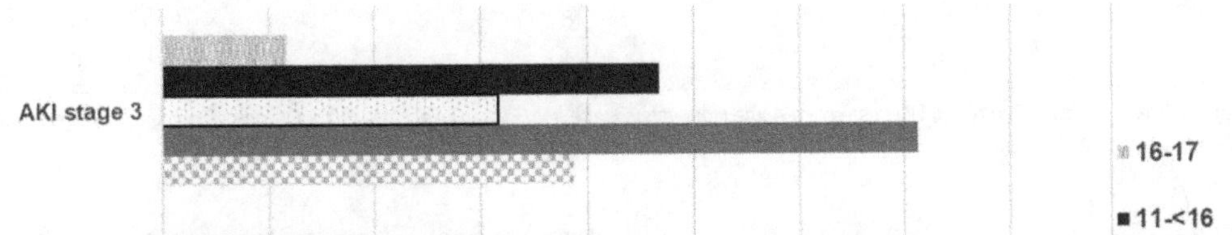

FIGURE 1 | Distribution of $n = 1,112$ children with AKI alerts shown as percentage of children in each age band by worst stage of AKI. Data by worst stage of AKI as indicated by maximal change in creatinine level from baseline using the National Health Service (NHS) AKI e-alert algorithm (16).

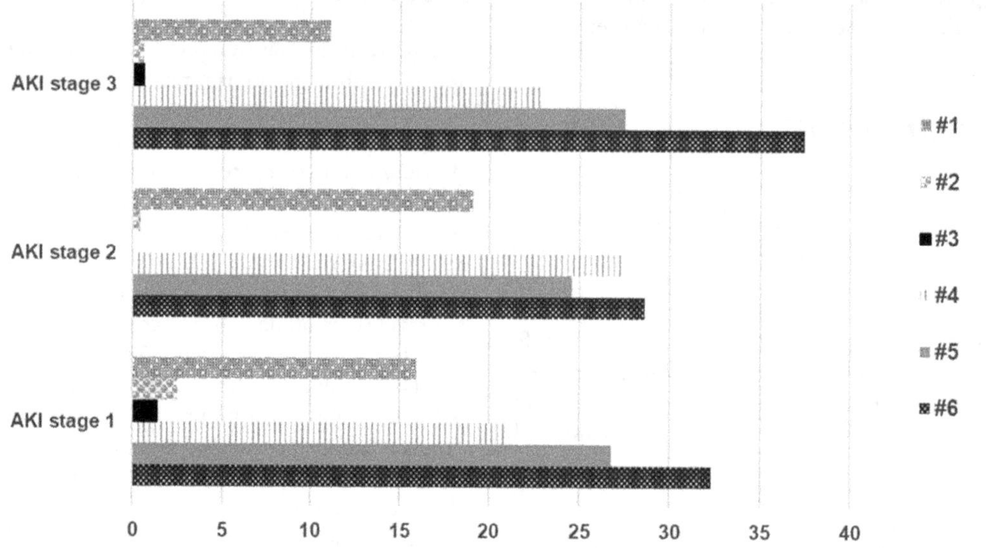

FIGURE 2 | Incidence of AKI alerts in $n = 1,112$ patients shown by percentage of children in each centre* by worst stage of AKI. Data by worst stage of AKI as indicated by maximal change in creatinine level from baseline using the National Health Service (NHS) AKI e-alert algorithm (16). *Centre #1, Leicester Royal Infirmary hospital; Centre #2, North Middlesex Hospital; Centre #3, Worcestershire Acute Hospitals; Centre #4, Bristol Royal Hospital for Children; Centre #5, Evelina London Children's Hospital; Centre #6, Royal Manchester Children's Hospital.

TABLE 2 | Clinical characteristics of randomly selected patients with AKI from five centres* identified retrospectively using National Health Service (NHS) AKI e-alert algorithm.

Centres	1	3	4	5	6
Number of patients, *n* (%)	29 (23.5%)	11 (8.9%)	28 (22.8%)	25 (20.3%)	30 (24.3%)
Age in years [median (IQR)], $n = 95$	2.0 (0.5, 3.3)	7.5 (0.6, 12.7)	No data available	2.3 (0.4, 6.6)	3.9 (1.8, 6.4)
Male, *n* (%)	15 (51.8%)	6 (54.6%)	14 (50%)	16 (64%)	17 (56.7%)
Creatinine in μmol/L at presentation [median (IQR)]	45 (36, 61)	46 (36, 85)	71 (51, 141)	44 (33, 86)	27 (21, 46)
Correctly identifed AKI, *n* (%)	3 (10.3%)	1 (9%)	11 (39%)	11 (44%)	6 (20%)
Management plan accounting for AKI					
Yes	4 (13.7%)	2 (18%)	13 (46.4%)	7 (28%)	6 (20%)
No	24	8	13	18	24
No information	1	1	2	0	0

**Centre #1, Leicester Royal Infirmary hospital; Centre #3, Worcestershire Acute Hospitals; Centre #4, Bristol Royal Hospital for Children; Centre #5, Evelina London Children's Hospital; Centre #6, Royal Manchester Children's Hospital.*

The median [IQR] age was 3.1 years (0.5, 6.6). AKI was correctly identified and a management plan following its identification was documented in 32 (26%) of patients. In 87 (71%) patients, AKI was not identified with no clinical notes highlighting this issue or no management plan for AKI; and for 4 (3%) patients there was no information available.

Data for patients in whom AKI was recognised ($n = 32$; AKI-R) was compared to those in whom AKI was not recognised ($n = 87$; AKI-NR) and their management plan following recognition reviewed (**Table 3**).

Median [IQR] age in years was the same in AKI-R and AKI-NR [3.1 (0.7, 6.4) vs. 3.1 (0.5,7.2), $p = 0.56$]. Boys were affected more in both groups AKI-R (59.3%) vs. AKI-NR (53.8%). Median [IQR] creatinine (μmol/L) was significantly higher in the AKI-R group compared to the AKI-NR group [103 (61,239) vs. 39 (29,57), $p < 0.0001$]. The largest number of AKI cases that were not recognised were admitted in General Paediatrics, followed by Cardiology, Intensive Care, and Oncology.

In terms of management of AKI, the risk of possible drug nephrotoxicity was considered in 59% in AKI-R group compared to 1% in AKI-NR group. A specialist nephrology opinion was sought in 37% vs. 1% in the AKI-R vs. AKI-NR group. 90% of the patients in AKI-R group were followed up in clinic compared to 55% in AKI-NR group (**Table 3**). Estimated glomerular filtration rate (eGFR) was rarely measured by non-renal specialties. At the time of discharge, serum creatinine had returned to baseline levels in 78% of patients. There was 1 death (3%) in the AKI- R group and none in the AKI-NR group.

TABLE 3 | Results of case note review for 119 of 123 patients for clinical management of recognised vs. unrecognised AKI during inpatient episode.

Demographics	AKI-Recognised	AKI-Not recognised
Number of patients (n = 123)^, n (%)	32 (26%)	87 (71%)
Age in years [median (IQR)]	3.1 (0.7,6.4)	3.1 (0.5,7.2)
Boys, n (%)	19 (59.3%)	49 (53.8%)
Creatinine in μmol/L at presentation [median (IQR)]^^	103 (61,239)	39 (29,57)
Patients admitted under		
Total	32	87
General Paediatrics	3	29
Cardiology	2	17
Neurology	0	2
Nephrology	13	1
Neonatology	2	1
Intensive care and ECMO	6	8
General surgery	0	2
Oncology	0	6
Specialty not known	6	21
Management		
Daily weight measurements n (%)	22 (69%)	13 (14%)
Twice daily weights, n (%)	4 (12%)	2 (2%)
Blood pressure measured, n (%)	31 (97%)	62 (68%)
Fluid balance, n (%)	29 (91%)	39 (43%)
Repeat creatinine measured, n (%)	31 (97%)	57 (63%)
Urine dipstick performed, n (%)	16 (50%)	13 (14%)
Renal Ultrasound scan performed, n (%)	15 (47%)	4 (4%)
Estimated GFR measured, n (%)	9 (28%)	1 (1%)
Role of drug related nephrotoxicity and AKI considered, n (%)	19 (59%)	1 (1%)
Paediatric Nephrology advice considered, n (%)	12 (37%)	1 (1%)
Follow up		
*OPD clinic review, n (%)	28 (90%)	50 (55%)
**GP review, n (%)	0	1 (1%)
Creatinine returned to baseline levels, n (%)		
Yes	25 (78%)	49 (54%)
No	5 (16%)	11 (12%)
Not re-measured	0	18 (20%)
No information	1 (3%)	13 (14%)
Died	1 (3%)	0

All patients identified retrospectively using National Health Service (NHS) AKI e-alert algorithm.
*^no, information available for 4 patients; ^^$P < 0.0001$; *OPD, outpatient department; **GP, general practitioner.*

DISCUSSION

This is the first multicentre study looking at the incidence and management of AKI in hospitalised children in selected English hospitals using a creatinine-based algorithm and includes a large data set of children over a 6 month period from both district general and teaching hospitals.

The number of studies of AKI in paediatric population are much less than in the adult population (20) and usually include small numbers of patients. Most of the paediatric studies are either single centre or, if multicentre, focused on high risk groups such as children in PICU whereas this study looked at the incidence of AKI among all hospitalised patients.

In this study here, the overall incidence of AKI was 10.8% which was similar to other studies (12, 21). This was less than the incidence reported in meta-analysis including studies across the world, that reported a pooled incidence of AKI in children of 33.7% (20). However, on inspecting the paediatric studies in the meta-analysis, 67% of the studies included patients in critical care or post cardiac surgery, and study numbers were generally small, therefore their results cannot be considered to represent the true incidence of AKI in all childhood admissions worldwide.

AKI stage 1 was the commonest stage across all ages in this study. The incidence of AKI was higher in the younger age group (~60% of AKI was in children under 6 years of age) which is similar to other studies (11, 21) but contrary to a large epidemiological study by Sutherland et al. where the highest incidence of AKI was seen in 15–18 year olds (10). However, Sutherland et al. used ICD-9-CM codes (International Classification of Diseases, Ninth Revision, Clinical Modification) applied at discharge rather than the creatinine-based criteria of AKIN or pRIFLE criteria for diagnosing AKI (10). Younger children tend to have lower serum creatinine values and therefore a small absolute change in the creatinine value could lead to identification of AKI using the AKIN or pRIFLE criteria but not with the ICD-9-CM coding system (10).

In this study reported here, the pRIFLE or AKIN criteria were not used by clinicians for routinely diagnosing AKI and so patients with a rise in creatinine from baseline but whose creatinine was still within the laboratory specified normal range were less likely to be recognised to have AKI. This includes the group of children who would be at risk of AKI (pRIFLE "R") and in whom appropriate intervention could be anticipated to prevent progression. It is important to note that in the sub-set of randomly selected patients who had case note review, 74% of patients with AKI were not recognised. Even in the group of children where AKI had been recognised (AKI-R), appropriate management was not implemented, highlighting the need for education and training among the medical staff.

The diagnosis of AKI is usually made by identifying increased serum creatinine with or without associated reduced urine output (17). Studies have shown that using a care bundle can improve the recognition of AKI which can lead to early initiation of treatment to reduce progression of AKI and so reduce morbidity and mortality (17, 18). The AKI alert algorithm was introduced across NHS England in 2015 to facilitate early diagnosis. In this study the data set was from a period before the introduction of the algorithm; further studies will be needed to examine if the early identification of AKI as a result of implementation of the NHS algorithm has led to improved recognition and management of AKI with a reduction in AKI related morbidity and mortality.

There are some important limitations to our study findings that need to be considered and include (i) Inherent biases related to the retrospective nature of such data; (ii) electronic alerts of AKI were based on serum creatinine values only and do not have any information regarding GFR or urine output. We recognise that in clinical practice and in widely established AKI criteria, urine output is integrated to facilitate early diagnosis and lack of these data are therefore likely to underestimate AKI, however we wished to examine the application of the NHS AKI e-alert algorithm in routine clinical practice; (iii) Although the algorithm is helpful for identifying AKI, we recognise in clinical practice use of creatinine alone may be misleading particularly in younger children who have physiologically low creatinine values; similar issues are likely to complicate evaluation in children with chronic illness and malnutrition; (iv) only one definition of AKI stage 3 was used. We recognise that sometimes an increase in serum creatinine may be $<3\times$ the baseline but the eGFR for the patient much worse and clinically significant; (v) In those patients in whom no creatinine values were available to compare an increase from a previous baseline, we used the upper limit of reference range as baseline creatinine. In those with a single high value we have not reported this as AKI here as per the algorithm and this may underestimate the true incidence of AKI in our cohort. Previous studies (22–24), have shown increased sensitivity in detecting AKI when using the lower reference limit or using back calculation to estimate the baseline creatinine from the Schwartz formula and defining baseline GFR as 120 ml/min/1.73m^2. Importantly, these approaches may categorise those with CKD as AKI but also overestimate the true incidence of AKI; furthermore back calculation requires the patient height. Despite this as shown in this study, there remain significant shortcomings in the recognition of AKI by non-renal physicians, with poor recording of urine output and/or of eGFR for hospitalised children receiving clinical care. A creatinine based algorithm embedded in hospital reporting systems is likely to be more effective in identifying AKI.

CONCLUSION

The incidence of AKI in this multicentre study was 10.8% with most patients under the age of 6 years and AKI stage 1 was the predominant stage across all ages. There remains an ongoing need for education and training of health professionals to improve recognition and management of patients with AKI. Timely recognition and optimal management of AKI is important to improve long term renal outcomes. Future studies will aim to determine the impact of the NHS AKI e-alert algorithm in the UK.

ETHICS STATEMENT

The study was registered with the corresponding authors institution as a multi-centre audit. This was a review of historical hospital results/records. No ethical approval was required following audit approval. Written informed consent from the participants' legal guardian/next of kin was not required to participate in this study in accordance with the national legislation and the institutional requirements.

AUTHOR CONTRIBUTIONS

SB: data collection, manuscript writing, final approval of the version to be published, and agreement to be accountable for all aspects of the work in ensuring that questions related to the accuracy or integrity of any part of the work are appropriately investigated and resolved. MS and DM: project leads, designing the project, data collection, analysis, manuscript writing, final approval of the version to be published, and agreement to be accountable for all aspects of the work in ensuring that questions related to the accuracy or integrity of any part of the work are appropriately investigated and resolved. JS, NM, HM, PH, AH, CS, WH, and RL: data collection from individual centres and approval of the final version.

ACKNOWLEDGMENTS

Preliminary results of this study were presented at the 48th Annual Scientific Meeting of the European Society for Paediatric Nephrology (ESPN) at Brussels and published as an abstract. JS, NM, SB, MS, and DM. Can early recognition of AKI in children be achieved by using an algorithm (preliminary results): on behalf of British Association for Paediatric Nephrology. Pediatr Nephrol. (2015) 30:1543.

REFERENCES

1. McCaffrey J, Dhakal AK, Milford DV, Webb NJ, Lennon R Recent developments in the detection and management of acute kidney injury. *Arch Dis Child.* (2017) 102:91–6. doi: 10.1136/archdischild-2015-309381
2. Andreoli, SP. Acute kidney injury in children. *Pediatr Nephrol.* (2009) 24:253–63. doi: 10.1007/978-3-540-76341-3_65
3. Eknoyan G. Emergence of the concept of acute renal failure. *Am J Nephrol.* (2002) 22:225–30. doi: 10.1159/000063766
4. Levi TM, de Souza SP, de Magalhães JG, de Carvalho MS, Cunha AL, de Oliveira Dantas JG et al. Comparison of the RIFLE, AKIN and KDIGO criteria to predict mortality in critically ill patients. *Rev Bras Ter Intensiva.* (2013) 25:290–6. doi: 10.5935/0103-507X.20130050
5. Chertow GM, Burdick E, Honour M, Bonventre JV, Bates DW. Acute kidney injury, mortality, length of stay, and costs in hospitalized patients. *J Am Soc Nephrol.* (2005) 16:3365–70. doi: 10.1681/ASN.2004090740
6. Ricci Z, Cruz D, Ronco C. The RIFLE criteria and mortality in acute kidney injury: a systematic review. *Kidney Int.* (2008) 73:538–46. doi: 10.1038/sj.ki.5002743
7. Mehta RL, Kellum JA, Shah SV, Molitoris BA, Ronco C, Warnock DG, et al. Acute kidney injury network: report of an initiative to improve outcomes in acute kidney injury. *Critical Care.* (2007) 11:R31. doi: 10.1186/cc5713
8. Chertow GM, Soroko SH, Paganini EP, Cho KC, Himmelfarb J, Ikizler TA, et al. Mortality after acute renal failure: models for prognostic stratification and risk adjustment. *Kidney Int.* (2006) 70:1120–6. doi: 10.1038/sj.ki.5001579
9. Slater MB, Anand V, Uleryk EM, Parshuram CS. A systematic review of RIFLE criteria in children, and its application and association with measures of mortality and morbidity. *Kidney Int.* (2012) 81:791–8. doi: 10.1038/ki.2011.466
10. Sutherland SM, Ji J, Sheikhi FH, Widen E, Tian L, Alexander SR, et al. AKI in hospitalized children: epidemiology and clinical associations in a

national cohort. *Clin J Am Soc Nephrol.* (2013) 8:1661–9. doi: 10.2215/CJN.00270113

11. Krishnamurthy S, Mondal N, Narayanan P, Biswal N, Srinivasan S, Soundravally R. Incidence and etiology of acute kidney injury in Southern India. *Indian J Pediatr.* (2013) 80:183–9. doi: 10.1007/s12098-012-0791-z
12. Jenssen GR, Hovland E, Bangstad HJ, Nygård K, Vold L, Bjerre A. The incidence and aetiology of acute kidney injury in children in Norway between 1999 and 2008. *Acta Pædiatr.* (2014) 103:1192–7. doi: 10.1111/apa.12742
13. Kaddourah A, Basu RK, Bagshaw SM, Goldstein SL. Epidemiology of acute kidney injury in critically Ill children and young adults. *N Engl J Med.* (2017) 376:11–20. doi: 10.1056/NEJMoa1611391
14. Greenberg JH, Coca S, Parikh CR. Long-term risk of chronic kidney disease and mortality in children after acute kidney injury: a systematic review. *BMC Nephrol.* (2014) 15:184. doi: 10.1186/1471-2369-15-184
15. Selewski DT, Charlton JR, Jetton JG, Guillet R, Mhanna MJ, Askenazi DJ, et al. Neonatal acute kidney injury. *Paediatrics.* (2015) 136:e463–73. doi: 10.1542/peds.2014-3819
16. NHS England patient safety alert: NHS/PSA/D/2014/010. Available online at: https://www.england.nhs.uk/patientsafety/wp-content/uploads/sites/32/2014/06/psa-aki2.pdf (accessed December 23, 2019).
17. Joslin J, Wilson H, Zubli D, Gauge N, Kinirons M, Hopper A, et al. Recognition and management of acute kidney injury in hospitalised patients can be partially improved with the use of a care bundle. *Clin Med.* (2015) 15:431–6. doi: 10.7861/clinmedicine.15-5-431
18. Tsui A, Rajani C, Doshi R, De Wolff J, Tennant R, Duncan N, et al. Improving recognition and management of acute kidney injury. *Acute Med.* (2014) 13:108–12.
19. Think Kidneys: Guidance for clinicians managing children at risk of, or with, acute kidney injury. Available online at: https://www.thinkkidneys.nhs.uk/aki/wp-content/uploads/sites/2/2016/05/Guidance__for__paediatric__patients__FINAL.pdf (accessed December 23, 2019).
20. Susantitaphong P, Cruz DN, Cerda J, Abulfaraj M, Alqahtani F, Koulouridis I, et al. World incidence of AKI: a meta-analysis. *Clin J Am Soc Nephrol.* (2013) 8:1482–93. doi: 10.2215/CJN.00710113
21. Mehta P, Sinha A, Sami A, Hari P, Kalaivani M, Gulati A, et al. Incidence of acute kidney injury in hospitalized children. *Indian Pediatrics.* (2012) 49:537–42. doi: 10.1007/s13312-012-0121-6
22. Zappitelli M, Parikh CR, Akcan-Arikan A, Washburn KK, Moffett BS, Goldstein SL. Ascertainment and epidemiology of acute kidney injury varies with definition interpretation. *Clin J Am Soc Nephrol.* (2008) 3:948–54. doi: 10.2215/CJN.05431207
23. Bagshaw SM, Uchino S, Cruz D, Bellomo R, Morimatsu H, Morgera S, et al. A comparison of observed versus estimated baseline creatinine for determination of RIFLE class in patients with acute kidney injury. *Nephrol Dial Transplant.* (2009) 24:2739–44. doi: 10.1093/ndt/gfp159
24. Siew ED, Matheny ME, Ikizler TA, Lewis JB, Miller RA, Waitman LR, et al. Commonly used surrogates for baseline renal function affect the classification and prognosis of acute kidney injury. *Kidney Int.* (2010) 77:536–42. doi: 10.1038/ki.2009.479

17

Interleukin-4 and Interleukin-13 Gene Polymorphisms in Children with Idiopathic Nephrotic Syndrome

Maysoun Al Rushood**, Amal A. Al-Eisa and Mohammad Z. Haider

Department of Pediatrics, Faculty of Medicine, Health Sciences Center, Kuwait University, Kuwait City, Kuwait

***Correspondence:**
Maysoun Al Rushood
maysoun.alrushood@ku.edu.kw

Background: Idiopathic Nephrotic syndrome (INS) is an immune-mediated disease in which a number of cytokines, including IL-4 and IL-13, have been implicated in the pathogenesis. Cytokine gene polymorphisms might affect their levels and activity. Therefore, may affect INS susceptibility and response to treatment. The aim of the study was to determine the association of IL-4 and IL-13 gene polymorphisms and INS susceptibility and their effects on steroid responsiveness in children.

Methods: The polymorphisms in IL-4 and IL-13 genes were detected by PCR-RFLP in 155 INS patients and 64 controls.

Results: A total of 132 steroid-sensitive (SS) and 23 steroid resistance (SR) INS patients; mean age 7.3 ± 4.0 years, were included. Male: Female ratio was 2:1. No significant statistical differences were detected in the frequency of CC, CT, and TT genotypes of IL-4 gene compared to controls ($P = 0.57$, 0.61, and 1.00, respectively). There was no significant difference in the T and C-allele frequencies, in SS and SR subgroups. Analysis of IL-13 gene polymorphism also did not show significant statistical differences in the frequency of QQ, RQ, and RR genotypes compared to controls ($P = 0.74$, 1.00, and 0.68, respectively). No significant difference was found in the Q and R-allele frequency. However, the heterozygous RQ genotype of the IL13 gene was significantly higher in SS INS patients compared to the SR INS cases ($P = 0.04$).

Conclusion: Our findings did not show an association between IL-4 and IL-13 gene polymorphisms and INS susceptibility. However, IL-13 RQ genotype was expressed more in children with INS who are steroid sensitive.

Keywords: interleukin-4, interleukin-13, nephrotic syndrome, gene polymorphisms, cytokine, steroids

INTRODUCTION

Idiopathic nephrotic syndrome (INS) is the most frequent form of nephrotic syndrome in children, representing more than 90% of cases between the age of 1 to 10 years (1). Immunological disturbances, especially T cell imbalance, have been implicated in the pathogenesis of the disease (1, 2). This association was suggested by the response to immunosuppressive treatment and the association between the disease with atopy and elevated serum IgE levels (1, 2).

T helper cells (Th2) with its signature cytokines such as IL-4 and IL-13 have been studied as potential important role players in the pathogenesis of the INS (3, 4). IL-4 is a Th2 cytokine produced by basophils, mast cells and activated TH2 cells (5), and plays an essential role in IgE regulation, Th2 differentiation, Th1 inhibition and induction and maintenance of allergy (6, 7). It might also act as an anti-tumor and an anti-inflammatory agent (8, 9).

On the other hand, IL-13 is an immunoregulatory protein produced by T-cells subsets, basophils, eosinophils and mast cells. It is believed to be an important mediator in allergic disease as its levels and genetic polymorphism variants have been shown to be associated with elevated serum IgE levels in atopic and asthmatic patients of different racial backgrounds (10–13).

Both IL-4 and IL-13 genes are located in a region of 140 kb on chromosome 5q31-33 that codes for a cluster of Th2 cytokines (10, 14). They share a common IL-4 receptor α chain (IL4 RA) in the multimeric IL-4 and IL-13 receptor complexes (15). Therefore, they share many biological activities that affect clinical conditions.

Gene Polymorphisms in the regulatory regions of these cytokines can influence the amount of cytokine produced as well as their biological activity and potency at their receptor sites (14). Cytokine gene polymorphism including that of IL-4 and IL-13 in nephrotic syndrome of children with an Arab race has not been explored previously. The aim of this study is to determine any association between IL-4 and cytokine IL-13 gene polymorphisms with the susceptibility to INS in Kuwaiti children and their effects on response to steroid treatment.

METHODS

Children less than 12 years of age with a confirmed diagnosis of Idiopathic nephrotic syndrome (INS) were included in this study. All had INS with a clinical and/or histopathological diagnosis of MCNS. Subjects were evaluated at a specialized pediatric nephrology clinic in Mubarak Al-Kabir University Hospital during the period 2012–2018. INS was defined as the presence of generalized edema, nephrotic- range proteinuria, hypoalbuminemia with or without hyperlipidemia (16). A total of 155 children were included. Patients were subdivided according to their response to steroids into steroid sensitive (SS) and steroid resistant (SR). Steroid responsiveness was defined as the disappearance of proteinuria (negative to trace in a urine dipstick for 3 consecutive days, or a urine protein/creatinine level of <0.2) within the first 4-week course of full dose prednisolone therapy (60 mg/M^2/day). Steroid resistance was defined as the persistence of proteinuria after a 4-week course of full dose prednisolone. Patients with poor compliance and not on regular follow-up were excluded as well as those with infrequent relapses. All SSNS patients were in full remission at the time of the study.

All patients underwent a thorough physical examination by an experienced pediatrician. A total of 64 age and gender- matched healthy children of the same ethnic background, were included as controls. All were examined by a senior pediatrician to exclude any renal disease. Controls were selected from patients visiting Hospital's Emergency Department for minor illnesses such as upper respiratory tract infection or acute gastroenteritis.

In all the study subjects (patients and controls), tests for blood urea, serum creatinine, total protein, albumin level and a complete lipid profile were carried out. Urine protein: creatinine ratio was also determined for all the study subjects.

At the end of the study, all SSNS patients had normal serum creatinine. Sixty-five percent of the patients were in remission for more than 6 months, while 35% continued to relapse, but less frequently, despite receiving second-line immunosuppressive treatment. For SSNS patients, renal biopsy was performed for steroid dependent patients and for those with frequent relapses (> 6 relapses/year) before initiating cytotoxic therapy.

Genetic study was done in 12 SRNS patients and they were NPHS1 negative. The genetic study for the rest of the SRNS patients was not available as it should be sent outside the country.

Genotyping of IL4 and IL13 Gene Polymorphisms

DNA was isolated from the peripheral leukocytes using a standard method (17). The genotypes were determined by PCR-RFLP (polymerase chain reaction-restriction fragment length polymorphism) method using the primers listed below (18, 19):

IL-4 Gene C590T Polymorphism

Forward primer: 5′-ACTAGGCTCACCTGATACG-3′
Reverse primer: 5′-GTTGTAATGCAGTCCTCCTG-3′

The PCR reactions were carried out in a total volume of 25 μl containing 100 ng of genomic DNA, 10 pmoles of each primer, 2 mM $MgCl_2$, 0.2 mM deoxynucleotides (dNTPs), 1 × buffer, and 2U of Taq DNA polymerase. The amplification was performed for 35 cycles with an annealing temperature of 58°C for 1 min for the IL-4 gene C590T polymorphism. The C—>T transition at codon 590 of the IL-4 gene abolished a restriction site for *Bsm*F1 in the T-allele. The polymorphism was identified by *Bsm*F1 restriction endonuclease digestion of the PCR-amplified fragment. The cleavage products were analyzed by 2% agarose gel electrophoresis and visualized under UV light after staining with ethidium bromide. The product sizes were 192 and 60 bp for the C-allele and 252 bp for the T-allele, respectively.

IL-13 Gene Polymorphism

The IL-13 gene polymorphisms R130Q (rs20541) and IL-13 gene promoter polymorphism (C- 1112T) was determined by PCR-RFLP methods described earlier (18, 19). The PCR primer sequences used were:

Sense primer: 5′-CTTCCGTGAGGACTGAATGAGAC GGTC-3′

Antisense primer: 5′-GCAAATAATGATGCTTTCGAAGTT TCAGTGGA-3′

For the R130Q polymorphism, amplification was carried out after denaturation at 94^{0}C for 5 min followed by 35 cycles of 94^{0}C for 45 s, 67^{0}C for 45 s and 72^{0}C for 30 s followed by an extension at 72^{0}C for 5 min. The PCR products were cleaved with restriction enzyme *Nla*IV (0.5 U) at 37^{0}C for 3 h and analyzed by agarose gel electrophoresis as described earlier. The expected cleavage products were 210 and 26 bp when a normal R130-genotype is present and in the case of mutant −130Q genotype the expected product size 178 bp, 32 and 26 bp, respectively.

Statistical Analysis

The genotypes were determined by gene counting and the data was analyzed using the Chi-squared test and the Fisher's exact test. Odds Ratio (OR) was calculated with 95% Confidence Interval (CI). *P*-values of 0.05 or less were considered as statistically significant.

Ethical approval was obtained from the Health Sciences Center Committee for the Protection of Human Subjects in Research, Kuwait University, as well as, Ministry of Health Ethics Committee. An informed consent was obtained from care givers of both patients and controls as per guidelines of the Committees.

RESULTS

The study included a total of 155 Kuwaiti children with INS. Of these, 132 were steroid-sensitive (SS) and 23 were steroid resistant (SR). The mean age in the INS patient group was 7.6 ± 4.3 years and Male: Female ratio was 2:1. The clinical and biochemical characteristics of INS patients and controls have been presented in **Table 1**. A total of 83 patients had history of atopy (53.5%), with some having more than one form of atopy. Asthma was reported in 53 patients (34%), eczema in 46 patients (27%), allergic conjunctivitis in 11 (7%), and allergic rhinosinusitis in 7 patients (4.5%). Food allergy was not reported in any patient. Atopy was not reported in any of the controls.

Genotype analysis of IL-4 gene polymorphism was inconclusive in 2 INS patients of the SS subgroup which were excluded from the statistical analysis for IL-4 gene polymorphism. From a total of 153 INS subjects and 64 controls, the CC genotype of IL-4 gene polymorphism was detected in 64% of the INS patients compared to 69.5% in the controls ($P = 0.57$). The heterozygous CT genotype was detected in 30% of INS patients compared to 25.5% in the controls ($P = 0.61$). The TT-genotype was detected in 6% of INS patients and in 5% of the controls ($P = 1.00$). The C-allele frequency in homozygous and heterozygous forms was found in 94% of INS patients compared to 95% of the controls ($P = 1.00$). The T-allele frequency in homozygous and heterozygous forms was found in 35.7% of INS patients compared to 30.5% of the controls ($P = 0.57$). **Table 2** summarized the gene and allele frequency of IL-4 gene polymorphism in both patients and controls. No significant difference was detected in any of the genotype frequencies between the SS and SR sub-groups when compared with each other or when compared to the controls (**Table 3**).

In the case of IL-13 gene polymorphism, genotyping was conclusive for all the 155 INS patients and 64 controls and the results have been presented in **Table 4**. The QQ genotype of IL-13 gene polymorphism was detected in 70.3% of the INS patients compared to 73.4% of the controls ($P = 0.74$). The heterozygous RQ genotype was detected in 25.8% of INS patients compared 28% of the controls ($P = 1.0$). The RR-genotype was detected in 3.9% of INS patients and 1.6% of the controls ($P = 0.68$). The Q-allele frequency in homozygous and heterozygous forms was found in 83.2% of INS patients compared to 86% of the controls ($P = 0.57$). The R-allele frequency in homozygous and heterozygous forms was found in 16.7% of INS patients compared to 14% of the controls ($P = 0.57$). When the genotype frequencies were compared between the SS and SR sub-groups, only the RQ genotype showed a statistically significant association with steroid sensitivity ($P = 0.04$; **Table 5**).

The data of SS patients and SR patients were studied separately and compared to controls. When IL-4 gene polymorphisms data of SR and SS patients were compared to controls separately, no significant differences in the genotype or allele frequencies were detected, as shown in **Tables 6, 7**.

Similarly, IL-13 gene polymorphisms data of SR and SS patients were compared to controls separately. No significant differences in the genotype or allele frequencies were detected, when each sub-group compared to controls, as shown in **Tables 8, 9**.

TABLE 1 | Clinical and laboratory data of Kuwaiti children with Idiopathic Nephrotic Syndrome (INS) and the controls.

Range		INS patients (n = 155)	Controls (n = 64)	Normal
Mean age (years)		7.6 ± 4.3	7.1 ± 3.7	
Gender	Male	104	42	
	Female	51	22	
Atopy (n)		83 (53.5%)	0 (0%)	
Mean serum creatinine (μmol/L)		47 ± 7	56 ± 8	(15–88)
Mean serum protein (g/L)		50 ± 2	73 ± 2	(68–80)
Mean serum albumin (g/L)		21 ± 3	34 ± 3	(30–40)
Mean serum cholesterol (mmol/L)		6.5 ± 0.4	3.2 ± 0.6	(3.1–5.2)
Mean UP: Cr ratio* (mg/mg)		2.8±0.7	0.02±0.05	(≤ 0.2)

UP, Urine Protein; Cr, Creatinine.

TABLE 2 | Interlukin-4 gene polymorphism in Kuwaiti children with INS and the controls.

Genotype	INS (%) n = 153	Controls (%) (n = 64)	Odds ratio (OR)	95% confidence Interval (CI)	P-values
CC	99 (64.71)	44 (68.75)	0.83	0.45–1.56	0.68
CT	45 (29.41)	17 (26.56)	1.15	0.59–2.22	0.79
TT	9 (5.88)	3 (4.69)	1.27	0.33–4.86	1.00
C allele	243/306	105/128	0.84	0.49–1.44	0.62
T allele	63/306	23/128	1.18	0.69–2.01	0.62

TABLE 3 | Comparison of IL-4 gene polymorphism genotype and allele frequencies between steroid sensitive (SS) and steroid resistant (SR) Kuwaiti INS patients.

Genotype	SS (%) n = 130	SR (%) (n = 23)	Odds ratio (OR)	95% confidence interval (CI)	P-values
CC	83 (63.85)	16 (69.57)	0.77	0.29–2.01	0.64
CT	40 (30.77)	5 (21.74)	1.60	0.55–4.61	0.46
TT	7 (5.38)	2 (8.69)	0.59	0.12–3.08	0.63
C allele	226/260	37/46	1.62	0.72–3.65	0.25
T allele	54/260	9/46	1.08	0.49–2.37	1.00

TABLE 4 | Genotype and allele frequencies of Interleukin-13 gene polymorphism in Kuwaiti children with INS and controls.

Genotype	INS (%) *n* = 155	Controls (%) (*n* = 64)	Odds ratio (OR)	95% confidence interval (CI)	*P*-values
QQ	109 (70.32)	47 (73.44)	0.86	0.45–1.65	0.74
RQ	40 (25.81)	16 (25.0)	1.04	0.53–2.04	1.00
RR	6 (3.87)	1 (1.56)	2.54	0.29–21.52	0.68
Q allele	258/310	110/128	0.81	0.45–1.45	0.57
R allele	52/310	18/128	1.23	0.69–2.20	0.57

TABLE 5 | Comparison of IL-13 gene polymorphism genotype and allele frequencies between steroid sensitive (SS) and steroid resistant (SR) Kuwaiti INS patients.

Genotype	SS (%) *n* = 132	SR (%) (*n* = 23)	Odds ratio (OR)	95% confidence interval (CI)	*P*-values
QQ	90 (68.18)	19 (82.60)	0.45	0.14–1.41	0.22
RQ	38 (28.79)	2 (8.70)	4.25	0.95–19.00	0.04
RR	4 (3.03)	2 (8.70)	0.33	0.05–1.90	0.22
Q allele	218/264	40/46	0.71	0.28–1.78	0.53
R allele	46/264	6/46	1.41	0.56–3.51	0.53

TABLE 6 | Comparison of IL-4 gene polymorphism genotype and allele frequencies between Steroid Sensitive (SS) patients and controls.

Genotype	SS (%) *n* = 130	Controls (%) (*n* = 64)	Odds ratio (OR)	95% confidence interval (CI)	*P*-values
CC	83 (63.85)	44 (68.75)	0.80	0.42–1.52	0.61
CT	40 (30.77)	17 (26.56)	1.23	0.63–2.40	0.66
TT	7 (5.38)	3 (4.69)	1.16	0.29–4.63	1.00
C allele	226/260	105/128	1.46	0.82–2.60	0.26
T allele	54/260	23/128	1.20	0.70–2.06	0.61

TABLE 7 | Comparison of IL-4 gene polymorphism genotype and allele frequencies between Steroid Resistant (SR) patients and controls.

Genotype	SR (%) (*n* = 23)	Controls (%) (*n* = 64)	Odds ratio (OR)	95% confidence interval (CI)	*P*-values
CC	16 (69.57)	44 (68.75)	1.04	0.37–2.92	1.00
CT	5 (21.74)	17 (26.56)	0.77	0.25–2.39	0.78
TT	2 (8.69)	3 (4.69)	1.94	0.30–12.40	0.60
C allele	37/46	105/128	0.90	0.38–2.12	0.83
T allele	9/46	23/128	1.11	0.47–2.62	0.83

TABLE 8 | Comparison of IL-13 gene polymorphism genotype and allele frequencies between Steroid Sensitive (SS) patients and controls.

Genotype	SS (%) *n* = 132	Controls (%) (*n* = 64)	Odds ratio (OR)	95% confidence interval (CI)	*P*-values
QQ	90 (68.18)	47 (73.44)	0.78	0.40–1.51	0.56
RQ	38 (28.79)	16 (25.0)	1.21	0.61–2.39	0.70
RR	4 (3.03)	1 (1.56)	1.97	0.22–17.99	1.00
Q allele	218/264	110/128	0.78	0.43–1.40	0.48
R allele	46/264	18/128	1.29	0.71–2.33	0.48

TABLE 9 | Comparison of IL-13 gene polymorphism genotype and allele frequencies between Steroid Resistant (SR) patients and controls.

Genotype	SR (%) (*n* = 23)	Controls (%) (*n* = 64)	Odds ratio (OR)	95% confidence interval (CI)	*P*-values
QQ	19 (82.60)	47 (73.44)	1.72	0.51–5.78	0.57
RQ	2 (8.70)	16 (25.0)	0.29	0.06–1.36	0.14
RR	2 (8.70)	1 (1.56)	6.00	0.52–69.62	0.17
Q allele	40/46	110/128	1.09	0.40–2.94	1.00
R allele	6/46	18/128	0.92	0.34–2.47	1.00

DISCUSSION

The immunopathogenesis of INS has been studied extensively during the recent years (1, 5, 10). The effects of various cytokines on the glomerular basement membrane in the kidneys is widely supported by many studies on different populations (1, 5, 10). IL-4 and IL-13 are two important mediators which have recently attracted attention in studies exploring the pathogenesis of INS. As many INS patients commonly develop atopy, and IL-4 and IL-13 are the major mediators involved in that process, it was not surprising to incriminate these two cytokines in the immune-pathogenesis of the INS. Several previous reports have demonstrated that both these cytokines share a number of biological activities including IgE isotope switching, CD23 induction and stimulation of eosinophils activity as they both share a common IL-4 receptor alpha chain (IL-4RA) in the multicentric IL-4 and IL-13 receptor complexes (5, 6, 8, 15).

In the present study, we did not find an association between IL-4 or IL-13 gene polymorphism and predisposition to INS in Kuwaiti Arab children.

Many previous studies reported conflicting results (2, 10, 20). When our findings were compared with other populations worldwide, our results were consistent with data obtained from Caucasians in the UK where IL-4 gene polymorphism was studied in 100 patients and 63 controls with no significant difference between allele distribution in INS patients and the controls (2). However, Kobayashi et al. (20) studied IL-4 gene polymorphism in 58 Japanese children and found that the frequency of the T allele was significantly lower in INS group than the controls. It has been previously reported that T allele of the 590C/T polymorphism was associated with increased IL-4 gene promoter activity (21, 22). Another study carried out in India on 150 children with INS, demonstrated that IL-4-C590T polymorphism may influence the prognosis and the clinical course of the disease (23).

Our study did not show any association between IL-13 gene polymorphism and susceptibility of children with an Arab racial background to INS. However, the RQ genotype was associated with steroid sensitivity.

These findings were consistent with studies reported in different other populations worldwide. Data in both Asian and Caucasian populations suggest that there is no association of IL-13 gene polymorphism with susceptibility to minimal change nephrotic syndrome (10, 24, 25). Similar results have been reported from British INS patients (24) as well as on German INS patients (25). In Singapore Asian children also, no significant association of IL-13 gene polymorphism with INS was detected (10).

The lack of association of both 1L-4 as well as IL-13 gene polymorphisms and INS reported in our study as well as other studies seems to be unexpectedly surprising knowing the previously documented effects of both these cytokines in kidneys. Many previous *in vivo* as well as *in vitro* studies had supported the important roles of both cytokines and their receptors in the pathogenesis of INS. Podocytes in the glomerular basement membranes in kidneys of express receptors for both interleukins IL-4 and IL-13 (26, 27). These cytokines have been shown *in vitro* to have direct effects on podocyte mediator production and barrier function (26–28). A mechanism whereby excess IL-13 might induce nephrotic syndrome is illustrated by changes in podocyte protein trafficking and proteolytic enzyme secretion seen when these cells are incubated with IL-4 or IL-13 *in vitro* (29).

Another intriguing animal study directly addressed the role of IL-13 by overexpressing it in the rats and reported that an MCN-like nephropathy was induced, with changes in podocyte structure and gene expression similar to those seen in human diseases (30).

Moreover, Van den Berg showed the presence of IL-13 receptors on glomerular epithelial cells, the stimulation of which, resulted in a decrease in the transepithelial electrical resistance suggesting a possible direct effect of this cytokine on the podocytes and its function in preserving circulatory albumin and preventing albuminuria, which is the hallmark of INS (27). It has been reported that children with nephrotic syndrome who had higher initial serum IgE levels, had higher relapsing rates, longer duration of steroid therapy before remission and higher serum IL-4 and IL-5 levels (31).

A dysfunctional glomerular filtration barrier characterizes nephrotic syndrome, the pathophysiology of which is highly complex. T cells, mainly Th2 and Th17, play an important role. The upregulation of specific cytokines (IL-4, IL-5, IL-9, and IL-13) was previously shown to promote the development of NS (32). Therefore, studying the gene polymorphisms of these cytokines is essential.

Our study might be limited by a relatively small sample size. It would be prudent to have the serum cytokine levels for correlation. Despite being a single center study, ours is the focal center for nephrotic syndrome in the entire country where all the complex cases are referred so it covers the whole country. Although we studied patients with the same ethnic background, it is actually a strength of our study because this type of genetic association has not been performed in any population in the Gulf Region. We studied the homozygous and the heterozygous genotypes. The allele frequencies in the homozygous and heterozygous forms were included.

In conclusion, we report no association between IL-4 and IL-13 gene polymorphisms and the predisposition of INS in Kuwaiti Arab children. Of note, IL-13 RQ genotype was expressed more in children with INS who are steroid sensitive. Further larger studies, involving samples of different ethnic backgrounds, are warranted to determine the genetic predisposition of INS, as well as, steroid responsiveness in children.

ETHICS STATEMENT

The studies involving human participants were reviewed and approved by Health Sciences Center committee for the protection of human subjects in research, Kuwait University, as well as, Ministry of Health ethics committee, Kuwait. Written informed consent to participate in this study was provided by the participants' legal guardian, patients and controls, as per the committees recommendations.

AUTHOR CONTRIBUTIONS

MA and AA-E: substantial contributions to conception and design. AA-E: acquisition of data. MH: gene studies and data analysis. MA and AA-E: interpretation of the results. MA and AA-E: drafting the article. AA-E and MH: revising it critically for important intellectual content. All authors: final approval of the version to be published.

ACKNOWLEDGMENTS

We thank Kuwait University for providing funds for this study. The assistance of Mrs. Asiya T. Ibrahim in the statistical analysis and of Mrs. Jalaja Sukumaran in the lab work is thankfully acknowledged.

REFERENCES

1. Davin JC. The glomerular permeability factors in idiopathic nephrotic syndrome. *Pediatric Nephrol.* (2016) 31:207–15. doi: 10.1007/s00467-015-3082-x
2. Parry RG1, Gillespie KM, Parnham A, Clark AG, Mathieson PW. Interleukin-4 and interleukin-4 receptor polymorphisms in minimal change nephropathy. *Clin Sci (Lond).* (1999) 96:665–8. doi: 10.1042/cs0960665
3. Ikeuchi Y, Kobayashi Y, Arakawa H, Suzuki M, Tamra K, Morikawa A. Polymorphisms in interleukin-4-related genes in patients with minimal change nephrotic syndrome. *Pediatr Nephrol.* (2009) 24:489–95. doi: 10.1007/s00467-008-1003-y
4. Cheung W, Wei CL, Seah CC, Jordan SC, Yap HK. Atopy, serum IgE, and interleukin-13 in steroid-responsive nephrotic syndrome. *Pediatr Nephrol.* (2004) 19:627–32. doi: 10.1007/s00467-004-1438-8
5. Fang X, Zhu Z, Yang S, Ji Y, Wang L. Association of IL-4 and IL-4 receptor gene polymorphisms with the risk, immunotherapeutic effects and prognosis of advanced renal cell carcinoma. *Int J Clin Exp Med.* (2016) 9:11449–57.
6. Luo Y, Ye Z, Li K, Chen R, Li S, Pang J. Associations between polymorphisms in the IL-4 and IL-4 receptor genes and urinary carcinomas: a meta-analysis. *Int J Clin Exp Med.* (2015) 15:1227–33.

7. Suppiah V, Goris A, Alloza I, Heggarty S, Dubois B, Carton H, et al. Polymorphisms in the interleukin-4 and IL-4 receptor genes and multiple sclerosis: a study in Spanish-Basque, Northern Irish and Belgian populations. *Int J Immunogenet.* (2005) 32:383–8. doi: 10.1111/j.1744-313X.2005.00542.x
8. Chu H, Wang M, Yan F, Zhong D, Shi D, Ma L, et al. Polymorphisms in the IL-13 and IL-4R genes are associated with the development of renal cell carcinoma. *Ann Oncol.* (2012) 23:2114–21. doi: 10.1093/annonc/mdr607
9. Banchereau J, Briere F, Galizzi JP, Miossec P, Rousset F. Human interleukin 4. *J Lipid Mediat Cell Signal.* (1994) 9:43–53.
10. Wei CL, Cheung W, Heng CK, Arty N, Chong SS, Lee BW, et al. Interleukin-13 genetic polymorphisms in Singapore Chinese children correlate with long-term outcome of minimal change disease. *Nephrol Dialysis Transplantation.* (2005) 20:728–34. doi: 10.1093/ndt/gfh648
11. Graves PE, Kabesch M, Halonen M, Holberg CJ, Baldini M, Fritzsch C, et al. A cluster of seven tightly linked polymorphisms in the IL-13 gene is associated with total serum IgE levels in three populations of white children. *J Allergy Clin Immunol.* (2000) 105:506–13. doi: 10.1067/mai.2000.104940
12. Liu X, Nickel R, Beyer K, Wahn U, Ehrlich E, Freidhoff LR, et al. An IL13 coding region variant is associated with a high total serum IgE level and atopic dermatitis in the German multicenter atopy study (MAS-90). *J Allergy Clin Immunol.* (2000) 106:167–70. doi: 10.1067/mai.2000.107935
13. Heinzmann A, Mao XQ, Akaiwa M, Kreomer RT, Gao PS, Ohshima K, et al. Genetic variants of IL-13 signaling and human asthma and atopy. *Hum Mol Genet.* (2000) 9:549–59. doi: 10.1093/hmg/9.4.549
14. Quirico-Santos T, Suppiah V, Heggarty S, Caetano R, Alves-Leon S, Vandenbroeck K. Study of polymorphisms in the interleukin-4 and IL-4 receptor genes in a population of Brazilian patients with multiple sclerosis. *Arq Neuropsiquiatr.* (2007) 65:15–9. doi: 10.1590/S0004-282X2007000100005
15. Shirakawa I, Deichmann KA, Izuhara I, Mao I, Adra CN, Hopkin JM. Atopy and asthma: genetic variants of IL-4 and IL-13 signaling. *Immunol Today.* (2000) 21:60–4. doi: 10.1016/S0167-5699(99)01492-9
16. Kidney Disease: Improving Global Outcomes (KDIGO) Glomerulonephritis Work Group. KDIGO Clinical Practice Guideline for Glomerulonephritis. *Kidney Inter Suppl.* (2012) 2:139–274.
17. Sambrook J, Fritsch EF, Maniatis T. *Molecular Cloning: A Laboratory Manual.* 2nd ed. New York, NY: Cold Spring Harbor Laboratory Press (1989).
18. Schotte H, Schiuter B, Rust S, Assmann G, Domschke W, Gaubitz M. Interleukin-6 promoter polymorphism (−174 G/C) in Caucasian German patients with systemic lupus erythematosus. *Rheumatology.* (2001) 40:393–400. doi: 10.1093/rheumatology/40.4.393
19. Tripathi G, Jafar T, Mandal K, Mahdi AA, Awasthi S, Sharma RK, et al. Does cytokine gene polymorphism affect steroid responses in idiopathic nephrotic syndrome? *Ind J Med Sci.* (2008) 62:383–91. doi: 10.4103/0019-5359.44017
20. Kobayashi Y, Arakawa H, Suzuki M, Takizawa T, Tokuyama K, Morikawa A. Polymorphism of interleukin-4 related genes in Japanese children with minimal change nephrotic syndrome. *Am J kidney Dis.* (2003) 42:271–6. doi: 10.1016/S0272-6386(03)00652-8
21. Jun TY, Lee KU, Pae CU, Chae JH, Bahk WM, Kim KS, et al. Polymorphisms of interleukin-4 promoter and receptor gene for schizophrenia in the Korean population. *Psychiatry Clin Neurosci.* (2002) 53:283–8. doi: 10.1046/j.1440-1819.2003.01118.x
22. Kawashima T, Nogushi E, Arinami T, Yamakawa-Kobayashi K, Nakagawa H, Otsuka F, et al. Linkage and association of an interleukin 4 gene polymorphism with atopic dermatitis in Japanese families. *J Med Genet.* (1998) 35:502–4. doi: 10.1136/jmg.35.6.502
23. Jafar T, Agrawal S, Mahdi A, Sharma RK, Awashti S, Agarwal GG. Cytokine gene polymorphism in idiopathic nephrotic syndrome children. *Ind J Clin Biochem.* (2011) 26:296–302. doi: 10.1007/s12291-011-0126-2
24. Gillespie KM, Anderson KL, Mathieson PW, Gillespie KM. Polymorphism not in the IL-13 gene promoter. *Science.* (1999) 286:1647. doi: 10.1126/science.286.5445.1647b
25. Tenbrock K, Schubert A, Stapenhorst L, Kemper MJ, Gellermann J, Timmermann K, et al. Type I IgE receptor, interleukin 4 receptor and interleukin 13 polymorphisms in children with nephrotic syndrome. *Clin Sci.* (2002) 102:507–12. doi: 10.1042/cs1020507
26. Parry RG, Gillespie KM, Mathieson PW. Effects of type 2 cytokines on cultured human glomerular epithelial cells. *Exp Nephrol.* (2001) 9:275–83. doi: 10.1159/000052622
27. Van den Berg JG, Aten J, Chand MA, Claessen N, Dijkink L, Wijdenes J, et al. Interleukin-4 and interleukin-13 act on glomerular visceral epithelial cells. *J Am Soc Nephrol.* (2000) 11:413–22.
28. Coers W, Vos JT, van der Meide PH, Van der Horst ML, Huitema S, Weening JJ. Interferon-gamma (INF-gamma) and IL-4 expressed during mercury-induced membranous nephropathy are toxic for cultured podocytes. *Clin Exp Immunol.* (1995) 102:297–307. doi: 10.1111/j.1365-2249.1995.tb03781.x
29. Van der Berg JG, Aten J, Annink C, Ravesloot JH, Weber E, Weening JJ. Interleukin-4 and interleukin-13 promote basolateral secretion of H(+) and cathepsin L by glomerular visceral epithelial cells. *Am J Physiol Renal Physiol.* (2002) 282:F26–33. doi: 10.1152/ajprenal.0102.2001
30. Lai KW, Wei CL, Tan LK, Tan PH, Chiang GS, Lee CG, et al. Overexpression of interleukin-13 induces minimal-change-like nephropathy in rats. *J Am Soc Nephrol.* (2007) 18:1476–85. doi: 10.1681/ASN.2006070710
31. Youn SY, Lim HH, Lee HJ. The clinical of steroid responsive nephrotic syndrome of children according to the serum immunoglobulin E levels and cytokines. *Yonsei Med J.* (2012) 53:715–22. doi: 10.3349/ymj.2012.53.4.715
32. Veissi S, Smeets B, Heuvel LP, Schreuder MF, Jansen J. Nephrotic syndrome in a dish: recent developments in modeling *in vitro*. *Pediatric Nephrol.* (2020) 35:1363–72. doi: 10.1007/s00467-019-4203-8

18

Altered B-Lymphocyte Homeostasis in Idiopathic Nephrotic Syndrome

Chen Ling[1], Xiaolin Wang[2,3], Zhi Chen[1], Jianfeng Fan[1], Qun Meng[1], Nan Zhou[1], Qiang Sun[1], Lin Hua[4], Jingang Gui[2,3] and Xiaorong Liu[1]*

[1] Beijing Key Laboratory of Pediatric Chronic Kidney Disease and Blood Purification, Department of Nephrology, National Center for Children's Health, Beijing Children's Hospital, Capital Medical University, Beijing, China, [2] Key Laboratory of Major Diseases in Children, Ministry of Education, Beijing Children's Hospital, Capital Medical University, Beijing, China, [3] Laboratory of Immunology, Beijing Pediatric Research Institute, Beijing Children's Hospital, Capital Medical University, Beijing, China, [4] School of Biomedical Engineering, Capital Medical University, Beijing, China

***Correspondence:**
Xiaorong Liu
lxrbch@sina.com

Background: B-cell-deleted therapy has been successfully used for children with idiopathic nephrotic syndrome (INS), suggesting that B cells may be involved in the pathogenesis of INS. B cells are a heterogenous population comprised of subpopulations distinguished by their phenotypes. However, few studies have focused on the alteration of B-cell homeostasis in INS.

Methods: We measured the levels of B-cell subsets in the blood of 87 INS children via flow cytometry, prior to treatment with steroids. INS patients were divided into steroid-sensitive nephrotic syndrome (SSNS) and steroid-resistant nephrotic syndrome (SRNS) groups based on their sensitivities to steroids after a one-month follow-up. Subsequently, we compared these INS patients with age- and sex-matched patients with relapse ($n = 35$) and remissions ($n = 32$), as well as healthy controls ($n = 75$).

Results: We found that 65 SSNS patients exhibited an altered peripheral-blood B-cell-subset distribution, with increased levels of total, transitional, memory, IgM (immunoglobulin M) memory and switched-memory B cells compared to 22 SRNS patients. The proportion of total B cells was significantly higher in the SSNS group (22.1 ± 6.7% L, $p < 0.001$) than in the SRNS, remission, and control groups. In contrast, the levels of B-cell subsets in SRNS patients were generally the same as those in remission patients and healthy controls. Patients in relapse presented elevated memory B cells compared to those in other groups. The area under the ROC (receiver operating characteristic) curve of transition B cells at initial onset for the prediction of SSNS was 0.907 (95% confidence interval, 0.835–0.979). The analysis rendered an optimal cut-off value of 2.05 (% Lymphocyte) corresponding to 79.1% sensitivity and 90.9% specificity.

Conclusions: We observed and verified that B-cell subsets are significantly altered in children with SSNS. We propose that elevated transitional B cells may be a promising marker for predicting successful immunosuppressive therapy during the initial onset of INS. Further research is needed to determine the function of memory B cells in INS.

Keywords: idiopathic nephrotic syndrome, B cells, children, transitional B cell, flow cytometry

INTRODUCTION

Idiopathic nephrotic syndrome (INS) is the most frequent glomerular disease during childhood. It is a clinical syndrome characterized by massive proteinuria, hypoalbuminemia, hyperlipidemia, and edema due to increased glomerular permeability. Although the role of B cells in several renal diseases is well-established (1), their contribution to the pathogenesis of INS is still being debated (2). The best supporting evidence for a role of B cells in INS comes from rituximab, a B-cell-specific antibody, which has been successfully used to treat patients with steroid-dependent or frequent relapse, and most of these patients have maintained remission in the absence of B cells (3–5). These findings imply that B cells are involved in the pathogenesis of INS.

B cells are a heterogeneous population that include different subsets characterized by their membrane phenotypes and/or cytokine-production profiles (6). B cells are capable of antibody production, antigen presentation, and immunomodulation. It has previously been reported—albeit debated—that CD19+ B cells increase during the acute phase of INS, but decrease to normal levels in the remission phase (7). It has also been reported that after treatment with rituximab, switched-memory B-cell recovery is associated with INS recurrence (8). In a recent study, elevated levels of memory B-cell subsets were considered to be closely related to the onset of INS (9). These studies suggest that different subpopulations of B cells play different roles in INS. However, few studies have focused on the alteration of B-cell homeostasis in children with INS.

Most INS is sensitive to prednisone treatment, and only a small number of patients exhibit steroid resistance (10). Steroid-resistant nephrotic syndrome (SRNS) is different from steroid-sensitive nephrotic syndrome (SSNS), and SRNS is currently recognized as a genetic disease or a disease due to other pathogenic factors. Therefore, we believe that SRNS and SSNS are also significantly different in terms of their corresponding subpopulations of B cells, and some B-cell subsets may serve as biomarkers for predicting one's sensitivity to steroid-therapy at the initial onset.

In the present study, we compared the distribution of B-cell subsets in the peripheral blood of SSNS and SRNS patients, as well as in healthy controls and in INS patients in relapse and remission. We hope that this investigation of altered B-cell subsets in INS may lead to the discovery of novel biomarkers for predicting INS-treatment responses.

MATERIALS AND METHODS

Patients

This study was conducted between March 2018 and March 2019 at the National Center for Children's Health in China. Children with active nephrotic syndrome during the initial onset were recruited for the collection of blood samples before the treatment with prednisone. These children were followed up for at least 4 weeks. Patients who achieved remission with prednisone (60 mg/m^2/day) within 4 weeks of treatment were classified as having SSNS, whereas those who did not respond were classified as having SRNS. Additionally, we included children with INS relapse and children with INS remission. Finally, 75 age- and sex-matched healthy children receiving routine medical examinations were included as healthy controls.

The diagnosis of INS was based on the presence of generalized edema, proteinuria (urine protein + + + or more by the heat-precipitation method and/or spot-urine protein/creatinine > 2 mg/mg), hypoalbuminemia (serum albumin < 2.5 g/dl) and hypercholesterolemia (serum cholesterol > 5.72 mmol/L). Patients were considered in relapse if they had edema, a serum albumin level of < 2.5 g/dl, and a urinary protein/creatinine (mg/mg) ratio of > 2.0, and they were considered to be in remission if they had no edema and their urinary protein/creatinine ratio was < 0.40 in a random urine sample.

Exclusion criteria were as follows: (1) age < 1 year old or > 10 years old; (2) positive family history of kidney disease; (3) systemic diseases, such as lupus and purpura; or (4) active infections, such as Epstein-Barr virus and cytomegalovirus.

Our treatment criterion followed the Improving Global Outcomes (KDIGO) guidelines of 2012 for kidney disease (11), which recommends the induction treatment of the initial episode of nephrotic syndrome in children with daily oral prednisone at 2 mg/kg/day (maximum 60 mg/day) for 4 weeks. No patients received or were ready to receive other forms of immunosuppression.

The study protocol was approved by the Capital Medical University Institutional Review Board, and informed consent was obtained from the parents or the authorized representative of each child.

Cell Isolation

The blood of each child was collected in the morning after 1–2 days of hospitalization, and 3 mL of blood was collected in a heparin-anticoagulation tube. Blood samples were placed in a 4–6°C refrigerator and were analyzed within 6 h. Peripheral-blood mononuclear cells (PBMCs) were isolated from heparinized blood using the Ficoll-Hypaque (Axis-Shield, Oslo, Norway) density-gradient centrifugation method. Freshly isolated heparin-anticoagulated blood diluted in phosphate-buffered saline (PBS, 1:1) was layered on the surface of Ficoll at a ratio of 2:1 and was centrifuged at 1,600 g for 20 min at 20°C, with no breaks. The cells were harvested from the Ficoll interface.

Flow Cytometry

To identify different B-cell subpopulations, PBMCs were stained with the following fluorochrome-conjugated antibodies: CD19-FITC (fluorescein isothiocyanate), CD24-PE (phycoerythrin), CD27-PE (phycoerythrin), CD38-PerCP (peridinin chlorophyll protein), IgM-APC (allophycocyanin), and IgD-PerCP (peridinin chlorophyll protein) (BD Biosciences, San Jose, CA, USA). The antibodies were then analyzed by a multicolor flow cytometer (FACSCalibur; BD

Biosciences). Gated events (30,000) on living lymphocytes were analyzed for each sample. Four-color data acquisition was performed by FACS Calibur, and data were analyzed with CellQuest analysis software (BD Biosciences, San Diego, CA, USA).

Subsets of gated $CD19^{+}$ (total) B cells were identified on the basis of the expression of surface markers as follows (**Figure 1**): transitional ($CD24^{high}CD38^{high}$), mature/naïve ($CD24^{low}CD38^{intermediate}$), and memory ($CD24^{high}$ $CD38^{-}$) or ($CD27^{+}$) B cells. Memory B-cell subclasses ($CD19^{+}CD27^{+}$) were also defined as IgM memory ($IgM^{+}IgD^{intermediate}$) or switched memory ($IgM^{-}IgD^{-}$) and they were expressed as the percentage of total circulating lymphocytes (8).

Statistical Analyses

Data were analyzed using SPSS v.19 (SPSS Inc., Chicago, IL, USA). Data are summarized as the mean ± SEM and median (interquartile range) for continuous variables, as well as the percentage and frequency for categorical variables. Statistically significant differences were analyzed using independent *t*-tests or Mann-Whitney *U* tests for continuous variables and chi-squared tests for categorical variables. A receiver operating characteristic (ROC) curve was constructed and the area under the ROC curve (AUC) was calculated to assess the predictive strength. Optimal cutoff points to maximize both sensitivity and specificity were also determined. Statistical tests were two-tailed, and a *P*-value of < 0.05 was considered statistically significant. Additionally, a *p*-value < 0.005 (i.e., 0.05/10) was used to indicate statistical significance after Bonferroni correction.

RESULTS

Baseline Characteristics of the Study Population

The demographic characteristics of the subjects enrolled are presented in **Table 1**. A total of 156 patients with nephrotic syndrome were included in the study and were divided according to the stages of their diseases. Eighty-seven patients at disease onset (before any immunosuppressive treatment) were further divided according to their responses to prednisone (SSNS = 65, SRNS = 22). Additionally, there were 35 patients in relapse and 32 patients in stable (at least 1 month) remission. There was no difference in age or gender among the groups. Compared with that of the remission group and the control group, the albumin level in the disease-onset group and the relapse group was lower and the 24-h urine-protein level was higher. Serum-creatinine levels were normal for all patients and healthy controls.

In the relapse group and the remission group, all patients were treated with PDN. No children were treated with other immunosuppressants at the time of enrollment. For the IgA and IgM levels, there were no statistically significant differences among the groups. Additionally, the IgG level at the remission period was significantly lower than that during the active and relapse periods. The IgE level was significantly higher in SSNS patients than in other groups. The total T-cell ratio did not differ significantly among groups, and the CD4/CD8 ratio was slightly higher in the SSNS group than in the other populations. The proportion of NK cells was significantly lower in SSNS and relapsed groups than in other groups, and children in the SSNS group had a lower proportion of NK cells than those in the relapsed group.

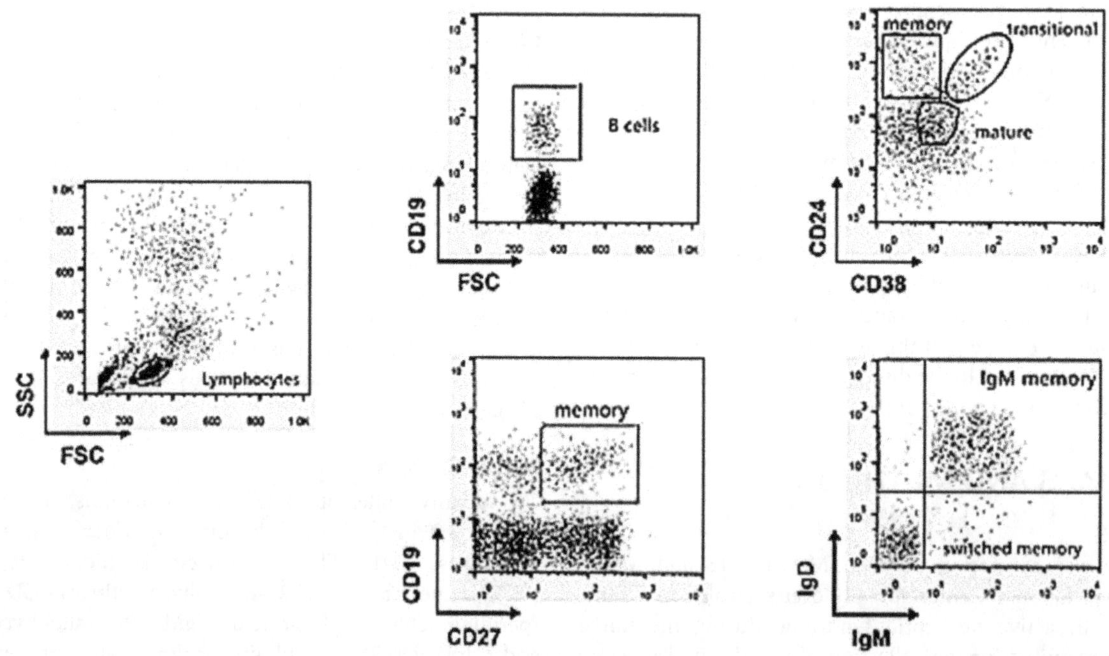

FIGURE 1 | Gating strategy to discriminate the different B cell subpopulations by multicolor flow cytometry analysis.

TABLE 1 | Characteristics of patients with nephrotic syndrome and controls.

Parameter	Onset		Relapse ($n = 35$)	Remission ($n = 3\ 2$)	Health controls ($n = 75$)
	SS ($n = 65$)	SR ($n = 22$)			
Age, years	5.2 ± 2.9	5.5 ± 4.3	5.6 ± 4.2	5.5 ± 2.8	5.2 ± 2.7
Sex, male	44 (67.7%)	16 (72.7%)	23 (65.7%)	22 (68.7%)	48 (64.0)%
Serum albumin, g/L	$18.1 \pm 5.8^{\ddagger\ddagger}$	$20.9 \pm 6.0^{\ddagger\ddagger}$	$23.2 \pm 8.3^{\ddagger\ddagger}$	$35.4 \pm 7.6^{\#\#,\dagger\dagger}$	–
Serum creatinine, g/L	32.8 ± 11.8	37.5 ± 15.7	37.2 ± 20.3	35.1 ± 7.0	–
24-h urine protein, mg/kg	$132.1 \pm 78.9^{\ddagger\ddagger}$	$148.1 \pm 103.5^{\ddagger\ddagger}$	$135.3 \pm 102.1^{\ddagger\ddagger}$	$13.2 \pm 9.5^{\#\#,\dagger\dagger}$	–
IgA, g/l	1.19 ± 0.78	1.10 ± 0.71	1.17 ± 0.62	1.31 ± 1.06	–
IgG, g/l	$3.07 \pm 2.9^{\#,\dagger,\ddagger\ddagger}$	$3.98 \pm 2.11^{\ddagger\ddagger}$	$4.24 \pm 2.41^{\ddagger\ddagger}$	$6.98. \pm 2.74^{\#\#,\dagger\dagger}$	–
IgM, g/l	1.57 ± 0.92	1.59 ± 0.94	1.50 ± 0.45	1.41 ± 0.57	–
IgE, g/l	216.2 (59.2, 537.8)$^{\#\#,\dagger,\ddagger\ddagger}$	90.6 (42.4, 284.0)	45.0 (20.1, 346.5)	76.2 (55.7, 104.09)	–
T cell, %L	70.9 ± 8.9	71.6 ± 7.2	71.5 ± 8.2	71.4 ± 5.3	–
CD4+ T, %L	40.5 ± 8.2	36.9 ± 8.4	36.8 ± 8.2	39.1 ± 4.2	–
CD8+ T, %L	$24.3 \pm 6.0^{\#,\dagger,\ddagger}$	29.9 ± 7.6	29.7 ± 7.0	27.9 ± 5.0	–
CD4/CD8,	$1.8 \pm 0.6^{\#,\dagger,\ddagger}$	1.3 ± 0.5	1.2 ± 0.5	1.4 ± 0.3	–
Nature kill, %L	$5.7 \pm 3.0^{\#\#,\dagger\dagger,\ddagger\ddagger}$	$8.0 \pm 4.1^{\ddagger\ddagger,\dagger}$	$6.5 \pm 3.8^{\ddagger\ddagger,\#}$	13.5 ± 3.3	–
B cell, %L	$22.1 \pm 6.7^{\#\#,\dagger,\ddagger\ddagger,**}$	$12.7 \pm 6.1^{\dagger}$	$18.5 \pm 7.4^{\#,\ddagger\ddagger,*}$	$13.7 \pm 3.3^{\dagger\dagger}$	$14.1 \pm 3.3^{\dagger}$
Transitional B, %L	$5.3 \pm 3.8^{\#\#,\dagger\dagger,\ddagger\ddagger,**}$	$2.0 \pm 1.5^{\ddagger}$	2.0 ± 1.8	$2.5 \pm 2.0^{\#}$	2.0 ± 1.4
Mature B, %L	$22.8 \pm 9.6^{*}$	$22.4 \pm 8.9^{\ddagger,*}$	$23.7 \pm 7.5^{\ddagger,*}$	$27.6 \pm 8.0^{\#,\dagger}$	$30.0 \pm 11.0^{\#,\dagger}$
Memory B, %L	$4.5 \pm 2.4^{\dagger\dagger,*}$	$3.5 \pm 2.0^{\dagger\dagger,*}$	$7.7 \pm 5.5^{\#\#,**,\ddagger\ddagger}$	$4.6 \pm 3.0^{\dagger\dagger,*}$	$2.8 \pm 1.5^{\dagger\dagger,\#,\ddagger}$
IgM memory B, %L	$1.5 \pm 0.8^{\dagger\dagger,\ddagger,*}$	$1.0 \pm 0.8^{\dagger\dagger}$	$1.9 \pm 0.9^{\#\#,\ddagger\ddagger,**}$	$0.9 \pm 0.5^{\dagger\dagger}$	$1.0 \pm 0.5^{\dagger\dagger}$
Switched memory B, %L	1.3 ± 0.8	$1.0 \pm 0.4^{\dagger\dagger}$	$1.4 \pm 0.5^{\#\#,\ddagger\ddagger,**}$	$1.0 \pm 0.3^{\dagger\dagger}$	$1.1 \pm 0.4^{\dagger\dagger}$

SS, steroid sensitive; SR, steroid resistant; Ig, Immunoglobulin; %L, Percentage of lymphocytes.
$^{\#}p < 0.005$; $^{\#\#}p < 0.001$, compared to SRNS patients at onset.
$^{\dagger}p < 0.005$; $^{\dagger\dagger}p < 0.001$, compared to patients in relapse.
$^{\ddagger}p < 0.005$; $^{\ddagger\ddagger}p < 0.001$, compared to patients in remission.
$^{*}p < 0.005$; $^{**}p < 0.001$, compared to controls.

B-Cell Subsets Are Significantly Altered in Children With SSNS

The proportion of total B cells was significantly higher in the SSNS group (22.1 ± 6.7% L, $p < 0.001$) than in the SRNS, remission, and control groups (**Figure 2**). Although prednisone was being applied, the children in the relapse group also had an increased proportion of total B cells compared with that in the SRNS, remission, and control groups (18.3 ± 5.5% L, $p < 0.005$). There were no statistically significant differences among the SRNS, remission and control groups in terms of the proportion of total B cells ($p > 0.005$).

The proportion of mature B cells did not differ significantly in SSNS, SRNS, and relapse groups ($p > 0.005$), but was slightly higher in the remission patients and healthy controls ($p < 0.005$).

The proportion of transition B cells was significantly higher in the SSNS group (5.3 ± 3.8% L, $p < 0.001$) than in the other groups, and was significantly lower in the relapse group and the remission group after treatment with PDN. These proportions were not different between the relapse, remission, and healthy control groups. There was no significant increase in the proportion of SRNS at the time of onset ($p > 0.005$).

Memory B cells did not increase significantly at the time of initial onset, but increased significantly in the relapse phase compared with those of other groups (7.7 ± 5.5% L, $p < 0.001$). This phenomenon was due to an increase in the proportion of IgM-memory B cells (1.93 ± 0.86% L) and switched-memory B cells (1.39 ± 0.51% L).

Transition B Cells as a Biomarker for SSNS

Transition B cells differed greatly in patients with newly diagnosed SSNS and SRNS. Hence, we attempted to use transition B cells as biomarkers to predict the outcome of PDN therapy. ROC curves were used to assess the potential utility of transition B-cell detection in patients with SSNS at the time of initial onset. The area under the ROC curve of transition B cells for the prediction of SSNS was 0.907 (95% confidence interval, 0.835–0.979). The analysis rendered an optimal cutoff value of 2.05% L corresponding to a 79.1% sensitivity and 90.9% specificity (**Figure 3**).

DISCUSSION

This cohort study from China confirmed that B-cell subsets are altered in an SSNS population in children. We tested 87 newly diagnosed INS children before any immunosuppressive treatment, and all patients were followed up for 1 month.

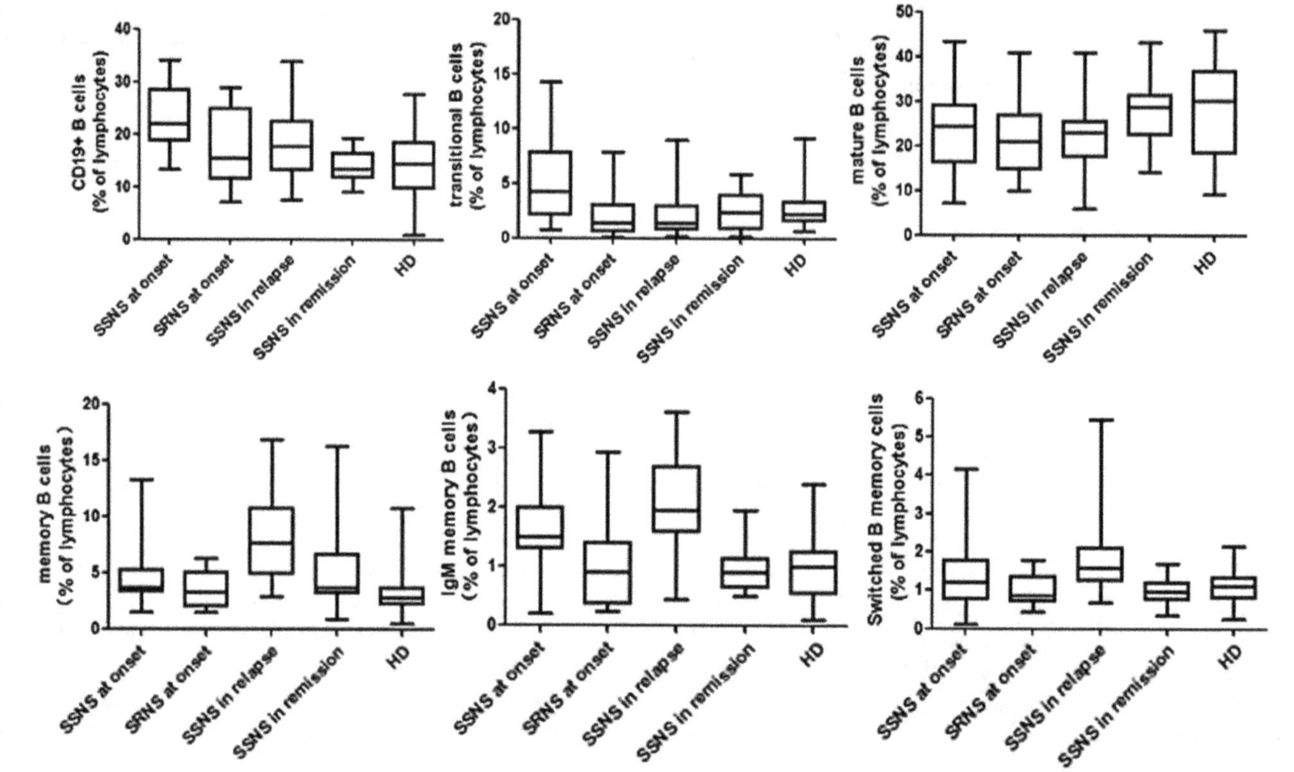

FIGURE 2 | Multicolor flow cytometry analysis is circulating B cell subsets in NS patients and controls. B cells cell subsets from patients at disease onset ($n = 87$, in which SSNS = 65, SRNS = 22), in relapse ($n = 35$), in remission ($n = 32$), and healthy controls ($n = 75$) were compared with each other. All of them were expressed as percentages of total lymphocytes. Each box plot represents the median and the 25th and 75th centiles.

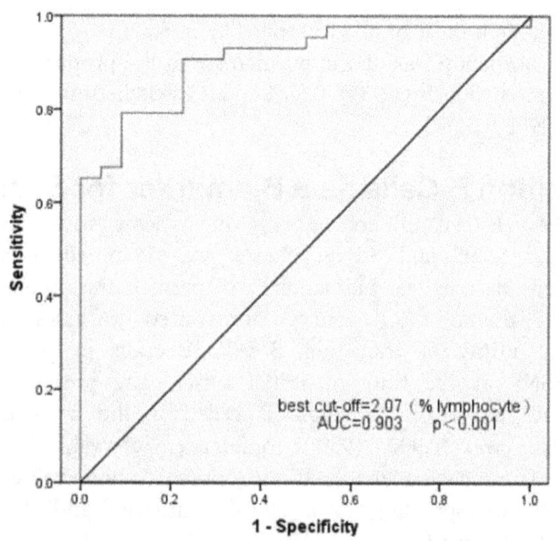

FIGURE 3 | Receiver operating characteristics (ROC) curve analysis for transitional B cell as a marker for the identification of SSNS.

Other groups were age- and sex-matched. According to the efficacy of prednisone, patients were divided into SSNS and SRNS groups.

An increased level of B cells has already been reported in SSNS, but conflicting results also exist (12). Colucci et al. suggested that prednisone treatment is the cause of these controversial conclusions (9). We confirmed the theory that $CD19^+$ B cells were significantly elevated in initial-onset NS children before steroid treatment, which is consistent with reports by Colucci et al. (9). We also observed an increase in B cells in the relapse group compared with that in the remission group, but this increase was not as high as that of the SSNS group during first onset, which may be related to the effects of immunosuppressive therapy.

We further compared the changes in B-cell subsets in SSNS and SRNS groups during the first onset. We found that transitional B cells ($CD19{+}CD24^{hi}CD38^{hi}$) were significantly elevated in the SSNS population compared to those in the SRNS population. This is consistent with the results reported in a previous study (9). When using a cut-off value of 2.05 (% of lymphocytes), transitional B cells allowed observers to distinguish SSNS from SRNS with an AUC of 0.907, an optimized sensitivity of 79.1%, and a specificity of 90.9%. This suggests that transitional B cells may be a biomarker for early screening for steroid-sensitive nephrotic syndrome.

It is worth mentioning that in recent years, some transitional B cells have been found to secrete the anti-inflammatory factors, interleukin-10 (IL-10) and transforming growth factor-β

(TGF-β), and to express inhibitory surface molecules, which are considered to have immunomodulatory effects (13). The importance of regulatory B cells has been shown in several autoimmune conditions. For example, a prolonged presence of transitional B cells has been associated with long-term non-relapsing of systemic lupus erythematosus (14). Moreover, transitional B lymphocytes are associated with protection from kidney-allograft rejection (15). The opposite result showed a positive correlation between CD38+CD19+ B cells and IL-10+CD19+ B cells and hepatitis B virus-associated membranous nephropathy (16). Our present study showed that transitional B cells exhibited a markedly abnormal increase in early disease, and that transitional B cells showed a markedly rapid and sustained decrease after steroid administration. Although our present study demonstrates that transitional B cells may be used as steroid-sensitive biomarkers in children with NS, it is necessary to further study the mechanisms of transition B-cell elevation and their role in the pathogenesis of SSNS.

Memory B cells are one of the focuses of current research on children with primary nephrotic syndrome. The first report by Colucci et al. showed that delayed reconstitution of memory B cells was protective against relapse after rituximab (8). This finding was partly confirmed by a study from India (17). However, Bhatia et al. observed that total B cells and memory B cells recovered earlier in relapsers, but Colucci et al. considered that this is related to the prolonged depletion of memory B cells rather than of total B cells. In our present study, memory B cells were significantly elevated in the relapse group and also in the SSNS group during onset. Overall, these phenomena may imply that memory B cells are involved in the pathogenesis of SSNS. One hypothesis of memory B cells in NS is that the Epstein-Barr Virus is able to establish latent benign infection in memory B cells that display phenotypes similar to those of antigen-selected memory B cells. A specific anti-EBNA1 antibody internalized in podocytes via the neonatal FC receptor might cross-react with a major podocyte protein (18). These possibilities have not been explored and should be investigated further.

The class conversion of immunoglobulins is the basis for the body to produce different classes of antibodies and serve different functions. We observed that SSNS had low IgG levels and high IgE levels. Following statistical analyses, we did not find any correlation between IgG and IgE with serum albumin and B-cell subsets. The role of antibodies in INS has been proposed by a number of clinical observations and experimental studies. Dantal et al. showed that a permeability factor inducing albuminuria may bind to an immunoglobulin and induce decreases of IgG (19). IgE is often associated with allergic diseases, and elevated IgE may be due to a response to elevated plasma IL-13 in allergic disease (20).

The current study also has limitations. First, although we showed that the percentage of transitional B cells appeared to be a marker of steroid sensitivity with reasonable sensitivity and specificity, this finding requires further verification in a separate group of recently diagnosed nephrotics. Second, although children in the relapsing and remission groups never received other immunosuppressive agents, their concurrent use of steroids may have had an effect on the levels of B cells and their subpopulations.

In conclusion, we validated that there is an alteration of B-cell subsets in children with SSNS, and that transition B cells may be a biomarker for SSNS during the initial onset before steroid treatment. Future studies should investigate the function of B-cell subsets at different periods of NS, which will help to further elucidate the pathogenesis of NS.

ETHICS STATEMENT

The study protocol was approved by Beijing Children's Hospital at Capital Medical University. All procedures performed in our studies were in accordance with these ethical standards. All parents of the individual participants included in the study provided written informed consent.

AUTHOR CONTRIBUTIONS

CL and XL designed the research. CL wrote the paper. ZC, QS, JF, QM, and NZ were responsible for collecting clinical pathology. LH was responsible for statistical processing. XW and JG completed the laboratory work.

REFERENCES

1. Hoffman W, Lakkis FG, Chalasani G. B Cells, antibodies, and more. *Clin J Am Soc Nephrol.* (2016) 11:137–54. doi: 10.2215/CJN.09430915
2. Colucci M, Corpetti G, Emma F, Vivarelli M. Immunology of idiopathic nephrotic syndrome. *Pediatr Nephrol.* (2018) 33:573–84. doi: 10.1007/s00467-017-3677-5
3. Iijima K, Sako M, Nozu K, Mori R, Tuchida N, Kamei K, et al. Rituximab for Childhood-onset Refractory Nephrotic Syndrome Study G Rituximab for childhood-onset, complicated, frequently relapsing nephrotic syndrome or steroid-dependent nephrotic syndrome: a multicentre, double-blind, randomised, placebocontrolled trial. *Lancet.* (2014) 384:1273–81. doi: 10.1016/S0140-6736(14)60541-9
4. Ravani P, Rossi R, Bonanni A, Quinn RR, Sica F, Bodria M, et al. Rituximab in children with steroid-dependent nephrotic syndrome: a multicenter, open-label, noninferiority, randomized controlled trial. *J Am Soc Nephrol.* (2015) 26:2259–66. doi: 10.1681/ASN.2014080799
5. Ruggenenti P, Ruggiero B, Cravedi P, Vivarelli M, Massella L, Marasà M, et al. Rituximab in steroid-dependent or frequently relapsing idiopathic nephrotic syndrome. *J Am Soc Nephrol.* (2014) 25:850–63. doi: 10.1681/ASN.2013030251
6. Perez-Andres M, Paiva B, Nieto WG. Human peripheral blood B-cell compartments: a crossroad in B-cell traffic. *Cytometry B Clin Cytometry.* (2010) 78(Suppl. 1):S47–60. doi: 10.1002/cyto.b.20547
7. Printza N, Papachristou F, Tzimouli V, Taparkou A, Kanakoudi-Tsakalidou F. Peripheral CD19+ B cells are increased in children with active steroid-sensitive nephrotic syndrome. *NDT Plus.* (2009) 2:435–6. doi: 10.1093/ndtplus/sfp087

8. Colucci M, Carsetti R, Cascioli S, Casiraghi F, Perna A, Ravà L, et al. B cell reconstitution after rituximab treatment in idiopathic nephrotic syndrome. *J Am Soc Nephrol.* (2016) 27:1811–22. doi: 10.1681/ASN.2015050523
9. Colucci M, Carsetti R, Cascioli S, Serafinelli J, Emma F,Vivarelli M. B cell phenotype in pediatric idiopathic nephrotic syndrome. *Pediatr Nephrol.* (2019) 34:177–81. doi: 10.1007/s00467-018-4095
10. Noone DG, Iijima K, Parekh R. Idiopathic nephrotic syndrome in children. *Lancet.* (2018) 392:61–74. doi: 10.1016/S0140-6736(18)30536-1
11. Lombel RM, Gipson DS, Hodson EM. Treatment of steroid-sensitive nephrotic syndrome: new guidelines from KDIGO. *Pediatr Nephrol.* (2013) 28:415–26. doi: 10.1007/s00467-012-2310-x
12. Lapillonne H, Leclerc A, Ulinski T, Balu L, Garnier A, Dereuddre-Bosquet N, et al. Stem cell mobilization in idiopathic steroid-sensitive nephrotic syndrome. *Pediatr Nephrol.* (2008) 23:1251–6. doi: 10.1007/s00467-008-0793-2
13. Oleinika K, Mauri C, Salama AD. Effector and regulatory B cells in immune-mediated kidney disease. *Nat Rev Nephrol.* (2019) 15:11–26. doi: 10.1038/s41581-018-0074-7
14. Anolik JH, Barnard J, Owen T, Zheng B, Kemshetti S, Looney RJ, et al. Delayed memory B cell recovery in peripheral blood and lymphoid tissue in systemic lupus erythematosus after B cell depletion therapy. *Arthritis Rheum.* (2007) 56:3044–56. doi: 10.1002/art.22810
15. Shabir S, Girdlestone J, Briggs D, Kaul B, Smith H, Daga S, et al. Transitional B lymphocytes are associated with protection from kidney allograft rejection: a prospective study. *Am J Transplant.* (2015) 15:1384–91. doi: 10.1111/ajt.13122
16. Liu Y, Wang H, Hu X, Qu Z, Zhang H, Crew R, et al. A higher frequency of IL-10-producing B cells in Hepatitis B virus-associated membranous nephropathy. *Clin Exp Pharmacol Physiol.* (2016) 43:417–27. doi: 10.1111/1440-1681.12552
17. Bhatia D, Sinha A, Hari P, Sopory S, Saini S, Puraswani M, et al. Rituximab modulates T- and B-lymphocyte subsets and urinary CD80 excretion in patients with steroid-dependent nephrotic syndrome. *Pediatr Res.* (2018) 84:520–6. doi: 10.1038/s41390-018-0088-7
18. Dossier C, Jamin A, Deschênes G. Idiopathic nephrotic syndrome: the EBV hypothesis. *Pediatr Res.* (2017) 81:233–9. doi: 10.1038/pr.2016.200
19. Dantal J, Godfrin Y, Koll R, Perretto S, Naulet J, Bouhours JF, et al. Anti-human immunoglobulin affinity immunoadsorption strongly decreases proteinuria in patients with relapsing nephrotic syndrome. *J Am Soc Nephrol.* (1998) 9:1709–15.
20. Abdel-Hafez M, Shimada M, Lee PY, Johnson RJ, Garin EH. Idiopathic nephrotic syndrome and atopy: is there a common link? *Am J Kidney Dis.* (2009) 54:945–53. doi: 10.1053/j.ajkd.2009.03.019

19

Rituximab for Steroid-Dependent or Frequently Relapsing Nephrotic Syndrome in Children

Xia Gao [1†], Yan Wang [2,3†], Zichuan Xu [1†], Huiying Deng [1], Huabin Yang [1] and Fu Zhong [1*]*

[1] Nephrology Department, Guangzhou Women and Children's Medical Center, Guangzhou, China, [2] Graduate School, Ningxia Medical University, Yinchuan, China, [3] Neonatology Department, Northwest Women and Children's Hospital, Xi'an, China

***Correspondence:**
Xia Gao
gaoxiagz@vip.163.com
Fu Zhong
zfbox@126.com

† These authors share first authorship

Objective: To explore the effectiveness and safety of rituximab (RTX) for steroid-dependent or frequently relapsing nephrotic syndrome *via* a systematic review and meta-analysis.

Methods: All the literature about RTX therapy for childhood nephrotic syndrome (NS) on PubMed, Web of Science, Cochrane Library, EMBASE, and Chinese biomedical literature database published before November 1, 2019, were conducted and selected according to the preset criteria. The Cochrane bias risk assessment tool was used to evaluate the quality of the literature included. The outcome data were analyzed by RevMan 5.3 software.

Results: There were six RCT studies that met the inclusion criteria with a moderate quality after evaluation. At the end of the treatment, the relapse rate of NS in the RTX group reduced significantly when compared with that in the control group [odds ratio (OR) = 0.11, 95% confidence interval (CI) (0.03, 0.43), $p = 0.001$]. The number of patients in the RTX group used less steroid or/and calcineurin inhibitors significantly than that in the control group [OR = 0.05, 95% CI (0.01, 0.28), $p = 0.0007$]. For children who were steroid-dependent, RTX treatment significantly reduced the dosage of the steroid, compared with that in control [standardized mean difference (SMD) = −1.49, 95% CI (−2.00, −0.99), $p < 0.00001$]. There was no significant reduction in protein excretion between the two groups [SMD = −0.33, 95% CI (−0.71, 0.04), $p = 0.08$]. Fewer serious adverse reactions of RTX in the six studies were reported and most adverse events were mild.

Conclusion: RTX is effective and safe for children with steroid-dependent or frequently relapsing nephrotic syndrome.

Systematic Review Registration: Identifier: CRD 42020150933. https://www.crd.york.ac.uk/prospero/. This review has been registered to the PROSPERO on 27 Feb 2020.

Keywords: rituximab, meta-analysis, systematic review, effect and safety, nephrotic syndrome

INTRODUCTION

The incidence of idiopathic nephrotic syndrome (NS) is 2–4 per 100,000 children (1). Prednisone is the core treatment for NS. There are still some patients who relapse when the steroid was withdrawn or tapering. According to their recurrence rate, these patients were classified as steroid-dependent nephrotic syndrome (SDNS) and frequently relapsing nephrotic syndrome (FRNS) (2, 3). The long-term use of steroids in children could result in serious adverse effects such as growth retardation, obesity, osteopenia, hypertension, and cataract (4). The SDNS or FRNS required a combined therapy of steroid and immunosuppressive agents, such as cyclophosphamide (5), cyclosporine A (CSA) (6), tacrolimus (TAC) (7), mycophenolate esters (8), and vincristine (VCR) (9). These immune suppressants brought the patients a higher remission rate, together with even more serious adverse reactions, such as renal toxicity, hyperglycemia, headache, and dyslipidemia (10).

Rituximab (RTX), a monoclonal antibody targeting the CD20 antigen of B lymphocytes, was first proposed to lymphoma (11) and rheumatoid arthritis (12). Recently, RTX was introduced to the relapsing NS (13–15) and brought the patients a long-lasting remission. Other findings suggested that RTX could also bring better benefits to children. In Guigonis's clinical trials (16), 22 patients were given RTX treatment. Nineteen children received remission. Additionally, there were some other case reports that showed that RTX induced remission in patients (17–20), whereas some studies reported no benefits of RTX to patients that were resistant to steroids and CNIs. Kari et al. (21) observed that in four children with steroid-resistant NS, after RTX protocol, only one child received a short remission and then relapsed, and the other three children showed little effects.

We aimed to evaluate the efficacy of RTX for SDNS or FRNS in children compared to the conventional treatment by meta-analysis and to summarize the adverse effects to evaluate the safety. The research was introduced as follows.

METHODS

Electronic Searches

A unified search strategy was adopted for the selected five databases to ensure consistency. The medical subject heading of the disease was restricted to Nephrotic Syndrome, the text words were Nephrotic Syndromes; Syndrome, Nephrotic; and Syndromes, Nephrotic; the medical subject heading of the intervention was RTX, and the text words were CD20 Antibody, Rituximab; Rituximab CD20 Antibody; Mabthera; IDEC-C2B8 Antibody IDEC C2B8 Antibody; IDEC-C2B8; IDEC C2B8; GP2013; and Rituxan. The subject heading of study type was Randomized Controlled Trial, and the text words were RCT; Random. Boolean operations were used to connect these subject words and text words to form search formulas. Two researchers checked the search results multiple times after independent searches and saved the search results in EndNote software.

Study Selection Criteria

The study type was restricted to the randomized controlled trial. We selected children with SDNS or FRNS who were younger than 18 years old. Two groups of patients were studied; one received any dose of RTX. The other was considered as the control, receiving conventional drugs, such as steroid and TAC/CSA. Since the use of RTX is only intended for non-genetic nephrotic syndrome, genetic nephrotic syndrome is not included in this study.

The main outcome was the relapse number. The secondary outcomes were the number of using steroids or/and calcineurin inhibitors, the dose of steroids, and the degree of proteinuria.

Literature Bias Evaluation

The risk of bias was evaluated by the Cochrane bias risk assessment tool of RevMan software. The risk of bias included selective bias, performance bias, detection bias, attrition bias, reporting bias, and other biases.

Data Extraction

Two researchers extracted relevant data to a pre-designed form independently. The disputed data were discussed with a third researcher. The extracted information included the following sections: (1) literature basic information, (2) baseline data, (3) interventions, and (4) outcomes. The extracted data were mostly represented by the mean and standard deviation (SD).

Data Analysis

The data analysis was performed by RevMan (version 5.3.5). For dichotomous variables, the odds ratio (OR) and 95% confidence interval (CI) were calculated. Continuous variables were analyzed by the standardized mean difference (SMD) and 95% CI. The Q-test and I^2 analysis were used to test the heterogeneity of the literature. When $p < 0.10$ in the Q-test or $I^2 > 50\%$ in I^2 analysis, the random-effect model was used; otherwise, the fixed-effect model was used. We then attempted to determine the source of heterogeneity, and subgroup analysis was continued if possible. $p < 0.05$ denotes that the difference was considered significant.

RESULTS

A total of 347 eligible articles were retrieved, namely, 42 from PubMed, 103 from Web of Science, 67 from the Cochrane Library, 103 from EMBASE, and 32 from the Chinese Biomedical Literature Database. A total of 146 duplicate articles were eliminated by Endnote software. After selecting the title and abstract, 190 articles were excluded. The remaining 11 articles were selected for further reading. Among them, studies from Webb et al. (22), Deble-Bertin et al. (23), and Sinha et al. (24) were excluded because these were cohort studies. Research from Basu et al. (25) was excluded due to the addition of TAC in the control group. The study of Kamei et al. (26) was a long-term follow-up observational study, which was excluded due to the lack of a control group. Finally, six articles (27–32) were included in our study, and the screening flow chart is shown in **Figure 1**. The general data of the study design is shown in **Table 1**, and the baseline data of the study patients are shown in **Table 2**.

After repeatedly reading the six articles, the Cochrane Bias Risk Assessment Tool was used to evaluate the RevMan software. The results of the included literature bias assessment are shown in **Figure 2**.

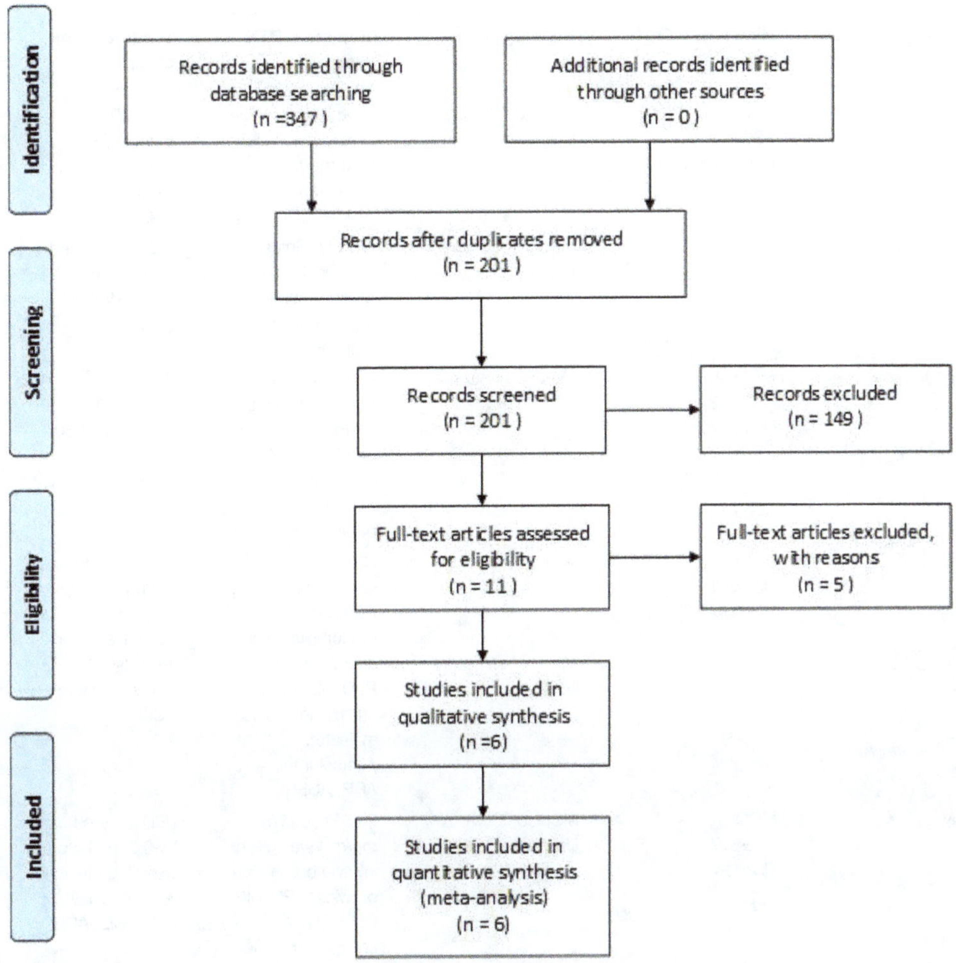

FIGURE 1 | The search results and selection details.

The Relapse Numbers

In this study, six studies reported the relapse number of NS in the RTX group and the control after the corresponding treatment. A total of 46 patients of 124 in the RTX group and 86 patients of 110 in the control relapsed, separately. RTX could significantly reduce the NS relapse during the observation period [OR 0.11, 95% CI (0.03, 0.43), $p = 0.001$]. The random-effect model was selected due to the large heterogeneity in this analysis ($I^2 = 66\%$, $p = 0.01$), and the results are shown in **Figure 3**.

The Number of Patients Using Steroids or/and CNI

In this study, there were two studies documenting the number of patients using steroids or/and CNI after the corresponding treatment. Twenty patients of 62 in the RTX group discontinued steroids or/and CNI and achieved remission. Only 1 patient of 43 in the control withdrew steroids or/and CNI. Thus, we concluded that RTX holds great potential of reducing steroids or/and CNI treatment [OR 0.05, 95% CI (0.01, 0.28), $p = 0.0007$]. The fixed-effect model was used according to the heterogeneity, which was acceptable ($I^2 = 14\%$, $p = 0.28$); the results are shown in **Figure 4**.

Steroid Dosage

Three studies recorded the steroid dosage after the corresponding treatment. Among them, the research from Ahn et al. (27) was excluded because of the large heterogeneity. The two remaining articles were included for further analyses and a total of 78 patients were studied, 39 in the RTX group and 39 in the control. The SMD was used for analysis due to the different units of steroids in the two research, which showed that the steroid dosage was significantly reduced after RTX treatment [SMD −1.49, 95% CI (−2.00, −0.99), $p < 0.00001$]. There was no obvious heterogeneity ($I^2 = 0\%$, $p = 0.77$) and the fixed-effect model was used; the results are shown in **Figure 5**.

Proteinuria Excretion

Three articles recorded urea protein excretion in 115 patients, of whom 58 were in the RTX group and 57 were in the

TABLE 1 | General information of the included studies.

References	Country	Histology RTX group	Histology con group	Treatment RTX group	Treatment con group	Follow-up
Ahn et al. (27)	Korea	MCD: 23 FSGS: 2 Unknown: 10	MCD: 8 FSGS: 1 Unknown: 7	RTX: a single dose of intravenous RTX (375 mg/m^2; maximum of 50 0 mg); PED; CNI	PED (60 mg/m^2/day, tapered by 25% every 4 weeks); CNI	12 M
Boumediene et al. (29)	France	MCD: 9 Unknown: 1	MCD: 11 FSGS: 1 Unknown: 1	RTX: two infusions at 1-week interval of Rituximab (375 mg/m^2); MMF: CNI; PED	PED (decreased every 2 weeks by 25%); MMF; CNI	6 M
Iijima et al. (28)	Japan	MCD: 21 FSGS: 2 Unknown: 1	MCD: 23 FSGS: 1	RTX: once weekly for 4 weeks (375 mg/m^2; maximum of 500 mg); MP; chlorpheniramine maleate; paracetamol	PED (60 mg/m^2/day, maximum of 80 mg/day, decreased every 2 weeks by 50%)	12 M
Magnasco et al. (30)	Italy	MCD: 3 FSGS: 10 Unknown: 2	MCD: 4 FSGS: 9 Unknown: 3	RTX: 375 mg/m^2, given intravenously twice (at randomization and after 2 weeks); PED; MP; CNI; chlorpheniramine maleate; paracetamol; ARB; ACEI	PED (median 0.42 mg/kg/day, after 30 days decreased every week by 0.3 mg/kg); CNI; ARB; ACEI	18 M
Ravani et al. (31)	Italy	MCD: 13 FSGS: 7 Unknown: 7	MCD: 6 FSGS: 10 Unknown: 116	Rituximab (375 mg/m^2) was given intravenously once or twice; ARB; MP; PED; CNI; ACEI; chlorpheniramine maleate; paracetamol	PED (tapered off by 0.3 mg/kg per week if proteinuria was <1 g/day); CNI; ACEI; ARB	12 M
Ravani et al. (32)	Italy	Unknown: 15	Unknown: 15	Rituximab (MabThera/RITUXAN;375 mg/m^2); PED; MP; chlorpheniramine maleate; paracetamol; ACEI; ARB; CNI; CYC	PED (tapered off by 0.3 mg/kg per week starting at 30 days); ACEI; ARB; CNI; CYC	12 M

MCD, minimal-change disease; FSGS, focal and segmental glomerular sclerosis; PED, prednisone; CNI, calcineurin inhibitors (cyclosporine or tacrolimus); MMF, mycophenolate mofetil; MP, methyl prednisone; ARB, angiotensin receptor inhibitor; ACEI, angiotensin-converting enzyme inhibitor; CYC, cyclophosphamide.

control group. Because the units of proteinuria were not uniform, the SMD was used for analysis. Compared with that in the control group, the proteinuria excretion in both RTX and control decreased, and the difference was not statistically significant [SMD −0.33, 95% CI (−0.71, 0.04), $p = 0.08$], as shown in the forest plot (**Figure 6**).

Safety

Adverse events, such as late-onset neutropenia, hypogammaglobulinemia, and increased risk of infections, have been rarely reported. Slight adverse reactions and infusion reactions were found in all included studies, which could be alleviated by reducing the speed of drug infusion or providing supportive treatment.

Publication Bias

In the main outcome of the relapse number, we used Stata software to evaluate publication bias. The results were as follows: $p = 0.060$ in the Begg test, $p = 0.022$ in the Egger test.

DISCUSSION

We included six randomized controlled trials. A total of 234 children were included and randomly assigned to the RTX group

TABLE 2 | Basic characteristics of included studies.

	Group	Ahn et al. (27)	Boumediene et al. (29)	Iijima et al. (28)	Magnasco et al. (30)	Ravani et al. (31)	Ravani et al. (32)
Sex (M/F)	RTX group	26/9	10/0	18/6	10/6	24/3	10/5
	Con group	13/3	6/7	16/8	9/6	19/8	11/4
Age (years)	RTX group	13.5 ± 5.0	11.1 ± 1.2	11.5 ± 5.0	8.5 ± 4.4	10.2 ± 4.0	6.9 ± 3.6
	Con group	12.5 ± 4.2	12.3 ± 1.0	13.6 ± 6.9	7.3 ± 3.7	11.3 ± 4.3	6.9 ± 3.1
Weight (kg)	RTX group	-	-	44.0 ± 18.6	31 ± 17	39.6 ± 15.2	30.0 ± 16
	Con group	-	-	47.5 ± 15.6	30 ± 17	45.5 ± 19.3	31.0 ± 41.0
Duration of NS (years)	RTX group	8.7 ± 4.9	-	7.9 ± 4.7	2.5 ± 8.4	5.7 ± 3.5	2.7 ± 2.4
	Con group	7.4 ± 4.9	-	8 ± 5.4	1.4 ± 5.6	7.8 ± 4.0	2.0 ± 2.5
Serum creatinine (μmol/L)	RTX group	-	-	39.8 ± 13.3	46.9 ± 30.9	48.6 ± 26.5	35.4 ± 17.7
	Con group	-	-	44.2 ± 15.9	48.6 ± 36.2	48.6 ± 17.7	36.2 ± 8.8
Serum albumin (g/dl)	RTX group	-	-	3.4 ± 0.6	2.4 ± 0.6	3.6 ± 0.9	3.8 ± 0.3
	Con group	-	-	3.4 ± 0.5	2.3 ± 0.5	3.2 ± 0.8	4.0 ± 0.4
Dose of prednisone (mg/kg/day)	RTX group	0.5 ± 0.4	-	-	0.5 ± 1.4	0.6 ± 0.4	0.6 ± 0.4
	Con group	0.3 ± 0.3	-	-	0.4 ± 0.8	0.6 ± 0.5	0.6 ± 0.5
CYC/TAC	RTX group	35/15	5/4	16/0	8/8	19/8	-
	Con group	16/6	6/3	16/0	7/8	19/8	-

CYC, cyclophosphamide; TAC, tacrolimus.

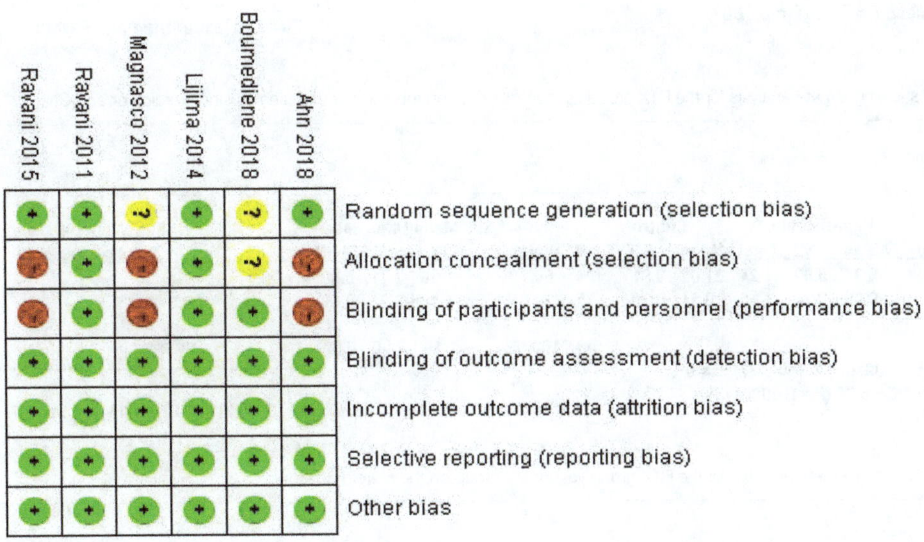

FIGURE 2 | Risk of bias summary.

(124 children) and the control group (110 children). We found that when compared to that in control, RTX could reduce the relapse number of NS, the use of steroids or/and calcineurin inhibitors, and the dosage of steroids, while RTX could not decrease the protein excretion. There were fewer reports of serious adverse reactions of RTX during the therapy, and most adverse events were mild and could be alleviated after stopping RTX or reducing the infusion speed.

As known, the immune disorder was an extremely important pathogenic factor for relapsing nephrotic syndrome (33). The T cell developed dysfunction and secreted some chemical mediators. These abnormal cytokines could change and damage the glomerular filtration membrane. The interest in B cell as a potential pathogenic factor for nephrotic syndrome resulted in reorganization in recent years. The B cells could express co-stimulatory molecules and cytokines, which induced activation and the dysfunction of T cell. RTX induced apoptosis and depletion of B cell, thus inhibiting the interaction between B cells and T cells and reducing the recurrence of nephrotic syndrome in children. Additionally, some research found that RTX had

Study or Subgroup	Experimental Events	Experimental Total	Control Events	Control Total	Weight	Odds Ratio M-H, Random, 95% CI
Ahn 2018	9	35	11	16	21.7%	0.16 [0.04, 0.58]
Boumediene 2018	1	10	13	13	10.1%	0.01 [0.00, 0.16]
Lijima 2014	17	24	23	24	15.7%	0.11 [0.01, 0.94]
Magnasco 2012	13	16	12	15	18.3%	1.08 [0.18, 6.44]
Ravani 2011	5	25	13	27	22.2%	0.27 [0.08, 0.93]
Ravani 2015	1	14	14	15	12.0%	0.01 [0.00, 0.10]
Total (95% CI)		**124**		**110**	**100.0%**	**0.11 [0.03, 0.43]**
Total events	46		86			

Heterogeneity: $Tau^2 = 1.65$; $Chi^2 = 14.52$, df = 5 (P = 0.01); $I^2 = 66\%$
Test for overall effect: Z = 3.23 (P = 0.001)

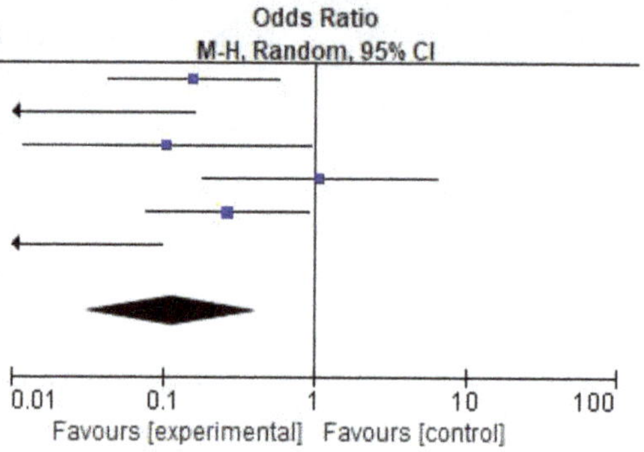

FIGURE 3 | Forest plot showing a meta-analysis for the RTX group vs. control group on the relapse numbers.

Study or Subgroup	Experimental Events	Experimental Total	Control Events	Control Total	Weight	Odds Ratio M-H, Fixed, 95% CI
Ahn 2018	30	35	16	16	17.3%	0.17 [0.01, 3.23]
Ravani 2011	10	27	26	27	82.7%	0.02 [0.00, 0.19]
Total (95% CI)		**62**		**43**	**100.0%**	**0.05 [0.01, 0.28]**
Total events	40		42			

Heterogeneity: $Chi^2 = 1.16$, df = 1 (P = 0.28); $I^2 = 14\%$
Test for overall effect: Z = 3.38 (P = 0.0007)

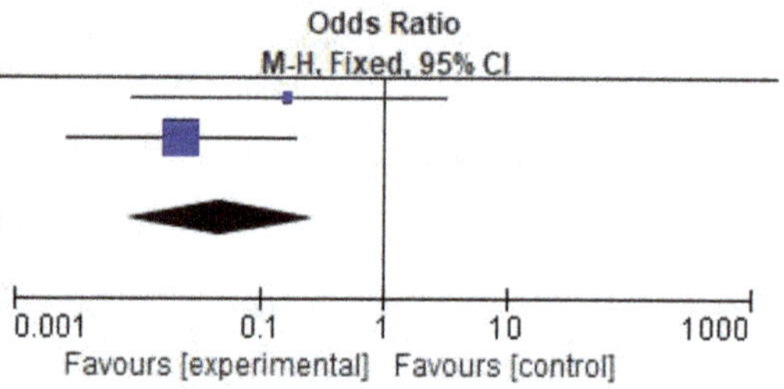

FIGURE 4 | Forest plot showing a meta-analysis for the RTX group vs. control group on the number of patients using steroids or/and CNI.

Study or Subgroup	Experimental Mean	Experimental SD	Experimental Total	Control Mean	Control SD	Control Total	Weight	Std. Mean Difference IV, Fixed, 95% CI
Lijima 2014	8.37	5.62	24	21.02	9.81	24	60.7%	-1.56 [-2.21, -0.90]
Ravani 2015	0.09	0.21	15	0.54	0.39	15	39.3%	-1.40 [-2.21, -0.59]
Total (95% CI)			**39**			**39**	**100.0%**	**-1.49 [-2.00, -0.99]**

Heterogeneity: $Chi^2 = 0.09$, df = 1 (P = 0.77); $I^2 = 0\%$
Test for overall effect: Z = 5.76 (P < 0.00001)

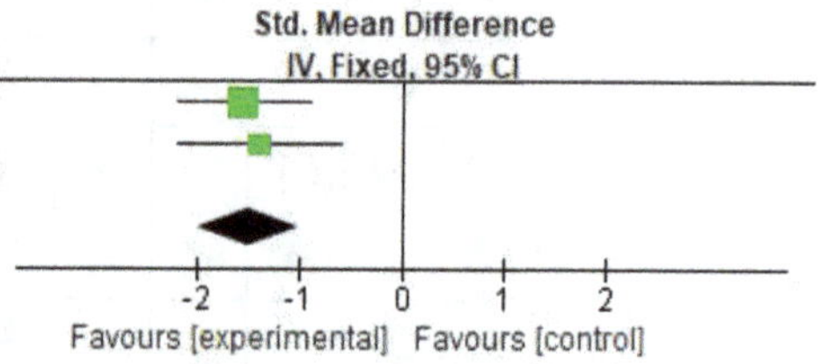

FIGURE 5 | Forest plot showing a meta-analysis for the RTX group vs. control group on the steroid dosage.

Study or Subgroup	Experimental Mean	Experimental SD	Experimental Total	Control Mean	Control SD	Control Total	Weight	Std. Mean Difference IV, Fixed, 95% CI
Magnasco 2012-1	2.7	4.593	9	3.9	4.37	7	14.0%	-0.25 [-1.25, 0.74]
Magnasco 2012-2	0.8	1.185	7	0.8	3.333	8	13.4%	0.00 [-1.01, 1.01]
Ravani 2011	0.11	0.177	27	0.36	0.5182	27	45.8%	-0.64 [-1.18, -0.09]
Ravani 2015	28	426.16	15	49	854.127	15	26.8%	-0.03 [-0.75, 0.69]
Total (95% CI)			**58**			**57**	**100.0%**	**-0.33 [-0.71, 0.04]**

Heterogeneity: $Chi^2 = 2.30$, df = 3 (P = 0.51); $I^2 = 0\%$
Test for overall effect: Z = 1.77 (P = 0.08)

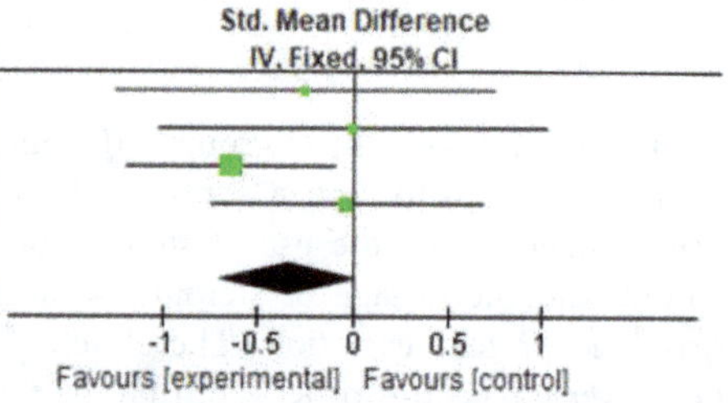

FIGURE 6 | Forest plot showing a meta-analysis for the RTX group vs. control group on the proteinuria excretion.

a protective effect on podocytes in a non-immune pathway (34). RTX could bind to the sphingomyelin phosphodiesterase acid-like 3b protein (SMPDL3b) in lipid rafts expressed on podocytes. The combination of RTX and SMPDL3b played a role in protecting the structure and function of podocytes because SMPDL3b was a key protein that regulated the cytoskeleton of the podocytes.

The research found that RTX holds great potential in reducing the relapses of NS compared with control. Kemper et al. (35) conducted a multicenter retrospective clinical trial and found that 69% of patients achieved long-term remission and 48% of patients stopped immune-suppressant treatments. Sun et al. (13) reported that RTX treatment showed an effective rate of 91.67%, and the number of relapses was significantly reduced ($p < 0.001$). Sellier-Leclerc et al. (19) showed that only 23% of the children relapsed during the treatment of RTX. After long-term observation, the number of relapses was only 37%.

We found a big heterogeneity in the number of relapses in the meta-analysis, with $I^2 = 66\%$, $p = 0.01$. We presumed that the different statistical time cutoffs could be the source of heterogeneity and performed a subgroup analysis by the different cutoffs, 3, 6, and 12 months. We did get a negative result; thus, considering the different cutoff could not be the source of the heterogeneity. We found another interesting difference among the studies included in the mate analysis; the dose of RTX was different. We hypothesized the dose of RTX as the variant and performed subgroup analysis, but could not find the sources of the heterogeneity, either. Last, we considered that the heterogeneity of the analysis would be caused by different experimental design methods, small sample sizes, and different outcome indicators.

Two articles in this study documented the number of patients who took steroids or/and CNI. The mate analysis showed a significant decrease in patients taking steroids or/and CNI after RTX treatment. In the research of Ito et al. (36), 41 of 53 (77%) SDNS/FRNS patients discontinued steroid successfully. Of 53 SDNS/FRNS patients, 17 (31%) stopped CSA. Guigonis et al. (16) found that 19 patients (85%) discontinued treatment with one or more immunosuppressive agents, with no recurrence and no additional immunosuppressive agents. These results indicated that RTX treatment could reduce the usage and the dosage of steroids and other immunosuppressants.

Three articles reported the dosage of steroids after the RTX therapy. In the research of Ahn et al. (27), a total of 61 patients were enrolled, 40 in the RTX group and 21 in the control, and the ratio was 2:1, which resulted in a huge heterogeneity, and the research was excluded. The heterogeneity could be reduced from 55 to 0%. The fixed-effect model was used to analyze the two remaining articles and the results showed the significantly reduced dosage of the steroid after RTX treatment. Sun et al. (13) recorded less steroid usage ($p = 0.014$) and less relapse ($p < 0.001$) in 12 children in the next 6 months after RTX treatment. Gulati et al. (37) studied 57 children, 12 of whom could discontinue one or more immunosuppressive agents. In the other eight patients, the dose of prednisone could be gradually reduced to 0.3–0.5 mg/kg every other day. Ahn et al. (27) and Iijima et al. (28) reported that the average days without steroid application were 141 and 211 days, respectively, and the toxic and side effects of long-term use of steroids for children were avoided.

As known, reducing proteinuria played a key role in NS treatments. Hofstra et al. (38) also found that proteinuria decreased significantly (2–3 g/day) within 2 weeks. Our analysis did not find a significant difference in the reduced proteinuria levels after RTX therapy. The following factors could be responsible for the result. First, the number of patients enrolled in the research was so limited and we needed a larger sample size for the evaluation of the effect of RTX. Secondly, there were big heterogeneities among the patients. Besides the differences in pathological types, children with early drug resistance and late drug resistance were enrolled in the research of Magnasco et al. (30). Last, the proteinuria was affected by a variety of factors. In the study of Dahan et al. (39), the serum albumin level can affect proteinuria.

Most patients tolerated the RTX treatment well. A review from Bonanni et al. (40) reported that the most common adverse event was rash, dyspnea, fever, cough, and infusion-related itching. All these adverse reactions could be well-controlled. Recently, anti-CD20 antibodies from human beings such as Ofatumumab were undergoing clinical research (41–43) and the adverse events remained to be further evaluated.

All the literature in our research showed good quality and held less bias in the Cochrane bias risk assessment. Stata software was applied to assess publication bias, and $p = 0.060$ in the Begg test and $p = 0.022$ in the Egger test. The Egger test result with a high $p = 0.022$ indicates that there was a publication bias, and the small size of the sample could be accounted for it.

There are some limitations. First, the length of remission before the relapse could be considered as an indicator of the drug efficacy. Second, the follow-up time of included studies was inconsistent and all were short. Third, the characteristics of baseline are different, and the age of the two studies (30, 32) is younger than other studies. Finally, RTX therapy has a higher cost than steroid and CNI treatment, and the economic benefits of RTX needed further evaluation. So, we needed much larger, long-term, comprehensive, and controlled studies to further evaluate the clinical value of RTX.

AUTHOR CONTRIBUTIONS

XG and FZ: guarantor of integrity of entire study and manuscript final version approval. XG and YW: study concepts. YW:

study design, statistical analysis, manuscript definition of intellectual content, and manuscript revision/review. HD: literature research. ZX: data acquisition and data analysis/interpretation. HY: manuscript preparation and manuscript editing. All authors contributed to the article and approved the submitted version.

REFERENCES

1. Beck L, Bomback AS, Choi MJ, Holzman LB, Waldman M. KDOQI US commentary on the 2012 KDIGO clinical practice guideline for glomerulonephritis. *Am J Kidney Dis.* (2013) 62:403–41. doi: 10.1053/j.ajkd.2013.06.002
2. Bhandari N, Shrestha D, Anand K, Pruthi PK. Role of rituximab in pediatric nephrotic syndrome. *Curr Med Res Pract.* (2014) 4:296–7. doi: 10.1016/j.cmrp.2014.11.010
3. Metz DK, Kausman JY. Childhood nephrotic syndrome in the 21st century: what's new? *J Padeiatr Child H.* (2015) 51:497–504. doi: 10.1111/jpc.12734
4. Kyrieleis H, Lowik MM, Pronk I, Cruysberg H, Kremer J, Oyen W, et al. Long-term outcome of biopsy- proven, frequently relapsing minimal-change nephrotic syndrome in children. *Clin J Am Soc Nephrol.* (2009) 4:1593–600. doi: 10.2215/CJN.05691108
5. Prasad N, Gulati S, Sharma RK, Singh U, Ahmed M. Pulse cyclophosphamide therapy in steroid-dependent nephrotic syndrome. *Pediatr Nephrol.* (2004) 19:494–8. doi: 10.1007/s00467-003-1404-x
6. Tejani A, Butt KH, Trachtman HO, Suthanthiran M, Rosenthal CJ, Khawar MR. Cyclosporine-induced remission of relapsing nephrotic syndrome in children. *J Pediatr.* (1987) 111:1056–62. doi: 10.1016/S0022-3476(87)80056-2
7. Loeffler K, Gowrishankar M, Yiu V. Tacrolimus therapy in pediatric patients with treatment-resistant nephrotic syndrome. *Pediatr Nephrol.* (2004) 19:281–7. doi: 10.1007/s00467-003-1370-3
8. Mendizábal S, Zamora I, Berbel O, Sanahuja MJ, Fuentes J, Simon J. Mycophenolate mofetil in steroid/cyclosporine-dependent/resistant nephrotic syndrome. *Pediatr Nephrol.* (2005) 20:914–9. doi: 10.1007/s00467-005-1877-x
9. Kausman JY, Yin L, Jones CL, Johnstone L, Powell HR. Vincristine treatment in steroid-dependent nephrotic syndrome. *Pediatr Nephrol.* (2005) 20:1416–9. doi: 10.1007/s00467-005-1940-7
10. Sinha A, Bagga A. Rituximab therapy in nephrotic syndrome: implications for patients' management. *Nat Rev Nephrol.* (2013) 9:154–69. doi: 10.1038/nrneph.2012.289
11. Coiffier B, Lepage E, Brière J, Herbrecht R, Tilly H, Bouabdallah R, et al. CHOP chemotherapy plus rituximab compared with CHOP alone in elderly patients with diffuse large-B-cell lymphoma. *New Engl J Med.* (2002) 346:235. doi: 10.1056/NEJMoa011795
12. Buch MH, Smolen JS, Betteridge N, Breedveld FC, Burmester G, Dorner T, et al. Updated consensus statement on the use of rituximab in patients with rheumatoid arthritis. *Ann Rheum Dis.* (2011) 70:909–20. doi: 10.1136/ard.2010.144998
13. Sun L, Xu H, Shen Q, Cao Q, Rao J. Efficacy of rituximab therapy in children with refractory nephrotic syndrome: a prospective observational study in Shanghai. *World J Pediatr.* (2014) 10:59–63. doi: 10.1007/s12519-014-0453-5
14. Prytuła A, Iijima K, Kamei K, Geary D, Gottlich E, Majeed A. Rituximab in refractory nephrotic syndrome. *Pediatr Nephrol.* (2010) 25:461–8. doi: 10.1007/s00467-009-1376-6
15. Kamei K, Ishikura K. Rituximab treatment for refractory steroid-resistant nephrotic syndrome. *Pediatr Nephrol.* (2016) 31:337–8. doi: 10.1007/s00467-015-3205-4
16. Guigonis V, Dallocchio A, Baudouin V, Dehennault M, Camus CHL, Afanetti M, et al. Rituximab treatment for severe steroid- or cyclosporine-dependent nephrotic syndrome: a multicentric series of 22 cases. *Pediatr Nephrol.* (2008) 23:1269–79. doi: 10.1007/s00467-008-0814-1
17. Smith GC. Is there a role for rituximab in the treatment of idiopathic childhood nephrotic syndrome? *Pediatr Nephrol.* (2007) 22:893–8. doi: 10.1007/s00467-006-0427-5
18. Nakayama M, Kamei K, Nozu K, Matsuoka K, Nakagawa A, Sako M, et al. Rituximab for refractory focal segmental glomerulosclerosis. *Pediatr Nephrol.* (2008) 23:481–5. doi: 10.1007/s00467-007-0640-x
19. Sellier-Leclerc A-L, Baudouin V, Kwon T, Macher M-A, Guérin V, Lapillonne H, et al. Rituximab in steroid-dependent idiopathic nephrotic syndrome in childhood-follow-up after CD19 recovery. *Nephrol Dial Transpl.* (2012) 27:1083–9. doi: 10.1093/ndt/gfr405
20. Fujinaga S, Hirano D, Nishizaki N, Kamei K, Ito S, Ohtomo Y, et al. Single infusion of rituximab for persistent steroid-dependent minimal-change nephrotic syndrome after long-term cyclosporine. *Pediatr Nephrol.* (2010) 25:539–44. doi: 10.1007/s00467-009-1377-5
21. Kari JA, El-Morshedy SM, El-Desoky S, Alshaya HO, Rahim KA, Edrees BM. Rituximab for refractory cases of childhood nephrotic syndrome. *Pediatr Nephrol.* (2010) 26:733–7. doi: 10.1007/s00467-011-1778-0
22. Webb H, Jaureguiberry G, Dufek S, Tullus K, Bockenhauer D. Cyclophosphamide and rituximab in frequently relapsing/steroid-dependent nephrotic syndrome. *Pediatr Nephrol.* (2016) 31:589–94. doi: 10.1007/s00467-015-3245-9
23. Delbe-Bertin L, Aoun B, Tudorache E, Lapillone H, Ulinski T. Does rituximab induce hypogammaglobulinemia in patients with pediatric idiopathic nephrotic syndrome? *Pediatr Nephrol.* (2013) 28:447–51. doi: 10.1007/s00467-012-2361-z
24. Sinha A, Bagga A, Gulati A, Hari P. Short-term efficacy of rituximab versus tacrolimus in steroid-dependent nephrotic syndrome. *Pediatr Nephrol.* (2012) 27:235–41. doi: 10.1007/s00467-011-1997-4
25. Basu B, Sander A, Roy B, Preussler S, Barua S, Mahapatra TKS, et al. Efficacy of rituximab vs. tacrolimus in pediatric corticosteroid-dependent nephrotic syndrome. *JAMA Pediatr.* (2018) 172:757–65. doi: 10.1001/jamapediatrics.2018.1323
26. Kamei K, Ishikura K, Sako M, Aya K, Tanaka R, Nozu K, et al. Long-term outcome of childhood-onset complicated nephrotic syndrome after a multicenter, double-blind, randomized, placebo-controlled trial of rituximab. *Pediatr Nephrol.* (2017) 32:2071–8. doi: 10.1007/s00467-017-3718-0
27. Ahn YH, Kim SH, Han KH, Choi HJ, Cho H, Lee JW, et al. Efficacy and safety of rituximab in childhood-onset, difficult-to-treat nephrotic syndrome: a multicenter open-label trial in Korea. *Medicine.* (2018) 97:e13157. doi: 10.1097/MD.0000000000013157
28. Iijima K, Sako M, Nozu K, Mori R, Tuchida N, Kamei K, et al. Rituximab for childhood-onset, complicated, frequently relapsing nephrotic syndrome or steroid-dependent nephrotic syndrome: a multicentre, double-blind, randomised, placebo-controlled trial. *Lancet.* (2014) 384:1273–81. doi: 10.1016/S0140-6736(14)60541-9
29. Boumediene A, Vachin P, Sendeyo K, Oniszczuk J, Zhang SY, Henique C, et al. NEPHRUTIX: a randomized, double-blind, placebo vs. Rituximab-controlled trial assessing T-cell subset changes in minimal change nephrotic syndrome. *J Autoimmun.* (2018) 88:91–102. doi: 10.1016/j.jaut.2017.10.006
30. Magnasco A, Ravani P, Edefonti A, Murer L, Ghio L, Belingheri M, et al. Rituximab in children with resistant idiopathic nephrotic syndrome. *J Am Soc Nephrol.* (2012) 23:1117–24. doi: 10.1681/ASN.2011080775
31. Ravani P, Magnasco A, Edefonti A, Murer L, Rossi R, Ghio L, et al. Short-term effects of rituximab in children with steroid- and calcineurin-dependent nephrotic syndrome: a randomized controlled trial. *Clin J Am Soc Nephro.* (2011) 6:1308–15. doi: 10.2215/CJN.09421010
32. Ravani P, Rossi R, Bonanni A, Quinn RR, Ghiggeri GM. Rituximab in children with steroid-dependent nephrotic syndrome: a multicenter, open-label, noninferiority, randomized controlled trial. *J Am Soc Nephro.* (2015) 26:2259–66. doi: 10.1681/ASN.2014080799
33. Berre LL, Bruneau S, Naulet J, Renaudin K, Buzelin F, Usal C, et al. Induction of T regulatory cells attenuates idiopathic nephrotic syndrome. *J Am Soc of Nephrol.* (2009) 20:57–67. doi: 10.1681/ASN.2007111244
34. Fornoni A, Sageshima J, Wei C, Merscher-Gomez S, Aguillon-Prada R, Jauregui AN, et al. Rituximab targets podocytes in recurrent focal segmental glomerulosclerosis. *Sci Transl Med.* (2011) 3:85ra46-85ra46. doi: 10.1126/scitranslmed.3002231

35. Kemper MJ, Jutta G, Sandra H, Krmar RT, Katalin D, Therese J, et al. Long-term follow-up after rituximab for steroid-dependent idiopathic nephrotic syndrome. *Nephrol Dial Transpl.* (2011) 27:1910–5. doi: 10.1093/ndt/gfr548
36. Ito S, Kamei K, Ogura M, Udagawa T, Fujinaga S, Saito M, et al. Survey of rituximab treatment for childhood-onset refractory nephrotic syndrome. *Pediatr Nephrol.* (2013) 28:257–64. doi: 10.1007/s00467-012-2319-1
37. Gulati A, Sinha A, Jordan SC, Hari P, Dinda AK, Sharma S, et al. Efficacy and safety of treatment with rituximab for difficult steroid-resistant and -dependent nephrotic syndrome: multicentric report. *Clin J Am Soc Nephrol.* (2010) 5:2207–12. doi: 10.2215/CJN.03470410
38. Hofstra JM, Deegens JK, Wetzels JF. Rituximab: effective treatment for severe steroid-dependent minimal change nephrotic syndrome? *Nephrol Dial Transpl.* (2007) 22:2100–2. doi: 10.1093/ndt/gfm128
39. Dahan K, Debiec H, Plaisier E, Cachanado M, Rousseau A, Wakselman L, et al. Rituximab for severe membranous nephropathy: a 6-month trial with extended follow-up. *J Am Soc Nephrol.* (2017) 28:348–58. doi: 10.1681/ASN.2016040449
40. Bonanni A, Calatroni M, D'Alessandro M, Signa S, Bertelli E, Cioni M, et al. Adverse events linked with the use of chimeric and humanized anti-CD20 antibodies in children with idiopathic nephrotic syndrome. *Brit J Clin Pharmaco.* (2018) 84:1238–49. doi: 10.1111/bcp.13548
41. Bonanni A, Rossi R, Murtas C, Ghiggeri GM. Low-dose ofatumumab for rituximab-resistant nephrotic syndrome. *BMJ Case Reports.* (2015) 2015:210208. doi: 10.1136/bcr-2015-210208
42. Basu B. Ofatumumab for rituximab-resistant nephrotic syndrome. *New Engl J Med.* (2014) 370:1268–70. doi: 10.1056/NEJMc1308488
43. Lundberg S, Westergren E, Smolander J, Bruchfeld A. B cell-depleting therapy with rituximab or ofatumumab in immunoglobulin A nephropathy or vasculitis with nephritis. *Clin Kidney J.* (2017) 10:20–6. doi: 10.1093/ckj/sfw106

20

Overview of Monogenic or Mendelian Forms of Hypertension

Rupesh Raina [1,2,3†], Vinod Krishnappa [2,4†], Abhijit Das [4], Harshesh Amin [5], Yeshwanter Radhakrishnan [6], Nikhil R. Nair [7] and Kirsten Kusumi [3]*

[1] Department of Nephrology, Cleveland Clinic Akron General, Akron, OH, United States, [2] Akron Nephrology Associates, Cleveland Clinic Akron General, Akron, OH, United States, [3] Department of Pediatric Nephrology, Akron Children's Hospital, Akron, OH, United States, [4] Department of Medicine, Northeast Ohio Medical University, Rootstown, OH, United States, [5] Department of Internal Medicine, Carolinas Health Care System Blue Ridge, Morganton, NC, United States, [6] Department of Internal Medicine, Cleveland Clinic Akron General, Akron, OH, United States, [7] Department of Biochemistry, Case Western Reserve University, Cleveland, OH, United States

Correspondence:
Rupesh Raina
rraina@akronchildrens.org;
raina@akronnephrology.com

These authors share first authorship

Monogenic or Mendelian forms of hypertension are described as a group of conditions characterized by insults to the normal regulation of blood pressure by the kidney and adrenal gland. These alterations stem from single mutations that lead to maladaptive overabsorption of electrolytes with fluid shift into the vasculature, and consequent hypertension. Knowledge of these various conditions is essential in diagnosing pediatric or early-onset adult hypertension as they directly affect treatment strategies. Precise diagnosis with specific treatment regimens aimed at the underlying physiologic derangement can restore normotension and prevent the severe sequelae of chronic hypertension.

Keywords: monogenic hypertension, Liddle syndrome, congenital adrenal hyperplasia, apparent mineralocorticoid excess, Gordon syndrome, familial hyperaldosteronism

INTRODUCTION

†

Hypertension is one of the most prevalent diseases in the world, affecting an estimated 34% of individuals at or above the age of 20 within the United States alone (1). In contrast, the prevalence of hypertension among individuals aged 12–19 in the United States is 4.11% (2). Treatment of high blood pressure is paramount for improving cardiovascular health and preventing long term morbidity and mortality, per the World Heart Federation (3). The significance of untreated hypertension is emphasized by the severity of end organ damage and extreme systemic sequelae in patients with longstanding disease. The majority of hypertension results from a combination of behavioral and environmental factors; however, various genetic mutations have been identified as distinct causes as well. These genetic forms of hypertension stem from gain- or loss-of-function mutations within the mineralocorticoid, glucocorticoid, or sympathetic pathways (4). The term, monogenic hypertension, is used to describe specific genetic hypertensive disorders which inhibit normal renal and/or adrenal blood pressure regulation. It is especially important to keep these rare conditions in mind when diagnosing hypertension in children, as the younger the child, the more likely that their hypertension is due to a secondary cause. Recent advancements in genetic sequencing methodology have provided further insight into these conditions.

Monogenic hypertension drives volume expansion by three distinct mechanisms: (1) excessive sodium ion reabsorption by hyperactive channels, (2) hyperstimulation of mineralocorticoid receptors due to alterations in steroid synthesis, and (3) excess mineralocorticoid synthesis causing volume expansion (5, 6). However, one could conceptualize the latter two mechanisms as indirect means of increasing salt reabsorption, which is the basis of the first mechanism. Monogenic hypertension is further classified based on serum renin and aldosterone levels. Low renin monogenic hypertension conditions can be further categorized by aldosterone level: low, normal, or high (**Table 1**). Another category is monogenic hypertension due to andrenergic/sympathetic excess. Treatment must be specific to each syndrome's unique derangements within the mineralocorticoid, glucocorticoid, or sympathetic pathways. However, as with all types of hypertension, treatment is aimed at the amelioration of cardiovascular morbidity and mortality associated with long standing high blood pressure. The various types of monogenic hypertension with specific evaluation and treatment considerations will be reviewed in this article. **Table 2** provides an overview of the causes of monogenic hypertension and their Online Mendelian Inheritance in Man (OMIM) numbers (7). **Figure 1** depicts the diagnostic evaluation for monogenic hypertension.

TABLE 1 | Basic classification scheme for causes of monogenic hypertension.

Low renin level	Low aldosterone levels	Liddle syndrome Congenital adrenal hyperplasia Apparent mineralocorticoid excess Gellers syndrome
	Normal aldosterone levels	Gordon syndrome (pseudohypoaldosteronism type II)
	High aldosterone levels	Familial hyperaldosteronism type I (glucocorticoid-remediable aldosteronism) Familial hyperaldosteronism type II Familial hyperaldosteronism type III Familial hyperaldosteronism type IV
Adrenergic/sympathetic excess	High metanephrine and normetanephrine levels	Familial pheochromocytoma
Vascular smooth muscle proliferation		Hypertension and brachydactyly syndrome

LOW ALDOSTERONE MONOGENIC HYPERTENSION

Case 1: A 10-year-old boy presented to the clinic with skeletal muscle weakness, paresthesia, nausea, and vomiting, all starting ~5–6 months ago. He had no significant past medical history and was previously healthy. His mother had been diagnosed with hypertension at the age of 20 years, but no other significant family history was noted. The patient was not currently on any medications and had no known drug allergies. On examination, the child was mildly lethargic. Blood pressure measured 164/92 mmHg in the arms and 183/112 mmHg in the legs. The rest of the general physical examination was unremarkable. The patient's height and weight were at the 50th and 62nd percentile, respectively, based on the WHO growth chart. Laboratory work up included complete blood count, electrolytes, thyroid profile, liver profile, urinalysis (UA), and abdominal imaging was obtained. The patient's electrolytes were significant for hypokalemia with serum potassium levels of 2.1 mEq/L (normal 3.5–5.0 mEq/L) as well as a mild metabolic alkalosis with serum bicarbonate of 31 mmol/L (normal 22–29 mmol/L). The remaining labs and imaging studies were unremarkable. The patient was started on spironolactone for the elevated blood pressure and potassium supplements for hypokalemia and was asked to return for a follow up visit in 2 weeks.

After 2 weeks, the patient returned to the clinic with no change in symptoms. Lab values remained the same despite appropriate medication adherence. Plasma renin, serum aldosterone, 11-beta-hydroxylase, and 17-alpha-hydroxylase were ordered. Lab values revealed suppressed plasma renin <1.0 ng/mL/h (normal 2.8–39.9 ng/mL/h) as well as low aldosterone level 8.2 ng/mL/h (normal >20 mg/mL/h). The plasma aldosterone to plasma renin ratio was greater than 30 ng/dL. The child was diagnosed with Liddle syndrome and was started on amiloride. At the next follow up visit, the patient's prior symptoms resolved, blood pressure had returned to the normal range based on age, sex, and height; and the hypokalemia had resolved.

LIDDLE SYNDROME

Genetics and pathogenesis: Liddle Syndrome is caused by an autosomal dominant (AD), gain-of-function mutation of the epithelial sodium channel (ENaC) present in the collecting duct. The ENaC beta and gamma subunits, SCNN1B and SCNN1G, respectively, are most commonly affected (4, 8). Mutation of these subunits disrupts expression of proline-rich regions of the cytoplasmic carboxyl terminus and results in loss of regulatory binding sites for Nedd4-2, a ubiquitin ligase necessary for the breakdown of ENaC (8–10). Thus, ENaC remains constitutively active with increased Na^+ reabsorption and subsequent intravascular volume expansion culminating in hypertension (**Figure 2**) (8, 11, 12). Liddle Syndrome-associated Na^+ reabsorption is independent of aldosterone, and a hallmark of the disease is the suppression of renin and aldosterone. Hypokalemia ensues as excess Na^+ is continually absorbed with extrusion of K^+ via the Na/K-ATPase pump (8, 13). Mild metabolic alkalosis is also seen, as the increased Na^+ reabsorption increases the net negativity of the lumen, causing an increase in H^+ extrusion via the renal outer medullary potassium (ROMK) channel and H^+-ATPase pump located on alpha-intercalated cells (10).

Epidemiology: Liddle's is rare with only 30 patients having been formally diagnosed since 2008; however, many nephrologists perceive that it is an under recognized cause of hypertension (14). Liddle's has an estimated prevalence of 1.5% with genetic testing in a Chinese population and was found to have a 6% prevalence in hypertensive patients among a study of US veterans in Louisiana (15, 16). Age of onset for hypertension is typically young, between late childhood and adolescence (17). Patients lacking a family history have also been noted, indicating that LS should always remain in the differential for early-onset hypertension irrespective of the family history (8).

TABLE 2 | Overview of the causes of monogenic hypertension and their OMIM genotype and phenotype numbers.

Condition	Mode of inheritance	OMIM phenotype number(s)	OMIM genotype numbers(s)	Cytogenetic loci	Pathophysiology	Management
Liddle syndrome	Autosomal dominant	177200	600760 (SCNN1B) 600761 (SCNN1G)	16p12.2	Hyperactive ENaC reabsorbs sodium at elevated levels, resulting in volume expansion and hypertension	Patients present with early onset HTN with hypokalemia non-responsive to conventional therapy. Genetic testing confirms the diagnosis. Use ENaC inhibitory agents: amiloride, triamterene.
Congenital adrenal hyperplasia	Autosomal recessive	202010 (type IV)	610613 (CYP11B1)	8q24.3	Defects in steroid synthesis cause buildup of intermediate metabolites with MR activity	Patients present with HTN at very young ages along with atypical sexual development. Glucocorticoid supplementation to suppress ACTH expression treats HTN; potentially add MR antagonists for better control. Therapy should also be individualized to address aspects of sexual dysfunction.
	Autosomal recessive	202110 (type V)	609300 (CYP17A1)	10q24.32		
Syndrome of apparent mineralocorticoid excess	Autosomal recessive	218030	614232 (HSD11B2)	16q22.1	HSD11B2 deficiency allows excess cortisol stimulation at the MR	Therapy uses MR antagonists to alleviate overactivity and may call for ACTH suppression with excess cortisol
Geller syndrome	Autosomal dominant	605115	600983 (NR3C2)	4q31.23	Genetic mutations in the MR alter its structure and binding affinities, allowing atypical stimulation by other steroids, especially progesterone	Presents by early adult life; most critical in pregnant women. Management would be with delivery of the child and subsequent monitoring. Spironolactone is to be avoided.
Gordon syndrome (pseudohypoaldosteronism type II)	Autosomal dominant	145260 (type IIA)	Unspecified	1q31-1q42	Mutations in regulatory proteins for the NCC channel allow for unchecked activity, causing subsequent electrolyte and fluid overabsorption	Thiazide diuretic therapy directly treats NCC hyperactivity.
	Autosomal dominant	614491 (type IIB)	601844 (WNK4)	17q21.2		
	Autosomal dominant	614492 (type IIC)	605232 (WNK1)	12p13.33		
	Autosomal recessive or dominant	614495 (type IID)	605775 (KLHL3)	5q31.2		
	Autosomal dominant	614496 (type IIE)	603136 (CUL3)	2q36.2		
Familial hyperaldosteronism type I (glucocorticoid-remediable aldosteronism)	Autosomal dominant	103900	610613 (CYP11B1)	8q24.3	Unequal crossing over between the CYP11B1 and CYP11B2 genes generates a chimeric product that is ACTH-sensitive and produces aldosterone	Treatment with glucocorticoids to reduce ACTH secretion, supplemented with MR antagonists if necessary. Patients should be screened regularly for HTN-induced cerebrovascular sequelae
Familial hyperaldosteronism type II	Autosomal dominant	605635	600570 (CLCN2)	3q27.1	Hyperplasia or benign neoplasia within the adrenal cortex results in excess aldosterone production	Medical management with MR antagonists with potential surgical resection
Familial hyperaldosteronism type III	Autosomal dominant	613677	600735 (KCNJ5)	11q24.3	Gain-of-function mutations in potassium channels allow adrenal cortical cells to depolarize and subsequently activate aldosterone synthase	Medical management with MR antagonists with potential surgical resection
Familial hyperaldosteronism type IV	Autosomal dominant	617027	607904 (CACNA1H)	16p13.3	Gain-of-function mutations in calcium channels delay inactivation of cells, allowing enhancing aldosterone synthase activity	Medical management with MR antagonists with potential surgical resection

(Continued)

TABLE 2 | Continued

Condition	Mode of inheritance	OMIM phenotype number(s)	OMIM genotype numbers(s)	Cytogenetic loci	Pathophysiology	Management
Familial pheochromocytoma	Autosomal dominant	171300	605995 (KIF1B) 185470 (SDHB) 613403 (TMEM127) 608537 (VHL) 600837 (GDNF) 164761 (RET) 602690 (SDHD) 154950 (MAX)	1p36.22 1p36.13 2q11.2 3p25.3 5p13.2 10q11.21 11q23.1 14q23.3	Neoplasia of the adrenal medulla generates heightened levels of norepinephrine and epinephrine	Medical management with catecholamine antagonists and other antihypertensives prior to surgical resection. Continuous monitoring and genetic testing may prove helpful with syndromic causes
Hypertension and Brachydactyly Syndrome	Autosomal dominant	112410	123805 (PDE3A)	12p12.2	Gain-of-function mutations generate increased cAMP levels causing enhanced vascular smooth muscle proliferation, accompanied by brachydactyly due to dysfunctional chondrogenesis	High concentration milrinone therapy with possible benefits from phosphodiesterase inhibitors to increase cGMP levels

Gene names are in parentheses next to the genotype number, where applicable. HTN, hypertension; ENaC, epithelial sodium channel; ACTH, adrenocorticotropic hormone; MR, mineralocorticoid receptor; NCC, sodium chloride cotransporter.

Work Up: A strong family history of hypertension, suppressed renin/aldosterone levels and response to ENaC antagonism is highly suggestive, but a definitive diagnosis requires genetic testing (16). Random aldosterone/renin ratio can be used as a screening test, and a ratio >30 excludes the diagnosis (when expressed in ng/dL for aldosterone and ng/dL/h for renin) (15). Renin is suppressed by both elevated sodium levels and volume expansion; aldosterone is often less suppressed, resulting in the increased aldosterone/renin ratio. Liddle syndrome is alternatively known as pseudohyperaldosteronism due to its similarity to hyperaldosteronism with hypertension, hypokalemia, and metabolic alkalosis (18).

Treatment: Treatment consists of direct ENaC inhibition with potassium-sparing diuretics such as amiloride or triamterene. Spironolactone is not useful as the genetically altered ENaC is independent of mineralocorticoid regulation (8). A low sodium diet is also important in managing hypertension and counteracting the altered ENaC physiology (19).

Case 2: A 10-year-old female presented with hirsutism, particularly on her face as well as the pubic area. She first noticed the hair development 2 months ago. Her past medical history is significant for menarche at the age of 8 with irregular menstrual periods accompanied by breast development. Her maternal aunt also went through puberty around the age of 7–8. The patient was not on any medications at the time of office visit. On examination, the patient was alert with no signs of distress. Her blood pressure measured 168 /104 mmHg on manual auscultation. She is currently Tanner stage II, though her clitoral folds were noted to be enlarged. She is at the 80 and 90th percentiles for height and weight, respectively. Pertinent labs including a complete metabolic panel, adrenal profile, and thyroid profile were obtained. Lab results showed hypokalemia as well as elevated levels of multiple hormone precursors and androgens [serum potassium 2.1 mEq/L (normal 3.5–5.0 mEq/L), serum deoxycorticosterone 21 ng/dL (normal 2–13 ng/dL), serum dehydroepiandrostenedione sulfate (DHEAS) 392 μg/dL (normal <160 μg/dL), serum testosterone, 82 ng/dL (normal 0–30 ng/dL)]. Based on presentation and laboratory findings, the patient was diagnosed with congenital adrenal hyperplasia due to 11β-hydroxylase deficiency. She was started on hydrocortisone with subsequent resolution of her hypertension and hypokalemia.

CONGENITAL ADRENAL HYPERPLASIA

Though 21α-hydroxylase deficiency is more common, 11β-hydroxylase deficiency (11OHD or CAH type IV) and 17α-hydroxylase deficiency (17OHD or CAH type V), are two subtypes of CAH known to cause monogenic hypertension (13). The respective enzymes regulate different steps in steroid synthesis, but 11OHD and 17OHD deficiency both cause elevated deoxycortisol and deoxycorticosterone levels. These intermediates have activity at the mineralocorticoid receptors. Unchecked mineralocorticoid activity leads to hypertension and hypokalemia. Both types are inherited in an autosomal recessive

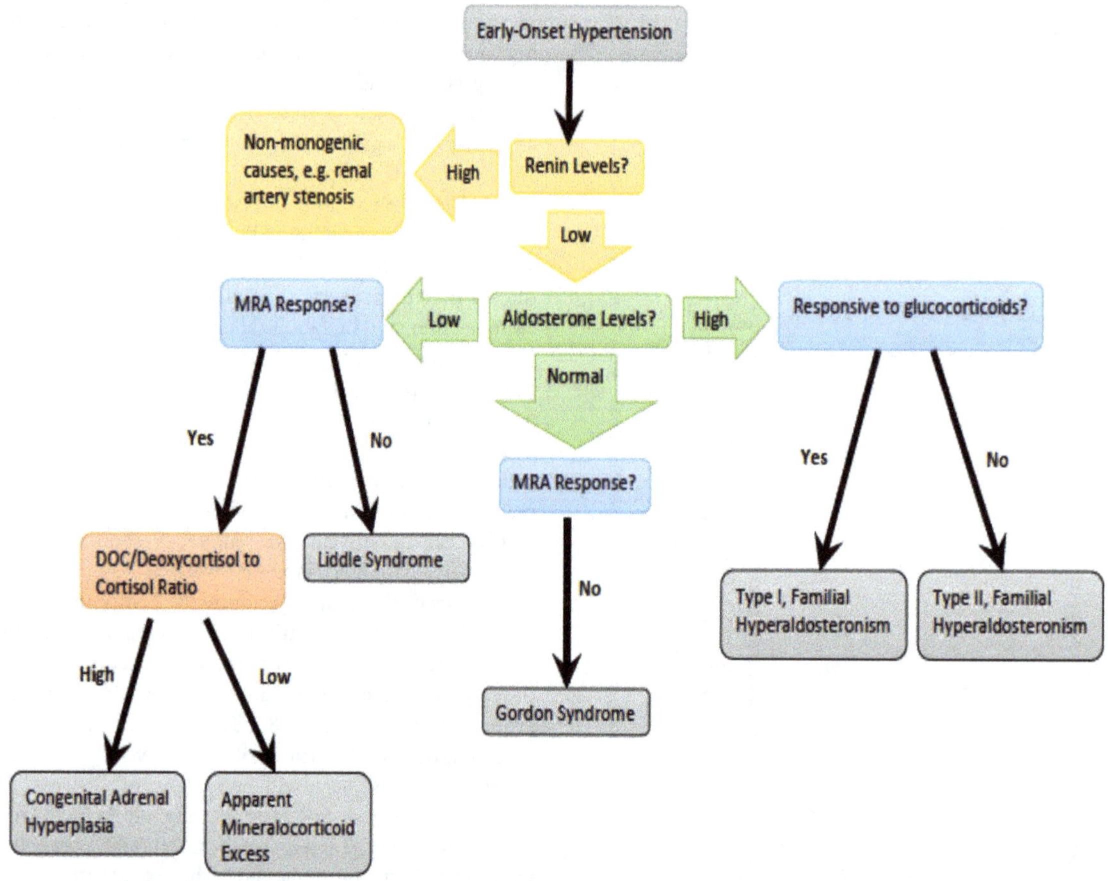

FIGURE 1 | Diagnostic evaluation for monogenic hypertension. DOC, deoxycorticosterone.

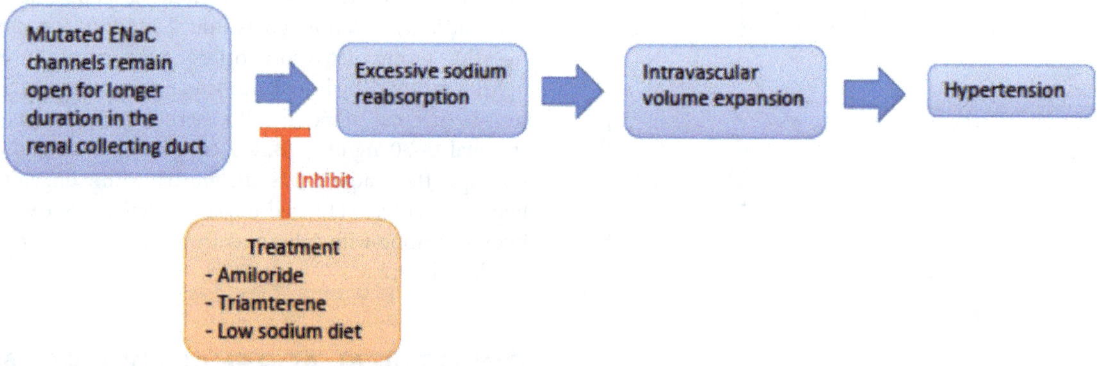

FIGURE 2 | An overview schematic of Liddle svndrome pathophysiology and treatment. ENaC, epithelial sodium channel.

(AR) fashion, stemming from inactivating mutations that prevent expression of the respective enzymes (20).

11β-Hydroxylase Deficiency

Genetics and Pathophysiology: CAH type IV, or loss of 11β-hydroxylase, prevents conversion of deoxycortisone and deoxycortisol into corticosterone and cortisol, respectively. Both deoxycortisone and deoxycortisol have weak activity at the mineralocorticoid receptor, but their accumulation in CAH type IV leads to significant mineralocorticoid activity and subsequent hypertension. As the conversion to glucocorticoids, androgens and estrogens are preserved, patients present with high levels of deoxycorticosterone, deoxycoritsol and androgens, mainly androstenedione and dehydroepiandrosterone (DHEA)

(**Figure 3**). This is a key factor in laboratory diagnosis after ACTH (adrenocorticotropic hormone) stimuation, as high levels of the androgens coupled with HTN prove helpful in differentiating 11OHD from other causes of CAH and monogenic hypertension (21).

Epidemiology: 11OHD is considered to be a rare condition that accounts for 5–8% of CAH cases (22). However, it has been seen with relatively high frequency among certain populations and accounts for 15% of CAH cases in Muslim and Jewish Middle Eastern populations (23). Detection of this disorder can be done by testing for 11β-hydroxylase activity or measuring tetrahydro-11-deoxycortisol in amniotic fluid or urine.

Workup: Like other CAH subtypes, 11OHD manifests with disorders of sexual development. Patients can potentially be identified at birth based on physical findings. Due to androgen accumulation, female infants undergo virilization, presenting with ambiguous genitalia at birth with enlarged clitoral folds (4). Androgen excess can also cause precocious puberty in both males and females. Regardless of variations in sexual development, patients present with hypertension at very young ages. Diagnosis relies on measuring levels of the adrenal steroid hormones to identify enzyme activity and defects. Further genetic testing for the CYP11B1 gene (cytogenetic locus 8q24.3) offers a definitive understanding of disease pathophysiology, guiding treatment (21).

Treatment: Treatment consists of glucocorticoid doses sufficient to decrease ACTH secretion, inhibiting stimulation of steroid synthesis and accumulation of mineralocorticoid receptor agonists. Spironolactone, amiloride, and calcium channel blockers may be further used to treat hypertension. Further considerations include individualized therapy to accommodate sexual development in patients and genital malformations in females may need surgical correction (24).

17α-Hydroxylase Deficiency

CAH type V, also known as P450C17α deficiency, manifests clinically as hypogonadism, hypokalemia, and hypertension. The gene, CYP17A1, located at cytogenetic locus 10q24.32 encodes 17α-hydroxylase with two key steroidogenic functionalities: 17α-hydroxylase and 17,20-lyase activity (21). Its 17α-hydroxylase function generates 17α-hydroxypregnenolone and 17α-hydroxyprogesterone, which can be converted to cortisol. These products of the 17α-hydroxylase are also substrates for the 17,20-lyase, which generates DHEA and androstenedione to serve as precursors for androgen and estrogen synthesis. This rare disorder thus blocks the production of cortisol as its direct precursors are not synthesized, shunting steroid production toward the mineralocorticoids (**Figure 3**). Since the blockage is so early in the pathway, there is very little production of sex hormones (23). Male patients have ambiguous external genitalia and may even exhibit a female phenotype, while females present with primary amenorrhea and delayed sexual development (6).

Workup: Steroid analysis upon ACTH-stimulation would lead to an appropriate diagnosis, showing atypically elevated levels of pregnenolone and progesterone relative to 17α-pregnenolone and 17α-progesterone, respectively.

Treatment: Treatment for these patients would be the same as type IV regarding hypertension with the addition of sex hormone therapy (6).

Case 3: A 10-month-old infant came to the clinic with severe hypertension. The patient had no significant past medical history. Lab results as well as imaging reveal severe hypokalemia, mild left ventricular hypertrophy (LVH), and nephrocalcinosis on renal ultrasound. Further metabolic lab studies showed low aldosterone and renin levels. A 24-h urine tetrahydrocortisol (THF) + allo-tetrahydrocortisol (5α-THF) to tetrahydrocortisone (THE) was collected when prior labs detected normal deoxycorticosterone, corticosterone, 18-hydroxydeoxycorticosterone, and 18-hydroxycortisol levels. The 24-h urine sample of THF + 5αTHF confirmed the diagnosis of syndrome of apparent mineralocorticoid excess (AME). The patient was started on amiloride with potassium supplements. A follow up visit in 2 weeks showed normalization of blood pressure as well as normalized potassium.

APPARENT MINERALOCORTICOID EXCESS

Genetics and pathophysiology: The syndrome of apparent mineralocorticoid excess (AME) is an autosomal recessive disease caused by an inactivating mutation of 11β-hydroxysteroid dehydrogenase type 2 (HSD11B2). The cytogenetic location is on chromosome 16q22.1 (4). The mineralocorticoid receptor's prototypical ligand is aldosterone, but cortisol is also able to bind and activate the receptor. Thus, the primary function of HSD11B2 is to prevent cortisol from binding to the mineralocorticoid receptor by catalyzing its metabolism to cortisone which does not have mineralocorticoid activity (6, 23). As cortisol is expressed at much higher physiologic levels than aldosterone, HSD11B2 function is critical to maintaining proper control over mineralicorticoid receptor activation. With this mutation, cortisol is not metabolized and is able to bind to the mineralocorticoid receptor, causing clinical features similar to pseudohyperaldosteronism (**Figure 4**). However, in this disorder the defect is at the level of the receptor itself rather than down stream at the ENaC channel. However, due to this similarlity both groups of patients typically present with hypokalemia, hypertension, and metabolic alkalosis (25).

Epidemiology: AME has been observed in many ethnic groups, including Caucasians, African Americans, Asians, and American Indians. This disease presents in early childhood. Severe phenotypes can present with low birth weight and failure to thrive, and if left untreated, these patients have high mortality rates (13).

Workup: The diagnosis is based on laboratory findings of hypokalemia, metabolic alkalosis, hyporeninemia, hypoaldosteronemia, and an elevated urinary cortisol to cortisone ratio by THF + 5αTHF to THE in a 24-h urine collection (26). It is important to rule out chronic excess licorice or carbenoxolone ingestion; as these cause similar symptoms due to inhibition of the same enzyme as in AME, but typically resolve once the offending agent is removed (24).

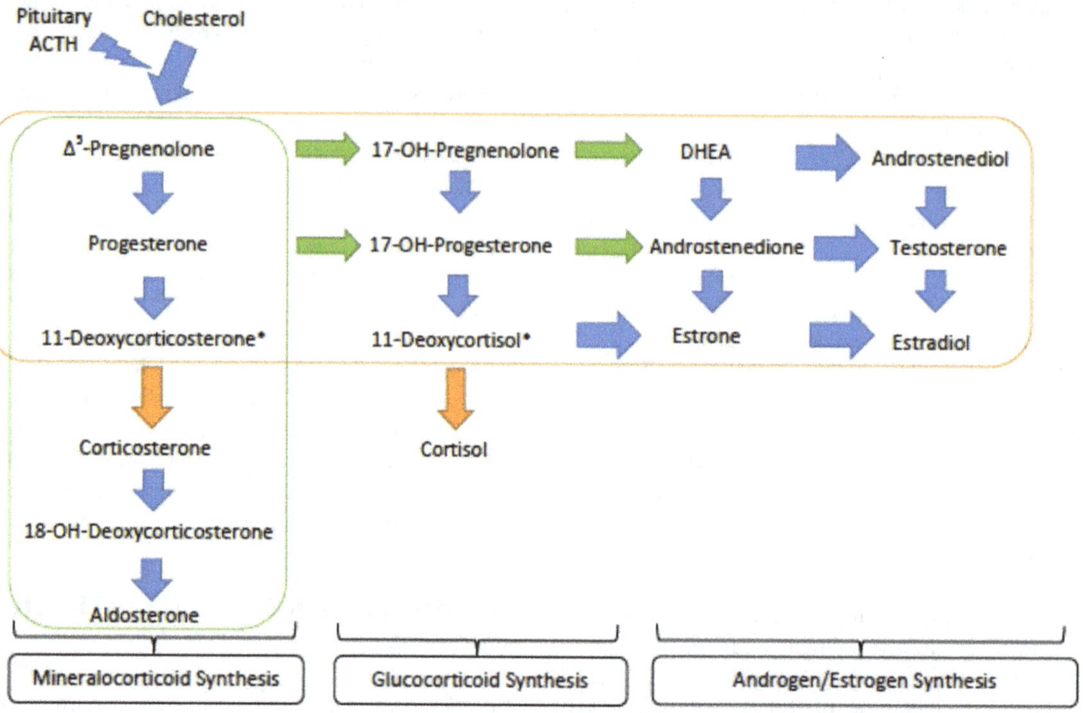

FIGURE 3 | An overview of the steroid synthesis pathways and the enzyme deficiences that lead to congenital adrenal hyperplasia (CAH) types IV and V. The orange arrows show the activity of 11β-hydroxylase (deficient 1 in type IV) while the orange rectangle surrounds the steroid hormones still produced in CAH type IV. The green arrows denote the activity of 17α-hydroxylase (deficient in type V) while the green rectangle encircles those hormones produced in CAH type V. ACTH - adrenocorticotropic hormone; DHEA - dihydroepiandrosterone. *These metabolites are active at the mineralocorticoid receptor and are important in generating hypertension.

Treatment: Treatment consists of mineralocorticoid receptor antagonists, such as spironolactone or eplerenone, along with potential potassium supplements and dietary sodium restriction (6, 24). Elevated cortisol levels may further warrant glucorticoid therapy to reduce ACTH-stimulated cortisol production and subsequent mineralocorticoid receptor stimulation (19, 27). Renal transplantation may be curative in some cases (28).

Case 4: A 17-year-old with a past medical history of hypertension came in for her routine checkup for her 34-week-old fetus. She had a family history of elevated blood pressure on her father's side. She complained of mild headaches for the past couple of weeks. On exam, her blood pressure was severely elevated. Laboratory testing including basic metabolic panel, thyroid function tests, and serum cortisol came back normal. Brain CT was normal. Her hypertension was attributed to pre-eclampsia and the patient was admitted for emergent C-section. After delivery, the patient's blood pressure was still mildly elevated and she received a dose of spironolactone. Two hours after taking the medication, her blood pressure worsened instead of improving. The patient was given other antihypertensives and her blood pressures improved. Genetic testing revealed a mutation of the mineralocorticoid receptor gene to confirm the diagnosis of Geller Syndrome.

GELLER SYNDROME

Geller syndrome, also referred to as constitutive activation of the mineralocorticoid receptor, results from a gain-of-function mutation on chromosome 4q31. Geller syndrome has an autosomal dominant inheritance pattern (17). This mutation within the mineralocorticoid receptor causes it to remain constitutively active due to changes to receptor sites that result in altered specificities to the steroid hormones. Steroid hormones, including progesterone, subsequently act as agonists of the mineralocorticoid receptor, as opposed to their normal antagonism (5).

The onset of hypertension starts before the age of 20 (17). It is essential to recognize this disease, as pregnancy can severely exacerbate the hypertension due to elevated progesterone levels. This causes activation of the mineralocorticoid receptors, though both aldosterone and renin are suppressed. Potassium levels are surprisingly normal in these patients. A clear diagnosis can be done by genetic testing for gene mutations in the mineralocorticoid receptor (17). Treatment is unlike many other causes of monogenic hypertension, as spironolactone is contraindicated and will worsen the disease. The mainstay for treatment during pregnancy is to deliver the fetus. Optimal management of non-pregnant females and males is not well-defined.

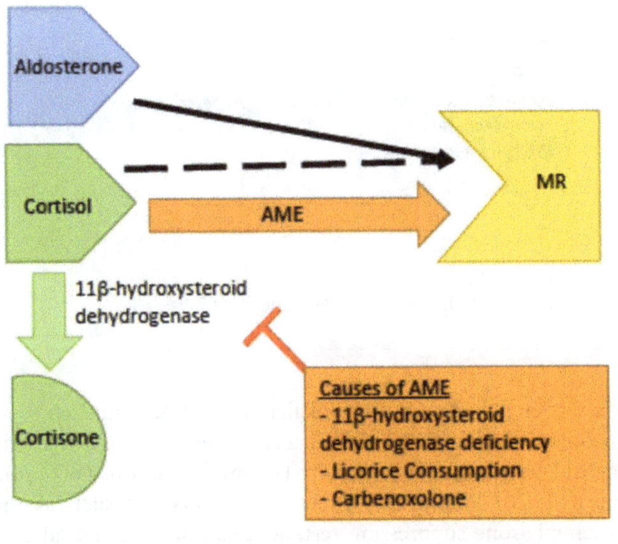

FIGURE 4 | A schematic of the pathophysiology of apparent mineralocorticoid excess (AME). The dashed black arrow indicates normal binding of cortisol to the mineralocorticoid receptor (MR) with conversion to cortisone by 11β-dehydrogenase.The orange arrow indicates AME. In AME, deficiency or inhibition of 11β -dehydrogenase leads to increased levels of cortisol increased cortisol-MR binding, and subsequent hyperactivity of the MR.

NORMAL ALDOSTERONE MONOGENIC HYPERTENSION

Case 5: A 9-year-old female was brought into the clinic by her mother for new onset dizziness and muscle weakness. The patient's height and weight were normal based on the WHO growth chart. Laboratory testing including chemistries were notable for severe hyperkalemia and hypocalcemia. All other lab values including PTH were normal. On exam her blood pressure was very elevated at 145/90 prompting renin and aldosterone testing. Renin levels were below normal and aldosterone was at the upper limits of normal. The patient was diagnosed with Gordon syndrome and she was started on a low dose thiazide.

Pseudohypoaldosteronism Type II (Gordon Syndrome)

Genetics and pathophysiology: Pseudohypoaldosteronism type II (PHAII), also referred to as Gordon syndrome, is autosomal dominant and affects the WNK serine-threonine kinase family (WNK1 and WNK4) (29). PHAII type B is due to a loss-of-function mutation of the WNK4 gene on chromosome 17q21.2, while PHAII type C results from gain-of-function mutation of the WNK1 gene on chromosome 12p12.3 (30). The most common clinical features seen are hyperkalemia, hyperchloremic metabolic acidosis, and normal-to-elevated levels of aldosterone. Mutation of the WNK genes leads to failure of endocytosis of the Na^{+}-Cl^{-} co-transporter (NCC). This loss of inhibitory regulation of NCC in the distal convoluted tubule causes hyperchloremic metabolic acidosis. More specifically, WNK4 activity directly inhibits NCC activity by reducing its expression on the extracellular membrane. In contrast, WNK1 inhibits WNK4 to reduce inhibition of NCC expression on the apical membrane. Thus, a loss-of-function in WNK4 or gain-of-function in WNK1 both generate a PHAII phenotype. The resulting increase in sodium reabsorption in the distal convoluted tubule inhibits normal sodium reabsorption downstream by ENaC (**Figure 5**). Without ENaC sodium reabsorption, ROMK potassium excretion as well as H-K exchange are both suppressed, driving the hyperkalemia and acidosis associated with Gordon's (13). Hypercalciuria is also found in these patients, and specifically hypercalciuria in the absence of elevated parathyroid hormone or serum calcium. The mechanism of urine calcium wasting is not completely understood, though multiple mechanisms have been postulated. WNK4 is known to modulate the activity of the transient receptor potential V5 channel (TRPV5), also located in the distal convoluted tubule. Decreased WNK4 function may thus decrease the normal inflow of calcium ions through TRPV5 in the DCT. Increased plasma sodium levels in PHAII may also inhibit the function of the Na^{+}/Ca^{2+} exchanger in the PCT. Ultimately, reduced calcium reabsorption places these patients at risk for urolithiasis and osteoporosis (31, 32).

Two additional genes, KLHL3 and CUL3, located at chromosome 5q31.2 and 2q36.2, respectively, have been identified as aiding WNK4 function; KLHL 3 mutations are implicated in PHAII type D, while CUL3 is implicated in PHAII type E (4, 33). Activation of WNK1 stimulates SGK1 (serum- and glucocorticoid-inducible protein kinase 1), which activates the NCC, increasing sodium reabsorption, and leading to hypertension (34).

Epidemiology: Hypertension generally manifests in adolescence to adulthood, but cases involving younger patients have been reported (31). It is important to note that Spitzer-Weinstein syndrome in children has similar clinical features, such as metabolic acidosis and hyperkalemia, and is thought to be an early presentation of Gordon syndrome (13). The prevalence of this disorder is unknown; only about 180 cases have been reported (31).

Workup: No criteria for the diagnosis of PHAII has been officially published. A clinical history and family history of a first-degree relative would aid in diagnosis, but a first degree-relative is not necessary. Molecular genetic testing is ideal for diagnosis, due to variation in severity and presentation.

Treatment: Electrolyte and blood pressure abnormalities can be treated with a low dose thiazide, which directly inhibits NCC hyperactivity. Patients should have routine follow up for assessment of electrolyte levels and blood pressure (31). Counseling patients to adhere to a low-sodium diet is an important consideration in long-term management of hypertension.

HIGH ALDOSTERONE MONOGENIC HYPERTENSION

Case 6: A 15-year-old boy presented to the emergency room with projectile vomiting, migraine and hypertension. The patient had no significant past medical or surgical history. A CT scan of the head showed that the patient had a minor bleed. A cerebral

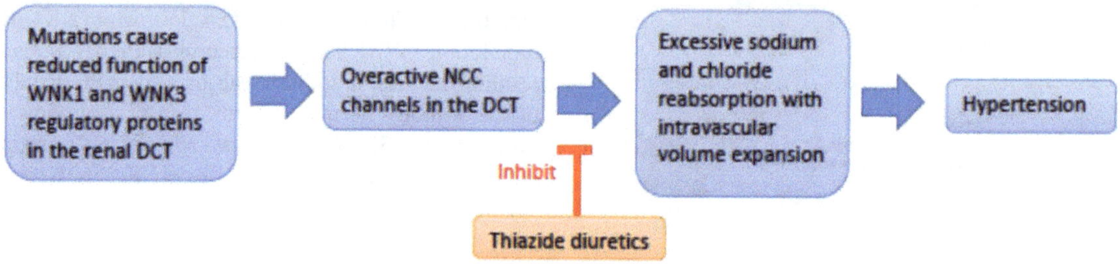

FIGURE 5 | An overview schematic of Gordon Syndrome pathophysiology and treatment. NCC is the sodium chloride co-transporter; DCT is the distal convoluted tubule.

angiogram showed rupture of a small aneurysm. Appropriate management, including acute blood pressure reduction, was performed and the patient survived. He presented to the clinic for a follow up visit. He is asymptomatic but still has elevated blood pressure, and laboratory testing demonstrates hypokalemia. All other labs are normal, except for low renin and elevated aldosterone levels. Adrenal vein sampling shows elevated levels of ACTH, and the patient is diagnosed with Familial Hyperaldosteronism type 1. The patient was started on dexamethasone and potassium supplements. Follow-up shows resolution of the hypertension.

Familial Hyperaldosteronism Type 1 (Glucocorticoid-Remediable Aldosteronism)

Genetics and pathophysiology: Inherited in an autosomal dominant fashion, familial hyperaldosteronism type 1 (FHT-I) is also also known as glucocorticoid-remediable aldosteronism (GRA) (20). This condition is due to alterations in the CYP11B1 (11β-hydroxylase) and CYP11B2 (aldosterone synthase) genes that lie adjacent to each other on chromosome 8q24.3 (13, 35). Unequal crossover between these genes results in a chimeric variant that incorporates regulatory elements of CYP11B1 with the coding sequence of CYP11B2 (**Figure 6**). As a result the gene is regulated by ACTH rather than angiotensin II, however, the gene still controls aldosterone secretion (36). Normally, aldosterone is secreted by the zona glomerulosa of the adrenal gland, but due to this chimeric gene, aldosterone is ectopically secreted from the adrenal zona fasciculata instead (37). Increased production of aldosterone drives the key clinical features of hypertension and hypokalemia in the setting of suppressed renin levels (20).

Epidemiology: Most patients with this disease present with severe hypertension in childhood or even infancy. These patients also suffer from a high incidence of intracerebral hemorrhage (11–18%) with a high associated mortality rate (61%) at an early age (31.7 ± 11.3 years) (38).

Workup: Brain imaging with computed tomography angiogram (CTA) or magnetic resonance angiography (MRA) may be warranted due to clinical presentation and a strong family history of cerebrovascular incidents and early onset of hypertension (39, 40). Due to high rates of cerebrovascular events in GRA patients, screening is recommended every 5 years after puberty (41). Hypokalemia is usually mild and few go on to develop metabolic alkalosis. The plasma aldosterone (ng/dL) to plasma renin activity (ng/mL/h) ratio usually > 30 (normal<20). Many other diagnostic modalities such as the dexamethasone suppression test, adrenal imaging, and adrenal vein sampling may help in distinguishing FHT-I from other forms of hyperaldosteronism (13).

Treatment: Treatment for FHT-I includes glucocorticoids which suppress ACTH, and thus prevent the secretion of aldosterone (36). If glucocorticoids do not reduce the blood pressure, then mineralocorticoid receptor antagonists, such as spironolactone, or sodium epithelium receptor antagonists, such as triamterene or amiloride, can be used as second line therapy (39).

Case 7: A 14-year-old female presented with back pain and muscle spasms. The patient has been complaining of muscle spasms for the past 2 months but she believed it was due to her menstrual cycle. She was initially sent to obstetrics/gynecology for exploratory laparoscopy to rule out endometriosis. The exploratory laparoscopy was negative for endometriosis but the patient was noted to be hypertensive. She has a family history of hypertension. Laboratory work up was benign. A CT scan was completed and an adrenal tumor was identified. Biopsy revealed that it was a benign adenoma. Plasma aldosterone (ng/dL) to plasma renin (ng/mL/h) ratio was well above normal (normal<20). The patient was diagnosed with familial hyperaldosteronism type 1. The patient was given glucocorticoids and asked to come back the following week. The following week, the patient still had the same complaints and elevated blood pressures. The patient was then given mineralocorticoid receptor antagonists which lead to resolution of her symptoms and hypertension. The patient's diagnosis was changed from familial hyperaldosteronism Type 1 to Type 2.

Familial Hyperaldosteronism Type 2

Familial Hyperaldosteronism type 2 (FHT-II) is similar to FHT-I in that ectopic aldosterone synthesis occurs due to the loss of negative feedback seen with physiologic aldosterone secretion (42). However, the aldosterone synthase gene is not controlled by ACTH as in FHT-I, causing a non-dexamethasone-suppressible form of hyperaldosteronism. FHT-II had previously been mapped to chromosome 7p22, but no specific gene at this locus has been identified as the cause of the disease (43, 44).

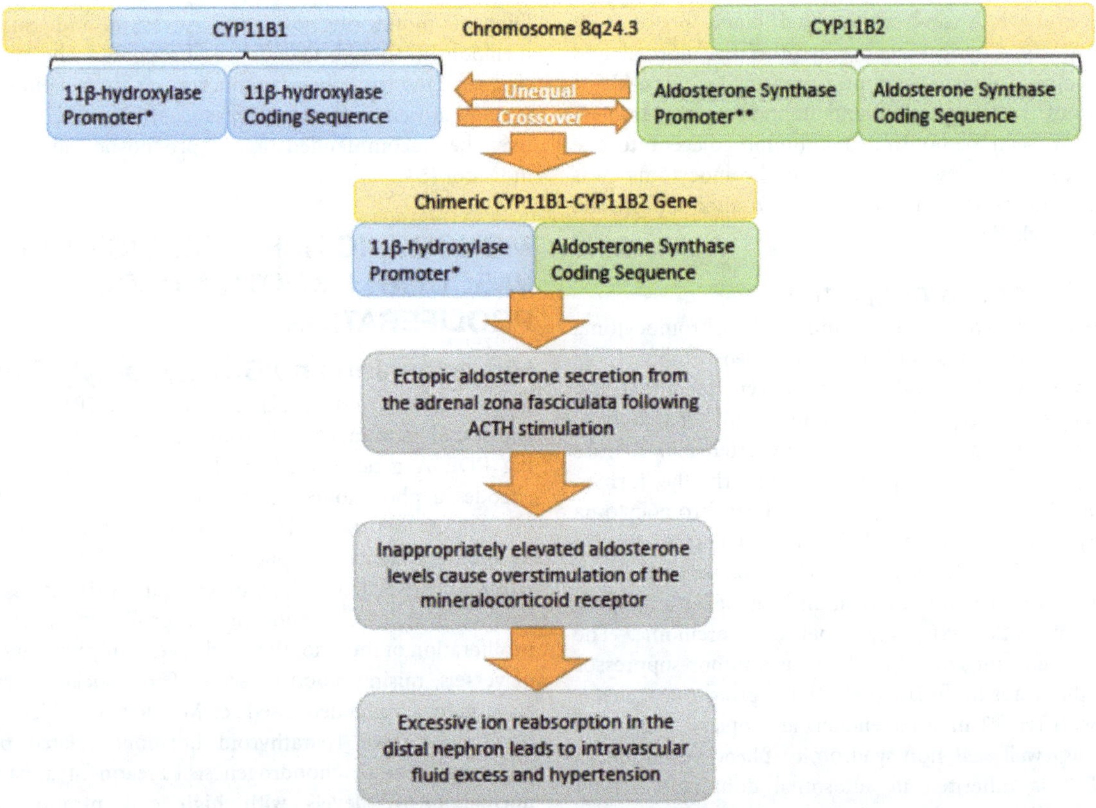

FIGURE 6 | An overview of the genetic pathophysiology of familial hyperaldosteronism type I. * Promoter responsive to adrenocotropic hormone (ACTH). **Promoter responsive to angiotensin II.

A recent study of patients diagnosed with FHT-II implicates gain-of-function mutations in the CLCN2 gene, encoding a chloride channel, ClC-2, located at chromosome 3q27.1 (45). The variant channels were shown *in vitro* to cause depolarization of adrenocortical cancer cell lines, leading to increased expression of aldosterone synthase and aldosterone production (45). FHT-II is characterized by bilateral adrenocortical disease and adenomas (42). The diagnosis of FHT-II should be confirmed by positive family history because FHT-II is clinically and biochemically indistinguishable from non-inherited primary aldosteronism (13). Genetic testing for CLCN2 mutations may prove helpful, though further work is needed to identify other possible causative genes (45). The mainstay of treatment for this disease is mineralocorticoid receptor antagonists or unilateral adrenalectomy (4).

Familial Hyperaldosteronism Type 3

Familial hyperaldosteronism type 3 (FHT-III) is an autosomal dominant condition caused by gain-of-function mutations in the KCNJ5 gene located at locus 11q24.3. KCNJ5 encodes a potassium channel, which loses its ionic selectivity in disease-causing variants to allow other cations, particularly sodium, to pass through. This allows for depolarization of the adrenal cortical cell, enhancing the expression of aldosterone synthase and subsequently raising aldosterone levels in patients (44). Treatment is similar to FHT-II and primary aldosteronism, ranging from mineralocorticoid antagonists to possible adrenalectomy depending on the severity of the hypertension (44, 46).

Familial Hyperaldosteronism Type 4

Familial hyperaldosteronism type 4 (FHT-IV) is an autosomal dominant condition caused by gain-of-function mutations in the CACNA1H gene located at chromosome 16p13.3 (44). CACNA1H encodes a transient opening calcium channel localized to the zona glomerulosa. The mutations implicated in FHT-IV cause the channel to be more likely to open at the baseline electrochemical gradient and remain open longer upon activation (47). These changes allow for greater influx of calcium ions, stimulating adrenal cortical cells and subsequently activating aldosterone synthase (47). As with other FHT types, treatment depends on the severity of the condition, possibly varying on the specific mutation, and ranges from medical management with mineralocorticoid antagonists to potential surgical adrenalectomy (46).

MONOGENIC HYPERTENSION DUE TO ADRENERGIC/SYMPATHETIC EXCESS

Case 8: A 7-year-old boy was brought to the clinic with a pounding headache. The child had also complained of palpitations for the past year. The patient had no other complaints and had been healthy since birth. The patient was noted to have a severely elevated blood pressure of 210 / 130 mmHg. Physical exam was otherwise normal and routine laboratory values showed no significant findings. Urine metanepharines were collected and found to be elevated. Abdominal CT scan demonstrated a tumor adjacent to the adrenal glands. The diagnosis of pheochromocytoma was made and the tumor was surgically removed after appropriate perioperative blockade.

Familial Pheochromocytoma

Genetics and pathophysiology: Familial pheochromocytoma describes increased susceptibility to pheochromocytoma due to a variety of well-documented genetic mutations. Pheochromocytoma typically presents with paroxysmal symptoms, such as episodes of severe hypertension. Release of norepinephrine and epinephrine, pariticularly the former, is above and beyond physiologic levels. Pheochromocytoma susceptibility can be inherited alone or as a part of several syndromes. Von Hippel-Lindau disease (VHL) is associated with bilateral pheochromocytomas, retinal and cerebellar angiomas, renal and pancreatic cysts, and renal cell carcinoma. The mutation is on chromosome 3p25.3 and is a tumor-suppressor gene defect that leads to disease (48). RET, a proto-oncogene, is associated with type 2 multiple endocrine neoplasia syndrome (MEN 2) as well as non-syndromic pheochromocytoma (49). MEN 2 is inherited in autosomal dominant fashion due to a mutation on chromosome 10q11.21. MEN 2 has two subtypes MEN 2A and 2B. MEN 2A is associated with pheochromocytoma, medullary carcinoma of the thyroid, and hyperparathyroidism while MEN 2B is associated with pheochromocytoma, medullary carcinoma of the thyroid, and mucosal neuromas (50). Pheochromocytoma has also been associated with neurofibromatosis type I, caused by mutations in the NF1 gene, located at chromosome 17q11.2 (51). Solitary pheochromocytomas have also been shown to contain mutations in the aforementioned genes. One study of solitary tumors reported that 86% contained copy number alterations in genes associated with familial pheochromocytoma; changes in NF1 were found to be the most frequent at 26% of the tumors studied (52).

Epidemiology: Initially pheochromocytomas were considered to have 10% familial and 90% sporadic development. New technology in genetic testing has demonstrated that pheochromocytomas are 50% sporadic with 15–25% due to germ line mutations (53).

Workup: Catecholamine metabolism studies such as plasma free metanephrines and urinary fractionated metanephrines allow for successful screening of the condition and can be monitored for treatment response (54).

Treatment: Per The Endocrine Society clinical practice guideline, the treatment of functional pheochromocytomas begins with initiation of antihypertensive therapy followed by tumor resection. Medical management prior to surgery, known as pre-operative blockade, utilizes alpha-adrenergic antagonists (e.g., phenoxybenzamine or doxazosin) as firstline therapeutics. Other antihypertensives, particularly dihydropyridines and beta-adrenergic antagonists, may be used supplementarily. Diligent monitoring of blood pressure and catecholamine metabolism should take place throughout the perioperative course. Due to pheochromocytoma's association with the various aforementioned neoplastic syndromes, genetic testing may be recommended as a prognostic and preventative indicator (54).

MONOGENIC HYPERTENSION DUE TO VASCULAR SMOOTH MUSCLE PROLIFERATION

Hypertension and Brachydactyly Syndrome

Hypertension and brachydactyly (HTNB) describes an autosomal dominant syndrome caused by a mutation in the PDE3A gene located at chromosome 12p12.2; this gene encodes a phosphodiesterase that hydrolyzes cAMP. Variants of PDE3A that cause HTNB exhibit a gain-of-function due to altered enzyme phosphorylation (21). The mutant PDE3A enzymes consequently decrease cellular cAMP levels in vascular smooth muscle cells, allowing for proliferation. Uncontrolled proliferation of the smooth muscle eventually narrows the lumen of vessels, raising blood pressure. The associated brachydactly also stems from decreased cAMP levels, which lower the levels of PTHrP (parathyroid hormone related protein), a key moderator of chondrogenesis. Treatment aims to restore normal cAMP levels with high concentration milrinone, and there is possible benefit to increasing cGMP levels with phosphodiesterase inhibitors (21).

CONCLUSION

Hypertension is known as the silent killer; if not managed properly, it can lead to progressive end organ damage and death. Essential hypertension is often the result of multiple patient factors including polygenic inheritance and environmental factors, such as diet and physical activity. Monogenic hypertension refers to specific genetic mutations that interfere with normal renal and adrenal regulation of blood pressure. All forms of monogenic hypertension have low renin and can be further classified by the levels of aldosterone. Accurate diagnosis may require further hormonal studies or genetic testing. It important to have a high level of clinical suspicion and precisely diagnose these patients, as treatment is often quite different from traditional patients with essential hypertension. Appropriate treatment can decrease the morbidity and mortality associated with uncontrolled hypertension. With future advancements in genetic testing modalities and treatment options, there is hope for earlier recognition and improved management of the various forms of monogenic hypertension.

AUTHOR CONTRIBUTIONS

All the authors are responsible for the literature review, drafting and revision of the manuscript, and approved the final version of the manuscript.

REFERENCES

1. Benjamin EJ, Virani SS, Callaway CW, Chamberlain AM, Chang AR, Cheng S, et al. Heart disease and stroke statistics-2018 update: a report from the American Heart Association. *Circulation.* (2018) 137:e67–492. doi: 10.1161/CIR.0000000000000558
2. Jackson SL, Zhang Z, Wiltz JL, Loustalot F, Ritchey MD, Goodman AB, et al. Hypertension among youths - United States, 2001-2016. *MMWR Morb Mortal Wkly Rep.* (2018) 67:758–62. doi: 10.15585/mmwr.mm6727a2
3. Yusuf S, Wood D, Ralston J, Reddy KS. The World Heart Federation's vision for worldwide cardiovascular disease prevention. *Lancet.* (2015) 386:399–402. doi: 10.1016/S0140-6736(15)60265-3
4. Burrello J, Monticone S, Buffolo F, Tetti M, Veglio F, Williams TA, et al. Is there a role for genomics in the management of hypertension? *Int J Mol Sci.* (2017) 18. doi: 10.3390/ijms18061131
5. Garovic VD, Hilliard AA, Turner ST. Monogenic forms of low-renin hypertension. *Nat Clin Pract Nephrol.* (2006) 2:624–30. doi: 10.1038/ncpneph0309
6. Simonetti GD, Mohaupt MG, Bianchetti MG. Monogenic forms of hypertension. *Eur J Pediatr.* (2012) 171:1433–9. doi: 10.1007/s00431-011-1440-7
7. Hamosh A. *Online Mendelian Inheritance in Man* [Online]. McKusick-Nathans Institute of Genetic Medicine, Johns Hopkins University School of Medicine (2018). Available online at: https://omim.org/about (accessed November 17, 2018).
8. Cui Y, Tong A, Jiang J, Wang F, Li C. Liddle syndrome: clinical and genetic profiles. *J Clin Hypertens.* (2017) 19:524–9. doi: 10.1111/jch.12949
9. Shimkets RA, Warnock DG, Bositis CM, Nelson-Williams C, Hansson JH, Schambelan M, et al. Liddle's syndrome: heritable human hypertension caused by mutations in the beta subunit of the epithelial sodium channel. *Cell.* (1994) 79:407–14. doi: 10.1016/0092-8674(94)90250-X
10. Gennari FJ, Hussain-Khan S, Segal A. An unusual case of metabolic alkalosis: a window into the pathophysiology and diagnosis of this common acid-base disturbance. *Am J Kidney Dis.* (2010) 55:1130–5. doi: 10.1053/j.ajkd.2009.11.028
11. Botero-Velez M, Curtis JJ, Warnock DG. Brief report: Liddle's syndrome revisited–a disorder of sodium reabsorption in the distal tubule. *N Engl J Med.* (1994) 330:178–81. doi: 10.1056/NEJM199401203300305
12. Martinez-Aguayo A, Fardella C. Genetics of hypertensive syndrome. *Horm Res.* (2009) 71:253–9. doi: 10.1159/000208798
13. Vehaskari VM. Heritable forms of hypertension. *Pediatr Nephrol.* (2009) 24:1929–37. doi: 10.1007/s00467-007-0537-8
14. Rossier BC, Schild L. Epithelial sodium channel: mendelian versus essential hypertension. *Hypertension.* (2008) 52:595–600. doi: 10.1161/HYPERTENSIONAHA.107.097147
15. Tapolyai M, Uysal A, Dossabhoy NR, Zsom L, Szarvas T, Lengvarszky Z, et al. High prevalence of liddle syndrome phenotype among hypertensive US Veterans in Northwest Louisiana. *J Clin Hypertens.* (2010) 12:856–60. doi: 10.1111/j.1751-7176.2010.00359.x
16. Wang LP, Yang KQ, Jiang XJ, Wu HY, Zhang HM, Zou YB, et al. Prevalence of Liddle syndrome among young hypertension patients of undetermined cause in a Chinese population. *J Clin Hypertens.* (2015) 17:902–7. doi: 10.1111/jch.12598
17. Melcescu E, Ca K. Syndromes of mineralocorticoid excess. In: Koch CA, Chrousos GP, editors. *Endocrine Hypertension: Underlying Mechanisms and Therapy.* Tolawa, NJ: Humana Press (2013) 33–50. doi: 10.1007/978-1-60761-548-4_2
18. Aziz DA, Memon F, Rahman A, Ali M. Liddle's Syndrome. *J Ayub Med Coll Abbottabad.* (2016) 28:809–11.
19. Melcescu E, Phillips J, Moll G, Subauste JS, Koch CA. 11Beta-hydroxylase deficiency and other syndromes of mineralocorticoid excess as a rare cause of endocrine hypertension. *Horm Metab Res.* (2012) 44:867–78. doi: 10.1055/s-0032-1321851
20. Ehret GB, Caulfield MJ. Genes for blood pressure: an opportunity to understand hypertension. *Eur Heart J.* (2013) 34:951–61. doi: 10.1093/eurheartj/ehs455
21. Aggarwal A, Rodriguez-Buritica D. Monogenic hypertension in children: a review with emphasis on genetics. *Adv Chronic Kidney Dis.* (2017) 24:372–9. doi: 10.1053/j.ackd.2017.09.006
22. White PC, Curnow KM, Pascoe L. Disorders of steroid 11 beta-hydroxylase isozymes. *Endocr Rev.* (1994) 15:421–38. doi: 10.1210/er.15.4.421
23. Izzo J, Sica D, Black H. *Hypertension Primer: The Essentials of High Blood Pressure: Basic Science, Population Science, and Clinical Management.* Philadelphia, PA: Lippincott Williams and Wilkins (2007).
24. Sahay M, Sahay RK. Low renin hypertension. *Indian J Endocrinol Metab.* (2012) 16:728–39. doi: 10.4103/2230-8210.100665
25. Luft FC. Monogenic hypertension: lessons from the genome. *Kidney Int.* (2001) 60:381–90. doi: 10.1046/j.1523-1755.2001.00810.x
26. Williams SS. Advances in genetic hypertension. *Curr Opin Pediatr.* (2007) 19:192–8. doi: 10.1097/MOP.0b013e32801e217c
27. Palermo M, Quinkler M, Stewart PM. Apparent mineralocorticoid excess syndrome: an overview. *Arq Bras Endocrinol Metabol.* (2004) 48:687–96. doi: 10.1590/S0004-27302004000500015
28. Palermo M, Cossu M, Shackleton CH. Cure of apparent mineralocorticoid excess by kidney transplantation. *N Engl J Med.* (1998) 339:1787–8. doi: 10.1056/NEJM199812103392414
29. Riepe FG. Clinical and molecular features of type 1 pseudohypoaldosteronism. *Horm Res.* (2009) 72:1–9. doi: 10.1159/000224334
30. Padmanabhan S, Caulfield M, Dominiczak AF. Genetic and molecular aspects of hypertension. *Circ Res.* (2015) 116:937–59. doi: 10.1161/CIRCRESAHA.116.303647
31. Ellison DH. Pseudohypoaldosteronism Type II. In: Adam MP, Ardinger HH, Pagon RA, Wallace SE, Bean LJH, Stephens K, Amemiya A, editors. *GeneReviews((R)).* Seattle, WA: University of Washington (1993).
32. Pathare G, Hoenderop JG, Bindels RJ, San-Cristobal P. A molecular update on pseudohypoaldosteronism type II. *Am J Physiol Renal Physiol.* (2013) 305:F1513–20. doi: 10.1152/ajprenal.00440.2013
33. Boyden LM, Choi M, Choate KA, Nelson-Williams CJ, Farhi A, Toka HR, et al. Mutations in kelch-like 3 and cullin 3 cause hypertension and electrolyte abnormalities. *Nature.* (2012) 482:98–102. doi: 10.1038/nature10814
34. O'shaughnessy KM. Gordon Syndrome: a continuing story. *Pediatr Nephrol.* (2015) 30:1903–8. doi: 10.1007/s00467-014-2956-7
35. Pascoe L, Curnow KM, Slutsker L, Connell JM, Speiser PW, New MI, et al. Glucocorticoid-suppressible hyperaldosteronism results from hybrid genes created by unequal crossovers between CYP11B1 and CYP11B2. *Proc Natl Acad Sci USA.* (1992) 89:8327–31. doi: 10.1073/pnas.89.17.8327
36. Stowasser M, Bachmann AW, Huggard PR, Rossetti TR, Gordon RD. Treatment of familial hyperaldosteronism type I: only partial suppression of adrenocorticotropin required to correct hypertension. *J Clin Endocrinol Metab.* (2000) 85:3313–8. doi: 10.1210/jcem.85.9.6834
37. Sutherland DJ, Ruse JL, Laidlaw JC. Hypertension, increased aldosterone secretion and low plasma renin activity relieved by dexamethasone. *Can Med Assoc J.* (1966) 95:1109–19.
38. Gates LJ, Benjamin N, Haites NE, Macconnachie AA, Mclay JS. Is random screening of value in detecting glucocorticoid-remediable aldosteronism within a hypertensive population? *J Hum Hypertens.* (2001) 15:173–6. doi: 10.1038/sj.jhh.1001152
39. Lee IS, Kim SY, Jang HW, Kim MK, Lee JH, Lee YH, et al. Genetic analyses of the chimeric CYP11B1/CYP11B2 gene in a Korean family with glucocorticoid-remediable aldosteronism. *J Korean Med Sci.* (2010) 25:1379–83. doi: 10.3346/jkms.2010.25.9.1379
40. Peng J, Liu Z, Luo C, Chen L, Hou X, Xiao L, et al. Treatment of cervical artery dissection: antithrombotics, thrombolysis, and endovascular therapy. *Biomed Res Int.* (2017) 2017:3072098. doi: 10.1155/2017/3072098
41. Litchfield WR, Anderson BF, Weiss RJ, Lifton RP, Dluhy RG. Intracranial aneurysm and hemorrhagic stroke in glucocorticoid-remediable aldosteronism. *Hypertension.* (1998) 31:445–50. doi: 10.1161/01.HYP.31.1.445
42. Torpy DJ, Gordon RD, Lin JP, Huggard PR, Taymans SE, Stowasser M, et al. Familial hyperaldosteronism type II: description of a large kindred and exclusion of the aldosterone synthase (CYP11B2) gene. *J Clin Endocrinol Metab.* (1998) 83:3214–8. doi: 10.1210/jc.83.9.3214
43. Fardella CE, Rodriguez H, Montero J, Zhang G, Vignolo P, Rojas A, et al. Genetic variation in P450c11AS in Chilean patients with

low renin hypertension. *J Clin Endocrinol Metab.* (1996) 81:4347–51. doi: 10.1210/jcem.81.12.8954040
44. Stowasser M, Wolley M, Wu A, Gordon RD, Schewe J, Stölting G, et al. Pathogenesis of familial hyperadolsteronism type II: new concepts involving anion channels. *Curr Hypertens Rep.* (2019) 21:1–10. doi: 10.1007/s11906-019-0934-y
45. Scholl UE, Stölting G, Schewe J, Thiel A, Tan H, Nelson-Williams C, et al. CLCN2 chloride channel mutations in familial hyperaldosteronism type II. *Nat Genet.* (2018) 50:349–54. doi: 10.1038/s41588-018-0048-5
46. Young WF. Primary aldosteronism: renaissance of a syndrome. *Clin Endocrinol.* (2007) 66:607–18. doi: 10.1111/j.1365-2265.2007.02775.x
47. Scholl UE, Stölting G, Nelson-Williams C, Vichot AA, Choi M, Loring E, et al. Recurrent gain of function mutation in calcium channel CACNA1H causes early-onset hypertension with primary aldosteronism. *eLife.* (2015) 4:e063115 doi: 10.7554/eLife.06315
48. Neumann HP, Wiestler OD. Clustering of features of von Hippel-Lindau syndrome: evidence for a complex genetic locus. *Lancet.* (1991) 337:1052–4. doi: 10.1016/0140-6736(91)91705-Y
49. Neumann HP, Bausch B, Mcwhinney SR, Bender BU, Gimm O, Franke G, et al. Germ-line mutations in nonsyndromic pheochromocytoma. *N Engl J Med.* (2002) 346:1459–66. doi: 10.1056/NEJMoa020152
50. Ishizaka Y, Itoh F, Tahira T, Ikeda I, Sugimura T, Tucker J, et al. Human ret proto-oncogene mapped to chromosome 10q11.2. *Oncogene.* (1989) 4:1519–21.
51. Ledbetter DH, Rich DC, O'connell P, Leppert M, Carey JC. Precise localization of NF1 to 17q11.2 by balanced translocation. *Am J Hum Genet.* (1989) 44:20–4.
52. Welander J, Larsson C, Backdahl M, Hareni N, Sivler T, Brauckhoff M, et al. Integrative genomics reveals frequent somatic NF1 mutations in sporadic pheochromocytomas. *Hum Mol Genet.* (2012) 21:5406–16. doi: 10.1093/hmg/dds402
53. Kaplan NM, Victor RG. *Kaplan's Clinical Hypertension.* Philadelphia, PA: Lippincott Williams and Wilkins (2009).
54. Lenders JW, Duh QY, Eisenhofer G, Gimenez-Roqueplo AP, Grebe SK, Murad MH, et al. Pheochromocytoma and paraganglioma: an endocrine society clinical practice guideline. *J Clin Endocrinol Metab.* (2014) 99:1915–42. doi: 10.1210/jc.2014-1498

21

Circulating *de novo* Donor Specific Antibodies and Carotid Intima-media Thickness in Pediatric Kidney Transplant Recipients

Kristen Sgambat[1*†], *Sarah Clauss*[2†] *and Asha Moudgil*[1†]

[1] *Department of Nephrology, Children's National Hospital, Washington, DC, United States,* [2] *Department of Cardiology, Children's National Hospital, Washington, DC, United States*

Correspondence:
Kristen Sgambat
ksgambat@childrensnational.org

†ORCID:
Kristen Sgambat
orcid.org/0000-0003-0795-3210
Sarah Clauss
orcid.org/0000-0002-1293-5757
Asha Moudgil
orcid.org/0000-0002-9376-6659

Background: The presence of circulating *de novo* donor specific anti-HLA antibodies (dnDSA) has been implicated in an immune-mediated form of accelerated systemic arteriosclerosis in adult heart and kidney transplant recipients, however this has not been previously investigated in pediatric kidney transplant recipients. Carotid intima-media thickness (CIMT) is a reliable method for detection of arteriosclerosis. We hypothesized that children who develop dnDSA after kidney transplant would have increased CIMT compared with those who remain dnDSA negative.

Methods: A prospective, controlled pilot cohort study of 38 transplant patients and 20 healthy controls was conducted to investigate the association between CIMT and development of dnDSA after kidney transplant. CIMT, anthropometrics, blood pressure and lipid panel were measured at 1, 18, and 30 months post-transplant. DSA was checked at 6, 12, 18, 24 and 30 months post-transplant. CIMT of DSA positive transplant recipients was compared to DSA negative and controls.

Results: Of the 38 transplant recipients, 7 patients developed dnDSA by 18–30 months post-transplant. Among 5 dnDSA positive patients who did not receive treatment for DSA prior to CIMT measurement (n=6 observations), the median CIMT was 0.505 mm (95% CI 0.454–0.560 mm) at 18–30 months post-transplant, compared to 0.455 mm (95% CI 0.440–0.470) in DSA negative transplant recipients ($n = 54$ observations of 30 patients) and 0.450 mm (95% CI 0.436–0.460) in the healthy controls (20 observations of 20 patients). Presence of dnDSA was independently associated with a 7.8% increase in CIMT compared to those without dnDSA (p=0.006), after adjusting for race, hypertension, dyslipidemia, and abdominal obesity.

Conclusions: Development of dnDSA was associated with increased CIMT, an indicator of arteriosclerosis, in a cohort of dnDSA positive pediatric kidney transplant recipients. The association between dnDSA and CIMT was independent of traditional CV risk factors, including hypertension, dyslipidemia, and abdominal obesity.

Keywords: donor specific antibodies, carotid intima-media thickness, cardiovascular, arteriosclerosis, pediatric, kidney transplant

INTRODUCTION

Pediatric kidney transplant recipients are at high risk for cardiovascular (CV) disease, the second leading cause of mortality in this population (1). Traditionally, factors such as hypertension, dyslipidemia, and obesity have been associated with increased CV risk in both the general population (2) and in kidney transplant recipients (3, 4). However, recently, the presence of circulating *de novo* donor specific anti-HLA antibodies (dnDSA) have been implicated in an immune-mediated form of accelerated systemic arteriosclerosis in adult heart and kidney transplant recipients (5, 6). In addition, one pediatric study has identified a link between dnDSA and antibody-associated arteriosclerosis in heart transplant recipients (7). This form of antibody-associated arteriosclerosis is a condition characterized by arterial inflammation and fibrointimal thickening of the arteries caused by endothelial activation, a pro-inflammatory and pro-coagulant state of the endothelial cells lining the lumen of the blood vessels.

The study by Loupy et al. demonstrated that the presence of circulating dnDSA was significantly associated with severe allograft arteriosclerosis, independent of traditional CV risk factors in adult kidney transplant recipients (5). In addition, patients with dnDSA-associated arteriosclerosis had decreased allograft survival, increased occurrence of major adverse cardiovascular events, and increased mortality.

Carotid-intima media thickness (CIMT) is one known reliable indicator of arteriosclerosis that can be utilized to assess CV risk in renal transplant recipients (1, 4). The association of dnDSA with arteriosclerosis and CV risk has not been previously investigated in pediatric kidney transplant recipients. Therefore, the aim of our pilot study was to investigate the effect of dnDSA on CIMT as a marker of arteriosclerosis in pediatric kidney transplant recipients, based on the hypothesis that the presence of circulating DSA promotes vascular proliferation resulting in increased CIMT.

PATIENTS AND METHODS

Patients and Controls

A prospective, controlled cohort study was conducted to investigate the association between CIMT and the development of dnDSA after kidney transplant. Children, 3–20 years of age, who received a kidney transplant between September 2010-January 2015 at Children's National Hospital in Washington DC were eligible to enroll in the study at the time of transplant. Patients with an estimated glomerular filtration rate (eGFR) <60 mL/min/1.73 m^2 at 1 month post-transplant, multi-organ transplant, or nephrotic-range proteinuria were excluded from the study.

Healthy children 3–20 years of age served as controls. The healthy control participants were recruited from the local pediatric community, reflecting similar environmental exposures to the transplant cohort, and the racial distribution of the control population was matched to that of the transplant group.

Approval was obtained from the IRB at Children's National Hospital (IRB protocol number 2024). Informed consent was obtained from all participants, and the study was conducted in accordance with the Helsinki Declaration of 1975.

Measurement and Classification of dnDSA

Transplant patients were monitored for development of dnDSA at 6, 12, 18, 24, and 30 months post-transplant, as well as for-cause. Donor-specific antibodies were tested using multiple solid phase assay platforms. In cases where flow panel reactive antibody (PRA) Screen was positive, both SAB (One Lambda, Inc., Canoga Park, CA, USA) and phenotype bead (LABScreen PRA assay by One Lamba, Inc.) assays were then performed. DSA was determined to be positive when mean fluorescence intensity (MFI) was >1000. DSA were further classified as weak if MFI was 1000–2000, strong if MFI was >2000–10,000, or very strong if MFI was >10,000.

For purposes of the study, transplant patients were classified as DSA positive (DSA+) if strong or very strong DSA was detected at 18 and/or 30 months post-transplant. Observations of CIMT at the time of DSA+ detection, prior to receiving any pharmacologic treatment for DSA or acute cellular-mediated rejection were included in the analysis. Any CIMT measurements performed after administration of treatment for DSA+ and/or acute cellular-mediated rejection, such as pulse methylprednisolone, alemtuzumab, rituximab, and bortezomib, were excluded from the analysis. CIMT measurements of patients with weak DSA (MFI >1000–2000) were also excluded from the analysis. Patients were classified as DSA negative (DSA-) if they never developed any dnDSA during the first 30 months post-transplant. In patients who were DSA+ at 18 months post-transplant but became DSA- by 30 months post-transplant, the 30 month data point was excluded from the analysis to minimize confounding effects of prior DSA positivity.

CIMT

CIMT was measured at baseline (0–1 months post-transplant), 18, and 30 months post-transplant in the transplant group, and at a single study visit in the healthy control group. CIMT was visualized using B-mode ultrasound imaging of the arterial far wall segments of the right and left common carotid arteries and carotid bulbs. Imaging was performed according to a standard protocol by a single pediatric sonographer using aiE33 xMatrix DS Ultrasound System (Philips North America Corporation, Andover, MA, USA). Intima-media thickness of the distal, mid-, and proximal segments of right and left common carotid arteries and carotid bulbs were analyzed by a pediatric cardiologist blinded to the clinical information. A composite of the eight measured segments was then created to represent the CIMT.

Abbreviations: CV, Cardiovascular; dnDSA, *De novo* donor specific antibody; DSA+, Donor specific antibody positive; DSA-, Donor specific antibody negative; CIMT, Carotid intima media thickness; eGFR, Estimated glomerular filtration rate; PRA, Panel reactive antibody; MFI, Mean fluorescence intensity; BMI, Body mass index; WHr, Waist to height ratio; CDC, Center for disease control; NHANES, National Health and Nutrition Examination Survey; HDL, High density lipoprotein; LDL, Low density lipoprotein; WC, Waist circumference; GEE, Generalized estimating equation; QIC, Quasi-likelihood under the independence model criterion; ESRD, End stage renal disease.

Traditional CV Risk Factors

Parameters traditionally used to evaluate CV risk, including BMI, waist-to-height ratio (WHr), fasting lipid panel, and blood pressure, were measured at 1, 18, and 30 months post-transplant in the transplant recipients. The children in the healthy control group had BMI, WHr, and blood pressure measured once, at the time of CIMT measurement. Presence of general obesity and abdominal obesity were assessed using BMI and WHr, respectively. Weight in kilograms and height in centimeters were measured and used to calculate BMI [weight (kg)/height(m^2)]. Participants were then classified as BMI-obese if they had a BMI $\geq$ 95th percentile-for-sex-and-age on the Center for Disease Control (CDC) growth charts (8). Waist circumference (WC) was measured using a Gulick II fiberglass tape measure (Country Technology, Gays Mills, WI) at the upper-most lateral border of the right ileum, according to standard National Health and Nutrition Examination Study (NHANES) procedures (9). WHr was calculated as a ratio of waist in centimeters divided by height in centimeters. Participants were then classified as WHr-obese if WHr $\geq$ 0.5 (10).

Cut-points for abnormal lipid parameters for high density lipoprotein (HDL), low density lipoprotein (LDL), and triglycerides were defined according to 2011 Guidelines for Cardiovascular Health and Risk Reduction in Children and Adolescents for children age 3–19 (11), and by the Adult Treatment Panel III criteria for those >19 years of age (12). Dyslipidemia was defined as the presence of at least one abnormal lipid parameter (HDL, LDL, or triglyceride). Hypertension was defined by diagnosis of hypertension (systolic and/or diastolic blood pressure >95th percentile for age-sex-and -height on 3 different occasions) and requiring antihypertensive medication (13). Estimated glomerular filtration rate (eGFR) was calculated using the updated Schwartz equation for children under 18 years of age and the MDRD equation was used for those $\geq$ 18 years of age.

Induction and Maintenance Immunosuppression

The transplant recipients received Thymoglobulin for induction immunosuppression, followed by maintenance immunosuppression with either with a steroid-withdrawal or steroid-based protocol, depending on their immunological risk. The steroid-withdrawal protocol was used for "standard immunological risk" patients, defined as those receiving their first transplant, with cPRA <20%, and ESRD diagnosis not due to autoimmune disorder or FSGS. The steroid-based protocol was used for "high immunological risk" patients, defined as those with history of a prior transplant, diagnosis of FSGS or autoimmune disorder, highly sensitized patients, or those with delayed graft function (as defined by need for dialysis in the immediate post-transplant period). The details of the induction therapy protocols have been previously published (14). Maintenance immunosuppression for those on the steroid-based protocol consisted of tacrolimus, mycophenolate mofetil (MMF), and prednisone, while those on the steroid-withdrawal received tacrolimus and MMF.

Statistical Analysis

Statistical analyses were conducted using Stata 14.0 (StataCorp LP, College Station, TX, USA). Analyses of the demographic and clinical characteristics of the study and control populations were conducted using Fisher's exact test for categorical variables and Wilcoxon rank-sum for continuous variables.

The median (95% CI) of the CIMT observations of the DSA+ and DSA- transplant groups at 18–30 months post-transplant and of the control group (single time point) are presented as descriptive statistics in the Results section and in graphical form in **Figure 1**. In order to establish a temporal reference point, the median CIMT of the DSA+ and DSA- transplant groups are also depicted at baseline (0–1 months post-transplant). Due to the longitudinal nature of the data, bivariate statistical tests of significance were not appropriate, and therefore **Figure 1** represents a descriptive presentation of the data only.

Unadjusted and adjusted linear regression models using generalized estimating equations (GEE) to account for repeated measures were used to evaluate association between CIMT and DSA status at 18–30 months post-transplant. Observations at 18 and/or 30 months post-transplant time points were included in the GEE regression analysis if both a CIMT measurement and a DSA measurement were performed at that time point. In total, 60 observations of 38 patients were included in this analysis. GEE regression analysis was selected due to its ability to account for the within-patient correlation inherent to longitudinal serial data, as well as the fact that this statistical method is robust to missing data (15). In addition, multivariable linear regression was performed at baseline (0–1 months post-transplant) to determine whether there was a pre-existing difference in CIMT between the two transplant groups prior to the onset of DSA. Due to the non-normal distribution of CIMT in the transplant group, all continuous CIMT data were log-transformed, and therefore results of the regression models are presented as a % change in CIMT. Quasi-likelihood under the independence model criterion (QIC) was used to determine the best-fit statistical model. The most robust multivariable model is reported and was adjusted for race, hypertension, dyslipidemia, and abdominal obesity by WHr.

Statistical Power Analysis

Ad-hoc power analysis indicates that the sample size of 60 observations of 38 patients provided 87% power to detect a significant association ($p < 0.05$) between dnDSA and CIMT using a 5-parameter regression model. The power analysis was based on a full model $R^2 = 0.52$, reduced model $R^2 = 0.44$, and change in $R^2 = 0.08$. Therefore, the study was adequately powered to detect the primary outcome measure, a significant association between CIMT and DSA, by GEE multiple regression analysis.

RESULTS

Study Population

Of 70 patients who received a kidney transplant at Children's National between September 2010 and January 2015, 61 patients met the study inclusion criteria. Of these 61 eligible patients, 43

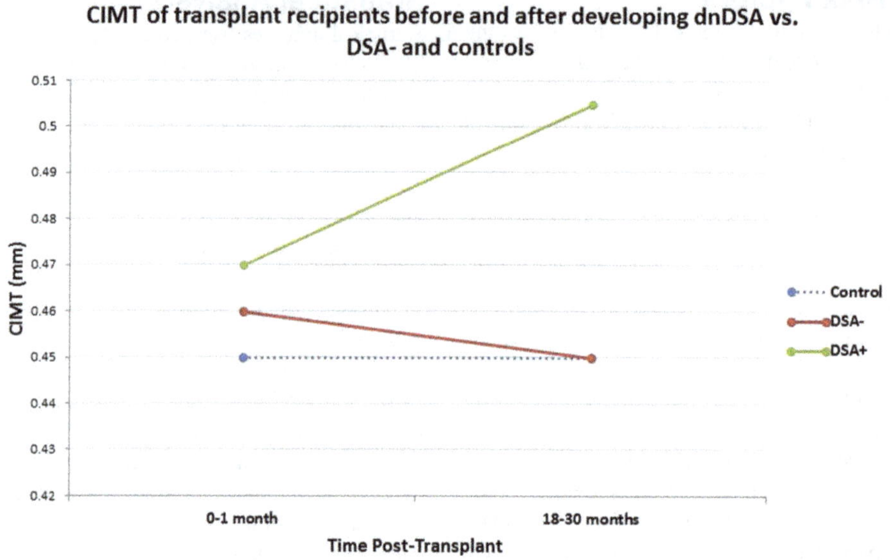

FIGURE 1 | Median CIMT observations of the group who remained DSA negative decreased from 0.460 to 0.455 mm between baseline (0–1 month) and 18–30 months, while CIMT increased from 0.470 to 0.505 mm in the group who developed dnDSA at 18–30 months post-transplant. Median CIMT of healthy controls was 0.450 mm (one measurement).

consented to enroll in the study, and 38 of these enrolled patients completed the required study procedures. In total, 38 transplant recipients contributed 60 observations of CIMT between 18 and 30 months post-transplant to the analysis.

Within the transplant group, 18.4% of patients (7/38) had developed strong or very strong dnDSA by 18–30 months post-transplant and were thus classified as DSA+ for purposes of the study. Of the 7 DSA+ patients, 2 patients received pharmacologic treatments for DSA+ acute cellular-mediated rejection prior to their 18 month CIMT imaging, and therefore were excluded from the analysis. One additional patient had weak dnDSA detected at 18 months and was therefore excluded from the analysis. Six observations (4 observations at 18 months and 2 at 30 months post-transplant) of the remaining 5 DSA+ patients who did not receive treatments prior to CIMT measurement were included in the analysis. Of a possible 60 CIMT observations of the 30 DSA- transplant patients at 18 and 30 months post-transplant, 54 observations were included in the analysis. The 6 observations of DSA- participants were missing for the following reasons: 2 patients moved out of the area after 18 months, 2 patients missed the 18 month study visit, and 2 patients missed the 30 month study visit.

In addition, 20 healthy children contributed 20 observations to the study (one CIMT observation per each control participant).

Characteristics of Patients and Controls

The demographics and clinical characteristics of the DSA+, DSA- and healthy control groups are summarized in **Table 1**. Among the transplant patients included in the dnDSA positive study group, antibody profiles included 3 patients with strong Class II, 1 with very strong Class II, and 1 with a combination of very strong Class I and II. There were no differences in the age or race distribution of the DSA+, DSA-, or control groups ($p > 0.05$). Male sex was more prevalent in the DSA- vs. the control group ($p = 0.02$), but did not differ between the DSA + and DSA − groups and also did not differ between the DSA + and control groups ($p > 0.05$). In addition, male gender was not significantly associated with CIMT in the multivariate analysis, as shown in **Table 2**. There were no differences in the proportion of patients with pre-emptive transplant or the mean duration of dialysis prior to transplant between DSA + and DSA- groups ($p > 0.05$). There were no statistical differences in prevalence of hypertension, dyslipidemia, BMI-obesity, abdominal obesity, steroid protocol or in eGFR between DSA+ and DSA- groups at 18 months post-transplant ($p > 0.05$).

CIMT

At 18–30 months post-transplant, DSA+ transplant recipients had median CIMT of 0.505 mm (95% CI 0.454–0.560 mm), compared to 0.455 mm (95% CI 0.440–0.470) in DSA- transplant recipients and 0.450 mm (95% CI 0.436–0.460) in the healthy controls. In order to visualize a temporal relationship between DSA and CIMT, we also examined the CIMT of the DSA+ and DSA- groups at baseline (0–1 months post-transplant), prior to development of DSA. As shown in **Figure 1**, the median CIMT of the group who remained DSA- during the first 30 months post-transplant decreased slightly from 0.460 mm (95% CI 0.430–0.490) to 0.455 mm (95% CI 0.440–0.470) between baseline and 18–30 months post-transplant, while the median of CIMT of the group who became DSA+ increased from 0.47 mm (95% CI 0.440–0.491) at baseline to 0.505 mm (95% CI 0.454–0.560 mm) over the same time period. Due to the longitudinal nature of the data, bivariate statistical comparison was not appropriate. As these CIMT comparisons are descriptive only in nature and do not account for other potentially confounding factors, unadjusted and adjusted multivariable regression analyses were performed.

ASSOCIATION OF DSA WITH CIMT

18–30 Months Post-transplant, Unadjusted Analysis

Results of the unadjusted GEE regression analysis showed that the presence of DSA and African American race were associated with increased CIMT in transplant recipients. As shown in **Table 2**, DSA positive transplant recipients had 10.2% thicker CIMT compared with DSA negative transplant recipients ($p = 0.03$), and CIMT was 9.4% thicker in the African American transplant recipients compared with non-African Americans ($p = 0.0001$), prior to adjusting for any covariates. The remaining variables, which included BMI-obesity, WHr-obesity, hypertension, dyslipidemia, sex, age, steroid therapy, and eGFR at the time of CIMT measurement were not significantly associated with CIMT in the unadjusted analysis. Duration of dialysis prior to transplant was also not significantly associated with CIMT at 18–30 months post-transplant.

18–30 Months Post-transplant, Adjusted Analysis

After adjusting for potential confounding factors, multivariable GEE analysis showed that the presence of DSA was independently associated with a 7.8% increase in CIMT compared to those transplant recipients without DSA ($p = 0.006$). In addition, African American race was independently associated with a 9.3% increase in CIMT among transplant recipients ($p = 0.0001$). As presented in **Table 3**, the best-fit multivariable model was adjusted for race, abdominal obesity, hypertension, and dyslipidemia. Abdominal obesity was associated with a 3.7% increase in CIMT, with borderline statistical significance ($p = 0.059$).

TABLE 1 | Demographics and clinical characteristics.

	Transplant group		Control group
	DSA+	DSA-	
Age at transplant (mean ± SEM)	12.5 ± 2.9 years	11.8 ± 0.8 years	11.6 ± 0.9 years
African American Race (%)	60%	53.3%	50%
Male (%)	40%	66.6%*	30%*
Duration of dialysis prior to transplant (mean ± SEM)	13.7 ± 5.6 months	23.8±0.4 months	NA
Pre-emptive transplant	40%	30%	NA
Hypertension (%)**	60%	66.6%	0%
Dyslipidemia (%)**	20%	30%	NA
BMI-Obesity (%) **	50%	36.7%	0%
Abdominal obesity (%)** (WHr≥0.5)	60.0%	53.3%	0%
Steroid protocol (%)‡	60.0%	53.3%	NA
eGFR at 18 months (mean ± SEM)	96.4± 14.8 ml/min/1.73m^2	96.6 ± 5.1 ml/min/1.73 m^2	NA
dnDSA	➢ 60% strong Class II ➢ 20% very strong Class II ➢ 20% very strong Class I and II	No DSA	NA

Categorical variables were compared by Fisher's exact test and continuous variables by Wilcoxon rank-sum. There were no differences in the age or race distribution of the DSA+, DSA-, or control groups (p > 0.05). Male sex was more prevalent in the DSA- vs. the control group (p = 0.02), but did not differ between the DSA + and DSA – groups and also did not differ between the DSA + and control groups (p > 0.05). There were no differences in any of the remaining variables between DSA + and DSA- groups (p > 0.05).*
***Proportion of patients affected at any point during the 18–30 month post-transplant time period.*
‡Indicates proportion of patients who received maintenance steroid therapy.

TABLE 2 | Association of variables with CIMT (unadjusted analysis).

Variable	% change in CIMT[a] (95% CI)	*p*-value
dnDSA	10.2% (3.3 to 17.1%)	0.03*
African American race	9.4% (6.2 to 12.6%)	0.0001*
Hypertension	1.4% (−2.0 to 4.5%)	0.42
Dyslipidemia	−1.1% (−3.7 to 1.4%)	0.17
Obesity by BMI	−3.9% (−7.1 to 1.0%)	0.13
Abdominal Obesity (WHr)	0.23% (−3.1 to 3.5%)	0.89
Dialysis duration	0.08% (−0.03 to 0.20%)	0.16
eGFR	−0.02% (−0.07 to 0.03%)	0.43
Steroid therapy	−1.4% (−5.6 to 2.7%)	0.51
Male sex	−1.0% (−5.7 to 3.6%)	0.66
Age	−0.4% (−3.7 to 2.9%)	0.80

**Significant association with CIMT by GEE linear regression, without adjusting for any covariates.*
[a]Due to non-normal distribution, continuous CIMT data were log-transformed, and therefore results are presented as a % change in CIMT.

TABLE 3 | Association post-transplant dnDSA with CIMT (adjusted analysis).

Variable	% change in CIMT[a] (95% CI)	*p*-value
dnDSA	7.8% (2.2 to 13.4%)	0.006*
African American race	9.3% (5.5 to 13.1%)	0.0001*
Abdominal Obesity (WHr)	3.7% (0.0 to 7.5%)	0.059
Hypertension	0.70% (−2.8 to 4.2%)	0.69
Dyslipidemia	−1.6% (−5.2 to 2.0%)	0.38

**Significant association with CIMT by GEE linear regression, adjusted for race, hypertension, dyslipidemia, and abdominal obesity by WHr (p < 0.05).*
[a]Due to non-normal distribution, continuous CIMT data were log-transformed, and therefore results are presented as a % change in CIMT.

Temporal Validation of Relationship of DSA and CIMT, Adjusted Analysis

Multivariable linear regression was also performed to establish a timeline of the relationship between DSA status and CIMT among the transplant recipients. Results of this analysis showed that at baseline, prior to development of any DSA, neither group of transplant recipients had increased CIMT (coefficient −0.7%, 95% CI −6.3 - 4.0%, $p = 0.81$). As in the 18–30 month analysis, this linear regression model was adjusted for race, abdominal obesity, hypertension, and dyslipidemia. The results of this analysis demonstrate that association of increase in CIMT with DSA+ patients did in fact develop after the onset of dnDSA, and not before.

DISCUSSION

This pilot study is the first to demonstrate that development of dnDSA is associated with an indicator of arteriosclerosis, evidenced by increased CIMT, in a cohort of DSA positive pediatric kidney transplant recipients. Transplant patients with dnDSA exhibited thicker CIMT in comparison to transplant recipients without dnDSA at 18–30 months post-transplant, while CIMT of DSA- transplant recipients was similar to that of healthy controls. The association between dnDSA and CIMT was independent of traditional CV risk factors, including hypertension, dyslipidemia, and abdominal obesity. Our data also showed a temporal relationship between development of dnDSA and increased CIMT, as the association was not present at the time of transplant, prior to development of dnDSA.

Antibody-associated arteriosclerosis was previously described by Loupy et al. in a population of adult kidney transplant recipients (5). This study showed that presence of circulating dnDSA was associated with arterial inflammation and complement fraction C4d deposition resulting in intimal thickening of the arteries, and higher levels of DSA correlated with greater severity of arteriosclerosis (5).

Our findings are also supported by studies of dnDSA-associated vasculopathy in adult and pediatric heart transplant recipients (6, 7), which showed that circulating dnDSA were associated with increased risk of coronary artery vasculopathy, allograft failure, and mortality. The mechanism of action for accelerated antibody-associated arteriosclerosis has been previously demonstrated in animal models, as direct administration of anti-HLA antibodies to vascular endothelium induces release of inflammatory cytokines and complement activation, resulting in intimal hyperplasia and vasculopathy (16, 17).

The study by Loupy et al. also showed that adults with antibody-associated arteriosclerosis had 2.5 and 4.1 fold increased risk of major adverse CV events compared to those with non-antibody associated arteriosclerosis and those without significant arteriosclerosis, respectively, independent of other CV risk factors. The authors hypothesized that complement activation and release of inflammatory agents triggered by circulating dnDSA trigger not only injury localized to the allograft, but also ignite a generalized systemic process of arteriosclerosis, similar to that seen in other autoimmune diseases (5).

As major adverse CV events are not common in children, we used CIMT, a well-validated indicator for the early detection of CV disease, to identify arteriosclerosis in our study population. It was interesting to note that at the time of transplant, all transplant recipients had similar CIMT. In the group that went on to develop dnDSA, CIMT increased from 0.470 mm at baseline to 0.505 mm at 18–30 months post-transplant, while the DSA negative group had a slight decrease in CIMT from 0.460 to 0.455 mm (similar to the median CIMT of healthy controls, 0.450 mm) over the same time period (**Figure 1**). Previous longitudinal cohort studies of CIMT in children with ESRD suggest that CIMT would be expected to remain stable or slightly improve over time after kidney transplantation (18, 19). The results of our study suggest that the DSA negative transplant recipients follow the expected pattern, exhibiting stable or slightly improved CIMT, achieving a median CIMT matching that of race-matched healthy controls by 18–30 months post-transplant, while children who develop dnDSA exhibit an increasing trend in CIMT over time post-transplant.

Our results indicate that CIMT of DSA+ transplant recipients is approximately 0.05 mm higher than those of DSA- patients and healthy controls. Due to the rarity of major CV events in children, the exact magnitude of increase in CIMT that corresponds to increase in CV risk is not known. However, literature indicates that in adults, each absolute increase in cIMT by 0.1 mm corresponds to an increase in risk of stroke by 13–18% and an increase in risk of myocardial infarction by 10–15% (20). Therefore, based on this data combined with meta-analyses of pediatric studies of CIMT, an absolute increase in of 0.05 mm in CIMT a child is expected to be clinically significant in terms of portending future CV risk (21). The lack of significant association between CIMT with hypertension, dyslipidemia, and BMI that was observed in our study is in agreement with that of other pediatric solid organ transplant populations, as reported in a recent meta-analysis (21). Abdominal obesity as measured by WHr demonstrated a stronger magnitude of association with increased CIMT among our transplant cohort than did BMI, with borderline statistical significance ($p = 0.059$). Prior studies suggest that WHr is likely a more sensitive indicator of CV risk than BMI in children with kidney disease (22), but further research is needed to investigate its relationship to CIMT.

Strengths of our study included a prospective study design with a healthy control group that was matched by race to the transplant recipients. Matched race distribution between the study and control groups is important due to the known association of increased CIMT in African American children compared to other races (23). This was a pilot study, and as such was limited by small sample size, particularly in the DSA+ group. Our study was sufficiently powered to detect the association between DSA and CIMT, however larger multicenter studies would be needed to investigate more granular associations such as the type and strength of anti-HLA antibodies with severity of arteriosclerosis. In addition, although we demonstrated a temporal relationship between DSA development and increased CIMT, we cannot prove causality in the absence of histologic evidence. Our study design did incorporate several measures to isolate the possible effects of dnDSA on CIMT from those of the treatments given to patients with dnDSA. We excluded CIMT measurements from DSA+ patients who had already received therapeutic interventions for DSA with concomitant acute cell mediated rejection. In addition, our statistical analysis controlled for possible side effects of maintenance steroid therapy, including obesity, dyslipidemia and hypertension during the first 30 months post-transplant. Larger studies of longer duration post-transplant would be needed to examine possible long-term effects of dnDSA on cardiovascular risk profile in patients with persistent DSA.

In summary, dnDSA was found to be associated with increased CIMT in a cohort of pediatric kidney transplant recipients. The novel finding identified in our pilot study should be followed up by larger studies to verify this association and to elucidate the mechanism, effects, and possible therapies to treat antibody-associated arteriosclerosis in kidney transplant recipients.

ETHICS STATEMENT

The studies involving human participants were reviewed and approved by Children's National Hospital Institutional Review Board. Written informed consent to participate in this study was provided by the participants' legal guardian/next of kin.

AUTHOR CONTRIBUTIONS

All authors (KS, SC, AM) contributed to the conception, design, data collection and analysis, as well as writing and revision of the manuscript for this study. In addition, AM, pediatric nephrologist and Director of Kidney Transplantation, was the PI of the study and oversaw all of the research and regulatory aspects of the study. Statistical analysis was performed by KS, and analysis of CIMT was performed by pediatric cardiologist, SC.

REFERENCES

1. Sethna CB, Merchant K, Reyes A. Cardiovascular disease risk in children with kidney disease. *Semin Nephrol.* (2018) 38:298–313. doi: 10.1016/j.semnephrol.2018.02.009
2. Woo KS, Chook P, Yu CW, Sung RY, Qiao M, Leung SS, et al. Effects of diet and exercise on obesity-related vascular dysfunction in children. *Circulation.* (2004) 109:1981–6. doi: 10.1161/01.CIR.0000126599.47470.BE
3. Jardine AG, Gaston RS, Fellstrom BC, Holdaas H. Prevention of cardiovascular disease in adult recipients of kidney transplants. *Lancet.* (2011) 378:1419–27. doi: 10.1016/S0140-6736(11)61334-2
4. Sgambat K, Clauss S, Moudgil A. Cardiovascular effects of metabolic syndrome after transplantation: convergence of obesity and transplant-related factors. *Clin Kidney J.* (2018) 11:136–46. doi: 10.1093/ckj/sfx056
5. Loupy A, Vernerey D, Viglietti D, Aubert O, Duong Van Huyen JP, Empana JP, et al. Determinants and outcomes of accelerated arteriosclerosis: major impact of circulating antibodies. *Circ Res.* (2015) 117:470–82. doi: 10.1161/CIRCRESAHA.117.306340
6. Kaczmarek I, Deutsch MA, Kauke T, Beiras-Fernandez A, Schmoeckel M, Vicol C, Sodian R, et al. Donor-specific HLA alloantibodies: long-term impact on cardiac allograft vasculopathy and mortality after heart transplant. *Exp Clin Transplant.* (2008) 6:229–35.
7. Tran A, Fixler D, Huang R, Meza T, Lacelle C, Das BB. Donor-specific HLA alloantibodies: Impact on cardiac allograft vasculopathy, rejection, and survival after pediatric heart transplantation. *J Heart Lung Transplant.* (2016) 35:87–91. doi: 10.1016/j.healun.2015.08.008
8. Kuczmarski RJ, Ogden CL, Grummer-Strawn LM, Flegal KM, Guo SS, Wei R, et al. CDC growth charts: United States. *Adv Data.* (2000) 2000:1–27.
9. (CDC). *CfDC: National Health and Nutrition Examination Survey Anthropometry Procedures Manual* (2009).
10. Ochoa Sangrador C, Ochoa-Brezmes J. Waist-to-height ratio as a risk marker for metabolic syndrome in childhood. A meta-analysis. *Pediatr Obes.* (2018) 13:421–32. doi: 10.1111/ijpo.12285
11. Expert Panel on Integrated Guidelines for Cardiovascular Health and Risk Reduction in Children and Adolescents, National Heart, Lung, and Blood Institute. Expert panel on integrated guidelines for cardiovascular health and risk reduction in children and adolescents: summary report. *Pediatrics.* (2011) 128 (Suppl. 5):S213–56. doi: 10.1542/peds.2009-2107C
12. National Cholesterol Education Program (NCEP) Expert Panel on Detection, Evaluation, and Treatment of High Blood Cholesterol in Adults (Adult Treatment Panel III). Third Report of the National Cholesterol Education Program (NCEP) Expert Panel on Detection, Evaluation, and Treatment of High Blood Cholesterol in Adults (Adult Treatment Panel III) final report. *Circulation.* (2002) 106:3143–421. doi: 10.1161/circ.106.25.3143
13. National High Blood Pressure Education Program Working Group on High Blood Pressure in Children and Adolescents. The fourth report on the diagnosis, evaluation, and treatment of high blood pressure in children and adolescents. *Pediatrics.* (2004) 114(2 Suppl. 4th Report):555–76. doi: 10.1542/peds.114.2.S2.555
14. Eid L, Tuchman S, Moudgil A. Late acute rejection: incidence, risk factors, and effect on graft survival and function. *Pediatr Transplant.* (2014) 18:155–62. doi: 10.1111/petr.12203
15. Ballinger GA. Using generalized estimating equations for longitudinal data analysis. *Organ Res Methods.* (2004) 7:127–50. doi: 10.1177/1094428104263672
16. Mitchell RN. Learning from rejection: what transplantation teaches us about (other) vascular pathologies. *J Autoimmun.* (2013) 45:80–9. doi: 10.1016/j.jaut.2013.05.006
17. Libby P, Zhao DX. Allograft arteriosclerosis and immune-driven angiogenesis. *Circulation.* (2003) 107:1237–9. doi: 10.1161/01.CIR.0000059744.64373.08
18. Litwin M, Wuhl E, Jourdan C, Niemirska A, Schenk JP, Jobs K, et al. Evolution of large-vessel arteriopathy in paediatric patients with chronic kidney disease. *Nephrol Dial Transplant.* (2008) 23:2552–7. doi: 10.1093/ndt/gfn083
19. Krmar RT, Balzano R, Jogestrand T, Cedazo-Minguez A, Englund MS, Berg UB. Prospective analysis of carotid arterial wall structure in pediatric renal transplants with ambulatory normotension and in treated hypertensive recipients. *Pediatr Transplant.* (2008) 12:412–9. doi: 10.1111/j.1399-3046.2007.00837.x
20. Lorenz MW, Markus HS, Bots ML, Rosvall M, Sitzer M. Prediction of clinical cardiovascular events with carotid intima-media thickness: a systematic review and meta-analysis. *Circulation.* (2007) 115:459–67. doi: 10.1161/CIRCULATIONAHA.106.628875
21. Al Nasser Y, Moura MC, Mertens L, McCrindle BW, Parekh RS, Ng VL, et al. Subclinical cardiovascular changes in pediatric solid organ transplant recipients: a systematic review and meta-analysis. *Pediatr Transplant.* (2016) 20:530–9. doi: 10.1111/petr.12689
22. Sgambat K, Roem J, Mitsnefes M, Portale AA, Furth S, Warady B, et al. Waist-to-height ratio, body mass index, and cardiovascular risk profile in children with chronic kidney disease. *Pediatr Nephrol.* (2018) 33:1577–1583. doi: 10.1007/s00467-018-3987-2
23. Chowdhury SM, Henshaw MH, Friedman B, Saul JP, Shirali GS, Carter J, et al. Lean body mass may explain apparent racial differences in carotid intima-media thickness in obese children. *J Am Soc Echocardiogr.* (2014) 27:561–7. doi: 10.1016/j.echo.2014.01.007

22

CMV-Associated Congenital Nephrotic Syndrome

Anju Jacob[1], *Shameer M. Habeeb*[1,2], *Leal Herlitz*[3], *Eva Simkova*[1,2], *Jwan F. Shekhy*[1], *Alan Taylor*[1,4], *Walid Abuhammour*[1,5], *Ahmad Abou Tayoun*[1,4,6] *and Martin Bitzan*[1,2*]

[1] Department of Pediatrics, Al Jalila Children's Specialty Hospital, Dubai, United Arab Emirates, [2] Kidney Centre of Excellence, Al Jalila Children's Speciality Hospital, Dubai, United Arab Emirates, [3] Department of Anatomic Pathology, Cleveland Clinic, Cleveland, OH, United States, [4] Al Jalila Genomics Center, Al Jalila Children's Specialty Hospital, Dubai, United Arab Emirates, [5] Section of Infectious Diseases, Al Jalila Children's Specialty Hospital, Dubai, United Arab Emirates, [6] Department of Genetics, Mohammad Bin Rashid University of Medicine and Health Sciences, Dubai, United Arab Emirates

***Correspondence:**
Martin Bitzan
martin.bitzan@ajch.ae

Background: Congenital nephrotic syndrome, historically defined by the onset of large proteinuria during the first 3 months of life, is a rare clinical disorder, generally with poor outcome. It is caused by pathogenic variants in genes associated with this syndrome or by fetal infections disrupting podocyte and/or glomerular basement membrane integrity. Here we describe an infant with congenital CMV infection and nephrotic syndrome that failed to respond to targeted antiviral therapy. Case and literature survey highlight the importance of the "tetrad" of clinical, virologic, histologic, and genetic workup to better understand the pathogenesis of CMV-associated congenital and infantile nephrotic syndromes.

Case Presentation: A male infant was referred at 9 weeks of life with progressive abdominal distention, scrotal edema, and vomiting. Pregnancy was complicated by oligohydramnios and pre-maturity (34 weeks). He was found to have nephrotic syndrome and anemia, normal platelet and white blood cell count, no splenomegaly, and no syndromic features. Diagnostic workup revealed active CMV infection (positive CMV IgM/PCR in plasma) and decreased C3 and C4. Maternal anti-CMV IgG was positive, IgM negative. Kidney biopsy demonstrated focal mesangial proliferative and sclerosing glomerulonephritis with few fibrocellular crescents, interstitial T- and B-lymphocyte infiltrates, and fibrosis/tubular atrophy. Immunofluorescence was negative. Electron microscopy showed diffuse podocyte effacement, but no cytomegalic inclusions or endothelial tubuloreticular arrays. After 4 weeks of treatment with valganciclovir, plasma and urine CMV PCR were negative, without improvement of the proteinuria. Unfortunately, the patient succumbed to fulminant pneumococcal infection at 7 months of age. Whole exome sequencing and targeted gene analysis identified a novel homozygous, pathogenic variant (2071+1G>T) in *NPHS1*.

Literature Review and Discussion: The role of CMV infection in isolated congenital nephrotic syndrome and the corresponding pathological changes are still debated. A search of the literature identified only three previous reports of infants with congenital nephrotic syndrome and evidence of CMV infection, who also underwent kidney biopsy and genetic studies.

Conclusion: Complete workup of congenital infections associated with nephrotic syndrome is warranted for a better understanding of their pathogenesis ("diagnostic triad" of viral, biopsy, and genetic studies). Molecular testing is essential for acute and long-term prognosis and treatment plan.

Keywords: Finnish-type nephrotic syndrome, *NPHS1*, cytomegalovirus, *Streptococcus pneumoniae*, case report, glomerulonephritis, infantile nephrotic syndrome

INTRODUCTION

Congenital nephrotic syndrome (CNS) is a rare disease with poor renal and overall outcome. It is defined by the occurrence of large proteinuria and hypoproteinemia, resulting in generalized edema during the first 3 months of life (1). The estimated incidence is 1–3 per 100,000 children worldwide (2–4). The etiology of the CNS is heterogeneous and may present as part of a genetic syndrome.

Congenital infections, particularly CMV and *Treponema pallidum* (syphilis), and occasionally *Toxoplasma gondii*, and other pathogens, have long been associated with rare instances of CNS (5–12). Although CMV and cytomegalic inclusions have been demonstrated (predominantly) in renal tubular epithelial cells of patients with various CMV-associated glomerulopathies (7, 13), the causative role and the pathomechanism of the virus in cases of glomerulonephritis and nephrotic syndrome are still debated (4, 10, 14).

Recent surveys revealed the presence of disease causing genetic variants in up to 80% of CNS cases (4, 10, 15, 16). *Bona fide* pathogenic variants commonly lead to profound structural and functional abnormalities of the podocyte and/or glomerular basement membrane that compromise the glomerular filtration barrier. The prototypic, "Finnish type" congenital nephrotic syndrome is due to biallelic pathogenic variants in *NPHS1* (17, 18). Genes occasionally involved in congenital or infantile nephrotic syndrome with overlapping clinical and histological phenotypes include *NPHS2* (podocin), *LAMB2 (beta2-laminin)*, and *WT1* (Wilms Tumor 1 transcription factor), among others (4).

Early subtle histological alterations, such as microcystic proximal tubular dilatation, eventually lead to nephron loss and end stage kidney disease (ESKD) by the age of 2–3 years (1, 15, 19, 20). The spectrum of histological changes encompasses diffuse mesangial sclerosis (DMS), focal segmental glomerulosclerosis (FSGS), membranous glomerulopathy, and minimal change disease that are largely determined by the type of mutation and age at biopsy (1, 4, 15, 20, 21). The long-term management of patients with CNS remains challenging and may require early nephrectomy to minimize the pervasive effects of massive proteinuria, and subsequent kidney transplantation (4, 18, 22, 23).

We hypothesized that previously postulated infectious etiologies of CNS cases are biased due to the lack of biopsies and—historically not feasible—comprehensive genetic studies.

Here, we report an infant with CNS and CMV infection and demonstrate the importance of timely and complete diagnostic workup, i.e., the tetrad of clinical findings and virological/infectious disease, histopathologic, and molecular genetic studies.

CASE DESCRIPTION

A 9-week-old male (ex 34 weeks gestational age, corrected age 3 weeks) had been referred to our Emergency Department with suspected surgical abdomen. He presented a 3-day history of non-bilious, non-bloody vomiting and a 2-week-history of increasing abdominal distention and scrotal swelling. The patient was the second child of his parents who are from Kerala, India, and distantly related (3rd degree cousins). The couple's firstborn son is healthy.

Pregnancy was complicated by moderate oligohydramnios and decreased fetal movements which led to urgent C-section. Mother denied fever or rash during pregnancy, and her urinalysis was normal.

Birth weight was 1970 g (20th weight percentile). The weight of the placenta is not known. APGAR was 8 and 8 after 1 and 5 min, respectively. He received CPAP and then oxygen via nasal cannula for a total of 3 days. A post-natal brain ultrasound study was reportedly normal, TSH was 12 mU/L, and he was discharged home after 6 days. Immunizations were up-to-date, including PCV13.

Clinical Exam

At presentation, the infant was alert, irritable, pale and grunting. He was normocephalic without dysmorphic features. There was no rash, no jaundice, no petechiae or ecchymoses. He was tachycardic at 175 beats per minute and tachypneic. The remainder of the cardiovascular and pulmonary findings was unremarkable. The abdomen was distended, tense and shiny with large ascites and no palpably enlarged liver or spleen. Substantial scrotal edema was noted. Weight (with edema) was 3.5 kg (0.01%, z score −3.83), length 52.5 cm (0.00%, z score −4.31), and head circumference 35.5 cm (0.04%, z score −3.35).

Investigations

At the time of admission, there was large proteinuria, hypoalbuminemia, and hypercholesterolemia, consistent with nephrotic syndrome. Nephrotic range proteinuria was defined as a spot urine protein-to-creatinine ratio of >0.23 g/mmol (corresponding to >2.0 g protein/g creatinine). For details and definitions, see **Table 1**). The hemoglobin (Hb) level dropped from 100 to 69 g/L over the first 10 days of admission, with inadequate reticulocyte response and normal serum ferritin and iron levels. Serum C3 and C4 concentrations, measured on

TABLE 1 | Laboratory results during the disease course[a].

Parameter	Reference ranges	Presentation (age 9 weeks)	Start VGC (age 10 weeks)	One month VGC (age 14 weeks)	Last results (age 7.4 months)
Urine protein (g/L)	g/L	>2.0 (4+)	>2.0 (4+)	17.2	12.2
U protein creatinine ratio, nephrotic range	>0.23 g/mmol (>2.0 g/g)	>0.4 [b] (>3.52 g/g)	>0.7 [b] (>6.92 g/g)	6.44 (56.94 g/g)	3.71 (32.75 g/g)
Hematuria (dipstick/microscopy)	Dipstick negative 0–3/HPF	Small -	Small -	3+ >35	3+ >35
Serum albumin	33–54 g/L	9	17 [c]	9	12
Total serum protein	51–73 g/L	24.5	33.2	25.5	-
Toxoplasma IgM/IgG		neg/neg	-	-	-
Rubella IgM/IgG		neg/neg	-	-	-
CMV IgM	<0.69 COI	4.56	-	-	-
CMV IgG	<0.49 U/mL	5.54	-	-	-
CMV PCR blood		positive	-	negative	-
CMV PCR urine		positive	-	negative	-
HSV 1 & 2 PCR blood		neg/neg	-	-	-
Syphilis (*T. pallidum*)		Neg	-	-	-
Hepatitis B (HBs) Ag	<1.0 COI	-	-	0.394	-
Anti-HBs Ab	<10 mIU/mL	<2.00	-	4.2 [d]	-
Anti-HBc Ab		Non-reactive	-	-	-
Hepatitis C (anti-HCV Ab)		Non-reactive	-	-	-
EBV PCR (blood)		negative	-	-	-
Hemoglobin	111–131 g/L	100 [e]	69 [f]	93	106
WBC	6.0–16.0 × 10^9/L	11.7	12.6	5.6	16.8
Absolute neutrophil count	1.00–6.00 × 10^9/L	1.62	0.79	0.79 [g]	4.8
Platelets	200–550 × 10^9/L	328	357	584 [h]	827
Serum IgG	3.09–15.73 g/L	<0.4	-	-	-
Serum IgA	0.08–0.58 g/L	0.11	-	-	-
Serum IgM	0.04–0.89 g/L	0.49	-	-	-
Serum C3	0.82–1.67 g/L	-	0.31	-	-
Serum C4	0.14–0.44 g/L	-	0.08	-	-
C-reactive protein (CRP)	0–2.80 mg/L	0.42	-	0.63	-
Cholesterol	2.1–3.8 mmol/L	10.4	-	-	10.4 [i]
ALT	0–57 U/L	17	11	12	10 [i]
AST	0–110 U/L	28	40	27	30 [i]
GGT	0–203 U/L	1036/519 [j]	226	161	61 [i]
Total bilirubin	0–20.52 μmol/L	9.75/41.55 [j]	13.68	< 2.39	< 2.39 [i]
25 OH D3	75–250 nmol/L	32.5	-	-	27.5 [l]
1,25 $(OH)_2$ D3	48–190 pmol/L	-	-	-	221 [l]
Intact PTH	1.6–6.7 pmol/L	10.8	-	-	11.3 [l]
TSH	0.73–8.35 mU/L	23.23	4.97 [k]	-	4.11 [m]
Free T4	11.9–25.6 pmol/L	7.1	22.2 [k]	-	12.4 [m]
Body weight	kg	3.50 [n]	3.20	4.05	5.22
WHO growth chart	Centile (z score)	0.01 (−3.83)	0.00 (−4.89)	0.00 (−4.01)	0.00 (−4.21)
Head circumference	cm	35.5	-	-	-
WHO growth chart	Centile (z score)	0.04 (−3.35)	-	-	-

[a] *COI cut-off index, HPF high power field, VGC valganciclovir, - not obtained at that indicated interval.*

[b] *Protein titration in urine was not available initially. See Kidney Disease Improving Global Outcomes (KDIGO) Clinical Practice Guideline for Glomerulonephritis (2012) for the definition of nephrotic-range proteinuria.*

[c] *Following albumin infusions.*

[d] *Measured 2 weeks after commencing after HBV vaccination.*

[e] *Normocytic anemia with inadequately low reticulocyte count (2.38%).*

[f] *Patient received RBC transfusion following this result.*

[g] *Subsequent neutrophil counts remained >2 × 10^9/L.*

[h] *Persistently elevated platelet counts following treatment with VGC and the suppression of detectable CMV DNA.*

[i] *Last measurement at age 5.1 months.*

[j] *Change from day 1 to day 3 of admission; direct bilirubin was about 20% of total bilirubin.*

[k] *Rise of serum bilirubin concentration prior to commencement of VGC treatment.*

[l] *Supplementation with 2,000 IU cholecalciferol daily.*

[m] *Measurements during L-thyroxin supplementation.*

[n] *edematous.*

day 11 of admission, were decreased. The concomitant direct agglutination (Coombs) test was negative. Secondary findings were hypogammaglobulinemia, hypothyroidism with elevated TSH and low free T4 levels, hypovitaminosis D, low-normal serum ionized calcium (1.17 mmol/L) and moderately elevated intact PTH. ALT and AST were normal. GGT and bilirubin concentrations peaked during the first few days after admission (see **Table 1**).

The ultrasound (US) scan showed enlarged kindeys with mildly increased cortical echogenicity. Liver and spleen were of normal size and echotexture. The brain US study was normal, except the presence of thalamostriate mineralizing vasculopathy.

Cardiac echography demonstrated a small perimembranous ventricular septal defect of 2–3 mm with left-to-right shunt and patent foramen ovale, none requiring specific interventions.

Infectious disease workup revealed anti-CMV IgM antibodies and CMV DNA (by PCR) in blood and urine. Maternal screening during pregnancy for toxoplasma (IgG and IgM), rubella (IgM), HIV 1 & 2 antibodies/P24 antigen, hepatitis B (HBsAg) and hepatitis C (antibodies), and syphilis was negative. Subsequent CMV testing showed high maternal serum concentrations of CMV IgG, but no anti-CMV IgM.

Treatment of the Patient

Treatment consisted of frequent albumin infusions, diuretics and ACE inhibition, with improvement of ascites and peripheral edema. He also received L-thyroxin, vitamin D and oral penicillin prophylaxis, low-dose acetyl salicylic acid, iron, and indomethacin. In addition, he was vaccinated against *Streptococcus pneumoniae* (PCV13, twice) and hepatitis B.

Valganciclovir treatment was initiated 9 days after presentation at a dose of 22 mg/kg/day. CMV DNA became undetectable in plasma and urine after 1 month of antiviral therapy, however proteinuria failed to improve (**Table 1**) strengthening the presumptive clinical diagnosis of a genetic form of congenital nephrotic syndrome.

The patient's energy and protein intake remained precariously inadequate. However, parents were reluctant to agree to g-tube insertion or (unilateral) nephrectomy. Tragically, at the age of 7.9 months, following a few days of lapsed penicillin administration due to vomiting and diarrhea, the patient succumbed to fulminant sepsis, within hours after arrival in the Emergency Department, caused by pan-sensitive *S. pneumoniae*.

Kidney Biopsy

A kidney biopsy was performed 15 days after hospitalization (6 days after initiation of VGC treatment) to differentiate the pathohistological changes underlying the nephrotic presentation (1, 2, 4, 12). The majority of the >100 sampled glomeruli showed mild mesangial hypercellularity with patent capillaries and normal glomerular basement membrane (GBM) contours. Ten percent of the glomeruli were globally sclerosed or segmentally scarred. Three glomeruli showed active cellular or fibrocellular crescents with proliferation in the Bowman space and focal ruptures of GBM. There was a patchy, mononuclear tubulointerstitial inflammatory infiltrate. Infiltrating interstitial lymphocytes stained positive for CD3 and CD20, respectively, indicating the presence of T- and B-cells. Trichrome staining showed fibrosis in <5% of the cortex. Arteries and arterioles were histologically normal. Immunohistochemical staining for CMV was negative. Routine immunofluorescence showed faint, likely non-specific staining for IgM and C3. Electron microscopy revealed diffuse podocyte foot process effacement with prominent microvillous transformation, but no immune-type deposits. Endothelial fenestrations were intact, and no viral or endothelial tubuloreticular inclusions were noted (**Figure 1**).

Genetic Studies

Genomic DNA, extracted from peripheral blood cells, underwent a series of ultra-sonication, chemical, and enzymatic steps to generate a sequencing-ready library of short fragments (300–400 bp) using the SureSelect^{XT} kit (Agilent, USA). RNA capture probes targeting all coding regions were used to enrich for whole exome regions using the SureSelect Clinical Research Exome V2 kit (Agilent, USA). The enriched library was then subjected to next generation sequencing (2 × 150 bp) using the SP flow cell and the NovaSeq platform (Illumina, USA). Sequencing data were then processed using an in-house custom made bioinformatics pipeline to retain high quality sequencing reads with at least 100X coverage across all coding regions. Rare variants in 99 genes associated with nephrotic syndrome (**Supplementary Table 1**) were filtered for analysis and interpretation using the American College of Medical Genetics and Genomics (ACMGG) Sequence variant interpretation guideline (24). Two variants in the *NPHS1* and the *ITSN2* genes met the ACMGG criteria for reporting. *NPHS1* encodes nephrin which is central for the integrity of the podocyte slit diaphragm. Pathogenic variants in *NPHS1* cause classical Finnish-type congenital nephrotic syndrome (17). The apparently homozygous 2071+1G>T variant in *NPHS1* (NM_004646.3) has not been previously reported in individuals with disease and is absent from large population studies such as the Genome Aggregation Database (genomAD) and the Greater Middle East (GME) Variome database. This variant occurs in the conserved region (±1,2) of the splice consensus sequence of the only known *NPHS1* transcript, and is predicted to cause altered splicing leading to an abnormal or absent protein (25). The mutation is apparently homozygous, although a large deletion of the second allele could not be ruled out since parental testing was not conducted.

A heterozygous c.2713G>A p. (Ala905Thr) missense variant was also reported in *ITSN2* (NM_006277.2), the gene encoding intersectin 2, a member of the guanine exchange factor (GEF) family of proteins that activate Cdc42. This variant was classified as uncertain due to lack of sufficient evidence supporting its clinical significance. Bi-allelic pathogenic variants in *ITSN2* have been reported as a novel cause of nephrotic syndrome (26). The identified variant is absent from large population studies such as the Genome Aggregation Database (gnomAD) and the Greater Middle East (GME) Variome database. Computational prediction tools did not provide evidence for or against pathogenicity. No variants were discovered in complement-related genes or genes associated with (other) immunodeficiencies.

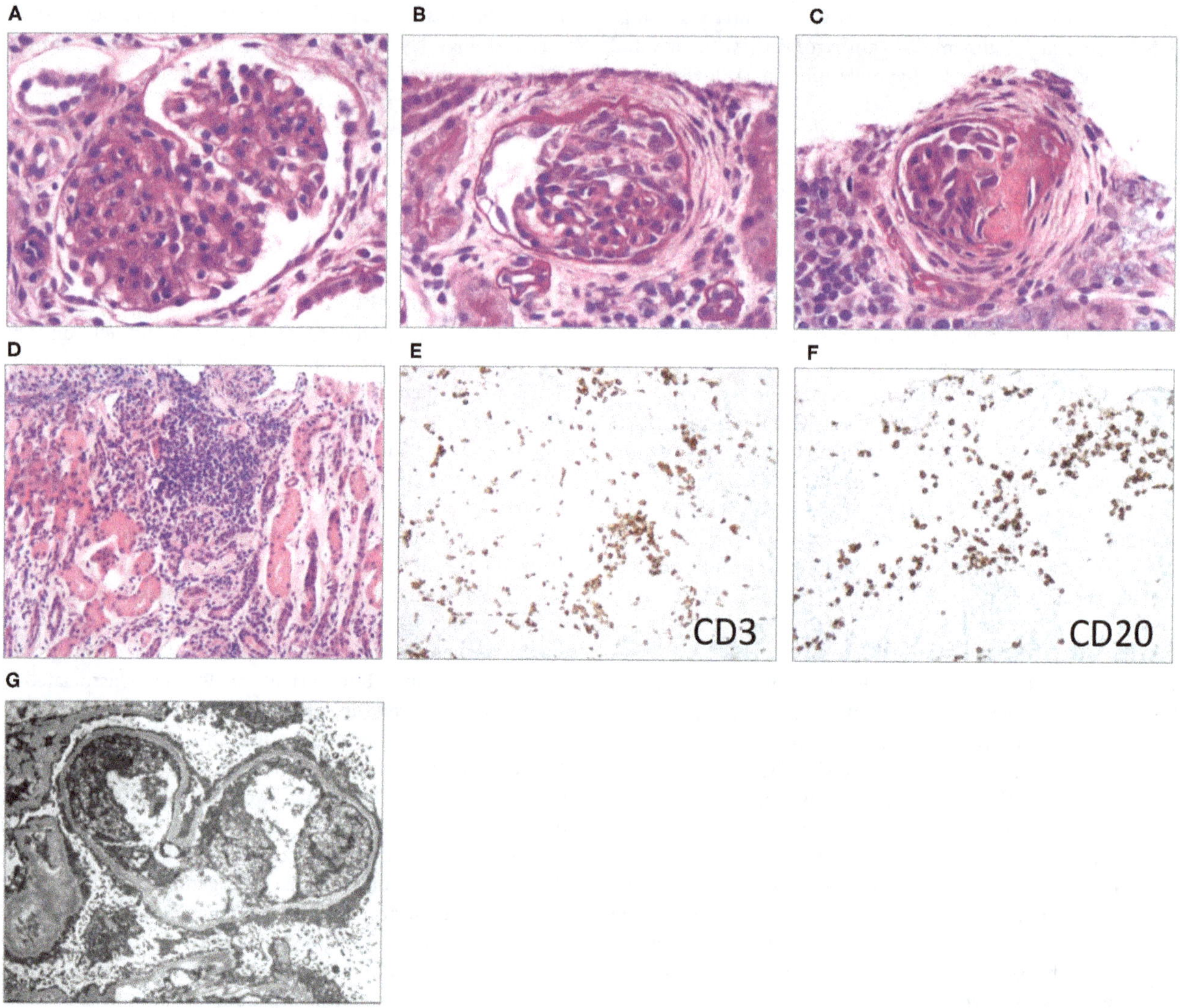

FIGURE 1 | Renal pathological presentation (kidney biopsy of the proband 15 days after admission). **(A–C)** Brightfield microscopy (PAS stain x600); **(D)** brightfield (H & E stain x200); **(E,F)** immunohistochemistry (x200); **(G)** electron microscopy. **(A)** Mesangial and endocapillary hypercellularity, **(B)** cellular crescent, **(C)** segmental scar/fibrous crescent, **(D–F)** interstitial infiltrates, **(G)** diffuse podocyte foot process effacement with prominent microvillous transformation.

SURVEY OF THE LITERATURE

CMV-Associated Congenital and Infantile Nephrotic Syndrome

Following the identification of a pathogenic *NPHS1* variant as the genetic cause of the patient's nephrotic syndrome, we wondered whether recognizable histopathological features would allow differentiating CMV-associated lesions (and CMV CNS) from CNS due to defined genetic variants. We therefore searched the available literature (PubMed and Google Scholar, without language restriction) for CMV-associated/infantile nephrotic syndrome with histological and genetic findings ("tetrad" of documented CMV infection and clinical features, kidney biopsy, and mutation screen).

Our survey identified only three cases with a complete tetrad: one patient with a homozygous *NPHS2* pathogenic variant, one patient with reported pathogenic variants in both *NPHS1* and *COL4A5* (however the number of variants and the phase of the variants in each gene was not detailed), and one with no detectable variants in *NPH1*, *NPH2*, and *WT1* (**Table 2**; patients #3, 7, and 6, respectively) (12, 14, 31). All three patients were treated with ganciclovir (GCV). Only patient #6 achieved sustained remission of proteinuria (31).

We then searched for reports of patients with CMV-associated congenital or infantile nephrotic syndrome, who also had a kidney biopsy. All identified cases (#1, 2, 4, 5) were treated with GCV (or GCV, followed by VGC), and all entered stable, proteinuria-free remission (**Table 2**). Mean antiviral treatment duration was 38 ± 27 (median 30) days; proteinuria improved substantially or disappeared after a mean of 20 ± 5 (median 19) days. The nephrotic syndrome was GCV-resistant in three cases (#3, 7, and 8). These patients were significantly younger at

TABLE 2 | CMV-associated congenital and infantile nephrotic syndrome (Literature review and proband).

#	Age onset Sex (gestation)	Pregnancy/ perinatal	Clinical presentation	Urinalysis Serum albumin	Infectious diagnostic	Treatment	Proteinuria after antiviral	Outcome	Genetic variants	References
1	5 mo F (39 w)	PBWR 0.2 (Maternal NS 8 mo in pregnancy (FSGS), resistant to Pred & POCY)	Normal at birth At 5 mo generalized edema At 6.5 mo fever, purpuric maculo-papular rash, hepatomegaly elevated ALT, LDH	Large proteinuria (>40 mg/m^2/h) Hypoalbuminemia (23 g/L)	At 5 mo CMV IgM+ (mat CMV IgM-, IgG+) (both Toxo, HSV, VZV, RV, Syph, HBV, HCV neg) (C3 &C4 N) At 6.5 mo CMV B-, U+, IgM+	At 5mo: High-dose Pred (ineffective) At 6.5mo GCV x 15 d	**Resolved** (proteinuria improved at 15d)	At 12 mo Clinically well, all symptoms resolved Sustained proteinuria remission, N renal function	ND	(27)
2	5 mo M (Term)	PBWR 0.19	Acute, generalized edema after URTI/vomiting US KUB normal	Large proteinuria (>40 mg/m^2/h) Hypoalbuminemia (6.9 g/L)	CMV IgM+, IgG+ (EBV, HBV/HBC, HIV, HSV, Syph, VZV neg) (mat CMV IgM-, IgG+)	Pred 60 x4w (ineffective), then oral GCV x12w	**Resolved** (remission at 4 w GCV)	Sustained proteinuria remission Stable at 17 mo FU	ND	(28)
3	45 d F (36 w)	Mild dysmorphic features Antenatal US large, echogenic kidneys) Ebstein anomaly	Generalized edema/ascites/pleural effusion Bilateral vitreitis Bilateral SNHL Increased renal echogenicity	Large proteinuria (170 mg/m^2/h) Hypoalbuminemia (22 g/L)	CMV U+, IgM+ (Toxo, RV, Syph, HBV, HCV, HIV neg) C normal	Daily IV Alb/ diuretic GCV (duration NR)	Persistent	Resolution SNHL & vitreitis 6 mo post-GCV ESRD at 21 mo	*NPHS2* [a]	(14)
4	57 d F (33 w)	Pregnancy uncomplicated Not dysmorphic	Generalized edema, HTN Respiratory symptoms Anemia 58 g/L, platelets 75/nL Enlarged, echogenic kidneys Brain cortical atrophy (no calcifications, no retinitis)	Large proteinuria (454 mg/m^2/h) Hypoalbuminemia (20 g/L) UA: WBC, RBC, gran casts	CMV IgG+, IgM- CMV PCR serum high (neg HBV/HCV, HSV1/2, RV, toxo Ab) (Mat CMV IgM-, IgG+)	Daily IV Alb & diuretics Captopril IV GCV x 3 w	**Resolved** Upc 0.079 g/mmol at 3w	Hematologic response, HTN resolved Remission >14 mo FU	ND	(29)
5	6 mo	NR	Persistent watery diarrhea Generalized edema & ascites Hb 107 g/L Plt 406/nL	Large proteinuria (28 g/L) Hypoalbuminemia (10 g/L)	CMV PCR (blood/urine?)	IV alb x 19d Captopril IV GCV x 2w, then VGC x 4w	**Resolved** Up low (CMV PCR neg) at 19d GCV/VGC	Resolution of colitis CMV PCR neg 19d Stable remission 1y	ND	(30)

TABLE 2 | Continued

#	Age onset Sex (gestation)	Pregnancy/ perinatal	Clinical presentation	Urinalysis Serum albumin	Infectious diagnostic	Treatment	Proteinuria after antiviral	Outcome	Genetic variants	References
6	5 mo M	Diamniotic twin pregnancy	Gastroenteritis Mild edema Large kidneys No dysmorphism/brain lesions Normal ophthalmological exam	Large proteinuria (Upc 7.83 g/mmol) Hypoalbuminemia (10.3 g/L) Normal GFR	CMV B-, PCR+ (EBV (PCR), HBV, HCV, HIV, Syph neg)	IV Alb x 16d Captopril x 16d IV GCV x 15d (from D15), then VGC x 15d	**Resolved** Up 0.15 g/L at 15d, Salb N	Sustained remission over 30 mo FU	Negative (*NPHS1*, *NPHS2, WT1*) [b]	(31)
7	15 d	NR	"asymptomatic"	Large proteinuria (3+, 2.82 g/mmol) Hypoalbuminemia (21.7 –>11.0 g/L) Normal cholesterol	CMV IgM+	GCV 10 x 4w	Partial remission (Upc 0.189, S-Alb 30.4 g/L)	CKD at 13mo (eGFR 55 mL/min/1.73m^2) Proteinuria 3+	*NPHS1*, *COL4A5* [c]	(12)
8	51 d M (34 w)	Oligohydramnios asymmetric IUGR	Ascites, scrotal edema FFT, developmental delay Anemia (100 69 g/L) GGT/mild hyperbilirubinemia Thalamostriate mineralizing vasculopathy	Large proteinuria (4+, 3.4 g/mmol) Microhematuria (15-20 RBC/HPF) Hypoalbuminemia (9 g/L) eGFR normal	CMV IgM+ CMV B-PCR+ CMV U-PCR+ (Toxo, RV IgM, Syph neg) Mat CMV IgG+, IgM- Low C3 &C4	Captopril VGC IV Alb/diuretic Pen-VK prophylaxis	persistent	CMV PCR neg 4 w post VGC, FFT Death pneumococcal sepsis at 7.9 mo	*NPHS1 (INTS2 – het)* [d]	This report

[a]*Homozygous for nonsense mutation c.412C<T (p.Arg138X), carrier status confirmed for both parents (14, 32).*
[b]*Testing was limited to the indicated genes. Methodological details are not reported.*
[c]*NPHS1 variant reported as c.2396G>T (p. Gly799Val) and c.1339G>A (p. Glu477Lys), COL4A5 variant not specified (12).*
[d]*Detail see Results section.*
CKD, chronic kidney disease; d, day(s); eGFR, estimated glomerular filtration rate (33); ESRD, end stage renal disease; FFT, failure to thrive; GGT, gamma glutamyl transferase; GCV, ganciclovir (IV); Hb, hemoglobin; HPF, high power field; HTN, hypertension, mo month(s); N, normal; NR, not reported; PBWR, placenta birthweight ratio; Plt, platelet(s); Upc, (urine protein-to-creatinine ratio), VGC, valganciclovir (oral); w, week(s).
SI unit conversion Upc (g/mmol) × 8.84 = g/g (reference range for nephrotic range proteinuria >0.23 g/mmol, corresponding to 2.0 g/g).

nephrotic syndrome onset (median 1.5, range 0.5–1.7 months) than GCV "sensitive" patients (median 5, range 1.9–6 months) ($P < 0.05$, unpaired t-test). There was no apparent difference in the presenting nephrotic features (urine protein excretion and serum albumin concentrations) between GCV/VGC responsive and refractory patients.

Kidney Biopsy Results in the Literature

Results of the biopsy survey are detailed in **Table 3**. In this analysis we included also patients without genetic results under the assumption that stable remission from CMV-associated nephrotic syndrome indicates the absence of podocyte gene mutations. We identified and evaluated eight patients (including our case) with a total of 9 biopsies. The biopsies of four of the five GCV "sensitive" (mutation "negative") patients (#1, 2, 4, and 6) (27–29, 31) revealed mild-moderate mesangial cell proliferation with or without (mesangial) matrix increase. One of these biopsies also demonstrated mesangial sclerosis (#4). This contrasts with the findings in patients with GCV "resistant" (mutation "positive") CNS (#3, 7, and 8) (12, 14), where light microscopic findings demonstrate a spectrum of normal-appearing glomeruli (#3a), glomerular sclerosis (#3b and 8) and occasional cellular or fibrocellular crescents, as well as focal mesangial proliferation (#7 and 8).

DISCUSSION

The presented case demonstrates features of classical (Finnish-type) congenital nephrotic syndrome (CNS) due to a homozygous *NPHS1* pathogenic variant, complicated by congenital CMV infection. There was no retinopathy or microcephaly, and apart from (non-specific) thalamostriate mineralizing vasculopathy (34, 35), the infant had no detectable cerebral abnormalities by ultrasound. However, he had substantial anemia (resulting in RBC transfusion), neutropenia (without thrombocytopenia) and temporary GGT and bilirubin elevation (without hepato- or splenomegaly). The C3 and C4 hypocomplementemia was surprising and deserves further inquiry in comparable cases of congenital/Finnish type nephrotic syndrome and of congenital CMV infections, whereas the extreme hypogammaglobulinemia resulted in all likelihood from massive protein loss via the disrupted glomerular filtration barrier.

Intrauterine or perinatal CMV exposure may have been responsible, at least in part, for the presenting signs and symptoms in our patient. However, there are no criteria to predict the role of CMV in this or similar patients' nephrotic syndromes. Due to health insurance reasons, we were unable to pursue early genetic testing. However, we proceeded with a kidney biopsy for diagnostic and therapeutic guidance (1, 4).

The histological findings were consistent with what has been described in CMV-related congenital nephrotic syndrome, including proliferative lesions and diffuse podocyte effacement. Lack of CMV detection (or inclusion bodies) in renal tissue makes it less likely that the virus was the direct cause of the observed morphological changes. Some of the demonstrated lesions may have arisen as part of the inflammatory and cytokine response of the host, albeit without virus or interferon-gamma-induced (endothelial) tubuloreticular arrays (36, 37). Interestingly, serum C3 and C4 protein levels were decreased during the early course, yet we failed to observe unequivocal immune deposits in the kidney biopsy.

Antiviral treatment was combined with supportive measures, mainly diuretic-assisted albumin infusions, thyroid hormone and vitamin D which controlled the profound edema and hormonal deficiencies. Persistence of large proteinuria and dependency on albumin infusions after the CMV PCR had become negative, favored a genetic cause of the nephrotic syndrome. Attempts to convince the parents to optimize nutrition (g-tube feeding) and (unilateral) nephrectomy to reduce protein losses (2, 4, 22) remained unsuccessful. Unfortunately, he succumbed to foudroyant pneumococcal sepsis at almost 8 months of age, despite repeat vaccination against *S. pneumoniae* and the prescription of antibiotic prophylaxis, which highlights the highly immunocompromised status of infants with severe nephrotic syndrome. We were eventually able to perform whole exome sequencing and can at least offer genetic counseling for the family.

The occurrence of NS in newborns with intrauterine exposure to CMV has been known since more than 50 years (7, 13). While infants with overwhelming congenital CMV disease demonstrate CMV invasion and proliferation in the kidney along with many other tissues (7), the mechanism of CMV-induced glomerular injury and podocytopathy is not well-defined. Previous studies have addressed direct, virus-mediated tissue injury and injury induced by the host immune response, such as T cell infiltration or immune complex formation (38, 39). However, the natural history and outcome of theses lesions has not been adequately documented, and there is a paucity of cases correlating virological and serological results with renal tissue and genetic studies.

The historical attribution of (severe) CNS to concurrent (congenital) CMV infection, including some of the histological changes, needs be revisited (4, 14). This notion does not negate the possible occurrence of (large) proteinuria and edema in newborns with severe, CMV-induced injuries, such as microcephaly or sensorineural hearing loss, with or without hepato- and splenomegaly and cytopenia.

Although the number of reported cases of CMV-associated CNS with a complete diagnostic "tetrad" is surprisingly small (**Table 2**), our analysis seems to confirm that an onset of nephrotic syndrome within 3 months of life predicts an underlying variant within podocyte or GBM-related genes, regardless of a coincidental CMV infection. In contrast, onset of nephrotic syndrome between 4 and 12 months and active CMV proliferation in previously asymptomatic infants appears to increase the likelihood of CMV as the remediable cause of the nephrotic syndrome. Neither the severity of proteinuria or hypoalbuminemia at presentation, nor (estimated) GFR or hematological parameters (anemia or thrombocytopenia)–where reported–appear to have discriminatory power in this small cohort.

Table 3 juxtaposes the histological findings of CMV-associated congenital and infantile NS. All but one patient demonstrating sustained remission of proteinuria following

TABLE 3 | Renal biopsy findings (Literature review and proband).

#	Onset/Bx (age in mo)	Glomerular compartment/BFM	IF/IH	EM	Tubulo-interstitial compartment	CMV-related findings	Genetic findings[a]	References
1	5/5.5	Enlarged glomeruli Mild mesangial cell proliferation	minimal mesangial IgM & C1q	Podocyte vacuolization w/o enlargement Foot process effacement Normal GBM Minor mesangial deposits Enlarged endothelial cells/single platelet thrombus/ scattered fibrin strands	NR	Endothelial tubulo-reticular arrays	ND	(27)
2	5/5	Mod mes cell & matrix increase in 25% of glomeruli w/o sclerosis	Diffuse mes IgM 2+	GBM normal	Normal w/o infiltrates or atrophy	No CMV inclusions Tissue PCR CMV+	ND	(28)
3a	1.5/<2	Normal-appearing glomeruli	NR/normal	NR	Normal (and normal vasculature)	Single inclusion body in distal tubule	*NPHS2*	(14)
3b	1.5/16	3/13 glomeruli globally sclerosed Remainder w/ mild mesangial proliferation & expansion	NR/normal	Foot process effacement	Normal (and normal vasculature)	Inclusion bodies absent Tissue CMV PCR & culture neg		
4	2/~2.3	Increased mes matrix & cell proliferation Some glomeruli w/ global, the remainder w/ seg mes sclerosis	Absent staining for IGs & C	NR	Focal tubular atrophy and fibrosis w/ tubular dilatation. Some tubules w/ Inflammatory infiltrates	Cytomegalic inclusion bodies in tubules and some glomeruli	ND	(29)
5	6/6	Mild endocapillary proliferation [b]	NR	NR	Atypical heavy tubular lesions, interstitial edema	NR	ND	(32)
6	5/5	Mild mes cell hypertrophy No mes sclerosis	NR	ND	Non-specific tubular lesions Interstitial edema	Absent viral cytopathic inclusions	Negative	(31)
7	0.5/2	Mild mesangial proliferation and Matrix increase. Multiple immature glomeruli with cellular crescents	Mesangial deposits of IgM (++) and C3 (+)	Mild mesangial cell/ matrix hyperplasia Podocyte foot process fusion Normal GBM No electron dense deposits	Vacuolar & granular degeneration tub epithelial cells, small focal atrophy Focal lymphoid interstitial mononuclear cells Eosinophil infiltrates w/ fibrosis Thickened small arterial walls	No CMV inclusions, CMV DNA neg	*NPHS1* *COL4A5*	(12)
8	1.7/2.6	Global or segmental sclerosis in 10% Focal mesangial proliferation Few cellular & fibrocellular crescents Mild cortical fibrosis (<5%)	Negative (non-specific trapping of IgM and C3)	Diffuse podocyte foot process effacement w/ microvillous transformation Intact endothelial fenestration	IF/TA Patchy, moderate tubule-interstitial infiltrates (CD3+, CD20+)	No endothelial tubulo-reticular arrays Staining for CMV negative	*NPHS1*	This report

[a]*Homozygous or compound heterozygous (except for COL4A5). For genetic details, see* ***Table 2****.*
[b]*Very brief pathology description.*
BFM, brightfield microscopy; Bx, kidney biopsy; C, complement; CKD, chronic kidney disease; d, day(s); EM, electron microscopy; ESRD, end stage renal disease; GCV, ganciclovir (IV); IF/IH, immunofluorescence/immuno histological stain; IF/TA, interstitial fibrosis/tubular atrophy; IG(s), immunoglobulin(s); mes, mesangial; mo, month(s); ND, not done; neg, negative; NR, not reported; w, week(s).

antiviral therapy, presented after 3 months of age. One of the common features of all patients with CMV-associated congenital or infantile nephrotic syndrome appears to be (usually mild) mesangial proliferation with or without matrix accumulation. Segmental and global glomerulosclerosis (40) and crescent formation is only noted in the two *NPHS1* patients. Given the paucity of completely defined cases and the heterogeneity of renal pathology among patients with autosomal recessive forms of CNS, the histological differentiation between CMV-induced congenital or infantile NS and patients with an underlying genetic variant remains challenging.

The *NPHS1* mutation identified in our patient is apparently homozygous, although a large deletion of the second allele could not be ruled out as parental testing was not possible. The recurrence risk would remain the same [25%] if the variant was homozygous, or compound heterozygous with a pathogenic deletion. Identifying the exact variant(s) allows for targeted variant analysis either prenatally or via *in vitro* fertilization and pre-implantation genetic diagnosis) for any future pregnancies.

The strength of this report is the complete characterization of the case and others identified in a comprehensive literature survey. Its limitation—and reason for publication—is the small number of fully described cases.

CONCLUSIONS

Genetic testing is warranted in all patients presenting with isolated or syndromic nephrotic syndrome immediately after birth or within the first 2–3 months of life, whether CMV is present or not. To further clarify the specific contributions of CMV and CMV disease to the histological changes in the kidney and severe, persistent nephrotic syndrome, a correlation (tetrad) of clinical and laboratory findings, kidney biopsy with all staining modalities and/or molecular tools, and genetic work-up are needed.

ETHICS STATEMENT

Written informed consent was obtained from the minors' legal guardian/next of kin for the publication of any potentially identifiable images or data included in this article.

AUTHOR CONTRIBUTIONS

AJ collected the data, reviewed the literature, and wrote the first draft of the manuscript. SH, ES, JFS, and AJ participated in the care of the patient. LH read and interpreted the kidney biopsy and provided the photographs. AT and AA were responsible for genetic counseling, performed whole exome sequencing, and analyzed and interpreted the molecular data. WA provided expert infectious disease consultation. MB supervised the care of the patient, reviewed all clinical and laboratory data, performed an independent comprehensive literature review, and wrote the final version of the manuscript. All authors critically reviewed and edited the manuscript.

ACKNOWLEDGMENTS

We thanked Dr. Muhammad Anwar for his help with the kidney biopsy and all physicians, nurses, and allied health professionals who contributed to the care and well-being of the described patient and his family.

REFERENCES

1. Habib R. Nephrotic syndrome in the 1st year of life. *Pediatr Nephrol.* (1993) 7:347–53. doi: 10.1007/BF00857534
2. Holmberg C, Laine J, Ronnholm K, Ala-Houhala M, Jalanko H. Congenital nephrotic syndrome. *Kidney Int Suppl.* (1996) 53:S51–6.
3. Holmberg C, Antikainen M, Ronnholm K, Ala Houhala M, Jalanko H. Management of congenital nephrotic syndrome of the Finnish type. *Pediatr Nephrol.* (1995) 9:87–93. doi: 10.1007/BF00858984
4. Reynolds BC, Oswald RJA. Diagnostic and management challenges in congenital nephrotic syndrome. *Pediatric Health Med Ther.* (2019) 10:157–67. doi: 10.2147/PHMT.S193684
5. Suskind R, Winkelstein JA, Spear GA. Nephrotic syndrome in congenital syphilis. *Arch Dis Child.* (1973) 48:237–9. doi: 10.1136/adc.48.3.237
6. Shahin B, Papadopoulou ZL, Jenis EH. Congenital nephrotic syndrome associated with congenital toxoplasmosis. *J Pediatr.* (1974) 85:366–70. doi: 10.1016/S0022-3476(74)80117-4
7. Beneck D, Greco MA, Feiner HD. Glomerulonephritis in congenital cytomegalic inclusion disease. *Hum Pathol.* (1986) 17:1054–9. doi: 10.1016/S0046-8177(86)80090-9
8. Roussel B, Pinon JM, Birembaut P, Rullier J, Pennaforte F. Congenital nephrotic syndrome associated with congenital toxoplasmosis. *Arch Fr Pediatr.* (1987) 44:795–7.
9. Niemsiri S. Congenital syphilitic nephrosis. *Southeast Asian J Trop Med Public Health.* (1993) 24:595–600.
10. Wang JJ, Mao JH. The etiology of congenital nephrotic syndrome: current status and challenges. *World J Pediatr.* (2016) 12:149–58. doi: 10.1007/s12519-016-0009-y
11. Kim YH, Song JH, Kim CJ, Yang EM. Congenital syphilis presenting with only nephrotic syndrome: reemergence of a forgotten disease. *J Korean Med Sci.* (2017) 32:1374–6. doi: 10.3346/jkms.2017.32.8.1374
12. Chen Y, Zhang Y, Wang F, Zhang H, Zhong X, Xiao H, et al. Analysis of 14 patients with congenital nephrotic syndrome. *Front Pediatr.* (2019) 7:341. doi: 10.3389/fped.2019.00341
13. Cozzutto C, Felici N. Unusual glomerular change in cytomegalic inclusion disease. *Virchows Arch A Pathol Anat Histol.* (1974) 364:365–9. doi: 10.1007/BF00432734
14. Frishberg Y, Rinat C, Feinstein S, Becker-Cohen R, Megged O, Schlesinger Y. Mutated podocin manifesting as CMV-associated congenital nephrotic syndrome. *Pediatr Nephrol.* (2003) 18:273–5. doi: 10.1007/s00467-003-1079-3
15. Sadowski CE, Lovric S, Ashraf S, Pabst WL, Gee HY, Kohl S, et al. A single-gene cause in 29.5% of cases of steroid-resistant nephrotic syndrome. *J Am Soc Nephrol.* (2015) 26:1279–89. doi: 10.1681/ASN.2014050489
16. Bierzynska A, McCarthy HJ, Soderquest K, Sen ES, Colby E, Ding WY, et al. Genomic and clinical profiling of a national nephrotic syndrome cohort advocates a precision medicine approach to disease management. *Kidney Int.* (2017) 91:937–47. doi: 10.1016/j.kint.2016.10.013
17. Kestila M, Lenkkeri U, Mannikko M, Lamerdin J, McCready P, Putaala H, et al. Positionally cloned gene for a novel glomerular protein–nephrin–is mutated in congenital nephrotic syndrome. *Mol Cell.* (1998) 1:575–82. doi: 10.1016/S1097-2765(00)80057-X
18. Jalanko H. Congenital nephrotic syndrome. *Pediatr Nephrol.* (2009) 24:2121–8. doi: 10.1007/s00467-007-0633-9
19. Machuca E, Benoit G, Nevo F, Tete MJ, Gribouval O, Pawtowski A,

et al. Genotype-phenotype correlations in non-Finnish congenital nephrotic syndrome. *J Am Soc Nephrol.* (2010) 21:1209–17. doi: 10.1681/ASN.2009121309

20. Trautmann A, Bodria M, Ozaltin F, Gheisari A, Melk A, Azocar M, et al. Spectrum of steroid-resistant and congenital nephrotic syndrome in children: the PodoNet registry cohort. *Clin J Am Soc Nephrol.* (2015) 10:592–600. doi: 10.2215/CJN.06260614
21. Kari JA, Montini G, Bockenhauer D, Brennan E, Rees L, Trompeter RS, et al. Clinico-pathological correlations of congenital and infantile nephrotic syndrome over twenty years. *Pediatr Nephrol.* (2014) 29:2173–80. doi: 10.1007/s00467-014-2856-x
22. Holtta T, Jalanko H. Congenital nephrotic syndrome: is early aggressive treatment needed? Yes. *Pediatr Nephrol.* (2020) 35:1985–90. doi: 10.1007/s00467-020-04578-4
23. Boyer O, Berody S. Congenital nephrotic syndrome: is early aggressive treatment needed?-No. *Pediatr Nephrol.* (2020) 35:1991–96. doi: 10.1007/s00467-020-04556-w
24. Li MM, Datto M, Duncavage EJ, Kulkarni S, Lindeman NI, Roy S, et al. Standards and guidelines for the interpretation and reporting of sequence variants in cancer: a joint consensus recommendation of the association for molecular pathology, American Society of Clinical Oncology, and College of American Pathologists. *J Mol Diagn.* (2017) 19:4–23. doi: 10.1016/j.jmoldx.2016.10.002
25. Abou Tayoun AN, Pesaran T, DiStefano MT, Oza A, Rehm HL, Biesecker LG, et al. Recommendations for interpreting the loss of function PVS1 ACMG/AMP variant criterion. *Hum Mutat.* (2018) 39:1517–24. doi: 10.1002/humu.23626
26. Ashraf S, Kudo H, Rao J, Kikuchi A, Widmeier E, Lawson JA, et al. Mutations in six nephrosis genes delineate a pathogenic pathway amenable to treatment. *Nat Commun.* (2018) 9:1960. doi: 10.1038/s41467-018-04193-w
27. Giani M, Edefonti A, Damiani B, Marra G, Colombo D, Banfi G, et al. Nephrotic syndrome in a mother and her infant: relationship with cytomegalovirus infection. *Pediatr Nephrol.* (1996) 10:73–5. doi: 10.1007/BF00863452
28. Berbel O, Vera-Sempere F, Cordoba J, Zamora I, Simon J. Cytomegalovirus nephrotic syndrome. *Nefrologia.* (2003) 23:451–3.
29. Besbas N, Bayrakci US, Kale G, Cengiz AB, Akcoren Z, Akinci D, et al. Cytomegalovirus-related congenital nephrotic syndrome with diffuse mesangial sclerosis. *Pediatr Nephrol.* (2006) 21:740–2. doi: 10.1007/s00467-006-0051-4
30. Zhang B, Fila M, Fakhoury M, Baudouin V, Deschenes G, Jacqz-Aigrain E, et al. Pharmacokinetics and dosage individualization of ganciclovir and valganciclovir in an infant with nephrotic syndrome associated with cytomegalovirus infection. *J Antimicrob Chemother.* (2014) 69:1150–1. doi: 10.1093/jac/dkt472
31. Hogan J, Fila M, Baudouin V, Peuchmaur M, Deschenes G, Niel O. Cytomegalovirus infection can mimic genetic nephrotic syndrome: a case report. *BMC Nephrol.* (2015) 16:156. doi: 10.1186/s12882-015-0152-z
32. Frishberg Y, Rinat C, Megged O, Shapira E, Feinstein S, Raas-Rothschild A. Mutations in NPHS2 encoding podocin are a prevalent cause of steroid-resistant nephrotic syndrome among Israeli-Arab children. *J Am Soc Nephrol.* (2002) 13:400–5.
33. Schwartz GJ, Munoz A, Schneider MF, Mak RH, Kaskel F, Warady BA, et al. New equations to estimate GFR in children with CKD. *J Am Soc Nephrol.* (2009) 20:629–37. doi: 10.1681/ASN.2008030287
34. Amir J, Schwarz M, Levy I, Haimi-Cohen Y, Pardo J. Is lenticulostriated vasculopathy a sign of central nervous system insult in infants with congenital CMV infection? *Arch Dis Child.* (2011) 96:846–50. doi: 10.1136/adc.2010.208405
35. Sisman J, Chalak L, Heyne R, Pritchard M, Weakley D, Brown LS, et al. Lenticulostriate vasculopathy in preterm infants: a new classification, clinical associations and neurodevelopmental outcome. *J Perinatol.* (2018) 38:1370–8. doi: 10.1038/s41372-018-0206-8
36. Hammar SP, Luu JY, Bockus DE, Remington FL, Luu JW, Friedman S, et al. Induction of tubuloreticular structures in cultured human endothelial cells by recombinant interferon alfa and beta. *Ultrastruct Pathol.* (1992) 16:211–8. doi: 10.3109/01913129209074562
37. Lee CJ, Suh KS, Kim KH, Chang YK, Na KR, Lee KW. The clinicopathologic significance of endothelial tubuloreticular inclusions in glomerular diseases. *Ultrastruct Pathol.* (2013) 37:386–94. doi: 10.3109/01913123.2013.814738
38. Stagno S, Volanakis JE, Reynolds DW, Stroud R, Alford CA. Immune complexes in congenital and natal cytomegalovirus infections of man. *J Clin Invest.* (1977) 60:838–45. doi: 10.1172/JCI108838
39. Platt JL, Sibley RK, Michael AF. Interstitial nephritis associated with cytomegalovirus infection. *Kidney Int.* (1985) 28:550–2. doi: 10.1038/ki.1985.163
40. Kuusniemi AM, Merenmies J, Lahdenkari AT, Holmberg C, Salmela K, Karikoski R, et al. Glomerular sclerosis in kidneys with congenital nephrotic syndrome (NPHS1). *Kidney Int.* (2006) 70:1423–31. doi: 10.1038/sj.ki.5001779

23

Persistent Abnormalities of Fatty Acids Profile in Children with Idiopathic Nephrotic Syndrome in Stable Remission

Stefano Turolo [1], Alberto C. Edefonti [1], William Morello [1], Marie-Louise Syren [2], Valentina De Cosmi [2,3], Luciana Ghio [1], Chiara Tamburello [1], Erika A. Demarco [4], Alfredo Berrettini [4*], Gianantonio Manzoni [4], Carlo Agostoni [2,3] and Giovanni Montini [1,2]*

[1] Pediatric Nephrology, Dialysis and Transplant Unit, Fondazione IRCCS Ca' Granda Ospedale Maggiore Policlinico, Milan, Italy, [2] Department of Clinical Sciences and Community Health, University of Milan, Milan, Italy, [3] Pediatric Intermediate Care Unit, Fondazione IRCCS Ca' Granda Ospedale Maggiore Policlinico, Milan, Italy, [4] Pediatric Urology Unit, Fondazione IRCCS Ca' Granda Ospedale Maggiore Policlinico, Milan, Italy

***Correspondence:**
Stefano Turolo
stefano.turolo@policlinico.mi.it
Alfredo Berrettini
alfredo.berrettini@policlinico.mi.it

Steroid-sensitive nephrotic syndrome is an immunological disorder mediated by still poorly defined circulating factor(s) that target the podocyte and damage the filtration barrier. Fatty acids (FA) have several biological roles and, in particular, are strictly involved in cell to cell communication, inflammatory processes and regulation of lymphocyte pools. Studies of FAs during INS have been mainly focused on biochemical changes during the phase of proteinuria; while no information is available about FA profile in patients with idiopathic nephrotic syndrome (INS) on stable remission. Aim of this study is to assess differences in blood FA profile between pediatric patients with INS during the phase of stable remission. Blood fatty acid profile of 47 pediatric patients on stable remission and 47 matched healthy controls were evaluated with gas chromatography. Patients with INS on stable remission had significantly higher levels of PUFA and omega-6 than controls (40.17 vs. 37.91% and 36.95 vs. 34.79%), lower levels of SFA and MUFA. Considering the single fatty acids, levels of omega-6 18:2n6 linoleic acid and omega-6 20:4n6 arachidonic acid were significantly higher in patients with INS than in controls (23.01 vs. 21.55%, p-value 0.003 and 10.37 vs. 9.65%, p-value 0.01). Moreover, patients with INS showed lower levels of SFA 14:0 (0.74 vs. 0.92%) and 18:0 (10.74 vs. 11.74%) and MUFA 18:1n9 oleic acid (18.50 vs. 19.83%). To the best of our knowledge this is the first study assessing FAs profile in children with INS in stable remission. In a population of 47 patients, we were able to demonstrate a higher blood level of linoleic and arachidonic acid, and consequently of omega-6 and PUFA, compared to controls. Persistently higher than normal levels of either linoleic or arachidonic acid, could be viewed as candidate biomarker for a state of risk of relapse in children with idiopathic nephrotic syndrome.

Keywords: idiopathic nephrotic syndrome (INS), fatty acids (FA), arachidonic acids, stable remission, omega-6 (ω-6) PUFA

INTRODUCTION

Childhood idiopathic nephrotic syndrome (INS) is characterized by the presence of heavy proteinuria (≥50 mg/kg/day), serum albumin <25 g/L, and edema (1–5). Children who respond to corticosteroids are defined as steroid-sensitive and have a favorable long-term prognosis; however, among them, those with relapsing episodes of proteinuria may require additional immunosuppressant therapy, which includes calcineurin inhibitors (6), mycophenolate mofetil, and more recently rituximab (7).

Steroid-sensitive nephrotic syndrome is an immunological disorder (1), mediated by still poorly defined circulating factor(s) that target the podocyte and damage the filtration barrier, causing proteinuria. There are some hypotheses on the genesis of the various proposed serum circulating factor(s) (8): T cells, B cells, and podocytes have been indicated as putative secretory cells (9), regulating B-lymphocytes homeostasis (10). A role of inflammation in childhood INS, driven by the activity of IL-17A (11) is supported by the fact that renal epithelial cells synthesize C-Reactive Protein (CRP) in a proteinuria independent manner (12); moreover, an increased expression of Tumor Necrosis Factor-α (TNF-α) in CD4-lymphocytes, with a concomitant decrease of expression of Interferon gamma (IFN-γ) in CD8-lymphocytes, regardless the proteinuria level (13), and an expression dysfunction of Toll Like Receptor-3 (TLR-3) (14) were observed in patients with INS.

Fatty acid metabolism is an emerging field of research in healthcare, not only under the nutritional aspect, but also within a more comprehensive and holistic approach, aimed at finding possible biomarkers for the cardiovascular risk (15, 16). Fatty acids have several biological roles and, in particular, are strictly involved in cell to cell communication, inflammatory processes and regulation of lymphocyte pools (17–21).

Fatty acids are compounds that can be classified either by chain length or saturation, resulting in the saturated fatty acid (SFA), monounsaturated fatty acid (MUFA), and polyunsaturated fatty acid (PUFA) categories.

PUFA include the essential fatty acids (EFAs) linoleic acid (18:2n6) and α-linolenic acid (18:3n3), which can be only taken with a diet (22). Among PUFA, the most relevant biologic role is played by the omega-3 and the omega-6 series, as they may regulate multiple gene expression and play a fundamental role in cell signaling and inflammation pathways (23, 24). In particular, the pivotal omega-6 arachidonic acid is released from membrane phospholipids when cells are under stress, and becomes the precursor of several pro-inflammatory bioactive compounds, like prostaglandins, thromboxanes, leukotrienes, lipoxines, epoxyeicosatrienoic acids, and hydroxyeicosatetranoic acids (21).

Studies of fatty acids during INS have been mainly focused on biochemical changes during the phase of proteinuria (25). While a decrease in palmitic and arachidonic acids and an increase of oleic acid have been described by Aldamiz Echevarria (26), Das found an increase in palmitic acid and a decrease of 18:0, alpha linolenic acid and EPA (27). This discrepancy may be explained by the fact that Das studied the effect of PUFA n3 supplementation on fatty acid levels, while Aldamiz Echevarria merely described the changes in fatty acid profile. Interestingly, for both authors the pivotal point was the change in the ratio between pro- and anti-oxidant PUFA metabolites, driving to a pro-inflammatory state. However, a pathogenetic meaning cannot be reasonably attributable to these observational findings.

If the changes in fatty acids levels during proteinuria are well-established, to the best of our knowledge no information is available about fatty acids profile in patients with INS on stable remission, although it is well-known that INS is characterized by periods of remission alternating with relapses of proteinuria, mainly in the course of infections, and that fatty acids are strictly involved in the inflammatory processes and in lymphocyte regulation.

The aim of this study is therefore to measure fatty acids levels in patients with INS on stable remission, comparing them to those of a group of matched healthy controls.

PATIENTS AND METHODS

The subjects participating in the study were enrolled according to the following criteria:

Patient group: (1) Pediatric patients with a previous diagnosis of idiopathic nephrotic syndrome, based on the following criteria: ratio of proteinuria to creatininuria UPr/UCr >2 mg/mg, and serum albumin <2.5 g/dl. (2) Steroid dependent or frequently relapsing course, according to the definition of the ISKDC: steroid dependent nephrotic syndrome is defined as steroid-sensitive NS with 2 or more consecutive relapses during tapering or within 14 days of stopping steroids; frequently relapsing NS is defined with 2 or more relapses within 6 months, or 4 or more relapses within a 12-months period. (3) Stable remission if UPr/UCr was <0.2 mg/mg, total serum protein >6.4 gr/dl, serum albumin >4 gr/dl (28), and duration of remission more than 30 days from the end of the nearest proteinuric event.

Control group: healthy controls matched for age and gender with neither concomitant inflammatory disease, nor a metabolic or genetic disease, enrolled from a group of children who performed a blood test in preparation to minor urologic corrective surgery.

Body Mass Index of both patients' and controls' groups was calculated, to exclude overweight or obese subjects from the study.

Patients' blood samples were collected for fatty acid profile, serum total protein, albumin, total cholesterol, and triglycerides during scheduled routine visits and obtained after parental consensus and following Helsinki declaration. Blood samples from controls were obtained after parental consensus. The related study protocol was approved by our local Ethical Committee.

Urine was collected from the first morning sample for urine protein and creatinine measurement and urine protein to creatinine ratio (mg/mg) was calculated.

Abbreviations: PUFA, polyunsaturated fatty acids; MUFA, monounsaturated fatty acids; SFA, saturated fatty acids; EFA, essential fatty acids; DHA, docoexaenoic acid; COX, cyclooxygenase; LOX, lipid oxygenase.

A 3-days dietary diary was collected in a random sample of 10 patients and 10 controls to assess differences in dietary fatty acid intake.

Blood samples were collected on Whatman 903 collection cards BHT (Sigma-Aldrich) pre-treated and stored at temperature of −20°C. Cards were cut and transferred into vials (one vial for each sample) for methylation as described by Marangoni et al. (29). Afterwards, 2 ml of KCl solution (Sigma Aldrich) and 330 μl hexane (Sigma-Aldrich) were added. Samples were first vortexed and then centrifuged 3,000 rpm for 10 min. Finally, hexane layer (the upper layer) was collected from each vial and transferred into gas chromatography vial for fatty acids profile evaluation with fast gas-chromatographer Master GC fast (Dani), equipped with a 15 m fused silica capillary column Omegawax^{TM} 100 (Supelco). The gas chromatography results were analyzed using Clarity software (Data Apex).

Fatty acids were evaluated as percent on the total of fatty acids; the obtained values were used for statistical analysis. Data are provided by clustering fatty acids on the basis of their saturation state (PUFA, MUFA, SFA) and considering among PUFA the omega-3 and omega-6 series.

The activity of the enzymes involved in FA synthesis pathway was evaluated by the product/precursor ratio (30).

Statistical analysis: *t*-test (SPSS 21.0 IBM) was conducted to assess differences in fatty acid profile between patients and controls after a normality test; a *p*-value $\leq$0.05 was considered significant.

In the absence of published data, the power of the test to calculate cohort sample size was not performed.

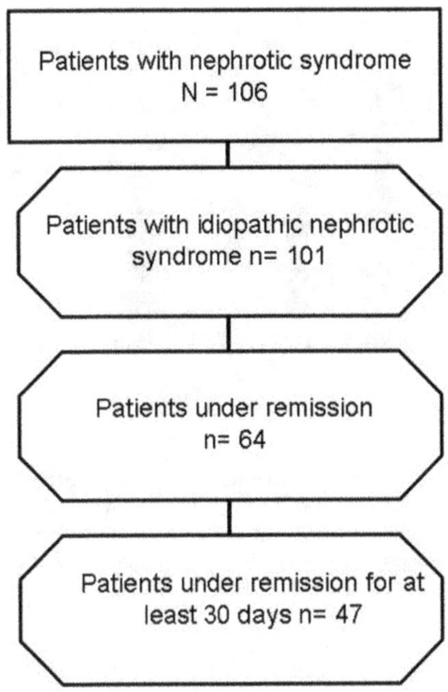

FIGURE 1 | Patients selection flow.

TABLE 1 | Fatty acids dietary intake (g/day) in a random sample of patients and healthy controls.

Fatty acids dietary intake		
	Patients (*n* = 10)	**Controls (*n* = 10)**
SFA	5.851	7.23
18:1n9	5.896	4.74
16:0	2.366	3.12
18:2 n-6	1.478	1.10
18:3 n-3	0.198	0.23
20:4 n-6	0.068	0.063
20:5 n-3	0.040	0.043
22:6 n-3	0.058	0.079

Values are expressed in g/day; dietary intake was calculated on the basis of a 3-days diary record.
n.s., not significant p-value at T-test.

RESULTS

Forty seven pediatric patients, aged 8 ± 4 years, 51% males, with steroid dependent or frequently relapsing nephrotic syndrome were enrolled into the study in the period 01/01/2016–31/12/2019 (**Figure 1**) and had a blood sampling for fatty acid profile during stable remission (median time elapsed from the nearest occurrence of proteinuria of 60 days, with a range of 32–150 days). Their serum total protein in remission was 7 ± 0.34 g/dl, serum albumin 4.7 ± 0.31 g/dl, and UPr/Cr 0.14 ± 0.04 mg/mg. Thirty-two out of 47 patients were in immunosuppressive therapy, 11 with cyclosporine A, 3 with tacrolimus, and 18 with mycofenolate mofetil.

Sixty healthy children matched for age and gender (age 8 ± 5 years, 51% males) were enrolled as a control group.

None of the patients and controls was overweight or obese. The two groups did not show any statistically significant difference in fatty acid intake at the analysis of the 3-days dietary diaries, as shown in **Table 1**, and their cholesterol and triglycerides levels were in the normal range.

Considering the main groups of fatty acids (**Figure 2**), patients with INS on stable remission had significantly higher levels of PUFA and omega-6 than controls (40.17 vs. 37.91% *p*-value 0.0004 and 36.95 vs. 34.79%, *p*-value 0.0005), with consequent lower levels of SFA (37.22 vs. 38.15%, *p*-value 0.02) and MUFA (22.57 vs. 23.94%, *p*-value 0.01). Omega-3 levels were not significantly different in the two groups (3.12 vs. 3.01%, *p*-value 0.53).

Considering the single fatty acids (**Figure 3** and **Table 2**), levels of omega-6 18:2n6 linoleic acid and omega-6 20:4n6 arachidonic acid were significantly higher in patients with INS during the phase of stable remission than in controls (23.01 vs. 21.55%, *p*-value 0.003 and 10.37 vs. 9.65%, *p*-value 0.01). Moreover, patients with INS, compared to healthy controls, showed significantly lower levels of SFA 14:0 (0.74 vs. 0.92%, *p*-value 0.008) and 18:0 (10.74 vs. 11.74%, *p*-value 0.00002) and MUFA 18:1n9 oleic acid (18.50 vs. 19.83%, *p*-value 0.011).

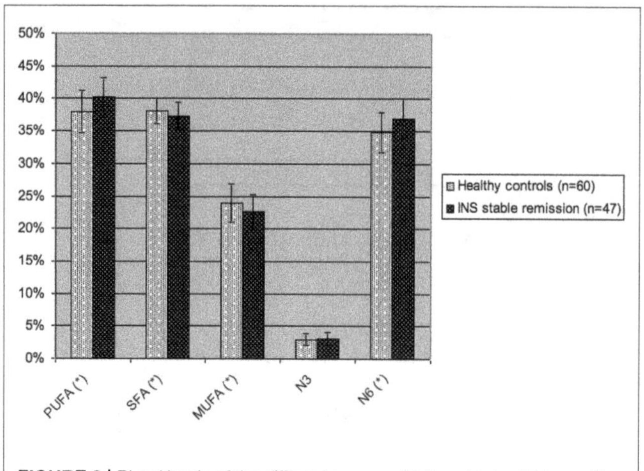

FIGURE 2 | Blood levels of the different groups of fatty acids in children with INS on stable remission and in healthy controls. PUFA, polyunsaturated fatty acids; SFA, saturated fatty acids; MUFA, monounsaturated fatty acids; N3, omega-3 fatty acids; N6, omega-6 fatty acids. Values are expressed as percent of total blood fatty acids. *p-value <0.05, statistically significant at *T*-test.

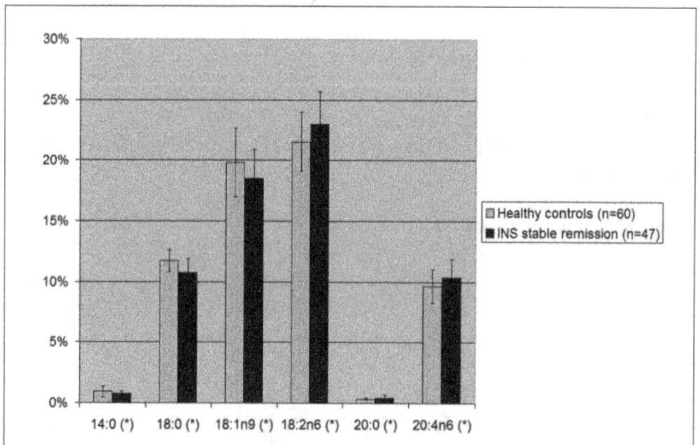

FIGURE 3 | Statistically significant single fatty acids blood levels in children with INS on stable remission and in healthy controls. 18:1n9, oleic acid; 18:2n6, linoleic acid; 20:4n6, arachidonic acid. *p-value <0.05 is statistically significant at *T*-test.

TABLE 2 | Blood levels of single fatty acids and different groups of fatty acids.

	Healthy controls		INS stable remission	
Fatty acid	**Average**	**s.d.**	**Average**	**s.d.**
14:0 (%)	0.92	0.43	0.74	0.23
16:0 (%)	22.61	1.36	22.94	1.37
16:1n7 (%)	0.92	0.29	1.01	0.31
18:0 (%)	11.74	0.92	10.74	1.12
18:1n9 (%)	19.83	2.85	18.50	2.40
18:1n7 (%)	1.26	0.16	1.25	0.21
18:2n6 (%)	21.55	2.43	23.01	2.69
18:3n6 (%)	0.27	0.13	0.30	0.12
18:3n3 (%)	0.22	0.09	0.22	0.06
20:0 (%)	0.34	0.07	0.42	0.23
20:3n9 (%)	0.12	0.04	0.11	0.05
20:3n6 (%)	1.59	0.28	1.58	0.39
20:4n6 (%)	9.65	1.37	10.37	1.52
20:5n3 (%)	0.28	0.16	0.32	0.21
22:0 (%)	1.03	0.20	1.05	0.24
22:4n6 (%)	1.22	0.31	1.14	0.41
22:5n6 (%)	0.50	0.25	0.62	0.38
22:5n3 (%)	0.60	0.14	0.62	0.15
24:0 (%)	1.52	0.29	1.47	0.43
22:6n3 (%)	1.91	0.63	1.90	0.70
24:1n9 (%)	1.68	0.33	1.55	0.44
PUFA	37.91	3.30	40.17	2.97
SFA	38.15	1.93	37.22	2.12
MUFA	23.94	2.88	22.57	2.63
Omega-3	3.01	0.84	3.12	1.03
Omega-6	34.79	3.11	36.95	3.08

Fatty acid levels are expressed as percent of total fatty acids. P-value calculated at T-test.

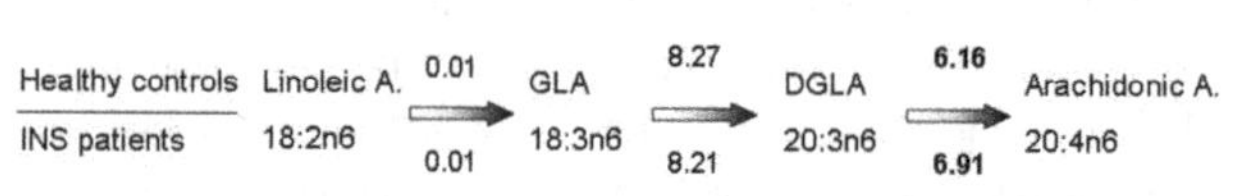

FIGURE 4 | Estimated enzymatic activity through omega-6 pathway. Estimated enzymatic activity from 18:2n6 linoleic acid (precursor) to 20:4n6 arachidonic acid (product). Numbers on the upper side of the figure indicate the estimated activity, calculated as the ratio of product to precursor, in healthy controls, while numbers on the lower side indicate the estimated activity in patients with INS under stable remission. Statistically significant data (*p*-value 0.03) are in bold. GLA, gamma linoleic acid; DGLA, dihomo gamma linoleic acid.

Finally, a significant increase in estimated enzymatic activity in the arachidonic acid synthesis pathway was found in the last step of the omega 6 pathway (**Figure 4**).

DISCUSSION

While previous reports have only been focused on the level of fatty acids in patients with proteinuria (26, 27), to the best of our knowledge this is the first study assessing FA profile in children with INS in stable remission. In contrast to the contradictory data on the fatty acids profile available in the literature (26, 27), we were able to demonstrate, in a population of 47 patients, a higher blood level of linoleic and arachidonic acid, and consequently of omega-6 and PUFA, compared to controls.

Immune system derangements resulting in an inflammatory state have been described during proteinuria in nephrotic syndrome and include a few mediators of inflammation, like IL17 A, TNF-α, IFN-γ, TLR-3, and CRP (11–14). Notably, for some of them, the expression was independent from the degree of proteinuria.

Our findings of high omega-6 levels, in particular arachidonic and linoleic acid, are on the same line and can be considered the expression of an inflammatory state, as it involves arachidonic acid (21). Indeed, omega-6 arachidonic acid is the precursor of several pro-inflammatory bioactive compounds, like eicosanoids (21).

However, such findings refer to patients in stable remission, not to patients with proteinuria, and this is the novelty of our study. A high blood level of arachidonic acid, and more generally omega-6 compounds, may be considered a biomarker of a persistent pro-inflammatory state in children with INS even during remission, possibly acting as co-factor involved in the relapse of proteinuria. Availability of larger pool of arachidonic acid, upon a trigger (for instance, an infection) could further contribute to activation of the omega 6 turnover, leading to increased synthesis of pro-inflammatory eicosanoids (the major end-products of arachidonic acid), possibly associated with relapsing proteinuria.

In our patients in stable remission, the high levels of arachidonic acid may be explained by an increase of the estimated enzymatic activity possibly supported by the described higher availability of linoleic acid, observed in the patients, but not in controls, in the last step of the omega 6 pathway, from DGLA to arachidonic acid.

The increased levels of arachidonic acid were associated with increased levels of linoleic acid, the arachidonic acid precursor. The increase in arachidonic and linoleic acid levels cannot be simply explained by a higher dietary intake of omega-6 in children with INS than in controls, as our 3-days dietary diary did not show any statistical difference between the two groups. On the contrary, the origin of the delta in linoleic acid levels between patients and controls could be explained in the first case by a different release from endogenous pools of fatty acids, as part of the general picture of non-communicable chronic diseases with inflammatory expression, in the second case by a reduced activity of metabolizing enzymes of linoleic acid LOX and COX in the patient's group (21). Furthermore, the fatty acids changes that we described did not depend on the use of immunosuppressive agents, as fatty acids levels are not affected by this group of medications (26).

Finally, the existing inverse correlation between blood levels of oleic acid and arachidonic acid (31) may account for the lower levels of MUFA oleic acid in patients than in controls. This association may be mechanistically explained by the biologic balance within families of unsaturated fatty acids (32, 33).

Considering the fatty acid profile described in the literature during the proteinuric phase (26, 27), and the data of this study relating to the remission phase, we can hypothesize that the imbalance of the PUFA n-3/PUFA n-6 ratio reported in the course of proteinuria is a phenomenon that persists even in the course of remission.

Strong points of this work are the homogenous and well-characterized cohort of patients and controls and the novelty of information about a so far scarcely investigated aspect of INS, with possible implications for the management of the disease.

A few limitations should also be recognized. First, the lack of direct measurement either of fatty acid metabolites or of the real enzymatic activity, possibly confirming our explanation of the mechanisms underlying fatty acids profile in patients with INS, otherwise based on the estimated product to precursor ratio. Second, the fact that the dietary record, as regards fatty acids intake, was performed only in 10 INS patients and 10 healthy controls, but the risk of potential inequality in fatty acids dietary intake in the two groups is low, considering that patients with INS on stable remission had no diet limitation and they came from the same geographical area as that of healthy, matched controls. The third limit is the absence of patients' fatty acids profile during relapse, that could help in better evaluating the fatty acids changes during remission, but this would imply longitudinal data, which were not available in all our patients. Also the absence in our series of infrequent relapser patients on full remission without immunosuppressive agents can be seen as a limit of our study, since their fatty acid profile might be similar to controls and serve as a proof of concept of the role of fatty acids as candidate biomarkers for a risk of relapse in children with INS.

In conclusion, our results suggest that patients with INS in stable remission could not be considered "healed," if they still show an abnormal fatty acid profile compared to that of healthy subjects. Persistently higher than normal levels of either linoleic or arachidonic acid, could be viewed as candidate biomarker for a state of risk of relapse in children with idiopathic nephrotic syndrome.

ETHICS STATEMENT

Ethical review and approval was not required for the study on human participants in accordance with the local legislation and institutional requirements. Written informed consent to participate in this study was provided by the participants' legal guardian/next of kin.

AUTHOR CONTRIBUTIONS

Material preparation, data collection, and analysis were performed by ST and M-LS. CT, ED, and AB selected and screened the subjects cohort. VD analyzed the dietary data. The first draft of the manuscript was written by ST. Manuscript was reviewed and edited by AE, LG, and WM. CA, GMa, and GMo critically revised the article and supervision. All authors contributed to the study conception and design, commented on previous versions of the manuscript, read, and approved the final manuscript.

REFERENCES

1. Noone DG, Iijima K, Parekh R. Idiopathic nephrotic syndrome in children. *Lancet*. (2018) 392:61–74. doi: 10.1016/S0140-6736(18)30536-1
2. Chanchlani R, Parekh RS. Ethnic differences in childhood nephrotic syndrome. *Front Pediatr*. (2016) 4:39. doi: 10.3389/fped.2016.00039
3. Pasini A, Benetti E, Conti G, Ghio L, Lepore M, Massella L, et al. The Italian Society for Pediatric Nephrology (SINePe) consensus document on the management of nephrotic syndrome in children: part I–diagnosis and treatment of the first episode and the first relapse. *Ital J Pediatr*. (2017) 43:41. doi: 10.1186/s13052-017-0356-x
4. Ariceta G. Clinical practice: proteinuria. *Eur J Pediatr*. (2011) 170:15–20. doi: 10.1007/s00431-010-1334-0

5. D'Agati VD, Kaskel FJ, Falk RJ. Focal segmental glomerulosclerosis. *N Engl J Med.* (2011) 365:2398–411. doi: 10.1056/NEJMra1106556
6. Vivarelli M, Massella L, Ruggiero B, Emma F. Minimal change disease. *Clin J Am Soc Nephrol.* (2017) 12:332–45. doi: 10.2215/CJN.05000516
7. Kallash M, Smoyer WE, Mahan JD. Rituximab use in the management of childhood nephrotic syndrome. *Front Pediatr.* (2019) 7:178. doi: 10.3389/fped.2019.00178
8. Stone H, Magella B, Bennett MR. The search for biomarkers to aid in diagnosis, differentiation, and prognosis of childhood idiopathic nephrotic syndrome. *Front Pediatr.* (2019) 7:404. doi: 10.3389/fped.2019.00404
9. Candelier JJ, Lorenzo HK. Idiopathic nephrotic syndrome and serum permeability factors: a molecular jigsaw puzzle. *Cell Tissue Res.* (2020) 379:231–43. doi: 10.1007/s00441-019-03147-y
10. Ling C, Wang X, Chen Z, Fan J, Meng Q, Zhou N, et al. Altered B-lymphocyte homeostasis in idiopathic nephrotic syndrome. *Front Pediatr.* (2019) 7:377. doi: 10.3389/fped.2019.00377
11. Cortvrindt C, Speeckaert R, Moerman A, Delanghe JR, Speeckaert MM. The role of interleukin-17A in the pathogenesis of kidney diseases. *Pathology.* (2017) 49:247–58. doi: 10.1016/j.pathol.2017.01.003
12. Shostak E, Krause I, Dagan A, Ben-Dor A, Keidar M, Davidovits M. Is serum CRP level a reliable inflammatory marker in pediatric nephrotic syndrome? *Pediatr Nephrol.* (2016) 31:1287–93. doi: 10.1007/s00467-016-3328-2
13. Guimarães F, Melo G, Cordeiro TM, Feracin V, Vieira ER, Pereira WF, et al. T-lymphocyte-expressing inflammatory cytokines underlie persistence of proteinuria in children with idiopathic nephrotic syndrome. *J Pediatr.* (2018) 94:546–53. doi: 10.1016/j.jped.2017.08.005
14. Jamin A, Dehoux L, Dossier C, Fila M, Heming N, Monteiro RC, et al. Toll-like receptor 3 expression and function in childhood idiopathic nephrotic syndrome. *Clin Exp Immunol.* (2015) 182:332–45. doi: 10.1111/cei.12659
15. Kim OY, Lee SM, An WS. Impact of blood or erythrocyte membrane fatty acids for disease risk prediction: focusing on cardiovascular disease and chronic kidney disease. *Nutrients.* (2018) 10:1454. doi: 10.3390/nu10101454
16. Marklund M, Wu J, Imamura F, Del Gobbo LC, Fretts A, de Goede J, et al. Biomarkers of dietary omega-6 fatty acids and incident cardiovascular disease and mortality. *Circulation.* (2019) 139:2422–36. doi: 10.1161/CIRCULATIONAHA.118.038908
17. Calder PC. Omega-3 fatty acids and inflammatory processes: from molecules to man. *Biochem Soc Trans.* (2017) 45:1105–15. doi: 10.1042/BST20160474
18. Brash AR. Arachidonic acid as a bioactive molecule. *J Clin Investig.* (2001) 107:1339–45. doi: 10.1172/JCI13210
19. Wei J, Gronert K. Eicosanoid and specialized proresolving mediator regulation of lymphoid cells. *Trends Biochem Sci.* (2019) 44:214–25. doi: 10.1016/j.tibs.2018.10.007
20. Hanna VS, Hafez E. Synopsis of arachidonic acid metabolism: a review. *J Adv Res.* (2018) 11:23–32. doi: 10.1016/j.jare.2018.03.005
21. Wang T, Fu X, Chen Q, Patra JK, Wang D, Wang Z, et al. Arachidonic acid metabolism and kidney inflammation. *Int J Mol Sci.* (2019) 20:3683. doi: 10.3390/ijms20153683
22. Echeverría F, Valenzuela R, Catalina Hernandez-Rodas M, Valenzuela A. Docosahexaenoic acid (DHA), a fundamental fatty acid for the brain: new dietary sources. *Prostaglandins Leukot Essent Fatty Acids.* (2017) 124:1–10. doi: 10.1016/j.plefa.2017.08.001
23. Koletzko B, Agostoni C, Bergmann R, Ritzenthaler K, Shamir R. Physiological aspects of human milk lipids and implications for infant feeding: a workshop report. *Acta Paediatr.* (2011) 100:1405–15. doi: 10.1111/j.1651-2227.2011.02343.x
24. Bennett M, Gilroy DW. Lipid mediators in inflammation. *Microbiol Spectr.* (2016) 4:10.1128/microbiolspec.MCHD-0035-2016. doi: 10.1128/microbiolspec.MCHD-0035-2016
25. Turolo S, Edefonti A, Syren ML, Marangoni F, Morello W, Agostoni C, et al. Fatty acids in nephrotic syndrome and chronic kidney disease. *J Renal Nutr.* (2018) 28:145–55. doi: 10.1053/j.jrn.2017.08.005
26. Das UN, Mohan IK, Raju TR. Effect of corticosteroids and eicosapentaenoic acid/docosahexaenoic acid on pro-oxidant and anti-oxidant status and metabolism of essential fatty acids in patients with glomerular disorders. *Prostaglandins Leukot Essent Fatty Acids.* (2001) 65:197–203. doi: 10.1054/plef.2001.0311
27. Aldámiz-Echevarría L, Vallo A, Aguirre M, Sanjurjo P, Gonzalez-Lamuño D, Elorz J, et al. Essential fatty acid deficiency profile in patients with nephrotic-range proteinuria. *Pediatr Nephrol.* (2007) 22:533–40. doi: 10.1007/s00467-006-0366-1
28. Ardissino G, Testa S, Daccò V, Viganò S, Taioli E, Claris-Appiani A, et al. Proteinuria as a predictor of disease progression in children with hypodysplastic nephropathy. Data from the Ital Kid Project. *Pediatr Nephrol.* (2004) 19:172–7. doi: 10.1007/s00467-003-1268-0
29. Marangoni F, Colombo C, Martiello A, Negri E, Galli C. The fatty acid profiles in a drop of blood from a fingertip correlate with physiological, dietary and lifestyle parameters in volunteers. *Prostaglandins Leukot Essent Fatty Acids.* (2007) 76:87–92. doi: 10.1016/j.plefa.2006.11.004
30. Marklund M, Morris AP, Mahajan A, Ingelsson E, Lindgren CM, Lind L, et al. Genome-wide association studies of estimated fatty acid desaturase activity in serum and adipose tissue in elderly individuals: associations with insulin sensitivity. *Nutrients.* (2018) 10:1791. doi: 10.3390/nu10111791
31. Høstmark AT, Haug A. The inverse association between relative abundances of oleic acid and arachidonic acid: a case of distribution dependent regulation? *Lipids Health Dis.* (2019) 18:123. doi: 10.1186/s12944-019-1067-7
32. Høstmark AT, Haug A. The inverse association between relative abundances of oleic acid and arachidonic acid is related to alpha-linolenic acid. *Lipids Health Dis.* (2014) 13:76. doi: 10.1186/1476-511X-13-76
33. Hayashi S, Satoh Y, Ogasawara Y, Dairi T. Recent advances in functional analysis of polyunsaturated fatty acid synthases. *Curr Opin Chem Biol.* (2020) 59:30–6. doi: 10.1016/j.cbpa.2020.04.015

24

A Novel Heterozygous Mutation of *CD2AP* in a Chinese Family with Proteinuria Leads to Focal Segmental Glomerulosclerosis

Yu-Xing Liu [1,2,3,4†], *Ai-Qian Zhang* [1†], *Fang-Mei Luo* [2,3], *Yue Sheng* [2,3], *Chen-Yu Wang* [2,3], *Yi Dong* [2,3], *Liangliang Fan* [1,2,3,4] *and Lv Liu* [4*]

[1] *Department of Obstetrics and Gynecology, The Third Xiangya Hospital of Central South University, Changsha, China,* [2] *Department of Cell Biology, The School of Life Sciences, Central South University, Changsha, China,* [3] *Hunan Key Laboratory of Animal for Human Disease, School of Life Sciences, Central South University, Changsha, China,* [4] *Department of Respiratory Medicine, Diagnosis and Treatment Center of Respiratory Disease, The Second Xiangya Hospital of Central South University, Changsha, China*

***Correspondence:**
Lv Liu
docliulv@csu.edu.cn

These authors have contributed equally to this work

Idiopathic focal segmental glomerulosclerosis (FSGS) is a relatively frequent kidney disorder that manifest clinically as proteinuria and progressive loss of renal function. Genetic factors play a dominant role in the occurrence of FSGS. CD2-associated protein (CD2AP) is an adapter molecule and is essential for the slit-diaphragm assembly and function. Mutations in the *CD2AP* gene can contribute to FSGS development. Here, we describe a Chinese family of four generations with unexplained proteinuria. The proband, a 12-year-old boy, was diagnosed as FSGS. Whole-exome sequencing (WES) revealed an unknown frameshift insertion mutation (p.K579Efs*7) of *CD2AP* gene that leads to a truncation of CD2AP protein. Bioinformatics strategies predicted that the novel mutation was pathogenic. The mutation was absent in either healthy family members or our 200 healthy controls. In summary, we used WES to explore the genetic lesion of FSGS patients and identified a novel mutation in *CD2AP* gene. This work broadens the mutation spectrum of *CD2AP* gene and provides data for genetic counseling to additional FSGS patients.

Keywords: FSGS, CD2AP, mutation, heterozygote, whole-exome sequencing

INTRODUCTION

Idiopathic focal segmental glomerulosclerosis (FSGS) is a relatively frequent kidney disorder that manifests clinically as proteinuria and progressive deterioration of renal function. FSGS is histologically characterized by focal and segmental glomerular sclerosis and foot-process effacement (1). As a leading cause of steroid-resistant nephrotic syndrome (SRNS), FSGS makes up about three quarters of the SRNS in children and adults and frequently leads to end-stage renal disease (2).

Genetic factors play a dominant role in the occurrence and development of FSGS. As a kind of podocytopathy, many FSGS-causing genes have been identified and are mainly expressed in glomerular podocytes. The proteins encoded by these genes are crucial for the maintenance of podocyte structure and function, including protein assembly of glomerular basement membrane (GBM) and podocyte skeleton (1). Over the past decades, at least 60 genes have been linked to

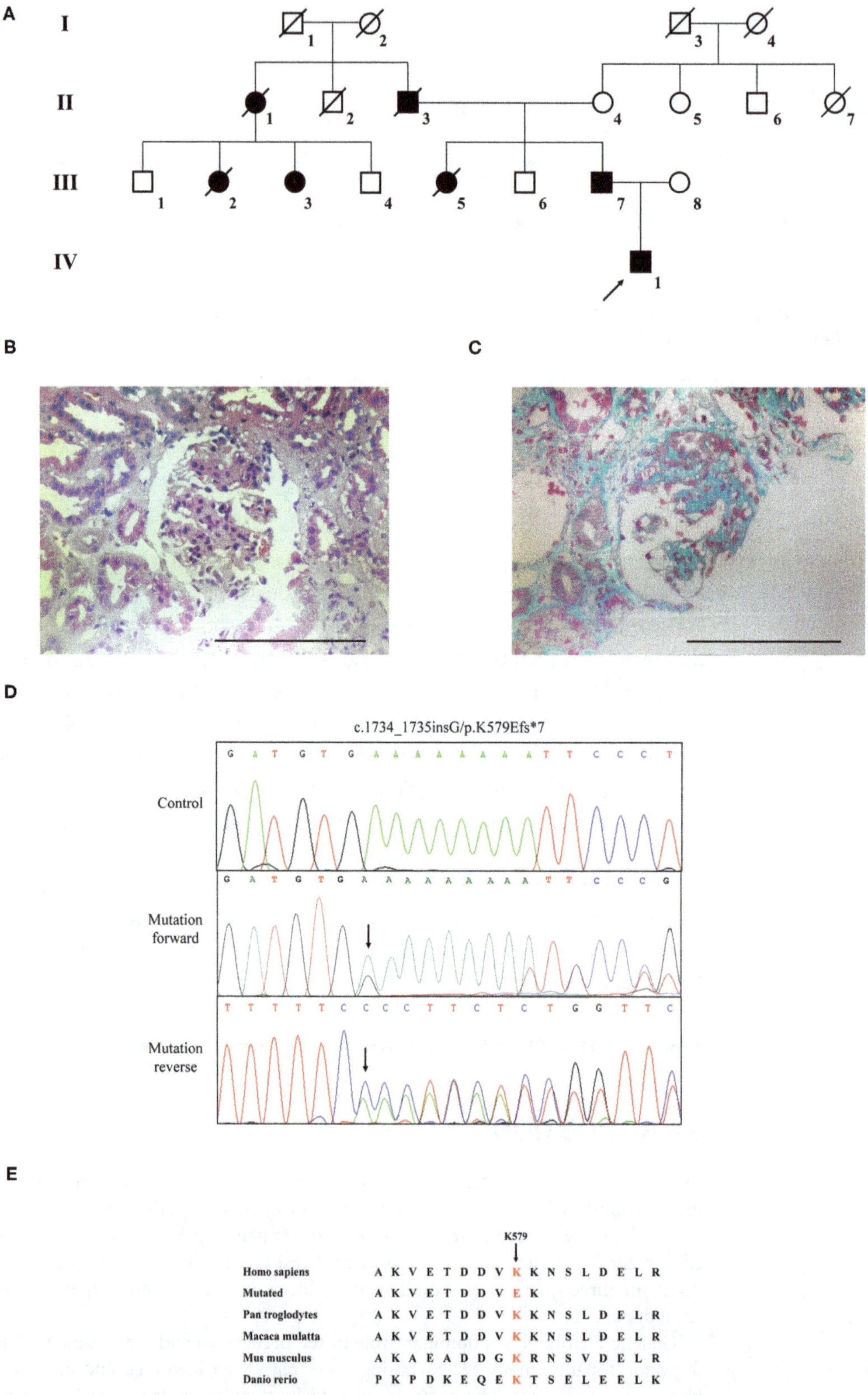

FIGURE 1 | The clinic and sequencing data of this FSGS family. **(A)** The pedigree of this FSGS family. Squares indicate male family members; circles, female members; black symbols, the affected members; white symbols, unaffected members; arrow, proband. **(B)** HE staining **(C)** Masson staining for renal biopsy of the proband (IV-1). **(D)** Sanger DNA sequencing chromatogram demonstrates a heterozygosity mutation (c.1734_1735insG/p.K579Efs*7) of *CD2AP* gene in affected members. **(E)** Alignment of multiple CD2AP protein sequences across species. Letters in red show the K579 site is evolutionarily conserved.

TABLE 1 | Clinical data of three patients in this family.

Subjects	IV-1 (proband)	III-3	III-7	Normal
Sex	M	F	M	/
Age (years)	12	49	40	/
Microscopic hematuria	1+	-	-	-
Proteinuria	2+	1+	1+	-
Uraemia	No	No	No	/
Blood creatinine (μmol/L)	149.0	128.3	168.5	M:<106; F:<86
Blood urea nitrogen (mmol/L)	8.81	11.04	8.52	1.8-7.1
Uric acid (μmol/L)	478.6	520.5	444.3	M:149-416; F:<89-357

F, female; M, male.

SRNS (3). Among them, ~20 pathogenic genes have been identified in FSGS patients (4). Genes such as collagen α3-5 (*COL4A3-5*), anillin actin binding protein (*ANLN*), inverted formin 2 (*INF2*), paired box 2 (*PAX2*), transient receptor potential cation channel 6 (*TRPC6*), α-actinin-4 (*ACTN4*), and podocin (*NPHS2*) show a higher mutation rate in FSGS patients (5–10). Moreover, mutations of CD2 associated protein (*CD2AP*) and Rho GTPase activating protein 24 (*ARHGAP24*) can also contribute to FSGS development (11, 12). With the development of sequencing technology, more causative genes, such as IFT139 (*TTC21B*), LIM homeobox transcription factor 1β (*LMX1B*), Integrin subunit β4 (*ITGB4*), and Nuclear RNA export factor 5 (*NXF5*), were found in rare FSGS (13–15). On account of high genetic heterogeneity and complicated hereditary constitution, the genetic etiology of primary FSGS remains obscure in many cases.

Herein, we investigate a Chinese family with unexplained proteinuria. The proband was diagnosed as FSGS. Using whole-exome sequencing (WES) technology in combined with bioinformatics strategies, we detected a previously unreported heterozygous mutation in *CD2AP*.

CASE PRESENTATION

Clinical Features

The Chinese family with four generations including 13 persons was described in this research (**Figure 1A**). Three living cases (IV1, III-3, and III-7) among the seven patients were enrolled in this family. Two hundred unrelated healthy subjects were collected as control subjects to exclude polymorphisms. The information of the healthy controls group has been provided in our previous study (16).

The proband (IV1) was a 12-year-old boy from Hunan Province in China. He visited our hospital because of an abnormal urine test. Physical examination showed lower extremity edema and hypertension. Laboratory examination showed high proteinuria (2+), high serum creatinine (149 μmol/L), blood urea nitrogen (8.81 mmol/L), and uric acid (478.6 μmol/L). Microscopic urine analysis indicated microscopic hematuria (1+). Since persistent proteinuria after 6 weeks of prednisone treatment (60 mg/m^2/day), the patient was considered as steroid resistant. Renal biopsy was carried out and revealed glomerulomegaly, segmental podocytes proliferation, and hypertrophic. The GBM characterized segmental thickening. Masson staining mesangial area showed mesophilic deposition (**Figures 1B,C**). Thus, the patient was diagnosed as FSGS. Family history survey showed his father (III-7) also suffered from proteinuria. One aunt (III-3) investigated proteinuria and had a similar 3-year history of lower extremity edema and high blood pressure. The proband's mother refused further medical examination because of divorce. The relevant clinical data of the patients in this family are provided in **Table 1**.

Genetic Analysis

WES yielded 9.13 Gb of data with 99.7% coverage of the target region and 99.1% of the target covered over 10×. In total, about 4,995 variants were detected in the proband. Data filtering were performed as our previous study (17). A set of 11 variants in 11 genes were detected (**Table 2**) and were further analyzed. Information including the inheritance pattern, OMIM clinical phenotypes, Toppgene function (18), and American College of Medical Genetics Classification (19) of these 11 genes has been shown in **Table 2**. No variants in other known FSGS-related genes were detected. Sanger sequencing was carried out in all family members. Co-segregation analysis shown that only a previously not described heterozygous mutation (c.1734_1735insG/p.K579Efs*7) in exon 16 of the *CD2AP* gene was observed in all three affected patients (III-3, III7, and IV-1) and excluded in the healthy members (**Figure 1D**). Family screening showed that the frameshift mutation was inherited *via* the paternal allele (**Figure 1A**). The newly identified mutation was absent in our 200 healthy controls. Alignment of CD2AP amino acid sequences revealed the affected amino acid was evolutionarily conserved (**Figure 1E**). In addition, Swiss-Model software (https://swissmodel.expasy.org/interactive) was utilized to explore the spatial configuration of this CD2AP mutation. As the results showed, a loss of almost all of the C-terminal in the K579Efs*7 mutated CD2AP protein was observed, in comparison with the wild type, as marked by the red frame in the figure (**Figure 2A**).

DISCUSSION

In the current research, we described a Chinese family with unexplained proteinuria. The proband was diagnosed as FSGS. Employing WES combined with bioinformatics strategies, a newly heterozygous mutation (p.K579Efs*7) of the *CD2AP* gene was detected. The frameshift mutation (p.K579Efs*7) locates in the exon 16 that alters the lysine codon at position 579 to a glutamic codon, and is expected to form a premature stop codon, leading to a truncated protein. Sanger sequencing confirmed that all 3 affected members in this FSGS family, including the proband's father (III-7) and his aunt (III-3), harbored the heterozygous frameshift mutation in *CD2AP*. The late patients' DNA was not available. Moreover, this heterozygous variant did not exist in the remaining unaffected family members. Given the segregation of the frameshift mutation with the disease phenotype and the degree of protein structure alteration, it was

TABLE 2 | Variants identified by WES in this family.

Gene	Transcript variant	Protein variant	SIFT	Polyphen-2	Mutationtaster	GnomAD	OMIM clinical phenotype	ToppGene function	American college of medical genetics classification
SLC28A1	NM_004213.4; c.1-16C>G	-	-	-	D	0.0189213	AR, uridine-cytidineuria	Purine nucleobase transport	pvs1, pm3, pp3
NEUROD1	NM_002500.4; c.34G>C	p.G12R	T	B	D	0.0015766	AD, type 2 diabetes mellitus	Pancreatic A cell fate commitment	ps1, pm2
TGM6	NM_198994.2; c.1171G>A	p.V391M	D	B	D	0.0096227	AD, spinocerebellar ataxia	Peptide cross-linking	ps1, pm1, pp3
CIDEC	NM_022094.3; c.457C>T	p.Q153*	-	-	D	-	AR, lipodystrophy	Lipid droplet organization	pvs1, pm1, pm2
TREM2	NM_018965.3; c.574G>A	p.A192T	T	B	P	0.000435114	AR, Polycystic lipomembranous osteodysplasia with sclerosing leukoencephalopathy	C-C chemokine receptor CCR7 signaling pathway	ps1, pm2, bp4
HOXA10	NM_018951.3; c.170A>G	p.Y57C	T	D	D	0.00121275	-	Proximal/distal pattern formation	ps1, pm2
CFTR	NM_000492.3; c.1666A>G	p.I556V	T	B	D	0.0471606	AR, Cystic fibrosis	Regulation of cyclic nucleotide-gated ion channel activity	ps1, pm1
PYGM	NM_005609.3; c.1860del	p.I621Sfs*37	-	-	D	-	AR, McArdle disease	Glucan catabolic process	pvs1, pm2
MCTP2	NM_018349.3; c.239del	p.S80Tfs*17	-	-	D	0.00364805	-	Calcium-dependent phospholipid binding	pvs1, pm2
XIRP2	NM_152381.5; c.3318_3319del	p.Y1107*	-	-	D	-	-	Muscle tissue morphogenesis	pvs1, pm2
CD2AP	NM_012120.2; c.1734dup	p.K579Efs*7	-	-	D	-	AD, Glomerulosclerosis, focal segmental	Transforming growth factor beta1 production	pvs1, pm2

B, begin; D, disease-causing; P, polymorphism; T, tolerated; AD, autosomal dominant; AR, autosomal recessive; bp, pathogenic benign; pp, pathogenic supporting; ps, pathogenic strong; pvs, pathogenic very strong; pm, pathogenic moderate.

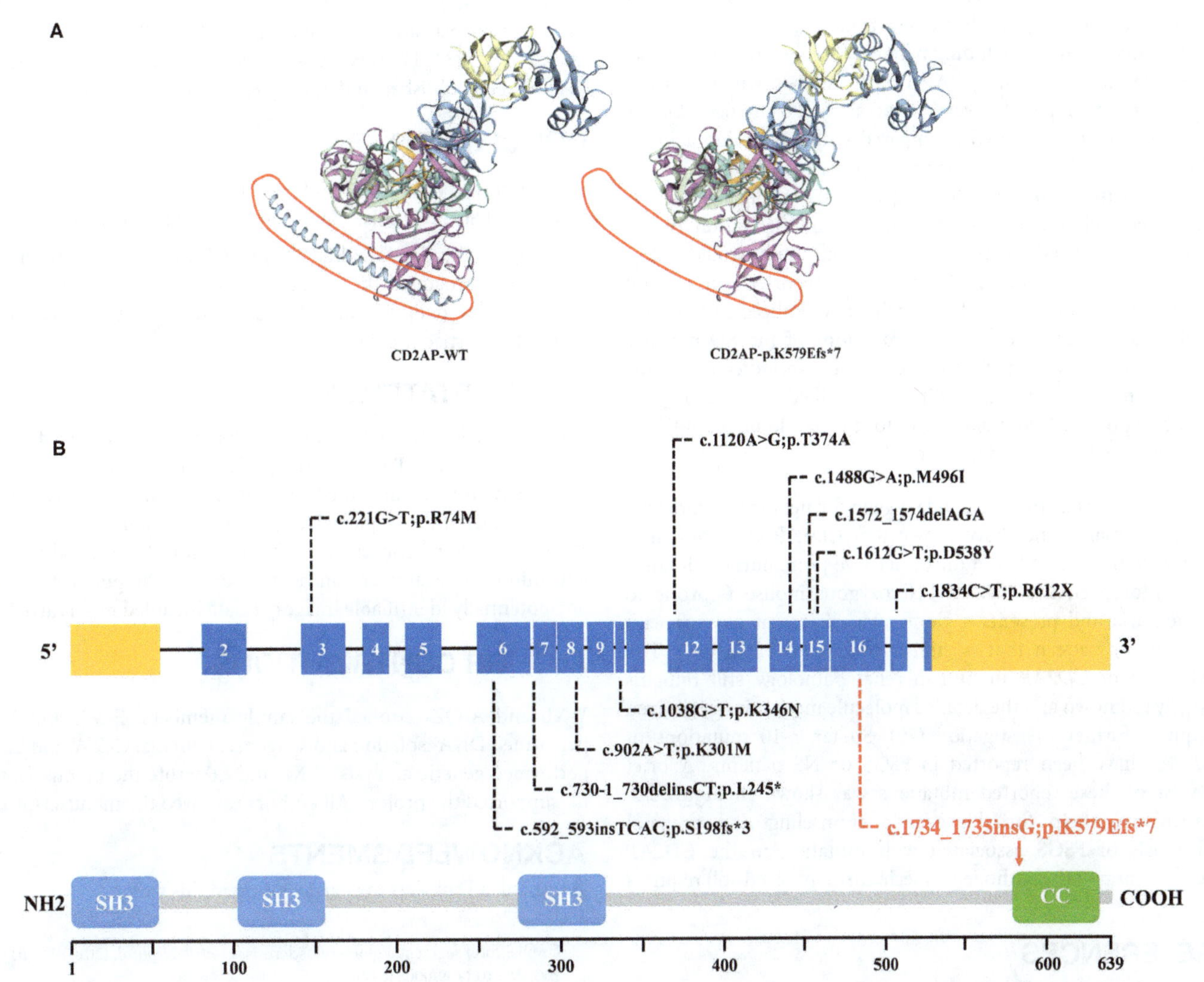

FIGURE 2 | The bioinformatics analysis of mutations. **(A)** Structure prediction of the mutant protein. The wild type CD2AP (CD2AP-WT) protein structure and the p.K579Efs*7 mutant CD2AP (CD2AP-p.K579Efs*7) protein structure were predicted by SWISS-MODEL online software. **(B)** Overview of all known and novel CD2AP mutations. The *CD2AP* gene is shown, with all known *CD2AP* mutations (black letters) and novel mutation (red letters). Blue rectangles indicate exons. Introns are not shown to scale. The CD2AP protein structure is shown. CC, coiled-coil domain; SH3, Src homology 3 domain.

highly considered that the mutation was responsible for the FSGS in this family.

FSGS is clinically characterized by proteinuria and progressive renal failure (1). In our study, all living patients (III-3, III7, and IV-1) in this family presented proteinuria, but definitive data on progression to end-stage renal failure were not available. In a previous report, Gigante et al. screened for changes in the *CD2AP* gene in a total of 80 Italian patients with idiopathic nephrotic syndrome. Three heterozygous mutations in *CD2AP* gene were found in three unrelated patients while there were no definitive data on renal failure in the reported patients (20). For the different molecular and pathogenesis bases of genetically associated FSGS and SRNS, the manifestation and prognosis are different (1). Thus, the genotype-phenotype relation between *CD2AP* gene and FSGS needs to be further investigated. Since most FSGS/SRNS patients with genetic factors do not respond to common treatment and show poor prognosis (1), the patients in this family were given the cyclosporine treatment according to the KDIGO 2012 guideline (21). And a follow-up visit has been scheduled in a few months to ensure the patients benefit from treatment.

CD2AP is prominently expressed in glomerular podocytes. It is an 80 kDa cytoplasmic protein which consists of four domains: three Src homology 3 (SH3) domains at the NH2 terminus and one coiled-coil domain at the COOH terminus (22). CD2AP was initially identified as a ligand for the T-cell-adhesion protein CD2. And it was also shown to bind to nephrin and podocin, thereby acting as an important component of the slit-diaphragm (SD) network (23). The three SH3 domains are essential for the interaction of CD2AP protein with CD2 (20). Recent reports exploring that phosphorylation of tyrosine residues within the SH3-1 domain may modify interactions between CD2AP and its binding partners, including nephrin (24). Furthermore, it has been demonstrated that CD2AP directly interacts with nephrin at the C-terminal region between amino acids 428 and 600 (25, 26). As shown in **Figures 2A,B**, compared with 639 amino acids in the wild type, the resulting truncated protein is 580 amino acids in length with an abnormal binding domain of nephrin, and lacks the coiled-coil domain that promotes homodimerization. In this case, the truncated CD2AP protein in our study would fail to bind to nephrin. Similarly, Gigante et al. reported a frameshift mutation (p.delE525) in *CD2AP*, which is localized in the same region, affects the ultrafiltration functions of the SD network and might lead to proteinuria (20). Thus, we indicate that the frameshift mutation (p.K579Efs*7) identified in *CD2AP* gene may be a potential candidate factor for the development of FSGS, consistent with the previous research.

CD2AP was a strong candidate gene for nephrotic syndrome (NS). Animal studies have shown that *CD2AP* knockout mice suffer from severe NS and die of massive proteinuria in infancy (27). Moreover, the *CD2AP* heterozygous mouse is prone to proteinuria and presents a glomerular disease at old age with a histology pattern that is similar to human FSGS (28). The relevance of *CD2AP* in human renal pathology still remains largely unknown and the detailed molecule mechanisms involved requires further investigation (20). So far, ~10 mutations of *CD2AP* have been reported in FSGS or NS patients. A brief review of these reported mutations was shown in **Figure 2B** which may help for the genetic counseling and prenatal diagnosis of FSGS associated with mutation in the *CD2AP* gene. Although the pathogenic mechanism involved still requires further investigation, our findings offer more evidence that *CD2AP* gene variant is significant in FSGS. Remarkably, the mutation (c.1734_1735insG/p.K579Efs*7) identified in this study has not been published and, therefore, is considered novel.

CONCLUSION

We applied WES to explore the genetic lesion in a Chinese FSGS family. A novel heterozygous mutation (c.1734_1735insG/p.K579Efs*7) of *CD2AP* was identified. Our study broadens the mutation spectrum of *CD2AP* gene and provides data for the clinical management and genetic counseling respect to FSGS.

ETHICS STATEMENT

The studies involving human participants were reviewed and approved by the Third Xiangya Hospital of Central South University. Written informed consent to participate in this study was provided by the participants' legal guardian/next of kin. Written informed consent was obtained from the individual(s), and minor(s)' legal guardian/next of kin, for the publication of any potentially identifiable images or data included in this article.

AUTHOR CONTRIBUTIONS

Y-XL and A-QZ enrolled the family members. F-ML and YS performed DNA isolation and sanger sequencing. C-YW and YD performed genetic analysis. Y-XL and LF wrote the manuscript. LL supported the project. All authors reviewed the manuscript.

ACKNOWLEDGMENTS

We thank all subjects for participating in this study.

REFERENCES

1. Liu J, Wang W. Genetic basis of adult-onset nephrotic syndrome and focal segmental glomerulosclerosis. *Front Med.* (2017) 11:333–9. doi: 10.1007/s11684-017-0564-1
2. Lowik M, Levtchenko E, Westra D, Groenen P, Steenbergen E, Weening J, et al. Bigenic heterozygosity and the development of steroid-resistant focal segmental glomerulosclerosis. *Nephrol Dial Transplant.* (2008) 23:3146–51. doi: 10.1093/ndt/gfn208
3. Saleem MA. Molecular stratification of idiopathic nephrotic syndrome. *Nat Rev Nephrol.* (2019) 15:750–65. doi: 10.1038/s41581-019-0217-5
4. Fan LL, Liu L, Luo FM, Du R, Wang CY, Dong Y, et al. A novel heterozygous variant of the COL4A4 gene in a Chinese family with hematuria and proteinuria leads to focal segmental glomerulosclerosis and chronic kidney disease. *Mol Genet Genomic Med.* (2020) 8:e1545. doi: 10.1002/mgg3.1545
5. Gast C, Pengelly RJ, Lyon M, Bunyan DJ, Seaby EG, Graham N, et al. Collagen (COL4A) mutations are the most frequent mutations underlying adult focal segmental glomerulosclerosis. *Nephrol Dial Transplant.* (2016) 31:961–70. doi: 10.1093/ndt/gfv325
6. Xie J, Hao X, Azeloglu EU, Ren H, Wang Z, Ma J, et al. Novel mutations in the inverted formin 2 gene of Chinese families contribute to focal segmental glomerulosclerosis. *Kidney Int.* (2015) 88:593–604. doi: 10.1038/ki.2015.106
7. Barua M, Stellacci E, Stella L, Weins A, Genovese G, Muto V, et al. Mutations in PAX2 associate with adult-onset FSGS. *J Am Soc Nephrol.* (2014) 25:1942–53. doi: 10.1681/ASN.2013070686
8. Zhang Q, Ma J, Xie J, Wang Z, Zhu B, Hao X, et al. Screening of ACTN4 and TRPC6 mutations in a Chinese cohort of patients with adult-onset familial focal segmental glomerulosclerosis. *Contrib Nephrol.* (2013) 181:91–100. doi: 10.1159/000348471
9. Gbadegesin RA, Hall G, Adeyemo A, Hanke N, Tossidou I, Burchette J, et al. Mutations in the gene that encodes the F-actin binding protein anillin cause FSGS. *J Am Soc Nephrol.* (2014) 25:1991–2002. doi: 10.1681/ASN.2013090976
10. He N, Zahirieh A, Mei Y, Lee B, Senthilnathan S, Wong B, et al. Recessive NPHS2 (Podocin) mutations are rare in adult-onset idiopathic focal segmental glomerulosclerosis. *Clin J Am Soc Nephrol.* (2007) 2:31–7. doi: 10.2215/CJN.02690806
11. Lowik MM, Groenen PJ, Pronk I, Lilien MR, Goldschmeding R, Dijkman HB, et al. Focal segmental glomerulosclerosis in a patient homozygous for a CD2AP mutation. *Kidney Int.* (2007) 72:1198–203. doi: 10.1038/sj.ki.5002469
12. Akilesh S, Suleiman H, Yu H, Stander MC, Lavin P, Gbadegesin R, et al. Arhgap24 inactivates Rac1 in mouse podocytes, and a mutant form is associated with familial focal segmental glomerulosclerosis. *J Clin Invest.* (2011) 121:4127–37. doi: 10.1172/JCI46458
13. Esposito T, Lea RA, Maher BH, Moses D, Cox HC, Magliocca S, et al. Unique X-linked familial FSGS with co-segregating heart block disorder is associated with a mutation in the NXF5 gene. *Hum Mol Genet.* (2013) 22:3654–66. doi: 10.1093/hmg/ddt215
14. Huynh CE, Bizet AA, Boyer O, Woerner S, Gribouval O, Filhol E, et al. A homozygous missense mutation in the ciliary gene TTC21B causes familial FSGS. *J Am Soc Nephrol.* (2014) 25:2435–43. doi: 10.1681/ASN.2013101126
15. Boyer O, Woerner S, Yang F, Oakeley EJ, Linghu B, Gribouval O, et al. LMX1B mutations cause hereditary FSGS without extrarenal involvement. *J Am Soc Nephrol.* (2013) 24:1216–22. doi: 10.1681/ASN.2013020171

16. Xiang R, Fan LL, Huang H, Cao BB, Li XP, Peng DQ, et al. A novel mutation of GATA4 (K319E) is responsible for familial atrial septal defect and pulmonary valve stenosis. *Gene.* (2014) 534:320–3. doi: 10.1016/j.gene.2013.10.028
17. Fan LL, Liu JS, Huang H, Du R, Xiang R. Whole exome sequencing identified a novel mutation (p.Ala1884Pro) of beta-spectrin in a Chinese family with hereditary spherocytosis. *J Gene Med.* (2019) 21:e3073. doi: 10.1002/jgm.3073
18. Kaimal V, Bardes EE, Tabar SC, Jegga AG, Aronow BJ. ToppCluster: a multiple gene list feature analyzer for comparative enrichment clustering and network-based dissection of biological systems. *Nucleic Acids Res.* (2010) 38:W96–102. doi: 10.1093/nar/gkq418
19. Richards S, Aziz N, Bale S, Bick D, Das S, Gastier-Foster J, et al. Standards and guidelines for the interpretation of sequence variants: a joint consensus recommendation of the American College of Medical Genetics and Genomics and the Association for Molecular Pathology. *Genet Med.* (2015) 17:405–24. doi: 10.1038/gim.2015.30
20. Gigante M, Pontrelli P, Montemurno E, Roca L, Aucella F, Penza R, et al. CD2AP mutations are associated with sporadic nephrotic syndrome and focal segmental glomerulosclerosis (FSGS). *Nephrol Dial Transplant.* (2009) 24:1858–64. doi: 10.1093/ndt/gfn712
21. Chen YM, Liapis H. Focal segmental glomerulosclerosis: molecular genetics and targeted therapies. *BMC Nephrol.* (2015) 16:101. doi: 10.1186/s12882-015-0090-9
22. Dustin ML, Olszowy MW, Holdorf AD, Li J, Bromley S, Desai N, et al. A novel adaptor protein orchestrates receptor patterning and cytoskeletal polarity in T-cell contacts. *Cell.* (1998) 94:667–77. doi: 10.1016/S0092-8674(00)81608-6
23. Takano T, Bareke E, Takeda N, Aoudjit L, Baldwin C, Pisano P, et al. Recessive mutation in CD2AP causes focal segmental glomerulosclerosis in humans and mice. *Kidney Int.* (2019) 95:57–61. doi: 10.1016/j.kint.2018.08.014
24. Tossidou I, Teng B, Worthmann K, Muller-Deile J, Jobst-Schwan T, Kardinal C, et al. Tyrosine phosphorylation of CD2AP affects stability of the slit diaphragm complex. *J Am Soc Nephrol.* (2019) 30:1220–37. doi: 10.1681/ASN.2018080860
25. Shih NY, Li J, Cotran R, Mundel P, Miner JH, Shaw AS. CD2AP localizes to the slit diaphragm and binds to nephrin *via* a novel C-terminal domain. *Am J Pathol.* (2001) 159:2303–8. doi: 10.1016/S0002-9440(10)63080-5
26. Schwarz K, Simons M, Reiser J, Saleem MA, Faul C, Kriz W, et al. Podocin, a raft-associated component of the glomerular slit diaphragm, interacts with CD2AP and nephrin. *J Clin Invest.* (2001) 108:1621–9. doi: 10.1172/JCI200112849
27. Shih NY, Li J, Karpitskii V, Nguyen A, Dustin ML, Kanagawa O, et al. Congenital nephrotic syndrome in mice lacking CD2-associated protein. *Science.* (1999) 286:312–5. doi: 10.1126/science.286.5438.312
28. Kim JM, Wu H, Green G, Winkler CA, Kopp JB, Miner JH, et al. CD2-associated protein haploinsufficiency is linked to glomerular disease susceptibility. *Science.* (2003) 300:1298–300. doi: 10.1126/science.1081068

25

The Monogenic Familial Steroid-Resistant Nephrotic Syndrome Caused by a Novel Missense Mutation of *NPHS2* Gene A593C in a Chinese Family

Ling Bai [1†], Jing Zhuang [2†], Changrong Zhang [2], Chen Lu [3], Xuefei Tian [4] and Hong Jiang [2*]*

[1] Department of Nephrology and Rheumatology, Children's Hospital of Xinjiang Uygur Autonomous Region, Urumqi, China, [2] Division of Nephrology, Department of Internal Medicine, People's Hospital of Xinjiang Uygur Autonomous Region, Urumqi, China, [3] Division of Nephrology, Department of Internal Medicine, The First Affiliated Hospital of Xinjiang Medical University, Urumqi, China, [4] Section of Nephrology, Department of Internal Medicine, Yale University School of Medicine, New Haven, CT, United States

***Correspondence:**
Xuefei Tian
xuefei.tian@yale.edu
Hong Jiang
jangh-yt@163.com

These authors have contributed equally to this work

Background: Pathogenic variants in the *NPHS2* gene encoding podocin in kidney podocytes are associated with autosomal recessive steroid-resistant nephrotic syndrome (SRNS) by disrupting podocyte function and the integrity of the glomerular filtration barrier. The outcome is generally poor by progressing into end-stage kidney disease (ESKD). With the help of gene diagnostics, we can further understand the role of podocin of podocytes in the development and progression of SRNS. However, the pathological mutation of *NPHS2* and clinical relevance remain further elusive.

Case Presentation: Two siblings, a 15-year-old girl and her 10-year-old younger brother from a consanguineous Chinese family, presented with nephrotic syndrome. Both of them developed progressive proteinuria starting from the 5-year-old of age. The renal pathological lesions for them revealed focal segmental glomerulosclerosis (FSGS). There was no response to the glucocorticoid, calcineurin inhibitors, and rituximab treatment. The female affected patient received the hemodialysis treatment due to ESKD in June 2020; the male patient was still in follow-up presenting with SRNS. The mutational screening of the two patients and their parents using Trio whole-exome sequencing showed the *NPHS2* gene *de novo* missense mutation in exon 5 (A593C), for which the two siblings were homozygous and their parents confirmed heterozygous asymptomatic carriers. No other SRNS-related gene variants with the SRNS were determined.

Conclusion: Pathological gene variants screening in children clinically suspected with SRNS might be helpful in the diagnosis as well as appropriate decisions on treatment strategies and prediction of prognosis.

Keywords: steroid-resistant nephrotic syndrome, mutation, *NPHS2*, genetic testing, focal segmental glomerulosclerosis

INTRODUCTION

Nephrotic syndrome (NS) is a common glomerular disease characterized by massive proteinuria, hypoalbuminemia, hyperlipidemia, and edemas. NS can be classified into hereditary, primary, and secondary types based on their etiologies. Meanwhile, the NS can be clinically divided into two types depending on the response of patients to the steroid therapy, including the steroid-sensitive NS (SSNS) and steroid-resistant NS (SRNS) (1, 2). Podocyte plays a crucial role in maintaining the integrity and stability of the glomerular filtration barrier (3); in children-onset and early adult-onset SRNS, mutation of more than 50 genes in the podocyte have been associated with two-third of these patients, especially nephrin (*NPHS1*), and podocin (*NPHS2*) (4–6). The SRNS is the second most cause leading to end-stage kidney disease (ESKD) in children.

The *NPHS2* (OMIM number 604766) is localized on chromosome 1q25-q31, it was first reported and mapped by linkage analysis in families with autosomal recessive SRNS in 2000, in which 10 different *NPHS2* mutations were identified (7). *NPHS2* comprises of 8 exons and encodes the 42 KD protein podocin with a 383-amino acid in the podocyte (8). Podocin localizes at the slit diaphragm in podocyte and is required for the maintenance of the integrity of the glomerular filtration barrier by interacting with nephrin, CD2AP, and TRPC6 et al., thereby orchestrating the mechanosensation signaling, cytoskeleton organization, and cell survival (9). The mutation of *NPHS2* has been reported to occur in 13% of patients that manifested with SRNS before 25 years of age and accounted for the 34% of all 27 common genes in podocytes causing SRNS (10). To date, many novel *NPHS2* gene mutations have been discovered and more genotype-phenotype correlations have been published, such as deletion c.988_989delCT, c.725C>T, c622G>A and c.928G>A et al. (11–13). With the advent of the latest next gene screening technology and the development of molecular genome database platforms, more and more pathogenic genetic mutations contributing to pediatric SRNS have been identified in recent years (14–16). In this study, we presented a case of two siblings from a consanguineous Chinese family with *NPHS2* mutation, whose renal histology showed focal segmental glomerulosclerosis (FSGS) and had no response to glucocorticoid, calcineurin inhibitors, and rituximab therapy. To the best of our knowledge, this is the first case report of the novel missense mutation of *NPHS2* in exon 5 (A593C) contributing to the SRNS. Our reports may help to further understand the pathogenesis of hereditary glomerulonephropathy caused by *NPHS2* mutation in podocytes, may help the clinicians to choose the proper treatment strategies and genetic and reproductive counseling.

CASE PRESENTATION

A 15-year-old Chinese girl was first diagnosed with proteinuria (2+) during a regular check-up at the age of 5 years old in 2011 but remained untreated until the age of 12 years old in 2018 when she was diagnosed with nephrotic syndrome. The child was transferred to our hospital for further evaluation. There was no abnormal birth and past medical history. Physical examination revealed edema, no skin rash or arthralgia, or gross hematuria. Laboratory studies indicated nephrotic syndrome without hematuria. Blood pressure and serum creatinine levels were normal. Screening of serum and urine from the patient excluded the presence of systemic lupus erythematosus (SLE), antineutrophil cytoplasmic antibody-associated vasculitis (AAV) et al. Since the proteinuria and hypoalbuminemia were resistant to the steroid treatment, prednisone 2 mg/kg per day for 8 weeks, a renal biopsy for her at the age of 12 years old was performed showing FSGS (**Figures 1A,B**). Based on pathological lesion assessment, intravenous methylprednisolone pulse, prednisone plus FK506 (blood trough levels 1.7–2.5 ng/ml), cyclosporine A, and rituximab were administered for 2 years. However, the patient presented persistent nephrotic syndrome and progressive renal failure. At the age of 14 years old in 2020, the patient started on hemodialysis because of ESKD.

Her sibling, a 10-year old Chinese boy, was diagnosed with proteinuria at the age of 5 years old in 2016 during a regular check-up. He was diagnosed with nephrotic syndrome at the age of 8 years old in 2019 and he was admitted to the hospital because of the exacerbating edema in the abdomen. There was no abnormal birth and past medical history. Screening of serum and urine from the patient excluded the presence of SLE, AAV et al. The renal biopsy of the patient at the age of 8 years old was carried out revealing FSGS (**Figures 1C,D**). The proteinuria and hypoalbuminemia were unresponsive to the treatment with prednisone (2 mg/kg per day) and cyclosporin A for 8 weeks, following by the treatment with several pulses of cyclophosphamide and methylprednisone. The patient is presently on non-immunosuppressive antiproteinuric treatment including the optimized renin-angiotensin system (RAS) blockade under the outpatient follow-up, with a relatively stable kidney function determined by serum creatinine (16.5–19.2 μmol/L).

There was a consanguineous family history of father and mother being first cousins for the two siblings, the parents do not present any symptoms of kidney disease.

Because of the SRNS of these two siblings and the consanguineous family history, genetic testing was recommended. All patients and their parents gave their consent for inclusion in this study. Genetic analysis for these two siblings and their parents was carried out by next-generation sequencing (NGS)-based Trio whole-exome sequencing (WES) (Chigene translational medical research center Co. Ltd., Beijing, China). Briefly, genomic DNA was isolated from peripheral blood leukocytes with EDTA as the anticoagulant, sequences of exons were captured using IDT probes (IDT xGen Exome research pane 1 v1.0) and sequenced using NGS sequencer Genome analyzer (NovaSeq 6000, PE150, Illumina). SRNS-related target variants identified by Trio WES were verified by Sanger sequencing (ABI 3730 DNA Analyzer). This revealed a novel missense mutation in exon 5 c.593 A>C (p. E198A) of the *NPHS2* gene, the two siblings were found to be homozygous and their parents were both heterozygous for this mutation. The result of minor allele frequency (MAF) of the *NPHS2* c.593 A>C missense mutation was <0.0005 in the general population, a

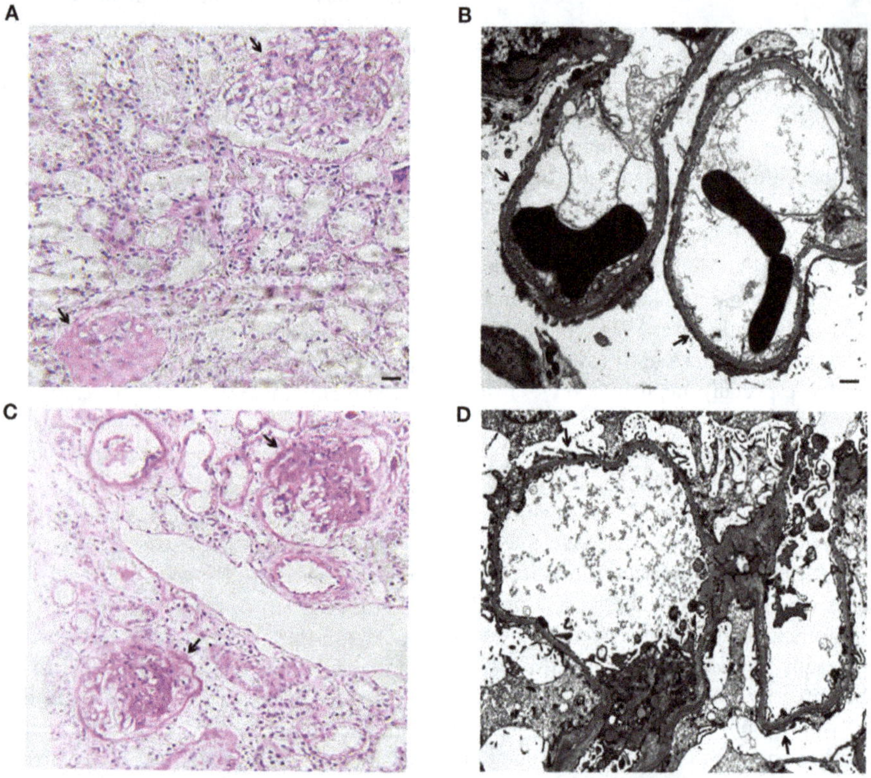

FIGURE 1 | Representative images of light microscopy and transmission electron microscopy (TEM) from the kidney biopsies of the elder sister at age 12 **(A,B)** and the younger brother at age 8 **(C,D)**. **(A)** Global or segmental glomerulosclerosis (arrow) in 23 of 38 glomeruli (Periodic Acid-Schiff staining. Scale bar: 50 μm). Immunofluorescence microscopy revealed negative for IgG, IgA, IgM, C3, C1q, kappa light chain, and lambda light chain in 2 glomeruli. **(B)** Representative TEM showed diffuse foot process effacement of the podocyte (arrow), partial irregularity of the glomerular basement membrane, foam cells, and no subendothelial and mesangial dense deposits (Scale bar: 1 μm). **(C)** Global or segmental glomerulosclerosis (arrow) in 7 of 33 glomeruli (Periodic Acid-Schiff staining. Scale bar: 50 μm). Immunofluorescence microscopy revealed mesangial IgM deposits (++) negative and negative results for IgG, IgA, C3, C1q, kappa light chain, and lambda light chain in 2 glomeruli. **(D)** Representative TEM showed diffuse foot process effacement of the podocyte (arrow), partial irregularity of the glomerular basement membrane, foam cells, and no subendothelial and mesangial dense deposits (Scale bar: 1 μm).

low-frequency mutation; the missense mutation results in the alanine instead of the glutamic acid in the 198th position of the amino acid sequence of the wild-type podocin (NM_014625). The missense mutation was not found in the normal control and was listed as "likely pathogenic" by ACMG (The American College of Medical Genetics and Genomics) 2015 guideline after analyzing the genotype-phenotype associated diseases database and genetic diagnostic platform. Novel missense mutation variants identified in this study were shown in **Figure 2**. The family cosegregation analysis of the phenotype-genotype for these two patients and their parents indicated the autosomal recessive inheritance type.

DISCUSSION

In this study, we described two siblings with SRNS who carried a novel homozygous missense mutation in exon 5 c.593 A>C (p. E198A) in the *NPHS2* gene, which encodes the podocin in the podocyte. No other mutations were found in the *NPHS2* gene or other SRNS-related genes such as *NPHS1*, *WT1*, *FN1*, *KANK2*, *BMP4*, and *PLOD1* et al. Their father and mother carried the same heterozygous missense mutation as the siblings. The parents showed no proteinuria, hematuria, or other abnormalities. It suggests that a missense mutation on both alleles in exon 5 c.593 A>C of the *NPHS2* gene is required for the development and progression of SRNS. The percentage of SNRS attributing to *NPHS2* variants varies from 12.7 to 29.5% (10, 17, 18). The *NPHS2* mutation usually presents the autosomal recessive form of hereditary SRNS, the phenotype is less severe than that of the SRNS caused by the *NPHS1* variants, which is one of the most common mutations resulting in the hereditary podocytopathy in children, and it encodes the nephrin in the podocyte. The onset age of patients with *NPHS1* mutation is at birth to 3 months, while it is later than 3 months at the onset age for the patients with *NPHS2* mutation (10, 19). The two siblings reported here both presented with SRNS and pathological lesions of FSGS, both of them were found proteinuria at 5 years old. Unfortunately, there were no medical records of their urinary analysis results in the past although their parent said that the two siblings were normal in appearance. Both of the two siblings

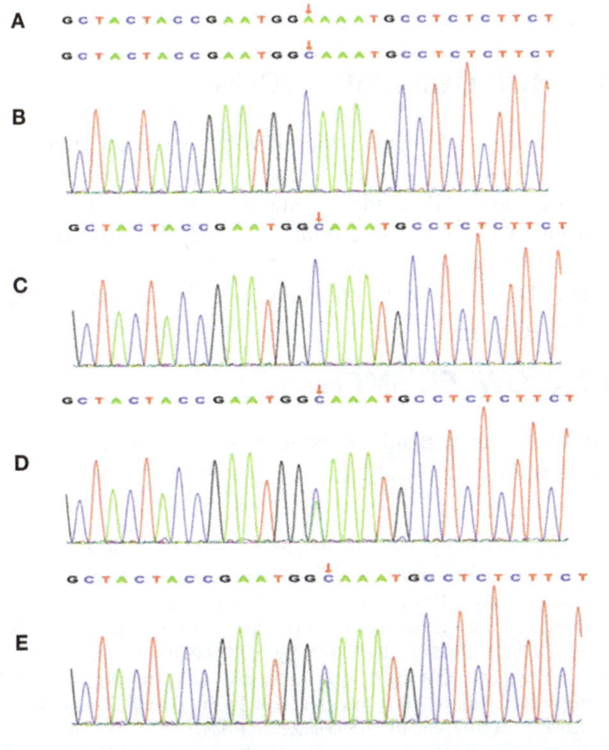

FIGURE 2 | A novel missense mutation in exon 5 (A593C) of the *NPHS2* gene was identified by Trio whole-exome sequencing in the affected individuals and family members. **(A)** normal control sequence. The affected elder sister **(B)** and the affected younger brother **(C)** carried the homozygous missense mutation in exon 5 (A593C) of the *NPHS2* gene. The father **(D)** and the mother **(E)** of the affected patients revealed the heterozygous missense mutation in exon 5 (A593C) of the *NPHS2* gene. The arrows indicate mutant positions.

failed to respond to steroid therapy and immunosuppressive agents, which did not have an impact on the etiological target of hereditary podocytopathy. It is worth noting, the longtime treatment with steroids and immunosuppressive agents causes side effects of drugs and increases the financial burdens to the family. The elder sister was started on hemodialysis at 14 years old due to ESKD, and the younger brother is currently on symptomatic treatment.

The underlying missense mutation of the *NPHS2* gene of patients in our study localized in the exon 5 encoding for the central part of the podocin consisting of 68 amino acids (from 179th amino acid to 246th amino acid), which suggests this area is of major importance for the proper function of podocin (20). Besides this mutation, two variants in exon 5 of the *NPHS2* gene have been reported to cause the SRNS (p.R229Q and p.A242V) in the population of Caucasians and Europeans (2). The c.593 A>C mutation of the *NPHS2* gene results in the alanine instead of the glutamic acid in the 198th position of the amino acid sequence of the podocin. Podocin is a membrane protein that is exclusively located in the slit diaphragm of the podocyte in the kidney (21). Podocin plays a critical role in the stability of the slit diaphragm and the maintenance of the integrity of the glomerular filtration barrier by forming a protein complex through co-localizing with other proteins such as nephrin, CD2-associated protein (CD2AP), zonula occludens-1(ZO-1), and transient receptor potential channel-6 (TRPC-6) et al., that ensure the stable anchorage of the membrane proteins of the slit diaphragm to the actin cytoskeleton in the podocyte (22, 23). These membrane multi-protein complexes localizing on the slit diaphragm in podocytes are capable of regulating the mechanosensation and cell signaling to maintain the integrity of the glomerular filtration barrier (23). The loss of the exon 5-coded central part, an essential component of the prohibitin homology domain, results in the podocin's inability to bind the cholesterol of the inner membrane of the cell (20) and abnormal distribution of podocyte-associated molecules (24). Nephrin is one of the most important components of the slit diaphragm in the podocyte, and nephrin exerts its role as the signal transducer through the phosphorylation of AP-1. The nephrin-activated AP-1 is augmented by podocin which is markedly attenuated by deletion of the prohibitin homology domain of podocin, thereby impairing the function of nephrin in podocytes (24, 25). Intriguingly, how does the replacement of glutamic acid in the 198th position of the amino acid sequence with the alanine lead to a significant loss of podocin function in podocytes, as observed in the family we described in this study, remains to be further determined.

SRNS caused by *NPHS2* mutation is believed to be a recessive inheritance disease requiring a mutation on both alleles coding for podocin, and these patients usually progress to an early onset of ESKD, such as the female patient reported here who started on hemodialysis at the age of 14 years old. Hence, it is very essential to adopt an appropriate therapeutic approach for these patients. Apart from the dialysis, burgeoning evidence has been furnished that renal transplantation may favor ESKD patients with genetic SRNS. In 2020, the results of 101 cases of kidney transplantation in children with SRNS in Italy reported that no disease recurrence was observed in all 41 genetic SRNS including *NPHS2* mutation compared to the idiopathic SRNS (59.5% recurrence) or unknown reasons SRNS patients (43.5% recurrence), during a median follow-up of 58.5 months (26). A cohort study in Germany involving 27 multiplex families (53 patients) and 25 patients with sporadic SRNS due to the *NPHS2* mutation showed these patients who underwent kidney transplantation did not develop recurrence of proteinuria (27). In the meantime, few reports suggested a risk of relapse in the SRNS due to *NPHS2* mutation (28, 29), however. the causative role of the *NPHS2* variants in these reports might be reconsidered with a further in-depth understanding of the pathogenic *NPHS2* variants in the SRNS; no anti-podocin antibodies have been detected in the tested *NPHS2* patients with disease recurrence after kidney transplantation (28, 30); many patients with disease recurrence showed an effective response to immunosuppression treatment (28, 29). The female patient with ESKD in this study has been recommended for kidney transplantation.

In conclusion, this paper reports an SRNS phenotype of familial NS with a pathological lesion of FSGS. Although the exact mechanism remains to be clarified, we offer evidence that the homozygous exon 5c.593 A>C (p. E198A) of the

NPHS2 gene plays a significant role in proper podocin protein function and its pathogenesis. The nephrologists are encouraged to do the genetic testing for these early-onset SRNS patients especially those with a positive family history, as it helps in their right diagnosis, proposes the appropriate therapeutic strategies, predicts the prognosis, and assists genetic and reproductive counseling.

ETHICS STATEMENT

The studies involving human participants were reviewed and approved by Medical Ethics Committee of People's Hospital of Xinjiang Uygur Autonomous Region. Written informed consent to participate in this study was provided by the participants' legal guardian/next of kin. Written informed consent was obtained from the individual(s), and minor(s)' legal guardian/next of kin, for the publication of any potentially identifiable images or data included in this article.

AUTHOR CONTRIBUTIONS

LB, JZ, and HJ made clinical data collection and were actively involved in the clinical care of the patients. XT, CL, and HJ made substantial contributions to the conception of the manuscript. HJ and CZ evaluated the renal pathology of the patients. XT, LB, and HJ drafted and edited the manuscript. All authors read and approved the final manuscript.

ACKNOWLEDGMENTS

We would like to thank the patients and their family for their participation in this study.

REFERENCES

1. Short versus standard prednisone therapy for initial treatment of idiopathic nephrotic syndrome in children. Arbeitsgemeinschaft fur Padiatrische Nephrologie. *Lancet.* (1988) 1:380–3.
2. de Almeida R, da Silva WC, Garbin HI, Itaquy TP, Dos Santos Pereira F, Garcia CD, et al. Prevalence of the NPHS2 variants p.R229Q, p.A242V, and p.R138Q in patients with focal segmental glomerulosclerosis. *Clin Nephrol.* (2020) 94:187–96. doi: 10.5414/CN110178
3. Tian X, Kim JJ, Monkley SM, Gotoh N, Nandez R, Soda K, et al. Podocyte-associated talin1 is critical for glomerular filtration barrier maintenance. *J Clin Inves.t.* (2014) 124:1098–113. doi: 10.1172/JCI69778
4. Kopp JB, Anders HJ, Susztak K, Podesta MA, Remuzzi G, Hildebrandt F, et al. Podocytopathies. *Nat Rev Dis Primers.* (2020) 6:68. doi: 10.1038/s41572-020-0196-7
5. Hinkes B, Vlangos C, Heeringa S, Mucha B, Gbadegesin R, Liu J, et al. Specific podocin mutations correlate with age of onset in steroid-resistant nephrotic syndrome. *J Am Soc Nephrol.* (2008) 19:365–71. doi: 10.1681/ASN.2007040452
6. Hinkes BG, Mucha B, Vlangos CN, Gbadegesin R, Liu J, Hasselbacher K, et al. Nephrotic syndrome in the first year of life: two thirds of cases are caused by mutations in 4 genes (NPHS1, NPHS2, WT1, and LAMB2). *Pediatrics.* (2007) 119:e907–19. doi: 10.1542/peds.2006-2164
7. Boute N, Gribouval O, Roselli S, Benessy F, Lee H, Fuchshuber A, et al. NPHS2, encoding the glomerular protein podocin, is mutated in autosomal recessive steroid-resistant nephrotic syndrome. *Nat Genet.* (2000) 24:349–54. doi: 10.1038/74166
8. Franceschini N, North KE, Kopp JB, McKenzie L, Winkler C. NPHS2 gene, nephrotic syndrome and focal segmental glomerulosclerosis: a HuGE review. *Genet Med.* (2006) 8:63–75. doi: 10.1097/01.gim.0000200947.09626.1c
9. Huber TB, Schermer B, Benzing T. Podocin organizes ion channel-lipid supercomplexes: implications for mechanosensation at the slit diaphragm. *Nephron Exp Nephrol.* (2007) 106:e27–31. doi: 10.1159/000101789
10. Sadowski CE, Lovric S, Ashraf S, Pabst WL, Gee HY, Kohl S, et al. A single-gene cause in 29.5% of cases of steroid-resistant nephrotic syndrome. *J Am Soc Nephrol.* (2015) 26:1279–89. doi: 10.1681/ASN.2014050489
11. Suvanto M, Patrakka J, Jahnukainen T, Sjostrom PM, Nuutinen M, Arikoski P, et al. Novel NPHS2 variant in patients with familial steroid-resistant nephrotic syndrome with early onset, slow progression and dominant inheritance pattern. *Clin Exp Nephrol.* (2017) 21:677–84. doi: 10.1007/s10157-016-1331-3
12. Sun L, Zhang X, Wang Z. NPHS2 gene polymorphism aggravates renal damage caused by focal segmental glomerulosclerosis with COL4A3 mutation. *Biosci Rep.* (2020) 41:BSR20203248. doi: 10.1042/BSR20203248
13. Riguetti MTP, Varela P, Fernandes DE, Polito MG, Casimiro FM, Pesquero JB, et al. Familial focal segmental glomerulosclerosis with late-onset presentation and R229Q/R291W podocin mutations. *Front Genet.* (2020) 11:533373. doi: 10.3389/fgene.2020.533373
14. Wang Y, Dang X, He Q, Zhen Y, He X, Yi Z, et al. Mutation spectrum of genes associated with steroid-resistant nephrotic syndrome in Chinese children. *Gene.* (2017) 625:15–20. doi: 10.1016/j.gene.2017.04.050
15. Sun S, Xu L, Bi Y, Wang J, Zhang Z, Tang X, et al. Early diagnosis of WT1 nephropathy and follow up in a Chinese multicenter cohort. *Eur J Med Genet.* (2020) 63:104047. doi: 10.1016/j.ejmg.2020.104047
16. Song X, Fang X, Tang X, Cao Q, Zhai Y, Chen J, et al. COQ8B nephropathy: early detection and optimal treatment. *Mol Genet Genomic Med.* (2020) 8:e1360. doi: 10.1002/mgg3.1360
17. Guaragna MS, Lutaif AC, Piveta CS, Souza ML, de Souza SR, Henriques TB, et al. NPHS2 mutations account for only 15% of nephrotic syndrome cases. *BMC Med Genet.* (2015) 16:88. doi: 10.1186/s12881-015-0231-9
18. Frishberg Y, Rinat C, Megged O, Shapira E, Feinstein S, Raas-Rothschild A. Mutations in NPHS2 encoding podocin are a prevalent cause of steroid-resistant nephrotic syndrome among Israeli-Arab children. *J Am Soc Nephrol.* (2002) 13:400–5. doi: 10.1681/ASN.V132400
19. Schoeb DS, Chernin G, Heeringa SF, Matejas V, Held S, Vega-Warner V, et al. Nineteen novel NPHS1 mutations in a worldwide cohort of patients with congenital nephrotic syndrome (CNS). *Nephrol Dial Transplant.* (2010) 25:2970–6. doi: 10.1093/ndt/gfq088
20. Relle M, Cash H, Brochhausen C, Strand D, Menke J, Galle PR, et al. New perspectives on the renal slit diaphragm protein podocin. *Mod Pathol.* (2011) 24:1101–10. doi: 10.1038/modpathol.2011.58
21. Tory K, Menyhard DK, Woerner S, Nevo F, Gribouval O, Kerti A, et al. Mutation-dependent recessive inheritance of NPHS2-associated steroid-resistant nephrotic syndrome. *Nat Genet.* (2014) 46:299–304. doi: 10.1038/ng.2898
22. Fukusumi Y, Miyauchi N, Hashimoto T, Saito A, Kawachi H. Therapeutic target for nephrotic syndrome: identification of novel slit diaphragm associated molecules. *World J Nephrol.* (2014) 3:77–84. doi: 10.5527/wjn.v3.i3.77
23. Benzing T. Signaling at the slit diaphragm. *J Am Soc Nephrol.* (2004) 15:1382–91. doi: 10.1097/01.ASN.0000130167.30769.55
24. Huber TB, Simons M, Hartleben B, Sernetz L, Schmidts M, Gundlach E, et al. Molecular basis of the functional podocin-nephrin complex: mutations in the NPHS2 gene disrupt nephrin targeting to lipid raft microdomains. *Hum Mol Genet.* (2003) 12:3397–405. doi: 10.1093/hmg/ddg360
25. Huber TB, Kottgen M, Schilling B, Walz G, Benzing T. Interaction with podocin facilitates nephrin signaling. *J Biol Chem.* (2001) 276:41543–6. doi: 10.1074/jbc.C100452200
26. Morello W, Puvinathan S, Puccio G, Ghiggeri GM, Dello Strologo L, Peruzzi L, et al. Post-transplant recurrence of

steroid resistant nephrotic syndrome in children: the Italian experience. *J Nephrol.* (2020) 33:849–57. doi: 10.1007/s40620-019-00660-9

27. Karle SM, Uetz B, Ronner V, Glaeser L, Hildebrandt F, Fuchshuber A. Novel mutations in NPHS2 detected in both familial and sporadic steroid-resistant nephrotic syndrome. *J Am Soc Nephrol.* (2002) 13:388–93. doi: 10.1681/ASN.V132388
28. Bertelli R, Ginevri F, Caridi G, Dagnino M, Sandrini S, Di Duca M, et al. Recurrence of focal segmental glomerulosclerosis after renal transplantation in patients with mutations of podocin. *Am J Kidney Dis.* (2003) 41:1314–21. doi: 10.1016/S0272-6386(03)00364-0
29. Billing H, Muller D, Ruf R, Lichtenberger A, Hildebrandt F, August C, et al. NPHS2 mutation associated with recurrence of proteinuria after transplantation. *Pediatr Nephrol.* (2004) 19:561–4. doi: 10.1007/s00467-003-1408-6
30. Bierzynska A, Saleem MA. Deriving and understanding the risk of post-transplant recurrence of nephrotic syndrome in the light of current molecular and genetic advances. *Pediatr Nephrol.* (2018) 33:2027–35. doi: 10.1007/s00467-017-3793-2

26

Dextran-Sulfate Plasma Adsorption Lipoprotein Apheresis in Drug Resistant Primary Focal Segmental Glomerulosclerosis Patients: Results from a Prospective, Multicenter, Single-Arm Intervention Study

Rupesh Raina[1,2†], Vinod Krishnappa[2,3†], Cheryl Sanchez-Kazi[4], Alejandro Quiroga[5], Katherine E. Twombley[6], Robert Mathias[7], Megan Lo[8], Ronith Chakraborty[2], Shefali Mahesh[9], Julia Steinke[10], Timothy Bunchman[11] and Joshua Zaritsky[12]*

[1] Department of Nephrology, Cleveland Clinic Akron General and Akron Children's Hospital, Akron, OH, United States, [2] Akron Nephrology Associates/Cleveland Clinic Akron General, Akron, OH, United States, [3] Northeast Ohio Medical University, Rootstown, OH, United States, [4] Department of Nephrology, Loma Linda University Children's Hospital, Loma Linda, CA, United States, [5] Department of Nephrology, Spectrum Health (Helen De Vos Children's Hospital), Grand Rapids, MI, United States, [6] Department of Pediatrics, Medical University of South Carolina, Charleston, SC, United States, [7] Department of Pediatrics, Nemours Children's Hospital, Orlando, FL, United States, [8] Department of Pediatrics, Children's Hospital of Richmond at VCU, Richmond, VA, United States, [9] Department of Nephrology, Akron Children's Hospital, Akron, OH, United States, [10] Division of Pediatric Nephrology, Dialysis and Transplantation, Helen Devos Children's Hospital and Clinics, Grand Rapids, MI, United States, [11] Pediatric Nephrology and Transplantation, Children's Hospital of Richmond, Virginia Commonwealth University, Richmond, VA, United States, [12] Nemours, A.I. duPont Hospital for Children, Wilmington, DE, United States

***Correspondence:**
Rupesh Raina
rraina@akronchildrens.org

† These authors share first authorship

Background: Focal segmental glomerulosclerosis (FSGS) causes end stage renal disease (ESRD) in significant proportion of patients worldwide. Primary FSGS carries poor prognosis and management of FSGS patients, refractory to standard treatments or resistant to steroids, remains a major challenge. Lipoprotein apheresis is a therapeutic approach for drug resistant primary FSGS and post-renal transplant primary FSGS recurrence.

Objectives: To examine the safety and probable benefit at 1, 3, 6, 12, and 24-months following completion of apheresis treatment using Liposorber® LA-15 system in patients with nephrotic syndrome (NS), due to refractory primary FSGS or primary FSGS associated NS, in post renal transplant children.

Material and Methods: Prospective, multicenter, single-arm intervention study using Liposorber® LA-15 system. Patients ≤21 years old with drug resistant or drug intolerant NS secondary to primary FSGS with glomerular filtration rate (GFR) ≥60 ml/min/1.73 m^2 or post renal transplant patients ≤21 years old with primary FSGS associated NS were included in the study. Each patient had 12 dextran-sulfate plasma adsorption lipoprotein apheresis sessions over a period of 9 weeks. All patients were followed up at 1, 3, 6, 12, and 24-months following completion of treatment.

Results: Of 17 patients enrolled, six were excluded from the outcome analysis (protocol deviations). Of the remaining 11 patients, all but one have completed apheresis treatments. Three patients were lost to follow-up immediately after completion of apheresis and excluded from outcome analysis. At one-month follow-up, 1 of 7 patients (14.3%) attained partial remission of NS while 2 of 4 subjects (50%) and 2 of 3 subjects (66.7%) had partial/complete remission at 3- and 6-months follow-up, respectively. One of two patients followed up for 12 months had complete remission and one patient had partial remission of NS after 24 months. Improved or stable eGFR was noted in all patients over the follow-up period.

Conclusion: The results of our multicenter study showed improvement in the response rates to steroid or immunosuppressive therapy and induced complete or partial remission of proteinuria in some of the patients with drug resistant primary FSGS. The main limitation of our study is the small number of subjects and high dropout rate.

Keywords: focal segmental glomerulosclerosis, lipoprotein apheresis, nephrotic syndrome, liposorber, proteinuria

BACKGROUND

Focal segmental glomerulosclerosis (FSGS) causes end stage renal disease (ESRD) in significant proportion of patients in the United States and worldwide (1, 2). FSGS is characterized by nephrotic or subnephrotic range proteinuria due to sclerosis and scarring of the glomerulus, which often progresses to ESRD (1, 3). Primary FSGS is idiopathic and commonly occurs in children and young adults, while secondary FSGS is frequently seen in older adults due to cytomegalovirus, human immunodeficiency virus (HIV) infection, systemic lupus erythematosus (SLE), sickle cell disease, hepatitis, reflux nephropathy, illicit drug use, and certain malignancies (1, 3). Pathology underlying FSGS is podocyte injury resulting in protein leak, capillary expansion, synechiae formation, and proliferation of mesangial matrix (3, 4). Proteinuria is the main presentation in FSGS and other symptoms are secondary to urinary protein loss, which include hypoalbuminemia, edema, hypertension, and hyperlipidemia (5, 6). Primary FSGS carries a poor prognosis as spontaneous remission is rare and it tends to rapidly progress to ESRD within 2–8 years in patients with persistent nephrotic range proteinuria (2, 7, 8).

The mainstay of treatment for primary FSGS is to control while preventing and decreasing the rate of progression to ESRD. Corticosteroids are most effective and commonly used treatment to induce remission of proteinuria in FSGS patients. However, remission rate is only 20–50% with steroid therapy for a mean duration of 3.7 ± 2 months (8, 9). Most steroid resistant FSGS patients develop ESRD (8). Furthermore, successful steroid therapy may come at the cost of severe adverse effects, such as growth impairment, hypertension, and immune suppression (6, 8). Steroid resistant or steroid intolerant FSGS patients can be treated with cyclophosphamide or a calcineurin inhibitor, but the response rates are very low (<25%) with significant complications (1, 8, 10). Moreover, long-term remission is uncertain in cyclophosphamide or calcineurin inhibitor responsive patients (1, 8).

FSGS recurs in 30–40% of renal transplant patients, and causes allograft injury in 20–30%, and graft loss in 40–50% of these patients (11). Furthermore, FSGS recurrence is the leading cause of graft failure in children and has the lowest 5-year graft survival rate for living donor renal transplant recipients compared to other renal disorders (7). Despite all the treatment options, management of FSGS patients, refractory to standard treatments or resistant to steroids, remains a major challenge. Lipoprotein apheresis therapy is used for drug resistant (corticosteroids and/or calcineurin inhibitors) primary FSGS and post-renal transplant primary FSGS reoccurrence. Lipoprotein apheresis selectively removes VLDL, LDL, and triglycerides without affecting serum HDL levels (12–14). Although underlying mechanism by which lipoprotein apheresis reduces proteinuria is unknown, several studies have shown that lipoprotein apheresis induces remission of drug resistant NS in FSGS patients (12, 14–19).

OBJECTIVES

The primary objective was to examine the safety and potential benefit of lipoprotein apheresis at 1 month following a 9-week

TABLE 1 | Demographics of patients.

	n (%)
Age (years)	
6–8	5 (29.4)
9–11	4 (23.5)
12–14	6 (35.3)
15–17	0
18–20	2 (11.8)
Sex	
Male	8 (47)
Female	9 (52.9)
Race/ethnicity	
Caucasian	9 (52.9)
African American	4 (23.5)
Hispanic/Latino	2 (11.8)
Unknown	2 (11.8)

course of dextran-sulfate plasma adsorption lipoprotein apheresis for the treatment of patients with primary FSGS associated NS, who are refractory or intolerant to standard therapy, or primary FSGS associated NS, in post renal transplant children. The secondary objective was to examine the safety and potential benefit of dextran-sulfate plasma adsorption lipoprotein apheresis at 3, 6, 12, and 24-months following apheresis treatment in the same patient population.

MATERIALS AND METHODS

Definitions Used in the Study

Nephrotic syndrome is defined as having a first morning void urine protein to creatinine ratio (UPCR) of >2 (g/g).

Drug resistant NS due to FSGS is defined as failure to attain partial or complete remission of NS with corticosteroids and/or calcineurin inhibitors (standard therapy) after at least 8 weeks of treatment in FSGS patients.

Drug intolerant NS due to FSGS is defined as patient not tolerating standard therapy due to severe adverse effects (such as growth impairment, hypertension, obesity, immune suppression, diabetes mellitus, etc.) with or without adequate clinical response.

Partial remission of NS is defined as first morning void sample UPCR of 0.2-2 (g/g) or decrease in UPCR $\geq$50% of initial screening value.

Complete remission of NS is defined as first morning void sample UPCR <0.2 (g/g).

Study Design

Prospective, multicenter, single-arm intervention study of dextran-sulfate plasma adsorption lipoprotein apheresis using Liposorber® LA-15 system. Liposorber® LA-15 system has been

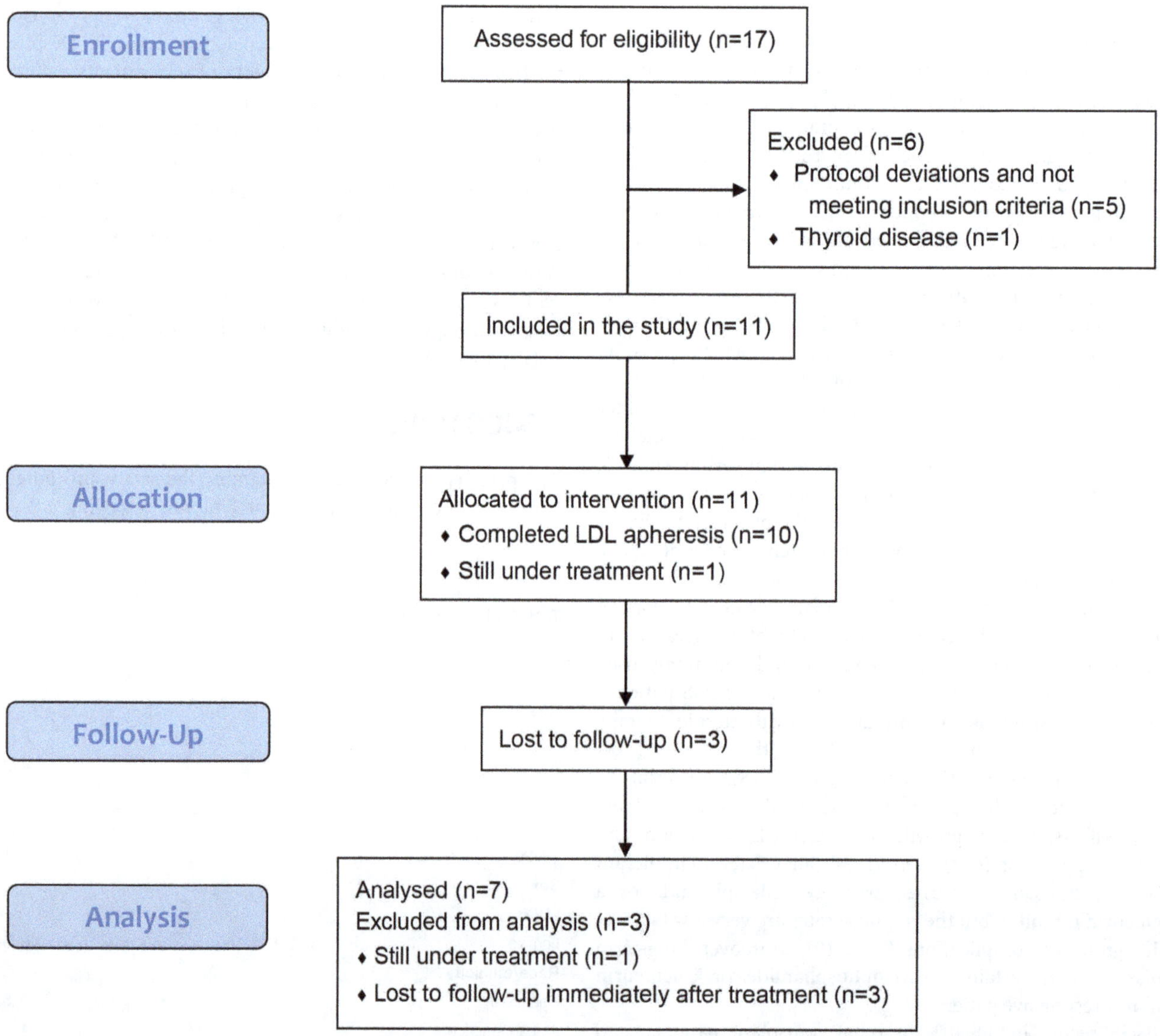

FIGURE 1 | CONSORT flow diagram.

TABLE 2 | Follow-up visit data and nephrotic syndrome status for study subjects.

Patient ID		Indication	Parameter	Baseline	After final treatment	1M F/U	3M F/U	6M F/U	12M F/U	24M F/U	Notes
NCH001	Patient 1	Post-transplant	NS	NS	Partial	Partial	Partial	Partial	Withdrawal		Withdrawal after 6-month F/U
			UPCR (g/g)	44.33	13.02	17.43	12.81	17.51			
			SCR (mg/dl)	0.8	0.4	0.6	0.6	0.6			
			eGFR (ml/min/1.73 m^2)	62.2	125.4	83.6	83.0	83.9			
			LDL (mg/dl)	60	71	269	344	498			
NDE001	Patient 2	Primary FSGS	NS	NS	NS	NA	NS		Withdrawal		Withdrawal after 3-month F/U
			UPCR (g/g)	8.11	3.84	Not performed	6.27				
			SCR (mg/dl)	0.7	0.7	0.7	0.8				
			eGFR (ml/min/1.73 m^2)	89.4	91.0	89.7	78.7				
			LDL (mg/dl)	212	30	181	189				
NDE002	Patient 3	Primary FSGS	NS	NS	NS	NS	Partial	Complete	Complete	Par	24-month F/U completed
			UPCR (g/g)	6.33	<5.0	3.33	0.90	0.18	0.08	0.36	
			SCR (mg/dl)	0.8	0.4	0.6	0.6	0.7	0.7	0.7	
			eGFR (ml/min/1.73 m^2)	84.9	172.2	112.9	114.3	98.3	100.3	100.4	
			LDL (mg/dl)	345	23	96	70	78	45	62	
NDE003	Patient 4	Post-Transplant Recurrence	NS		Not performed			Withdrawal			Withdrawal after final treatment (w/o F/U)
			UPCR (g/g)	5.05							
			SCR (mg/dl)	0.6							
			eGFR (ml/min/1.73 m^2)	95.8							
			LDL (mg/dl)	73							
NDE004	Patient 5	Primary FSGS	NS	NS			Excluded				Excluded from the study
			UPCR (g/g)	8.16							
			SCR (mg/dl)	0.7							
			eGFR (ml/min/1.73 m^2)	72.9							
			LDL (mg/dl)	N/A							
NDE005	Patient 6	Post-Transplant Recurrence	NS	NS	NS			Withdrawal			Withdrawal after final treatment (w/o F/U)
			UPCR (g/g)	19.52	25.58						
			SCR (mg/dl)	0.8	1.3						
			eGFR (ml/min/1.73 m^2)	76.6	47.1						
			LDL (mg/dl)	64	47						
ACH001	Patient 7	Primary FSGS	NS	NS							Excluded from the study
			UPCR (g/g)	1.05			Excluded				
			SCR (mg/dl)	1.9							
			eGFR (ml/min/1.73 m^2)	39.8							
			LDL (mg/dl)	165							

(Continued)

TABLE 2 | Continued

Patient ID		Indication	Parameter	Baseline	After final treatment	1M F/U	3M F/U	6M F/U	12M F/U	24M F/U	Notes
ACH002	Patient 8	Primary FSGS	NS	NS	NS	Partial	Complete	Partial	Complete	Complete	24-month F/U completed
			UPCR (g/g)	1.98	0.71	0.39	0.10	0.42	0.17	0.16	
			SCR (mg/dl)	0.3	0.3	0.4	0.4	0.4	0.4	0.5	
			eGFR (ml/min/1.73 m^2)	170.7	170.3	129.1	129.8	130.1	132.2	109.4	
			LDL (mg/dl)	126	26	98	91	115	179	95	
ACH003	Patient 9	Primary FSGS	NS	NS	NS	NS	NS	NS	NS		Withdrawal after 12-month F/U
			UPCR (g/g)	1.81	3.48	2.67	2.11	4.01	3.78	Withdrawal	
			SCR (mg/dl)	1.2	1.2	1.4	1.2	1.4	2.2		
			eGFR (ml/min/1.73 m^2)	60.0	60.0	51.9	60.9	52.5	33.9		
			LDL (mg/dl)	96	21	98	86	138	143		
ACH004	Patient 10	Primary FSGS	NS				Excluded				Excluded from the study
			UPCR (g/g)	0.08							
			SCR (mg/dl)	1.2							
			eGFR (ml/min/1.73 m^2)	158.5							
			LDL (mg/dl)	103							
ACH006	Patient 11	Post-Transplant Recurrence	NS	NA							
			UPCR (g/g)	Not performed							Under treatment
			SCR (mg/dl)	0.7							
			eGFR (ml/min/1.73 m^2)	72.7							
			LDL (mg/dl)	132							
LLU001	Patient 12	Post-Transplant Recurrence	NS	NS	NS	NS		Withdrawal			Withdrawal after 1-month F/U
			UPCR (g/g)	4.78	3.01	3.66					
			SCR (mg/dl)	2.1	0.5	0.4					
			eGFR (ml/min/1.73 m^2)	84.7	103.8	129.8					
			LDL (mg/dl)	N/A	4	81					
LLU002	Patient 13	Primary FSGS	NS	NS	NS	NS		Withdrawal			Withdrawal after 1-month F/U
			UPCR (g/g)	4.1	5.21	4.58					
			SCR (mg/dl)	0.3	0.3	0.3					
			eGFR (ml/min/1.73 m^2)	153.0	159.1	160.8					
			LDL (mg/dl)	N/A	7	110					
LLU003	Patient 14	Post-Transplant Recurrence	NS	NS	NS	Partial	Partial	Partial	Partial	Partial	24-month F/U completed
			UPCR (g/g)	1.09	1.66	1.49	0.70	0.67	0.37	0.34	
			SCR (mg/dl)	0.8	1.0	1.0	0.9	0.9	0.9	1.1	
			eGFR (ml/min/1.73 m^2)	78.0	13	65.3	69.3	69.3	69.3	71.7	
			LDL (mg/dl)	44	13	100	78	86	115	103	

(Continued)

TABLE 2 | Continued

Patient ID		Indication	Parameter	Baseline	After final treatment	1M F/U	3M F/U	6M F/U	12M F/U	24M F/U	Notes
HDV001	Patient 15	Primary FSGS	NS	NA	NA						Withdrawal after final treatment (w/o F/U)
			UPCR (g/g)	Not performed	Not performed			Withdrawal			
			SCR (mg/dl)	0.7	0.6						
			eGFR (ml/min/1.73 m^2)	83.2	98.8						
			LDL (mg/dl)	56	27						
CHS001	Patient 16	Primary FSGS	NS	NS	NA	NA	NS	NS	NS		12-month F/U completed
			UPCR (g/g)	5.42	Not performed	Not performed	12.51	8.83	2.77		
			SCR (mg/dl)	0.9	0.6	0.4	0.3	0.3	0.3		
			eGFR (ml/min/1.73 m^2)	60.3	89.5	134.2	179.0	183.0	191.4		
			LDL (mg/dl)	N/A	15	389	370	350	163		
CHS002	Patient 17	Primary FSGS	NS	NS	NS	NS		Withdrawal			Withdrawal after 1-month F/U
			UPCR (g/g)	28.04	8.33	38.4					
			SCR (mg/dl)	0.3	0.4	0.5					
			eGFR (ml/min/1.73 m^2)	216.1	163.5	130.8					
			LDL (mg/dl)	>DL*4	>DL*4	14					

NS, nephrotic syndrome; F/U, follow up; UPCR, urine protein to creatinine ratio; SCR, serum creatinine; eGFR, estimated glomerular filtration rate; LDL, low density lipoprotein.

described in the **Appendix A** (20). The study is registered on Clinical Trials.gov, which is a resource provided by the U.S. National Library of Medicine, and the number is as following: NCT02235857. The clinical sites (see **Appendix A**) have their Institutional Review Board (IRB) approval and they have been updated annually. Following FDA approval of the Liposorber® LA-15 system and the study plan in October 2013, the study was initiated in July 2014 with the enrollment completion in August 2018, expected follow up completion in October 2020, and expected final report submission in January 2021. Total duration of the study from initiation to completion of follow up will be 76 months. IRB approvals for the study from the respective clinical sites have been obtained. Informed consent from the patients or legal guardians of minor children (age <18 years) and assent from the children who can understand the language and procedure have been obtained. Sample size was calculated considering both primary safety and primary potential benefit objectives ($n = 30$). A maximum of 35 subjects from 3 to 10 sites will be enrolled in the study.

Study Population

Inclusion criteria: Patients ≤21 years old with drug resistant or drug intolerant NS secondary to primary FSGS with glomerular filtration rate (GFR) ≥60 ml/min/1.73 m^2 or post renal transplant patients ≤21 years old with primary FSGS associated NS. Patients with refractory or recurrent NS due to FSGS were also included if standard therapy was contraindicated. *Exclusion criteria:* Patients were excluded if they are >21 years old, pregnant, lactating or plan to conceive before completion of the study, unable to sign informed consent or adhere to follow up schedule, participating in another interventional study and weight <18 kgs. Patients were also excluded if they are on angiotensin converting enzyme (ACE) inhibitors that cannot be withheld for 24 h before each apheresis session, presently on other antihypertensives which cannot be withheld on the day of apheresis, life expectancy less than the study endpoint or medical condition that interferes with study schedule and outcome, known allergies to dextran sulfate or heparin or ethylene oxide, receiving vitamin K antagonists, severe hemophilia or hemorrhage diathesis, severe gastrointestinal ulcers, uncontrolled hypotension or hypertension, decompensated heart failure or valvular disease, unstable angina, acute myocardial infarction, uncontrolled cardiac arrhythmias, severe apoplexy, unresolved infection, hepatic or thyroid abnormalities.

Study Protocol

Eligible patients were started on lipoprotein apheresis using Liposorber® LA-15 system. Each patient had a total of 12 apheresis sessions (twice/week for 3 weeks then once/week for 6 weeks) over a period of 9 weeks. Patients received medications at the discretion of the treating physician or as per institution's standard of care. Few exceptions were: ACE inhibitors should not be given for at least 24 h before each apheresis session (to avoid bradykinin release), other antihypertensives should be withheld on the day of each apheresis treatment until completion of the session. No initiation, discontinuation or routine

TABLE 3 | Trends in eGFR and UPCR.

	Baseline eGFR (ml/min/1.73 m^2)	Last eGFR (ml/min/1.73 m^2)	Δ eGFR (ml/min/1.73 m^2)	Trend	Baseline UPCR	Last UPCR	Δ UPCR	Trend
Patient 1	62	84	+22	Increase	44.3	17.5	−26.8	Decrease
Patient 2	89	79	−10	Stable	8.1	6.3	−1.8	Stable
Patient 3	85	100	+15	Increase	6.3	0.4	−5.9	Decrease
Patient 12	85	130	+45	Increase	4.8	3.7	−1.1	Stable
Patient 13	153	161	+8	Stable	4.1	4.6	+0.5	Stable
Patient 16	60	191	+131	Increase	5.4	2.8	−2.6	Decrease
Patient 17	28	38	+10	Increase	216	131	−85	Decrease

eGFR, estimated glomerular filtration rate; UPCR, urine protein to creatinine ratio.

changes in dosages of immunosuppressives (e.g., corticosteroids, calcineurin inhibitors, etc.), ACE inhibitors or angiotensin receptor blockers (ARBs) for 2 weeks before first apheresis treatment until 1 month following last apheresis treatment unless deemed absolutely medically necessary. Initiation of low dose corticosteroids (<0.3 mg/kg or <15 mg/day whichever is lower) can be considered for edema during the study period and was not interpreted as treatment failure. All the patients were followed up at 1, 3, 6, 12, and 24 months following the last apheresis session, and data was being collected as per **Appendix A**.

Patient Participation Endpoints

All enrolled patients are expected to participate in the study for 24 months following last apheresis session. Participation will end if subject completes all the scheduled 24 month follow up visits, is lost to follow up, withdraws from the study, has reoccurrence of NS during 24 months follow up period, conceives during the study, requires plasmapheresis, develops ESRD, achieves complete remission at the time of baseline, death or study closure.

Study Endpoints

The primary potential benefit endpoint was the percentage of subjects with partial or complete remission at 1-month post treatment, and the primary safety endpoint s the rate of device or procedure related serious adverse events (SAEs) happening during apheresis treatments and until 1 month after last apheresis session. Secondary endpoints were complete or partial remission or persistent NS at 1, 3, 6, 12, and 24 months following last apheresis session, and percentage of subjects who attained partial or complete remission at the 3, 6, 12, and 24 months follow up visits. Secondary endpoints also include incidence of adverse events (AEs) during apheresis treatments, incidence of all AEs and SAEs within 3, 6, 12, and 24 month follow up, and percentage of subjects showing an increase or decrease in lab values including percent change from baseline and at 1, 3, 6, 12, and 24 months follow up.

Statistical Analysis

Clinically relevant baseline variables will be tabulated. Continuous variables will be reported as means and standard deviations and categorical variables will be reported as percents. Covariate analysis may be performed to identify predictors of SAEs and/or remission. Covariate analysis will also be performed with transplant status (i.e., pre-transplant, post-transplant) as a variable to identify additional predictors of SAEs and/or remission. Survival analysis techniques such as Kaplan-Meier or Cox Proportional Hazards will be incorporated if censoring of data occurs. Descriptive analysis of clinical parameters of NS (UPCR, serum total serum creatinine, eGFR, and LDL) stratified by the status of medication change (Yes vs. No) was provided.

RESULTS

A total of 17 patients from 6 sites have been enrolled into the study. The majority of the patients are Caucasians (52.9%) with the maximum number in the age group 12–14 years (6/17, 35.3%) followed by 6–8 years (5/7, 29.4%) (**Table 1**). Of 17 patients, six were excluded from the outcome analysis; one patients who did not start treatment due to thyroid disease and five who received treatment but did not meet inclusion/exclusion criteria (protocol deviations due to UPCR <2) (**Figure 1**). Of remaining 11 patients, 10 had completed 12 apheresis treatments over a period of 9 weeks and one is still receiving apheresis treatments (**Table 2**). Of the 10 patients who completed apheresis treatments, three patients were lost to follow-up immediately after completion of apheresis and were excluded from outcome analysis (**Table 2**).

One of the seven patients (14.3%) attained partial remission of NS at the 1-month follow-up visit and one patient whose UPCR data was missing during 1-month follow-up, had NS at the 3-month follow-up visit. Furthermore, 2 of 4 subjects (50%) and 2 of 3 subjects (66.7%) had partial/complete remission at 3- and 6-months following lipoprotein apheresis, respectively (**Table 2**). One out of two patients who were followed for 12 months had complete remission while one patient who was followed up for 24-months had partial remission of NS. Trends in eGFR and UPCR before (baseline) and after treatment are tabulated in **Table 3**. Improvement or stable eGFR was noted in all the patients (7/7, 100%) over the follow-up period. Details of steroids and immunosuppressive therapies are listed in **Table 4**. Reported side effects were nausea, vomiting, diarrhea, abdominal pain, fever/infection, pharyngitis, headache, lightheadedness,

TABLE 4 | Experimental subject's medication list.

	Medications at enrollment	During the course of LDL apheresis treatment
Patient 1	Prednisone Mycophenolate mofetil Tacrolimus Amlodipine Losartan	No medication
Patient 2	Prednisone Tacrolimus Pravastatin Lisinopril	Losartan (Before 2nd session)
Patient 3	Prednisone Tacrolimus Losartan	No medication
Patient 4	Prednisone Losartan Lisinopril Mycophenolate mofetil	No medication
Patient 5	Data not available as treatment not started due to thyroid disease	N/A
Patient 6	Prednisone Valganciclovir Ketoconazole Bactrim Tacrolimus Amlodipine	Prednisone (Before 2nd session) Cyclophosphamide (Before 3rd session) Tacrolimus (Before 4th session) Amlodipine (Before 7th session) Mycophenolate mofetil (Before 9th session) Metolazone (Before 11th session)
Patient 7	Prednisone Pravastatin Tacrolimus Valsartan Amlodipine	No medication
Patient 8	Prednisone Cyclosporine Mycophenolate mofetil Lisinopril	Prednisone (Before 2nd and 12th session) Mycophenolate mofetil (Before 11th session)
Patient 9	Cyclosporine Simvastatin Enalapril Chlorothiazide Amlodipine	Losartan Amlodipine (Before 9th session)
Patient 10	Data not available as treatment was not performed	N/A
Patient 11	Prednisone Pravastatin Mycophenolate mofetil Cyclosporine Valacyclovir Clonidine Cozaar Amlodipine Bactrim Aranesp	Aranesp (Before 2nd session) Methylprednisolone (Before 8th session)
Patient 12	No medication	No medication
Patient 13	No medication	Tacrolimus (Before 6th session)
Patient 14	No medication	Mycophenolate mofetil (Before 10th session)

(Continued)

TABLE 4 | Continued

	Medications at enrollment	During the course of LDL apheresis treatment
Patient 15	Prednisone Mycophenolate mofetil Tacrolimus Amlodipine Isradipine Labetalol	Tacrolimus (Before 3rd, 7th, 9th, 10th session)
Patient 16	Prednisone Mycophenolate mofetil Simvastatin Amlodipine Isradipine	Simvastatin (Before 12th session)
Patient 17	Prednisone Amlodipine	Cyclosporine (Before 5th, 7th, and 9th session) Prednisone (Before 8th, 9th, and 10th session) Losartan Amlodipine (Before 8th session) Mycophenolate mofetil (Before 12th session)

malaise, hypotension, leg cramps, allergic reaction, pneumonia, bacteremia, and anemia.

DISCUSSION

Our study showed that partial/complete remission rates of NS at 1, 3, 6, 12, and 24-month follow-up after completion of lipoprotein apheresis treatment were 14.3, 50, 66.7, 50, and 100%, respectively with stable or improvement in eGFR in all the patients. Management of steroid resistant primary FSGS is a challenge to date and bear poor prognosis given <25% response rate with uncertain long-term outcomes in patients treated with cyclophosphamide and calcineurin inhibitor therapy (1, 8, 10). Lipoprotein apheresis has been shown to improve the response rates to steroid or immunosuppressive therapy and induce complete or partial remission of proteinuria with histological recovery from the disease (12–19, 21–23). The mechanism by which lipoprotein apheresis produces favorable effects on the outcomes of primary FSGS is poorly understood, however, several theories have been put forth (24); (1) Improvement in macrophage function due to decrease in lipotoxic effect on glomeruli/interstitium as a result of reduction in lipid levels, (2) Better response to steroids and calcineurin inhibitor therapy as a result of lowering lipid levels, (3) improvement in endothelial dysfunction due to decrease in vascular cell adhesion molecule-1 (VCAM-1), (4) Better blood flow due to the removal of fibrinogen and other anticoagulants, (5) Vasodilation due to fall in thromboxane A2 levels and rise in the levels of vascular endothelial growth factor (VEGF), nitric oxide, bradykinin, and endothelial derived growth factor, (6) Anti-inflammatory effect due to reduction in LDL oxidation, C-reactive protein, intercellular adhesion molecule-1 (ICAM-1) and P-selectin, and (7) Reduced levels of vascular permeability factor in the circulation (24).

In the US, Liposorber LA-15® system received Humanitarian Device Exemption approval from FDA for lipoprotein apheresis in the treatment of primary FSGS in both adults and children who are refractory to standard treatment, have a GFR ≥60 mL/min/1.73 m^2, or are post-renal transplantation (25). Our study showed reduced remission rate at 1-month follow-up (14.3 vs. 64%) compared to a study by Hattori et al. (12). However, the limitation of our study is the small number of subjects and high dropout rate. Hattori et al. studied effectiveness of lipoprotein apheresis monotherapy vs. combination of lipoprotein apheresis with prednisolone therapy in 11 children with NS secondary to primary FSGS unresponsive to cyclosporine (CsA) and steroids (12). Lipoprotein apheresis alone did not have significant impact on lowering LDL levels or reducing proteinuria, however, significant reductions were noted in total cholesterol and triglycerides levels. Combination therapy of lipoprotein apheresis with prednisolone induced partial/complete remission of NS in 7 of 11 (64%) children at 1 month following lipoprotein apheresis. Of these seven children, five achieved complete remission and had normal renal function at median of 4.4 years after lipoprotein apheresis, and remaining two had partial remission at 1 month after lipoprotein apheresis (stable renal function at 4.5 years follow up in one patient while the other one eventually developed ESRD after 7.8 years) (12).

The prospective observational survey on the long-term effects of lipoprotein apheresis on drug-resistant nephrotic syndrome (POLARIS) showed remission of NS (urine protein <1.0 g/day) in 21 of 44 (47.7%) patients followed for 2 years (26). Clinical parameters immediately after lipoprotein apheresis therapy that contributed significantly for favorable outcome were serum total protein (4.9 ± 0.7 g/dl), serum albumin (2.9 ± 0.8 g/dl), serum creatinine (1.2 ± 0.7 mg/dl), eGFR (61 ± 27.2 ml/min/m^2), urine protein (1.7 ± 1.8 g/day), triglycerides (240.2 ± 156.3 mg/dl), total cholesterol (194.3 ± 65.6 mg/dl), LDL (83.1 ± 60.4 mg/dl), HDL (66.5 ± 18.3 mg/dl), fibrinogen (271.1 ± 77.2 mg/dl), and thrombin-antithrombin III complex (14.7 ± 38.6 ng/ml) (26). In addition, published literature has revealed few case studies showing remission of NS following dextran-sulfate plasma adsorption lipoprotein apheresis along with steroid and immunosuppressive therapies in children with drug resistant FSGS (14, 18, 19).

Available evidence from the published literature shows that lipoprotein apheresis enhances response rates to steroids and CsA in both adult and pediatrics NS patients as the effectiveness of lipoprotein apheresis monotherapy in the treatment of NS is not known (12, 16, 17, 21, 26). This is because VLDL and LDL decreases glucocorticoid receptor binding sites and impede glucocorticoid actions (24). Due to this, combination of lipoprotein apheresis with CsA or steroids or both is recommended by the Japanese Society of Pediatric Nephrology (27). In our study, most of the patients were on steroids and immunosuppressive therapies (**Table 4**). Additionally, maximum benefit can be achieved by starting lipoprotein apheresis early in the course of the disease process as response rates are better in patients with highly selective proteinuria and presence of advanced interstitial fibrosis indicates poor prognosis (12). Besides these benefits, a recent retrospective analysis involving five adult patients showed that lipoprotein apheresis prevented recurrence of FSGS in renal transplant recipients (28). Two sessions of lipoprotein apheresis was administered to all patients before renal transplantation except one patient who had single session (28). Survival of renal graft was noted in all patients without FSGS recurrence during 2–22 months of observation period following renal transplantation (28).

Common side effects that are associated with extracorporeal circulation can be encountered during lipoprotein apheresis, however, there are no serious adverse effects reported (27). ACE inhibitors should be discontinued during lipoprotein apheresis to avoid hypotensive events and shock (27). Restricting the use of lipoprotein apheresis therapy to children who weigh >30 kg is also recommended due to consumption of a significant amount of blood by the extracorporeal circuit (27). However, the lower weight limit for lipoprotein apheresis treatments for our study was recently set to 18 kg.

CONCLUSION

FSGS is the main cause of ESRD among children with a high recurrence rate. Primary FSGS carries a poor prognosis as spontaneous remission is rare and it more rapidly progresses to ESRD. Despite all the available treatments, management of FSGS patients refractory to standard treatments remains a major challenge. Lipoprotein apheresis therapy may be beneficial for drug resistant (corticosteroids and/or calcineurin inhibitors) primary FSGS and post-renal transplant primary FSGS reoccurrence. Results of our multicenter study showed partial remission rate of NS was 14.3% at 1-month following lipoprotein apheresis. Furthermore, partial/complete remission rates at 3 and 6-month follow-ups were 50 and 66.7%, respectively. In addition, all patients showed stable or improved eGFR during the follow-up period. The main limitation of our study is small number of subjects and high dropout rate.

AUTHOR CONTRIBUTIONS

RR, VK, CS-K, AQ, KT, RM, ML, SM, and JZ contributed to the conception and design of the study. RR, VK, CS-K, AQ, KT, RM, ML, RC, SM, JS, TB, and JZ helped organize the database and wrote sections of the manuscript. All authors contributed to manuscript revision and read and approved the submitted version.

ACKNOWLEDGMENTS

We thank Ms. Jennifer Clark, Medical Writer, Akron Children's Hospital for her assistance in language editing. We also thank Lena Nemer for her contributions in reviewing the manuscript.

REFERENCES

1. Rosenberg AZ, Kopp JB. Focal segmental glomerulosclerosis. *Clin J Am Soc Nephrol.* (2017) 12:502–17. doi: 10.2215/CJN.05960616
2. Gipson DS, Trachtman H, Kaskel FJ, Greene TH, Radeva MK, Gassman JJ, et al. Clinical trial of focal segmental glomerulosclerosis in children and young adults. *Kidney Int.* (2011) 80:868–78. doi: 10.1038/ki.2011.195
3. Jefferson JA, Shankland SJ. The pathogenesis of focal segmental glomerulosclerosis. *Adv Chronic Kidney Dis.* (2014) 21:408–16. doi: 10.1053/j.ackd.2014.05.009
4. Reidy K, Kaskel FJ. Pathophysiology of focal segmental glomerulosclerosis. *Pediatr Nephrol.* (2007) 22:350–4. doi: 10.1007/s00467-006-0357-2
5. Franceschini N, North KE, Kopp JB, McKenzie L, Winkler C. NPHS2 gene, nephrotic syndrome and focal segmental glomerulosclerosis: a HuGE review. *Genetics Med.* (2006) 8:63–75. doi: 10.1097/01.gim.0000200947.09626.1c
6. Korbet SM. Treatment of primary FSGS in adults. *J Am Soc Nephrol.* (2012) 23:1769–76. doi: 10.1681/ASN.2012040389
7. *North American Pediatric Renal Trials and Collaborative Studies 2008 Annual Report: Renal Transplantation, Dialysis, Chronic Renal Insufficiency.* (2008). p. 14–11.
8. Korbet SM. The treatment of primary focal segmental glomerulosclerosis. *Renal Failure.* (2000) 22:685–96. doi: 10.1081/JDI-100101956
9. Rydel JJ, Korbet SM, Borok RZ, Schwartz MM. Focal segmental glomerular sclerosis in adults: presentation, course, and response to treatment. *Am J Kidney Dis.* (1995) 25:534–42. doi: 10.1016/0272-6386(95)90120-5
10. Tarshish P, Tobin JN, Bernstein J, Edelmann CM Jr. Cyclophosphamide does not benefit patients with focal segmental glomerulosclerosis. A report of the International Study of Kidney Disease in Children. *Pediatr Nephrol.* (1996) 10:590–3. doi: 10.1007/s004670050167
11. Fine RN. Recurrence of nephrotic syndrome/focal segmental glomerulosclerosis following renal transplantation in children. *Pediatr Nephrol.* (2007) 22:496–502. doi: 10.1007/s00467-006-0361-6
12. Hattori M, Chikamoto H, Akioka Y, Nakakura H, Ogino D, Matsunaga A, et al. A combined low-density lipoprotein apheresis and prednisone therapy for steroid-resistant primary focal segmental glomerulosclerosis in children. *Am J Kidney Dis.* (2003) 42:1121–30. doi: 10.1053/j.ajkd.2003.08.012
13. Muso E, Yashiro M, Matsushima M, Yoshida H, Sawanishi K, Sasayama S. Does LDL-apheresis in steroid-resistant nephrotic syndrome affect prognosis? *Nephrol Dialysis Transplant.* (1994) 9:257–64.
14. Hattori M, Ito K, Kawaguchi H, Tanaka T, Kubota R, Khono M. Treatment with a combination of low-density lipoprotein aphaeresis and pravastatin of a patient with drug-resistant nephrotic syndrome due to focal segmental glomerulosclerosis. *Pediatr Nephrol.* (1993) 7:196–8. doi: 10.1007/BF00864397
15. Muso E, Mune M, Yorioka N, Nishizawa Y, Hirano T, Hattori M, et al. Beneficial effect of low-density lipoprotein apheresis (LDL-A) on refractory nephrotic syndrome (NS) due to focal glomerulosclerosis (FGS). *Clin Nephrol.* (2007) 67:341–4. doi: 10.5414/CNP67341
16. Muso E, Mune M, Fujii Y, Imai E, Ueda N, Hatta K, et al. Significantly rapid relief from steroid-resistant nephrotic syndrome by LDL apheresis compared with steroid monotherapy. *Nephron.* (2001) 89:408–15. doi: 10.1159/000046112
17. Muso E, Mune M, Fujii Y, Imai E, Ueda N, Hatta K, et al. Low density lipoprotein apheresis therapy for steroid-resistant nephrotic syndrome. Kansai-FGS-Apheresis Treatment (K-FLAT) Study Group. *Kidney Int Suppl.* (1999) 71:S122–5. doi: 10.1046/j.1523-1755.1999.07130.x
18. Oto J, Suga K, Matsuura S, Kondo S, Ohnishi Y, Inui D, et al. Low-density lipoprotein apheresis in a pediatric patient with refractory nephrotic syndrome due to focal segmental glomerulosclerosis. *J Anesth.* (2009) 23:284–7. doi: 10.1007/s00540-008-0726-z
19. Kawasaki Y, Suzuki S, Matsumoto A, Takano K, Suyama K, Hashimoto K, et al. Long-term efficacy of low-density lipoprotein apheresis for focal and segmental glomerulosclerosis. *Pediatr Nephrol.* (2007) 22:889–92. doi: 10.1007/s00467-006-0426-6
20. FDA. *LIPOSORBER LA-15 SYSTEM Operator's Manual.* New York, NY (2013).
21. Yokoyama K, Sakai S, Sigematsu T, Takemoto F, Hara S, Yamada A, et al. LDL adsorption improves the response of focal glomerulosclerosis to corticosteroid therapy. *Clin Nephrol.* (1998) 50:1–7.
22. Muso E, Mune M, Hirano T, Hattori M, Kimura K, Watanabe T, et al. Immediate therapeutic efficacy of low-density lipoprotein apheresis for drug-resistant nephrotic syndrome: evidence from the short-term results from the POLARIS Study. *Clin Exp Nephrol.* (2015) 19:379–86. doi: 10.1007/s10157-014-0996-8
23. Tojo K, Sakai S, Miyahara T. Therapeutic trial of low density lipoprotein apheresis (LDL-A) in conjunction with double filtration plasmapheresis (DFPP) in drug-resistant nephrotic syndrome due to focal glomerular sclerosis (FGS). *Progr Clin Biol Res.* (1990) 337:193–94.
24. Kobayashi S. Applications of LDL-apheresis in nephrology. *Clin Exp Nephrol.* (2008) 12:9–15. doi: 10.1007/s10157-007-0003-8
25. Muso E, Mune M, Hirano T, Hattori M, Kimura K, Watanabe T, et al. A prospective observational survey on the long-term effect of LDL apheresis on drug-resistant nephrotic syndrome. *Nephron Extra.* (2015) 5:58–66. doi: 10.1159/000437338
26. Okada T, Takahashi H, Ogura M, Nakao T, Shimizu T. [Complete remission of steroid-resistant minimal-change nephrotic syndrome by cyclosporin after additional low-density lipoprotein apheresis treatment]. *Nihon Jinzo Gakkai Shi.* (1996) 38:46–51.
27. Ishikura K, Matsumoto S, Sako M, Tsuruga K, Nakanishi K, Kamei K, et al. Clinical practice guideline for pediatric idiopathic nephrotic syndrome 2013: medical therapy. *Clin Exp Nephrol.* (2015) 19:6–33. doi: 10.1007/s10157-014-1030-x
28. Sannomiya A, Murakami T, Koyama I, Nitta K, Nakajima I, Fuchinoue S. Preoperative low-density lipoprotein apheresis for preventing recurrence of focal segmental glomerulosclerosis after kidney transplantation. *J Transpl.* (2018) 2018:1–5. doi: 10.1155/2018/8926786

APPENDIX

Appendix A: IRB approval has been given by the following institutions.

Name of the Hospital	State	Principal Investigator	Address
Akron Children's Hospital	OH	Dr. Rupesh Raina	130 W. Exchange Street Akron, OH 44302
Nemours/Alfred I. duPont Hospital	DE	Dr. Joshua Zaritsky	1600 Rockland Road, ARB 211 Wilmington, DE 19803
Loma Linda University Health	CA	Dr. Cheryl Sanchez-Kazi	11234 Anderson St. Room B-726 Loma linda, CA 92336
Medical University of South Carolina	SC	Dr. Katherine Twombley	135 Rutledge Avenue. Charleston, SC 29425
Helen DeVos Children's Hospital/ Spectrum Health	MI	Dr. Alejandro Quiroga	100 Michigan NE, Mail Code 038 Grand Rapids, MI 49503
Children's Hospital of Richmond at VCU	VA	Dr. Megan Lo	1000 E. Broad St., Richmond, VA 23219

27

Home Albumin Infusion Therapy, Another Alternative Treatment in Patients with Congenital Nephrotic Syndrome of the Finnish Type

Eugènia Serramontmany [1], Marina Muñoz [2], Aurora Fernández-Polo [1], María Morillo [3], Laura Gómez-Ganda [1], Carme Cañete-Ramírez [1] and Gema Ariceta [2]*

[1] *Pharmacy Department, Vall d'Hebron University Hospital, Barcelona, Spain,* [2] *Pediatric Nephrology Department, Vall d'Hebron University Hospital, Barcelona, Spain,* [3] *Nursery Department, Vall d'Hebron University Hospital, Barcelona, Spain*

***Correspondence:**
Eugènia Serramontmany
eserramontmany@vhebron.net

Background: Congenital nephrotic syndrome of the Finnish type (CNF) is a rare, severe glomerular disease caused by mutations in the NPHS1 gene, which codes for nephrin. It is characterised by massive proteinuria and severe edoema. Progression to end-stage kidney failure occurs during early childhood and the only curative treatment is kidney transplantation. Nowadays, patients need aggressive medical treatment, which includes daily albumin infusions (for months) until they get clinical stability to receive transplant.

Objective: In our paediatric hospital, we implemented a multidisciplinary program for the home infusion of albumin with outpatient follow-up. The aim of the study was to assess the safety and efficacy of this program for the first four years of its implementation.

Material and Methods: Retrospective observational study of CNF paediatric patients treated with home albumin infusion therapy from March 2014 to July 2018 at a tertiary care paediatric hospital. Information on albumin administration was obtained from the electronic prescription assistance program and details on clinical and care-related variables from the hospital's electronic information systems.

Results: Four patients with CNF received albumin infusions for 18, 21, 22 months, and 3 years. The treatment was safe, and the complication rates were to be expected considering the severity of disease. Patients required a median of two hospital admissions a year (19 in total); 47% due to catheter-related complications, but there were just three catheter infections.

Conclusions: In our experience, home albumin infusion therapy is safe and effective and helps to improve children health and quality of life.

Keywords: congenital nephrotic syndrome, finnish type, CNF, NPHS1, albumin, home albumin infusion therapy

INTRODUCTION

Nephrotic syndrome is the most common primary glomerular disease in the paediatric population. It is characterised by a glomerular lesion that leads to massive proteinuria (urine protein/creatinine ratio >2 mg/mg), resulting in hypoalbuminemia and generalised edoema. Nephrotic syndrome can be idiopathic or hereditary. Younger patients are more likely to have the hereditary form, and genetic diagnosis is recommended in all young patients with nephrotic syndrome who fail to respond to conventional treatment (1, 2). The most severe subgroup of nephrotic syndrome is congenital nephrotic syndrome (CNS), which is characterised by disease onset within the first 3 months of life, resistance to corticosteroids and immunosuppressive agents, and a very poor prognosis (3–5).

The prototype of severe hereditary nephrotic syndrome is CNS of the Finnish type (CNF) (OMIM: #256300), which, as its name suggests, is particularly prevalent in Finland, where it has an incidence of 1 case per 8,200 live births (4). However, CNF has been described in populations of different ethnic backgrounds around the world. It is an autosomal recessive disorder caused by loss-of-function mutations in the NPHS1 gene, leading up to alterations to the glomerular filtration barrier, responsible for the massive proteinuria typically seen in CNS (6, 7). Albumin is the main protein lost, but larger plasma proteins, such as immunoglobulins, may also be lost. Protein loss is correlated with hypoalbuminemia, severe malnutrition, hyperlipidemia, and an increased risk of thrombosis and infection (7).

Unlike idiopathic nephrotic syndrome, CNF is caused by a structural alteration. As such, it is resistant to corticosteroids and immunosupressants, and these treatments can even be harmful considering that patients are highly susceptible to infection (8).

As CNF is rare and challenging to manage, most patients are treated in specialised hospitals. Although prognosis has improved thanks to the introduction of early kidney transplantation and advances in dialysis techniques (9), patients still require an aggressive treatment approach to ensure that they survive until they attain an adequate weight and height for kidney transplantation (8).

In a study of 41 children diagnosed with CNF between 1953 and 1982, a team from the University of Minnesota led by Mahan et al. (10) found that all the children diagnosed before 1971 (before the introduction of early kidney transplantation) died. Those diagnosed later, however, showed 2-year survival rates of 82%.

As kidney transplantation is the only curative treatment for CNF, medical treatment is necessary to sustain good health and appropriate growth and development until the child is ready to undergo kidney transplantation (11). The goal of treatment thus is to control clinical manifestations to maintain clinical stability and prevent complications until the child attains a sufficient weight and height for transplantation.

The specific treatment aims are to control proteinuria and massive edoema through a high-calorie and high-protein diet and to prevent intercurrent infections and thromboembolic complications (3–12).

Various palliative treatments exist to control massive proteinuria and sustain clinical stability until the child is ready to undergo kidney transplantation.

The classic treatment for CNF, established by a group of Finnish experts two decades ago, is elective bilateral nephrectomy followed by dialysis until the moment of transplantation. This aggressive approach is justified by the presence of severe *NPHS1* mutations in the Finnish population (4, 5).

A more conservative approach, used at our hospital and other centres, consists of repeated intravenous albumin infusions associated with unilateral nephrectomy and/or treatment with antiproteinuric drugs to ensure clinical stability and normal glomerular filtration, thereby postponing the need for dialysis and transplantation and increasing the chances of success (11, 13–15).

This approach compensates for the massive loss of proteins and maintains intravascular oncotic pressure through daily intravenous infusions of albumin 20% (1 g/kg/day) in combination with furosemide (0.5 mg/kd/day) through a central venous catheter (CVC). In addition to a high-calorie and high-protein diet, patients are concomitantly prescribed drugs such as indomethacin (1–3 mg/kg/day) and angiotensin-converting enzyme inhibitors, to reduce glomerular filtration rate, and consequently proteinuria, and control severe edoema (15, 16).

Patients who remain clinically stable usually need to follow the above treatment for several months, i.e., until they are ready to undergo kidney transplantation. During this time, they typically need to be hospitalised or to make daily visits to the hospital for albumin infusions. This can have a major impact on the child's development and on family quality of life (5).

There have been growing reports of home infusion therapy programs being used in different fields that have proven to be both safe and effective. Examples are parenteral nutrition programs and antibiotic therapy programs for patients with cystic fibrosis (17, 18).

At our hospital we launched a multidisciplinary program for the home administration of intravenous albumin for children with CNF who only needed to be in hospital to receive this treatment. Apart from improving patient and family quality of life and favouring the children's personal and social development, the potential benefits of shortening hospital stays also included cost savings and a reduced risk of hospital-acquired infections.

The aim of this study was to assess the safety and efficacy of a home albumin infusion therapy program for paediatric patients with CNF from a tertiary care hospital during the first 4 years of the program and to evaluate associated morbidity.

METHOD

The program was launched by the paediatric nephrology, pharmacy, and nursing departments in March 2014 to educate and train relatives and caregivers of patients with CNF in home albumin infusion therapy. The goal was to promote outpatient care and minimise hospital stays. The program targeted clinically stable patients whose only reason for being in hospital was to

TABLE 1 | Interventions by the nursing in the home albumin infusion therapy program.

Actions	Pre-discharge	Discharge	Weekly follow-up visits for first 6 months	Twice-monthly follow-up visits after first 6 months
Primary caregiver training	Three training sessions on the knowledge, skills, and abilities needed for proper CVC[1] care and albumin infusion	Evaluation of knowledge, skills, and abilities acquired via a checklist	- Consolidation of good home care practises - Clarification of doubts	- Consolidation of good home care practises - Clarification of doubts
Broviac® CVC monitoring	- Supervision of primary caregiver CVC handling - Training in technique for albumin infusion in a sterile environment	Verification of CVC securement and functioning	- CVC dressing - Entry-point dressing - Assessment of permeability reflux	- CVC dressing - Entry-point dressing - Assessment of permeability reflux
Blood tests			Capillary blood sampling	Capillary blood sampling
Anthropometric characteristics			Weight, height, waist circumference, and blood pressure	Weight, height, waist circumference, and blood pressure
Warning signs and actions	- Training in detection of local and systemic warning signs - Actions: differentiation between contact with assigned nurse (Monday to Friday 9:00–17:00) and emergency visits	- Review of knowledge acquired: detection of local and systemic warning signs - Consolidation of knowledge about when and how to act		
Contact person	Ward nurse and assigned nurse	- Assigned nurse from Monday to Friday 9:00–17:00 - Emergency department	- Assigned nurse from Monday to Friday 9:00–17:00 - Emergency department	- Assigned nurse from Monday to Friday 9:00–17:00 - Emergency department

[1]*CVC, Central venous catheter.*

receive intravenous albumin and furosemide infusions. They were admitted to the program once their albumin infusion needs were reduced to a single daily infusion through a Broviac® CVC. This type of catheter was chosen to avoid the need for direct injections at home. Albumin was delivered by small, long-duration infusion pumps (Alaris™ GH Plus syringe pump from BD), provided by the hospital, that can be transported in dedicated backpacks to facilitate administration.

A multidisciplinary team formed by paediatric nephrologists, nursing staff, and pharmacists designed a series of health education and training sessions to teach the children's parents or caregivers to prepare and administer the albumin infusions in a sterile environment using the home infusion pumps.

Prior to discharge, parents also required to learn basic central line care skills to minimise risk of infection. There were also taught about warning signs (local signs in the area of the catheter and general signs such as edoema or fever) that they would need to watch for at home (**Table 1**). The nursing team evaluated the suitability of the home through a visit. In cases where the patient lived far from the hospital, the nursing team worked with the social worker of the area to assess the home.

Once the home program was launched, the multidisciplinary team worked together to ensure that the follow-up visits with the different teams coincided to minimise the number of scheduled visits to the hospital.

The nursing staff also set up communication channels with the patients' primary care teams to optimise management and follow-up. Weekly visits with nursing staff and members of the paediatric nephrology team were also arranged to coincide. The aim of these visits was to cheque weight, height, waist circumference, blood pressure, CVC securement and dressings, and to adjust overall treatment as necessary. The protocol also envisaged a switch to twice-monthly visits after an initial period of 6 months (**Table 1**).

Medical supplies, ordered through an online system, were sent to the patient's home on a monthly basis, ensuring thus that the caregivers only needed to pick up the medication from the hospital pharmacy twice a month. These trips were designed to coincide with the follow-up visits.

This was a retrospective observational study of paediatric patients with genetically confirmed CNF treated with home albumin infusion therapy from March 2014 (launch of program) to July 2019 at a tertiary care paediatric university hospital.

Information was collected on biodemographic characteristics (sex, age, and weight); clinical data (date of diagnosis, infusion-related complications, and date of kidney transplantation); and care-related variables (number of CVC dressing changes, hospital admissions, and successive visits to the outpatient clinic to cheque the catheter).

Information on albumin administration and dosage was obtained from the Electronic Prescription Assistance Program used in our centre. Details on clinical and care-related variables were obtained from the hospital's electronic information systems.

RESULTS

Four patients, all boys, were included in the home albumin infusion therapy program. They were from four unrelated

TABLE 2 | Clinical and demographic characteristics of patients.

	Patient			
	1	**2**	**3**	**4**
Age at diagnosis, days	2	71	23	7
Genetic diagnosis	c.1379G>A (p.Arg460Gln) Homozygosity	c.[1379G>A] + [2883G>A] (p.[Arg460Gln]+[Trp961*]) Compound heterozygosity	c.1135C>T(p.Arg379Trp) Homozygosity	c.3250_3251insG (p.Val1084Glyfs*12) Homozygosity
Post-diagnosis hospital stay, days	192 (6.5 months)	43 (1.5 months)	71 (2 months and 1 week)	83 (2.5 months)
Age at start of home albumin infusion therapy	6.5 months	4 months	2 months and 24 days	2 months and 23 days
Serum albumin at start of home albumin infusion therapy (g/dl)	2.7	2	2.18	2.1
Proteinuria prior to home albumin infusion therapy (mg/dl)*	3607.8	618	2,381	3,859
Time receiving home albumin infusion therapy	1 year and 6 months	3 years and 6 months	1 year and 10 months	1 year and 9 months
Age at time of kidney transplantation	2 years and 2 months	4 years and 10 months	2 years and 1 month	2 years
Dialysis before transplantation	No	No	No	No
Estimated glomerular filtration rate at time of kidney transplantation, mL/min (Schwartz equation)	15.55	19.5	6.82	14.57
Weight at the day of kidney transplantation, kg	10.4	18.9	11.1	11.5
Height at the day of kidney transplantation, cm	82.5	110.5	85	84
Weight percentile at the day of kidney transplantation	6.7	40	18.4	30.8
Height percentile at the day of kidney transplantation	2.3	44	18.4	11.5
First placement of *Broviac* CVC[1], days	33	18	18	13
Number of CVC[1]	5	3	2	3
Current glomerular filtration rate, mL/min (Schwartz equation)	106.42	36.87	121.31	103.77
Current creatinine level, mg/dL	0.39	1.12	0.32	0.39
Mechanical complications of CVC[1]s	2	3	3	1
Catheter-associated infections	1	1	0	2
Other complications: pyelonephritis	0	1	0	1
Number of hospital admissions from diagnosis to transplantation	7	5	4	5
Number of admissions due to CVC complications	3	4	1	3

[1] *CVC, central venous catheter; NA, not applicable.*

**The value corresponds to the last determination prior to hospital discharge (1–2 months before discharge).*

families, although three of them had a history of consanguinity. Two patients had been diagnosed with CNF during the first week of life and the other two were diagnosed between the ages of 1 and 2 months. The clinical diagnosis of CNF was confirmed genetically in all cases. Home albumin infusion therapy was started before the age of 4 months in all patients except the first boy recruited, who started when he was 6.5 months old (patient #1 in **Table 2**). The children were discharged from hospital when they required just a single daily infusion of albumin for <6 h. Median hospital stay during the children's first admission was 83 (range 43–192) days (**Table 2**).

All the patients had a suitable family and home environment. Two of the families were Moroccan and two were Spanish. They were from very different sociocultural backgrounds, but this had no influence on their ability to acquire the necessary knowledge and skills covered in the training sessions. We also observed no association between lower sociocultural level and an increased rate of complications.

Albumin 20% was daily administered intravenously at a dose of 1 g/kg over 4 h (0, 1–0.5 ml/min). Furosemide (0.5 mg/kg/day) was administered as two doses: 50% halfway through the albumin infusion and 50% at the end. In all cases the drugs were delivered by a continuous-flow syringe pump through a *Broviac®* CVC (**Table 2**).

All the patients were also treated with high doses of indomethacin, and the antiproteinuric drug captopril.

The home infusion treatment goal (serum albumin levels of around 2 g/dL) was achieved in all cases and edoema was well-controlled. The median number of outpatient follow-up visits with the nursing staff and the paediatric nephrology team was 56 (range 48–96). Nursing advice was given by telephone on a median of 8 (range 2–14) occasions. Overall, 176 visits were made to the hospital pharmacy [median 44 (range 34–62) per patient] and 68 home medical supply deliveries were made [median 17 (range 6–36)].

A median of 3 (range 2–5) CVC changes per patient was required; these were due to partial dislodgement, breakage, or blockage (**Table 2**). Twenty one hospital admissions were required over the study period. This corresponds to a median of 2.5 admissions per patient per year; 52.4% of the admissions were due to CVC complications.

One of the admissions was due to infection of the CVC exit site by methicillin-resistant *Staphylococcus aureus* and required treatment with topical mupirocin and oral co-trimoxazole for 14 days. The same patient was admitted on two other occasions for catheter-related sepsis, caused by *Enterococcus cloacae* in one case (treated with meropenem) and methicillin-sensitive *S. aureus* in the other (treated with cloxacillin). One additional patient admitted due a respiratory infection episode and catheter exit site infection, was treated with oral cefadroxil as no germen was isolated. Of the remaining admissions, two were due to influenza B virus (in two vaccinated patients), two were due to acute pyelonephritis, and one was due to kidney failure resulting from acute gastroenteritis. One patient with hyporexia also required admission for percutaneous endoscopic gastrostomy (**Table 2**).

All patients, aged 24, 25, 26 months, and 4 years and 10 months, respectively, were discharged from the program when they underwent kidney transplantation and currently, they remain with functional grafts. In every case they received preemptive kidney transplantation without prior dialysis. The patient who was managed with medical treatment up to almost 5 years of age, had a less severe *NHPS1* mutation (**Table 2**).

DISCUSSION

Based on our experience, the home albumin infusion therapy program implemented at our hospital is safe and effective. The complication rates observed were no higher than expected considering the patients' condition, and none of the complications were related to the administration of albumin. None of the patients experienced life-threatening events and they progressed favourably up to the moment of kidney transplantation. The program resulted in shorter hospital stays. The patients were discharged home after the age of 4–6 months and remained in the program until they underwent transplantation (at ~2 years of age). Management by a multidisciplinary team formed by nursing staff, paediatric nephrologists, nutritionists, and pharmacists ensured the efficacy of treatment. One patient started home therapy later than the others (at 6.5 months of age) even though he had been diagnosed with CNF at just 2 days of age. This was because he was the first patient included and his parents needed to provide care to another child of theirs who had recently undergone kidney transplantation because of same disease.

Home infusion therapy programs for paediatric patients are increasingly being used in different fields, and based on the reports in the literature, they do not result in a significant increase in CVC-related complications. In addition, they have a favourable impact on patient and family quality of life as they reduce hospital admission times and enable a faster return to normal life (19).

Our results are consistent with those reported by a team at the North Children's Hospital in the UK, which has been running a paediatric home albumin infusion program for 25 years. Based on their experience with seven children with CNF, their program is safe and has not resulted in an increased rate of catheter-related complications (20).

We have already included four children since the launch of our program just 4 years ago. Like the UK program, our home albumin infusion therapy program is safe and has not resulted in any serious complications. Considering their risk profile (young age, chronic hypoalbuminemia, hypogammaglobulinemia, daily catheter use, etc.), patients with CNF can be expected to experience a high number of complications, as described by many specialist hospitals (8). In our series, there were very few infection-related complications (one entry-point infection and two cases of sepsis), attesting to the quality of nursing care provided and the success of the training sessions in which caregivers were taught how to administer the drug in a sterile environment. There were no thrombotic complications, although it should be noted that home infusion of alteplase has been found to significantly reduce the risk of intraluminal thrombosis (21). We, however, do not have any experience in this area.

Although we observed a high number of hospital admissions ($N = 21$) over the study period, again, this is to be expected given the severity of the patients' condition. Moreover, over half of the admissions were due to events unrelated to the albumin infusion program, such as viral infections and/or morbidity associated with the primary kidney disease. No life-threatening events occurred.

Further, with our conservative therapeutic approach, we avoided potential complications associated with early dialysis initiation children with CNF (5, 9), mainly in those patients who maintained native kidney renal function for extended period of time, as described (8).

It should be noted that implementation of the program increased the outpatient care burden for both the paediatric nephrologist and nursing teams, who had to closely monitor the patients, and the hospital pharmacists, who had to dispense the medications required and arrange for other supplies to be sent to the patients' homes.

This type of home programs is, especially, important in the current state of the SARS- CoV-2 pandemic since they allow reducing patient's or relative's exits from the home and hospital visits, thus reducing the possibility of contagion. In this scenario, recently another infant boy with CNF has successfully entered at the home albumin infusion therapy program in our centre.

Limitations

The main limitation of this study is the small number of patients admitted to the program, but again, this is to be expected given the rarity of the disease. Nonetheless, the results obtained suggest that the program results in substantially shorter hospital stays and improved quality of life without compromising treatment efficacy and patient safety. Although we did not undertake a formal study of the impact of the program on quality of life, both the patients and their parents reacted very positively to being able to continue treatment at home.

A second limitation of our study is that we were unable to compare the economic impact of the home program with in-hospital care and treatment, as we did not have a control group.

Conclusions

Based on our experience, a paediatric home albumin infusion therapy program run under the supervision of an expert team is both safe and effective. In our opinion, this treatment modality should be offered to all paediatric patients with CNF who have reached the requirement of a single daily dose of albumin within the framework of a structured caregiver training program. We observed no significant increase in catheter-related complications, adverse drug effects, or albumin infusion reactions.

Our home albumin infusion therapy program allows patients and their families to continue treatment in the comfort of their home. It favours growth and development (and may even improve general health), reduces the need for long hospital stays, and offers an opportunity to optimise healthcare resource utilisation. Finally, it can reduce the psychological and social sequelae associated with this disease in early childhood.

AUTHOR CONTRIBUTIONS

ES, AF-P, MMo, LG-G, and CC-R: data collection. ES, MMu, AF-P, LG-G, and CC-R: data analysis. ES, MMu, and AF-P: manuscript writing. AF-P and GA: review. All authors contributed to the article and approved the submitted version.

REFERENCES

1. Asociación Española de Pediatría. *P. Anales de pediatría continuada: APC*. Vol. 12. Doyma (2014). p. 17–24. Available online at: https://www.elsevier.es/es-revista-anales-pediatria-continuada-51-articulo-sindrome-nefrotico-el-primer-ano-S1696281814701623 (accessed November 13, 2018).
2. Lovric S, Ashraf S, Tan W, Hildebrandt F. Genetic testing in steroid-resistant nephrotic syndrome: when and how? *Nephrol Dial Transplant*. (2016) 31:1802–13. doi: 10.1093/ndt/gfv355
3. Anton M, Rodriguez LM. *Nefrología Pediátrica. Manual Práctico*. AENP Asociación Española de Nefrología Pediátrica; Panamericana, Madrid (2011).
4. Jalanko H. Congenital nephrotic syndrome. *Pediatr Nephrol*. (2009) 24:2121–8. doi: 10.1007/s00467-007-0633-9
5. Holmberg C, Antikainen M, Riinnholm K, Ala-houhala M, Jalanko H. Management of congenital nephrotic syndrome of the Finnish type. *Pediatr Nephrol*. (1995) 9:87–93. doi: 10.1007/BF00858984
6. Hinkes BG, Mucha B, Vlangos CN, Gbadegesin R, Liu J, Hasselbacher K, et al. Nephrotic syndrome in the first year of life: two thirds of cases are caused by mutations in 4 genes (NPHS1, NPHS2, WT1, and LAMB2). *Pediatrics*. (2007) 119:e907–19. doi: 10.1542/peds.2006-2164
7. Büscher AK, Weber S. Educational paper: the podocytopathies. *Eur J Pediatr*. (2012) 171:1151–60. doi: 10.1007/s00431-011-1668-2
8. Dufek S, Holtta T, Trautmann A, Ylinen E, Alpay H, Ariceta G, et al. Management of children with congenital nephrotic syndrome: challenging treatment paradigms. *Nephrol Dial Transplant*. (2018) 1369–77. doi: 10.1136/archdischild-2017-084620.23
9. Dufek S, Ylinen E, Trautmann A, Alpay H, Ariceta G, Aufricht C, et al. Infants with congenital nephrotic syndrome have comparable outcomes to infants with other renal diseases On behalf of the ESPN Dialysis Working Group. *Pediatr Nephrol*. (2019) 34:649–655. doi: 10.1007/s00467-018-4122-0
10. Mahan JD, Mauer MS, Sibley RK, Vernier RL. Congenital nephrotic syndrome: evolution of medical management and results of renal transplatation. *J Pediatr*. (1984) 105:549–57. doi: 10.1016/S0022-3476(84)80418-7
11. Kim MS, Primack W, Harmon WE. Congenital nephrotic syndrome: preemptive bilateral nephrectomy and dyalisis before renal transplantation. *J Am Soc Nephrol*. (1992) 3:260–3.
12. Álvarez SD. Síndromes nefróticos congénitos y hereditarios. *Rev Cubana Pediatr*. (2011) 83:87–102.
13. Mattoo TK, Al-Sowailem AM, Al-Harbi MS, Mahmood MA, Katawee Y, Hassab MH. Nephrotic syndrome in 1st year of life and the role of unilateral nephrectomy. *Pediatr Nephrol*. (1992) 6:16–8. doi: 10.1007/BF00856821
14. Kovacevic L, Reid CJ, Rigden SP. Management of congenital nephrotic syndrome. *Pediatr Nephrol*. (2003) 18:426–30. doi: 10.1007/s00467-003-1131-3
15. González DC, Rodríguez JDG, López VMN, Martín-govantes JFLJ. Evaluación de las estrategias terapéuticas en el síndrome nefrótico congénito tipo finlandés. *Anales Pediatría*. (2006) 65:561–8. doi: 10.1157/13095849
16. Papez KE, Smoyer WE. Recent advances in congenital nephrotic syndrome. *Curr Opin Pediatr*. (2004) 16:165–70. doi: 10.1097/00008480-200404000-00009
17. Chicharro L, Planas M, Vélez C, José AS. El soporte nutricional en el ámbito de la hospitalización a domicilio. *Nutr Hosp*. (2009) 24:93–6.
18. Girón RM, Cisneros C, Al Nakeeb Z, Hoyos N, Martínez C, Ancochea J. Eficiencia del tratamiento antibiótico intravenoso domiciliario en la fibrosis quística. *Med Clin*. (2006) 127:567–71. doi: 10.1157/1309 3998
19. Moore DL, Bortolussi R, Society CP, Diseases I. Home intravenous therapy: accessibility for Canadian children and youth | Position statements and practice points | Canadian Paediatric Society. *Paediatr Child Health*. (2011) 16:105–9. doi: 10.1093/pch/16.2.105
20. Reynolds BC, Pickles CW, Lambert HJ, Ognjanovic M, Crosier J, Johnson SA, et al. Domiciliary administration of intravenous albumin in congenital nephrotic syndrome. *Pediatr Nephrol*. (2015) 30:2045–50. doi: 10.1007/s00467-015-3177-4
21. Gong M, He X, Song J, Zhao B, Shi W, Chen G, et al. Catheter-directed thrombolysis with a continuous infusion of low-dose alteplase for subacute proximal venous thrombosis: efficacy and safety compared to urokinase. *Clin Appl Thromb*. (2018) 1333–9. doi: 10.1177/1076029618775514

28

Complete Remission of C1q Nephropathy Treated With a Single Low-Dose Rituximab, a Reality or Coincidence?

Rui Ma [1,2], *Dengyan Wu* [1,2], *Zhiqin He* [1,2], *Qian Chang* [1,2] *and Yonghong Yang* [1,2,3*]

[1] Department of Pediatric Nephrology, Lanzhou University Second Hospital, Lanzhou, China, [2] Department of Nephrology, Gansu Children's Hospital, Lanzhou, China, [3] Department of Pediatrics, Children's Hospital of Xi'an International Medical Center, Xi'an, China

***Correspondence:**
Yonghong Yang
yhyangyh@126.com

C1q nephropathy is a glomerulopathy that is characterized by large amount of C1q deposits in the glomerular mesangium. It is a diagnosis of exclusion after ruling out systemic lupus erythematosus and membranoproliferative glomerulonephritis by systemic and serological examination. The pathogenesis of C1q nephropathy is unclear. In addition, there is very little generalizability in the treatment and prognosis for pediatric C1q nephropathy due to diversities in clinical manifestations and pathological types. Rituximab is a human/mouse chimeric monoclonal antibody against CD20, which is primarily used for treating lymphomas and, most recently, has been used to treat certain kidney diseases including C1q nephropathy. In this report, we used one quarter of the typical dose of rituximab for lymphoma treatment to achieve complete remission in a C1q nephropathy patient, significantly reducing deposition of immune complexes and glomerular damage. This case indicates that dosage reconsiderations may be necessary for rituximab in treatment of pediatric C1q nephropathy.

Keywords: C1q nephropathy, nephrotic syndrome, rituximab, complete remission, B lymphocyte depletion

INTRODUCTION

C1q nephropathy is characterized by large amounts of mesangial immunoglobulin and complement deposition with predominant appearance of C1q, after exclusion of systemic lupus erythematosus and membranoproliferative disease (1). The incidence of C1q nephropathy varies in different reports ranging from 0.2 to 16% with no gender differences (1–4). It is speculated that complement activation and glomerular antigen–antibody complex formation underlie pathogenesis of C1q nephropathy, with additional involvement of alternative complement pathway and lectin pathway (5).

The clinical manifestations of C1q nephropathy are diverse. Most of the patients present with nephrotic syndrome, some with acute or chronic glomerulonephritis, and, occasionally, the only presentation may be hematuria. The disease also presents with various nephropathologies, the most common being minimal change nephropathy, focal segmental glomerulosclerosis nephropathy, and immune complex-mediated mesangial proliferative glomerulonephritis (5). These distinctions are especially important, as prognosis of C1q nephropathy in patients depends on their pathological type and clinical manifestations. Notably, children with C1q nephropathy have higher rate of recurrence and shorter recurrence interval compared to nephrotic syndrome without C1q deposition (6). There are no disease-specific treatment guidelines for C1q nephropathy. Currently, treatment guideline for C1q nephropathy follows the general guidelines for treatment of primary nephrotic syndrome, with corticosteroid as first-line treatment. If a patient is corticosteroid-dependent or corticosteroid-resistant, a second-line medication, e.g., cyclosporine, is selected with criteria based on patient condition. Of interest to the case presented here, a small number of cases have reported the efficacy of rituximab for treating C1q nephropathy, with significant improvement of renal function and clinical manifestations (7–10). Rituximab is a human/mouse chimeric monoclonal antibody targeting CD20 (11). It was originally used to treat B-cell non-Hodgkin's lymphoma but has since been widely used in autoimmune anemia, rheumatic diseases, and more recently used for the treatment of autoantibody-related kidney diseases, including antineutrophil cytoplasmic antibodies (ANCA)-associated nephritis and membranous nephropathy (12–14). The target of rituximab is CD20, a tetra-transmembrane protein expressed in pre-B cells. Rituximab depletes B cells via direct signal-induced apoptosis, complement-dependent cytotoxicity, antibody-dependent cell-mediated cytotoxicity, and antibody-dependent phagocytosis (11, 12, 14). Depletion of B cells results in the reduction in antibody and immune complex formation and, ultimately, reduces C1q deposition.

The standard dosage of rituximab for treating nephrotic syndrome is adapted from existing guidelines for lymphoma treatment (10, 12, 15, 16). No disease-specific guidelines has been made available for treatment of C1q nephropathy using rituximab. In this report, we show complete remission achieved via a significantly reduced dose of rituximab in a pediatric patient with C1q nephropathy. Our results suggest the need for further investigation into disease-specific dosage for C1q nephropathy, especially in the pediatric setting, with benefits of lower risks of adverse events as well as cost considerations in uninsured and underinsured patients.

CASE PRESENTATION

The patient is a 7-year-old Asian girl who was diagnosed with nephrotic syndrome in June 2017 in a local primary care clinic before transferring care to our department 9 months later. Prior to diagnosis, patient was healthy, with no significant birth history and no history of surgery, trauma, or blood transfusion. The patient visited the local clinic due to cold/flu-like symptoms, swelling eyelids and lower limbs, and abdominal pain that was eventually diagnosed as nephrotic syndrome. No family history was reported. Based on the records provided by the patient's parents, the patient underwent a course of oral corticosteroid, and subsequently, urine protein was negative, indicating corticosteroid-sensitive response. However, patient's urine protein increased once again after tapering corticosteroid, and her steroid dosage was increased. Subsequently, her urinalysis was once again negative for protein, but each time steroid taper was attempted, patient relapsed with significant proteinuria. Although her disease was progressively steroid dependent, corticosteroid was discontinued per the request of the patient's parents after several courses due to concern for adverse effects of long-term therapy. Instead, the patient was switched to traditional Chinese medicine (ingredients unknown) for nearly 4 months (**Figure 1A**). During the treatment with traditional Chinese medicine alone, the patient visited her local primary care clinic for several urinalyses that consistently demonstrated 3+ proteinuria and occult blood. Meanwhile, the patient showed progressive clinical decline with severe complications including urinary tract infections, systemic edema, shortness of breath,

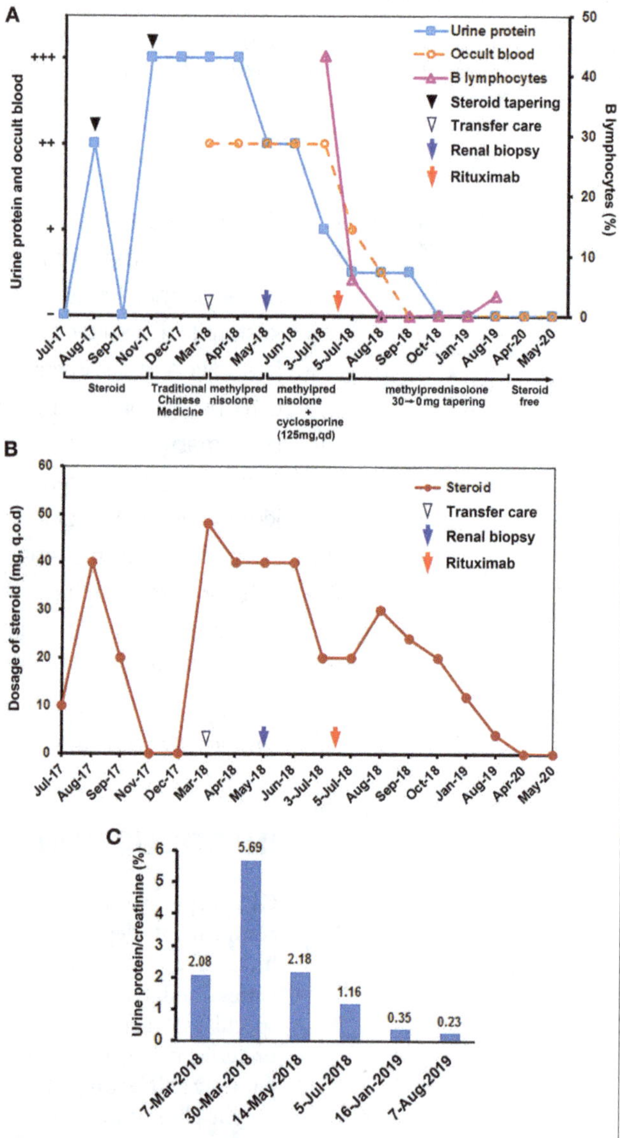

FIGURE 1 | The clinical course for the C1q nephropathy patient. **(A)** Selected urinalysis results and clinical course for the patient. Proteinuria and urinary occult blood have been negative for >18 months since administration of rituximab, indicating long-term remission. No relapse occurs after withdrawing maintenance dose of corticosteroid. **(B)** The course of steroid treatment is shown for corresponding time points in **(A)**. **(C)** Urinary protein/creatinine ratios during the care provided by us.

frequent urination, and dysuria. Due to significant disease progression, patient was referred to our hospital in March 2018.

On presentation to our hospital, the patient was admitted to the Pediatric Intensive Care Unit (PICU) and found to have a fungal infection, heart failure, hypertension, ascites, and persistent oliguria. Routine examination and laboratory tests showed body weight of 33 kg, body surface area of 1.11 m^2, serum albumin of 14.3 g/L, total cholesterol of 20.78 mol/L, and triglyceride of 11.13 mmol/L, indicating hypoproteinemia and hyperlipidemia. Renal function tests showed serum uric acid of 545 μmol/L, creatinine of 121.0 μmol/L, blood urea nitrogen (BUN) of 22.4 mmol/L, and glomerular filtration rate (GFR) of 37.86 ml/min, indicating azotemia and renal dysfunction. Initial treatment included correcting electrolyte disorder, diuresis, anticoaglutant therapy, and fluconazole (3.6 mg/kg) for fungal treatment. During this time, she was also treated with methylprednisolone (2 mg/kg daily) and aldehyde oxystarch, without significant efficacy (**Figures 1A,B**). Therefore, the patient underwent continuous renal replacement therapy (CRRT) with significant improvement of disease. Laboratory tests showed blood creatinine of 46 μmol/L, BUN of 10 mmol/L, and GFR of 99.59 ml/min. Patient was then transferred from PICU to our department for subsequent therapy. Autoimmune antibody panel was ordered, and all resulted negative. These included antinuclear antibody (ANA), antidouble-stranded DNA (anti-dsDNA), anti-Smith, antihistone antibody (AHA), anti-Sjögren's-syndrome-related antigen A (anti-SSA), anti-SSB, rheumatoid factor, ANCA, cardiolipin autoantibody, antimitochondrial antibody (AMA), smooth muscle antibody (SMA), anticentromere antibody, and antibasement membrane antibody. With negative immunological workup, we recommended a renal biopsy, but this was declined by her parents at that time with concerns regarding invasiveness of biopsy. During that admission, patient experienced repeated hypertension that was difficult to control on nifedipine and, subsequently, developed convulsions accompanied by right hemiplegia concerning for hypertensive encephalopathy. She subsequently underwent aggressive sodium nitroprusside (1–5 μg/kg/min), diuretic (spironolactone 20 mg and hydrochlorothiazide 10 mg daily), and steroid therapy (methylprednisolone 40 mg, q.o.d). Following these, her blood pressure returned to normal, neurological symptoms resolved, and systemic edema also improved. Laboratory tests showed that urine protein and occult blood decreased to 2+, blood creatinine was 42.0 μmol/L, and hypoproteinemia was corrected. Patient was discharged with continuation on methylprednisolone (40 mg daily in divided doses), losartan potassium (20 mg daily), and spironolactone (20 mg daily).

During her outpatient follow-up, patient's urine protein consistently returned 2–3+, suggesting steroid resistance. The need for tissue diagnosis via biopsy was reiterated, but patient's family continued to refuse at that time. Therefore, cyclosporine 5 mg/kg PO was added to her regimen. Subsequent labs showed improved proteinuria without significant decrease in serum creatinine despite the addition of cyclosporine. Due to frequency of relapses, renal biopsy was discussed again with the patient's parents for which consent was given in May 2018,

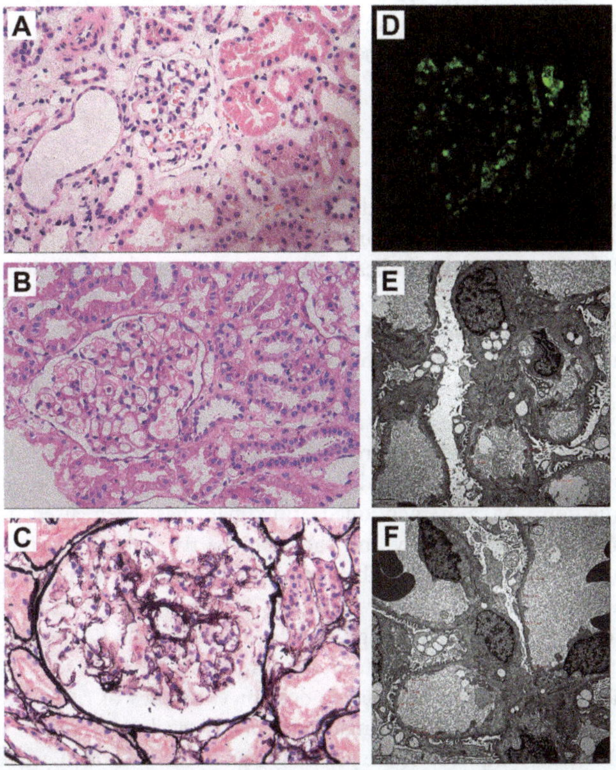

FIGURE 2 | Pathology evaluation for the C1q nephropathy patient. **(A)** Hematoxylin–eosin staining shows increased number of cells in glomerulus. No glomerular crescent, focal segmental glomerular sclerosis, and fibrosis are noted. However, renal tubule dilation and vacuolar degeneration of epithelial cells are present, and renal interstitium is slightly infiltrated with inflammatory cells, indicating a minimal change disease (MCD). **(B)** Periodic acid–Schiff (PAS) staining shows no remarkable cellular proliferation of mesangium and stroma. **(C)** Periodic Schiff–methenamine (PASM) staining shows normal capillary loops and no significantly thickened basement membrane. **(D)** Immunofluorescent staining confirms large amount of C1q deposition. **(E,F)** Transmission electron microscopy shows vacuolar degeneration of epithelial cells, podocyte foot processes effacement, proliferation of mesangium and stroma, and thin basement membrane.

and microscopy results were consistent with C1q nephropathy (**Figures 2A–F**).

Based on the pathological findings, a trial of rituximab was initiated after lymphocyte subset analysis showed B lymphocyte ratio of 43.2%. The patient received a single intravenous dose of 100 mg rituximab (93 mg/m^2). During infusion, patient experienced facial flushing but no other significant discomfort. B lymphocyte subset fell to 6.1% after 1 day. After 2 weeks of rituximab treatment, B cells were completely depleted, and renal function was significantly improved with a GFR of 93 ml/min (**Figure 1A**). Patient was then given prednisone starting at 30 mg every other day and gradually tapered at a rate of 5 mg/month. At 1-year follow-up in August 2019, patient presented with symptoms of urinary tract infection. Urinalysis at that time showed 4+ white blood cells (WBCs) but was negative for protein and blood. Serum tests showed normal kidney function and 3.30% of total B lymphocyte subset. At present, patient has maintained normal kidney function off steroid therapy and has had no relapses since rituximab therapy. The treatment courses and selected laboratory results are shown in **Figure 1**.

DISCUSSION

Although C1q nephropathy currently has no discrete clinical considerations from nephrotic syndrome, its pathogenesis and disease course do indicate disparate treatment guidelines. Patients with C1q nephropathy are frequently steroid dependent, more likely to relapse, and have a shorter recurrence period than nephrotic syndrome patients with no C1q deposition (4).

Typically, pathological findings in children with nephrotic syndrome are mostly small lesions, and in these cases, steroid therapy is preferred. If treatment is inefficacious, an immunosuppressor is added, with risk of detriment to renal function. As aforementioned, rituximab has been used to treat C1q nephropathy and shown to partially restore kidney function (9). At present, the dose of rituximab for treating C1q nephropathy is based on guidelines for lymphoma treatment, i.e., four doses of 375 mg/m^2 at weekly intervals (7). Recent studies reported complete remission for patients with C1q nephropathy by using a single dose or two doses of rituximab at 375 mg/m^2 (8, 10). In malignant disease such as lymphoma, abnormal lymphocytes are generally significantly elevated, while the number of lymphocytes in C1q nephropathy does not have similar magnitude of elevation. Therefore, we posited that the dosage of rituximab for treating C1q nephropathy may not need to be as high as that for lymphoma. Several studies have used low-dose rituximab (a fixed dose of 100 mg) to treat adult patients with idiopathic autoimmune hemolytic anemia and primary immune thrombocytopenia and showed comparable efficacy of standard dose (17, 18).

In this case, we reported the first successful use of a single low dose of rituximab (100 mg or 93 mg/m^2) for C1q nephropathy treatment, a quarter that of the dosage indicated for lymphoma. After treatment, our patient has shown normal renal function, negative urine protein, and occult blood for >18 months and is currently steroid-free, suggesting that successful remission was achieved at this significantly reduced dosage. The side effects of rituximab have not been clarified, with some occurring early in administration, including nausea, rash, and bronchospasm, although adverse effects can be minimized by controlling infusion rate (15). Viral infections and pyelonephritis accompanied by neutropenia can also occur during the rituximab treatment (15). As shown in the literature, low-dose rituximab may reduce risks of severe side effects such as neutropenia and pulmonary toxicity (19). A lower dose can also be cost saving and shortens infusion time, which are important considerations in making biologics accessible to indigent populations. In the setting of good treatment efficacy with better controlled adverse effect profile, reduced dosage treatment with rituximab in C1q nephropathy warrants additional examination.

Our report features only one case, which is a limitation presented by the rarity of C1q nephropathy in our practice. Although the response of this patient to such a low dose of rituximab may occur on occasion and could be race dependent, the overall outcomes for this patient is remarkable. These results suggest that the dosage of rituximab for treating pediatric nephrotic syndrome, particularly C1q nephropathy, may be significantly reduced. To further investigate, a prospective case-controlled clinical trial recruiting larger, more diverse populations will be needed.

Although the pathogenesis of C1q nephropathy still remains unclear, it is speculated that complement activation and glomerular antigen–antibody complex formation play a central role. Studies show that C1q molecules have affinity to various substances including DNA, RNA, viral proteins, Gram-negative bacteria, and various immune cells (5). C1q has been demonstrated to enhance B-cell response to antigens, which underlies the reason for use of rituximab to deplete B cells and reduce deposition of immune complexes. Previous studies have suggested that dosage of rituximab should be determined according to serum CD19 level, which is expressed in pre-B cells prior to differentiation (10). This method of quantitatively metered administration may be a focus of clinical trials in the future. Some Literatures also report that rituximab is less effective in patients with hormones and cyclosporine-dependent nephrotic syndrome (12). In consideration of increased complications with multidrug treatment, administration of rituximab in the early stages for steroid-dependent patients can effectively prevent progression of disease while also mitigating the myriad of harmful side effects of steroid treatment. There are also some reports suggesting that subcutaneous injection of rituximab is more time saving and less labor intensive compared to intravenous administration (11, 13). In addition, rituximab can be subcutaneously injected with recombinant human hyaluronidase that increases the dispersion and absorption of rituximab (11). Given the multitude of areas for development, we expect to continue investigating the mode of administration and dosage of rituximab to achieve maximum efficacy and minimize adverse outcomes.

ETHICS STATEMENT

The studies involving human participants were reviewed and approved by the Ethical Committee of Lanzhou University Second Hospital. Written informed consent to participate in this study was provided by the participants' legal guardian/next of kin.

AUTHOR CONTRIBUTIONS

RM collected the data and prepared the manuscript. DW participated in the patient's care. ZH collected and analyzed the data. QC participated in the patient's clinical care. YY participated in the patient's care, supervised the study, analyzed the data, and wrote the manuscript. All authors contributed to the article and approved the submitted version.

Hospital Cuiying Science and Technology Innovation Project (CY2017-MS16), and the Science and Technology Development Plan of Chengguan District, Lanzhou City, Gansu Province (2017KJGG0050).

ACKNOWLEDGMENTS

The authors thank the patient and her family for facilitating this work.

REFERENCES

1. Jennette JC, Hipp CG. C1q nephropathy: a distinct pathologic entity usually causing nephrotic syndrome. *Am J Kidney Dis.* (1985) 6:103–10. doi: 10.1016/S0272-6386(85)80150-5
2. Markowitz GS, Schwimmer JA, Stokes MB, Nasr S, Seigle RL, Valeri AM, et al. C1q nephropathy: a variant of focal segmental glomerulosclerosis. *Kidney Int.* (2003) 64:1232–40. doi: 10.1046/j.1523-1755.2003.00218.x
3. Iskandar SS, Browning MC, Lorentz WB. C1q nephropathy: a pediatric clinicopathologic study. *Am J Kidney Dis.* (1991) 18:459–65. doi: 10.1016/S0272-6386(12)80114-4
4. Abu-Shahin N, Al-Khader A, Qattan D, Akl K. C1q nephropathy among children with nephrotic syndrome: ten-year experience from a pediatric nephrology unit. *Turk J Pediatr.* (2018) 60:14–21. doi: 10.24953/turkjped.2018.01.003
5. Devasahayam J, Erode-Singaravelu G, Bhat Z, Oliver T, Chandran A, Zeng X, et al. C1q nephropathy: the unique underrecognized pathological entity. *Anal Cell Pathol.* (2015) 2015:490413. doi: 10.1155/2015/490413
6. Gunasekara VN, Sebire NJ, Tullus K. C1q nephropathy in children: clinical characteristics and outcome. *Pediatr Nephrol.* (2014) 29:407–13. doi: 10.1007/s00467-013-2692-4
7. Sinha A, Nast CC, Hristea I, Vo AA, Jordan SC. Resolution of clinical and pathologic features of C1q nephropathy after rituximab therapy. *Clin Exp Nephrol.* (2011) 15:164–70. doi: 10.1007/s10157-010-0377-x
8. Yang YH, Lee WS, Cheng CY. C1q nephropathy in a patient complicated with nephrotic syndrome and refractory to steroid therapy. *J Microbiol Immunol Infect.* (2020) 53:183–5. doi: 10.1016/j.jmii.2019.06.005
9. Bitzan M, Ouahed JD, Krishnamoorthy P, Bernard C. Rituximab treatment of collapsing C1q glomerulopathy: clinical and histopathological evolution. *Pediatr Nephrol.* (2008) 23:1355–61. doi: 10.1007/s00467-008-0781-6
10. Ramachandran R, Bharati J, Jha V. Successful treatment of C1q nephropathy with CD19 targeted Rituximab therapy. *Nephrology.* (2017) 22:265. doi: 10.1111/nep.12757
11. Pierpont TM, Limper CB, Richards KL. Past, present, and future of rituximab-the world's first oncology monoclonal antibody therapy. *Front Oncol.* (2018) 8:163. doi: 10.3389/fonc.2018.00163
12. Ravani P, Bonanni A, Rossi R, Caridi G, Ghiggeri GM. Anti-CD20 antibodies for idiopathic nephrotic syndrome in children. *Clin J Am Soc Nephrol.* (2016) 11:710–20. doi: 10.2215/CJN.08500815
13. MacIsaac J, Siddiqui R, Jamula E, Li N, Baker S, Webert KE, et al. Systematic review of rituximab for autoimmune diseases: a potential alternative to intravenous immune globulin. *Transfusion.* (2018) 58:2729–35. doi: 10.1111/trf.14841
14. Musette P, Bouaziz JD. B cell modulation strategies in autoimmune diseases: new concepts. *Front Immunol.* (2018) 9:622. doi: 10.3389/fimmu.2018.00622
15. Ravani P, Ponticelli A, Siciliano C, Fornoni A, Magnasco A, Sica F, et al. Rituximab is a safe and effective long-term treatment for children with steroid and calcineurin inhibitor-dependent idiopathic nephrotic syndrome. *Kidney Int.* (2013) 84:1025–33. doi: 10.1038/ki.2013.211
16. Iijima K, Sako M, Nozu K. Rituximab for nephrotic syndrome in children. *Clin Exp Nephrol.* (2017) 21:193–202. doi: 10.1007/s10157-016-1313-5
17. Zaja F, Vianelli N, Volpetti S, Battista ML, Defina M, Palmieri S, et al. Low-dose rituximab in adult patients with primary immune thrombocytopenia. *Eur J Haematol.* (2010) 85:329–34. doi: 10.1111/j.1600-0609.2010.01486.x
18. Barcellini W, Zaja F, Zaninoni A, Imperiali FG, Battista ML, Di Bona E, et al. Low-dose rituximab in adult patients with idiopathic autoimmune hemolytic anemia: clinical efficacy and biologic studies. *Blood.* (2012) 119:3691–7. doi: 10.1182/blood-2011-06-363556
19. Pavanello F, Zucca E, Ghielmini M. Rituximab: 13 open questions after 20 years of clinical use. *Cancer Treat Rev.* (2017) 53:38–46. doi: 10.1016/j.ctrv.2016.11.015

Permissions

All chapters in this book were first published by Frontiers; hereby published with permission under the Creative Commons Attribution License or equivalent. Every chapter published in this book has been scrutinized by our experts. Their significance has been extensively debated. The topics covered herein carry significant findings which will fuel the growth of the discipline. They may even be implemented as practical applications or may be referred to as a beginning point for another development.

The contributors of this book come from diverse backgrounds, making this book a truly international effort. This book will bring forth new frontiers with its revolutionizing research information and detailed analysis of the nascent developments around the world.

We would like to thank all the contributing authors for lending their expertise to make the book truly unique. They have played a crucial role in the development of this book. Without their invaluable contributions this book wouldn't have been possible. They have made vital efforts to compile up to date information on the varied aspects of this subject to make this book a valuable addition to the collection of many professionals and students.

This book was conceptualized with the vision of imparting up-to-date information and advanced data in this field. To ensure the same, a matchless editorial board was set up. Every individual on the board went through rigorous rounds of assessment to prove their worth. After which they invested a large part of their time researching and compiling the most relevant data for our readers.

The editorial board has been involved in producing this book since its inception. They have spent rigorous hours researching and exploring the diverse topics which have resulted in the successful publishing of this book. They have passed on their knowledge of decades through this book. To expedite this challenging task, the publisher supported the team at every step. A small team of assistant editors was also appointed to further simplify the editing procedure and attain best results for the readers.

Apart from the editorial board, the designing team has also invested a significant amount of their time in understanding the subject and creating the most relevant covers. They scrutinized every image to scout for the most suitable representation of the subject and create an appropriate cover for the book.

The publishing team has been an ardent support to the editorial, designing and production team. Their endless efforts to recruit the best for this project, has resulted in the accomplishment of this book. They are a veteran in the field of academics and their pool of knowledge is as vast as their experience in printing. Their expertise and guidance has proved useful at every step. Their uncompromising quality standards have made this book an exceptional effort. Their encouragement from time to time has been an inspiration for everyone.

The publisher and the editorial board hope that this book will prove to be a valuable piece of knowledge for researchers, students, practitioners and scholars across the globe.

List of Contributors

Corina Nailescu and Marcia L. Shew
Department of Pediatrics, Indiana University, Riley Hospital for Children, Indianapolis, IN, United States

Raoul D. Nelson
Department of Pediatrics, University of Utah, Primary Children's Hospital, Salt Lake City, UT, United States

Priya S. Verghese
Department of Pediatrics, University of Minnesota Masonic Children's Hospital, Minneapolis, MN, United States

Katherine E. Twombley
Department of Pediatrics, Medical University of South Carolina Children's Hospital, Charleston, SC, United States
Department of Pediatrics, Medical University of South Carolina, Charleston, SC, United States

Aftab S. Chishti
Department of Pediatrics, Kentucky Children's Hospital, University of Kentucky, Lexington, KY, United States

Michele Mills
Department of Pediatrics, C. S. Mott Children's Hospital, University of Michigan, Ann Arbor, MI, United States

John D. Mahan
Department of Pediatrics, Nationwide Children's Hospital, The Ohio State University, Columbus, OH, United States

James E. Slaven
Department of Biostatistics, Indiana University, Indianapolis, IN, United States

Cheryl L. Tran
Division of Pediatric Nephrology, Department of Pediatrics, Mayo Clinic, Rochester, MN, United States

David T. Selewski
Division of Pediatric Nephrology, Department of Pediatrics, Medical University of South Carolina, Charleston, SC, United States

Gia J. Oh
Division of Nephrology, Department of Pediatrics, Stanford University, Stanford, CA, United States

Jonathan P. Troost
Michigan Institute for Clinical and Health Research, University of Michigan, Ann Arbor, MI, United States

Susan F. Massengill
Levine Children's Hospital at Atrium Health, Charlotte, NC, United States

Samhar I. Al-Akash
Driscoll Children's Hospital, Corpus Christi, TX, United States

Shefali Mahesh
Division of Nephrology and Dialysis, Akron Children's Hospital, Akron, OH, United States

Rasheda Amin
Pediatric Specialists of Virginia, Fairfax, VA, United States
Department of Pediatrics, George Washington University, Washington, DC, United States

Isa F. Ashoor
Division of Nephrology, Department of Pediatrics, Louisiana State University, New Orleans, LA, United States

Rahul Chanchlani
Division of Pediatric Nephrology, Department of Pediatrics, McMaster University, Hamilton, ON, Canada

Mahmoud Kallash
Division of Nephrology, Nationwide Children's Hospital, Columbus, OH, United States

Robert P. Woroniecki
Division of Pediatric Nephrology and Hypertension, Stony Brook Children's Hospital and Renaissance School of Medicine, Stony Brook, NY, United States

Debbie S. Gipson
Division of Pediatric Nephrology, Department of Pediatrics, University of Michigan, Ann Arbor, MI, United States

Silvia Martín Ramos
Hospital Universitario Central de Asturias, Oviedo, Spain

Marta Gil-Calvo
Hospital Clínico Universitario de Santiago, Santiago de Compostela, Spain

Virginia Roldán and Ana Castellano Martínez
Hospital Universitario Puerta del Mar, Cádiz, Spain

Fernando Santos
Hospital Universitario Central de Asturias, Oviedo, Spain
Instituto de Investigación Sanitaria del Principado de Asturias, Oviedo, Spain
Universidad de Oviedo, Oviedo, Spain

Fen-fen Ni, Shi-lei Jia, Ran-ran Chen, Li-bing Liu, Cheng-rong Li and Xiao-Jie Gao
Department of Nephrology, Shenzhen Children's Hospital, Shenzhen, China

Guang-lei Liu
The Fifth Affiliated (Zhuhai) Hospital of Zunyi Medical University, Zhuhai, China

Jun Yang
Department of Immunology, Shenzhen Children's Hospital, Shenzhen, China

Ayo Matory
Division of Nephrology, Departments of Pediatrics and Medicine, Duke University Medical Center, Durham, NC, United States

Jennifer D. Varner, Megan Chryst-Stangl, Guanghong Wu, Brandon Lane and Gentzon Hall
Division of Nephrology, Departments of Pediatrics and Medicine, Duke University Medical Center, Durham, NC, United States
Duke Molecular Physiology Institute, Duke University Medical Center, Durham, NC, United States

Rasheed Gbadegesin
Division of Nephrology, Departments of Pediatrics and Medicine, Duke University Medical Center, Durham, NC, United States
Duke Molecular Physiology Institute, Duke University Medical Center, Durham, NC, United States
Department of Pediatrics, Duke University, Durham, NC, United States

Christopher Imokhuede Esezobor
Department of Pediatrics, College of Medicine of the University of Lagos, Lagos, Nigeria

Adaobi Solarin
Department of Pediatrics, Lagos State University Teaching Hospital, Ikeja, Nigeria

Asiri Abeyagunawardena
Department of Pediatrics, University of Peradeniya, Peradeniya, Sri Lanka

Tracy E. Hunley
Division of Nephrology, Department of Pediatrics, Vanderbilt University, Nashville, TN, United States

Jen Jar Lin
Department of Pediatrics, Wake Forest Baptist Medical Center, Winston Salem, NC, United States

David Howell
Department of Pathology, Duke University Medical Center, Durham, NC, United States

Siddharth Shah and M. Asope Elder
Department of Pediatrics, Norton Children's and University of Louisville, Louisville, KY, United States

Jessica Hata
Department of Pathology, Norton Children's and University of Louisville, Louisville, KY, United States

Jitendra Meena, Georgie Mathew, Pankaj Hari, Aditi Sinha and Arvind Bagga
Division of Nephrology, Department of Pediatrics, ICMR Center for Advanced Research in Nephrology, All India Institute of Medical Sciences, New Delhi, India

Tetyana L. Vasylyeva
Department of Pediatrics, Texas Tech University Health Sciences Center, Amarillo, TX, United States

María E. Díaz-González de Ferris
UNC Transition Program, Manning Drive N.C. Children's Hospital, The University of North Carolina, Chapel Hill, NC, United States

David S. Hains
Division of Pediatric Nephrology, Indiana University School of Medicine, Indianapolis, IN, United States

Jacqueline Ho
UPMC Children's Hospital of Pittsburgh, University of Pittsburgh, Pittsburgh, PA, United States

Lyndsay A. Harshman
Division of Pediatric Nephrology, Department of Pediatrics, University of Iowa Stead Family, Iowa City, IA, United States

Kimberly J. Reidy
Department of Pediatrics, Montefiore Medical Center, Albert Einstein College of Medicine, Children's Hospital at Montefiore, Bronx, NY, United States

Tammy M. Brady
Division of Pediatric Nephrology, Johns Hopkins University School of Medicine, Baltimore, MD, United States

Daryl M. Okamura
Center for Developmental Biology and Regenerative Medicine, Seattle Children's Hospital, University of Washington, Seattle, WA, United States

Dmitry V. Samsonov
New York Medical College, Valhalla, NY, United States

Scott E. Wenderfer
Renal Section, Baylor College of Medicine, Texas Children's Hospital, Houston, TX, United States

Erum A. Hartung
Division of Nephrology, Children's Hospital of Philadelphia, Perelman School of Medicine of the University of Pennsylvania, Philadelphia, PA, United States

Xin Xiang and Shi-Yuan Qiu
Ministry of Education Key Laboratory of Child Development and Disorders, Department of Nephrology, National Clinical Research Center for Child Health and Disorders, China International Science and Technology Cooperation Base of Child development and Critical Disorders, Children's Hospital of Chongqing Medical University, Chongqing, China
Chongqing Key Laboratory of Pediatrics, Chongqing, China

Mo Wang
Ministry of Education Key Laboratory of Child Development and Disorders, Department of Nephrology, National Clinical Research Center for Child Health and Disorders, China International Science and Technology Cooperation Base of Child development and Critical Disorders, Children's Hospital of Chongqing Medical University, Chongqing, China
Chongqing Key Laboratory of Pediatrics, Chongqing, China
Department of Nephrology, Children's Hospital of Chongqing Medical University, Ministry of Education Key Laboratory of Child Development and Disorders, National Clinical Research Center for Child Health and Disorders, China International Science and Technology Cooperation Base of Child Development and Critical Disorders, Chongqing Key Laboratory of Pediatrics, Chongqing, China
Western Pediatric Development Union, Chongqing, China

Evgenia Gurevich and Eytan Israel
Soroka University Medical Center, Ben-Gurion University of the Negev, Beersheba, Israel
Division of Pediatrics, Ben-Gurion University of the Negev, Beersheba, Israel

Yael Segev
Department of Microbiology and Immunology, Ben-Gurion University of the Negev, Beersheba, Israel

Daniel Landau
Department of Microbiology and Immunology, Ben-Gurion University of the Negev, Beersheba, Israel
Department of Pediatrics B, Schneider Children's Medical Center, Sackler School of Medicine, Tel Aviv University, Tel Aviv, Israel

Andrea Pasini, Cristina Bertulli, Claudio La Scola and Francesca Mencarelli
Nephrology and Dialysis Unit, Department of Pediatrics, IRCCS Azienda Ospedaliero-Universitaria di Bologna, Bologna, Italy

Luca Casadio
Unità Operativa Complessa of Paediatrics and Neonatology, Local Health Authority of Romagna, Ravenna, Italy

Ciro Corrado and Silvio Maringhini
Pediatric Nephrology Unit, Children's Hospital "G. Di Cristina", A.R.N.A.S. "Civico", Palermo, Italy

Alberto Edefonti and Antonio P. Mastrangelo
Pediatric Nephrology, Dialysis and Transplant Unit, Fondazione Ca' Granda Istituto di Ricovero e Cura a Carattere Scientifico Ospedale Maggiore Policlinico, Milan, Italy

Luciana Ghio
Pediatric Nephrology, Dialysis and Transplant Unit, Fondazione Ca' Granda Istituto di Ricovero e Cura a Carattere Scientifico Ospedale Maggiore Policlinico, Milan, Italy
Pediatric Nephrology, Dialysis and Transplant Unit, Fondazione IRCCS Ca' Granda Ospedale Maggiore Policlinico, Milan, Italy

GianMarco Ghiggeri
Division of Nephrology, Dialysis, Transplantation, Laboratory on Pathophysiology of Uremia, Istituto G. Gaslini, Genoa, Italy

Mario Giordano and Giovanni Messina
Nephrology Unit, Giovanni XXIII Children's Hospital, Bari, Italy

Cristina Malaventura
Section of Pediatrics, Department of Medical Sciences, University of Ferrara, Ferrara, Italy

Marco Materassi and Paola Romagnani
Nephrology and Dialysis Unit, Meyer Children's Hospital, Florence, Italy

Elena Monti
Specialty School of Paediatrics - Alma Mater Studiorum, Università di Bologna, Bologna, Italy

Giuseppe Puccio
Retired, Palermo, Italy

Giovanni Montini
Pediatric Nephrology, Dialysis and Transplant Unit, Fondazione Ca' Granda Istituto di Ricovero e Cura a Carattere Scientifico Ospedale Maggiore Policlinico, Milan, Italy
Giuliana and Bernardo Caprotti Chair of Pediatrics, Department of Clinical Sciences and Community Health, University of Milano, Milan, Italy
Pediatric Nephrology, Dialysis and Transplant Unit, Fondazione IRCCS Ca' Granda Ospedale Maggiore Policlinico, Milan, Italy
Department of Clinical Sciences and Community Health, University of Milan, Milan, Italy

Rezan Topaloğ lu, Bora Gülhan, Kübra Çelegen, Mihriban İnözü and Ali Düzova
Division of Pediatric Nephrology, Department of Pediatrics, School of Medicine, Hacettepe University, Ankara, Turkey

Mutlu Hayran
Department of Preventive Oncology, School of Medicine, Hacettepe University, Ankara, Turkey

Fatih Ozaltin
Division of Pediatric Nephrology, Department of Pediatrics, School of Medicine, Hacettepe University, Ankara, Turkey
Nephrogenetics Laboratory, School of Medicine, Hacettepe University, Ankara, Turkey
Center for Biobanking and Genomics, School of Medicine, Hacettepe University, Ankara, Turkey

Azriyanti Anuar Zaini, Nurshadia Samingan and Muhammad Yazid Jalaludin
Pediatric Unit, Faculty of Medicine, University of Malaya, Kuala Lumpur, Malaysia

Yam Ngo Lim, Yok Chin Yap, Mirunalini Appadurai, Sangeet Sidhu and Chee Sing Lai
Pediatric Institute of the Hospital, Kuala Lumpur, Malaysia

Karmila Abu Bakar
Pediatric Unit, Faculty of Medicine, University of Malaya, Kuala Lumpur, Malaysia
Pediatric Institute of the Hospital, Kuala Lumpur, Malaysia

Khairunnisa Khalil
Pediatric Institute of the Hospital, Kuala Lumpur, Malaysia
Paediatric Nephrology Unit, Institute of Paediatrics, Kuala Lumpur, Malaysia

Hengci Zhang, Cheng Zhong, Lin Shi and Jiacheng Li
Department of Nephrology, Children's Hospital of Chongqing Medical University, Ministry of Education Key Laboratory of Child Development and Disorders, National Clinical Research Center for Child Health and Disorders, China International Science and Technology Cooperation Base of Child Development and Critical Disorders, Chongqing Key Laboratory of Pediatrics, Chongqing, China
Western Pediatric Development Union, Chongqing, China

Shiyuan Qiu
Department of Nephrology, Children's Hospital of Chongqing Medical University, Ministry of Education Key Laboratory of Child Development and Disorders, National Clinical Research Center for Child Health and Disorders, China International Science and Technology Cooperation Base of Child Development and Critical Disorders, Chongqing Key Laboratory of Pediatrics, Chongqing, China
Pediatric Internal Medicine Department, Chongqing You You Baobei Women's and Children's Hospital, Chongqing, China

Tao Zhang and Xiaoping Zhu
Western Pediatric Development Union, Chongqing, China
Department of Pediatrics, The Affiliated Hospital of Guizhou Medical University, Guiyang, China

Kyle W. Freischlag
School of Medicine, Duke University, Durham, NC, United States

Vivian Chen, Shashi K. Nagaraj, Annabelle N. Chua, Delbert R. Wigfall, John W. Foreman and Eileen T. Chambers
Department of Pediatrics, Duke University, Durham, NC, United States

Dongfeng Chen
Department of Pathology, Duke University, Durham, NC, United States

Deepak Vikraman
Department of Surgery, Duke University, Durham, NC, United States

Sheetal Bhojani and Heather Maxwell
Royal Hospital for Children, Glasgow, United Kingdom

Jelena Stojanovic and Nabil Melhem
Evelina London Children's Hospital, London, United Kingdom

Peter Houtman and Angela Hall
Leicester Royal Infirmary, Leicester, United Kingdom

Cheentan Singh
North Middlesex University Hospital NHS Trust, London, United Kingdom

Wesley Hayes
Bristol Royal Hospital for Children, Bristol, United Kingdom

Rachel Lennon
Royal Manchester Children's Hospital, Manchester, United Kingdom

Manish D. Sinha
Evelina London Children's Hospital, London, United Kingdom
Kings College London, London, United Kingdom

David V. Milford
Birmingham Women's and Children's Hospital, Birmingham, United Kingdom

Maysoun Al Rushood, Amal A. Al-Eisa and Mohammad Z. Haider
Department of Pediatrics, Faculty of Medicine, Health Sciences Center, Kuwait University, Kuwait City, Kuwait

Chen Ling, Zhi Chen, Jianfeng Fan, Qun Meng, Nan Zhou, Qiang Sun and Xiaorong Liu
Beijing Key Laboratory of Pediatric Chronic Kidney Disease and Blood Purification, Department of Nephrology, National Center for Children's Health, Beijing Children's Hospital, Capital Medical University, Beijing, China

Xiaolin Wang and Jingang Gui
Key Laboratory of Major Diseases in Children, Ministry of Education, Beijing Children's Hospital, Capital Medical University, Beijing, China
Laboratory of Immunology, Beijing Pediatric Research Institute, Beijing Children's Hospital, Capital Medical University, Beijing, China

Lin Hua
School of Biomedical Engineering, Capital Medical University, Beijing, China

Xia Gao, Zichuan Xu, Huiying Deng, Huabin Yang and Fu Zhong
Nephrology Department, Guangzhou Women and Children's Medical Center, Guangzhou, China

Yan Wang
Graduate School, Ningxia Medical University, Yinchuan, China
Neonatology Department, Northwest Women and Children's Hospital, Xi'an, China

Rupesh Raina
Department of Nephrology, Cleveland Clinic Akron General, Akron, OH, United States
Akron Nephrology Associates, Cleveland Clinic Akron General, Akron, OH, United States
Department of Pediatric Nephrology, Akron Children's Hospital, Akron, OH, United States
Akron Nephrology Associates/Cleveland Clinic Akron General Medical Center, Akron, OH, United States
Department of Nephrology, Akron Children's Hospital, Akron, OH, United States
Department of Nephrology, Cleveland Clinic Akron General and Akron Children's Hospital, Akron, OH, United States

Kirsten Kusumi
Department of Pediatric Nephrology, Akron Children's Hospital, Akron, OH, United States

Vinod Krishnappa
Akron Nephrology Associates, Cleveland Clinic Akron General, Akron, OH, United States
Department of Medicine, Northeast Ohio Medical University, Rootstown, OH, United States
Northeast Ohio Medical University, Rootstown, OH, United States

Abhijit Das
Department of Medicine, Northeast Ohio Medical University, Rootstown, OH, United States

Harshesh Amin
Department of Internal Medicine, Carolinas Health Care System Blue Ridge, Morganton, NC, United States

Yeshwanter Radhakrishnan
Department of Internal Medicine, Cleveland Clinic Akron General, Akron, OH, United States

Nikhil R. Nair
Department of Biochemistry, Case Western Reserve University, Cleveland, OH, United States

Kristen Sgambat and Asha Moudgil
Department of Nephrology, Children's National Hospital, Washington, DC, United States

Sarah Clauss
Department of Cardiology, Children's National Hospital, Washington, DC, United States

Anju Jacob and Jwan F. Shekhy
Department of Pediatrics, Al Jalila Children's Specialty Hospital, Dubai, United Arab Emirates

Shameer M. Habeeb, Eva Simkova and Martin Bitzan
Department of Pediatrics, Al Jalila Children's Specialty Hospital, Dubai, United Arab Emirates
Kidney Centre of Excellence, Al Jalila Children's Speciality Hospital, Dubai, United Arab Emirates

Leal Herlitz
Department of Anatomic Pathology, Cleveland Clinic, Cleveland, OH, United States

Alan Taylor
Department of Pediatrics, Al Jalila Children's Specialty Hospital, Dubai, United Arab Emirates
Al Jalila Genomics Center, Al Jalila Children's Specialty Hospital, Dubai, United Arab Emirates

Walid Abuhammour
Department of Pediatrics, Al Jalila Children's Specialty Hospital, Dubai, United Arab Emirates
Section of Infectious Diseases, Al Jalila Children's Specialty Hospital, Dubai, United Arab Emirates

Ahmad Abou Tayoun
Department of Pediatrics, Al Jalila Children's Specialty Hospital, Dubai, United Arab Emirates
Al Jalila Genomics Center, Al Jalila Children's Specialty Hospital, Dubai, United Arab Emirates
Department of Genetics, Mohammad Bin Rashid University of Medicine and Health Sciences, Dubai, United Arab Emirates

Stefano Turolo, Alberto C. Edefonti and Chiara Tamburello
Pediatric Nephrology, Dialysis and Transplant Unit, Fondazione IRCCS Ca' Granda Ospedale Maggiore Policlinico, Milan, Italy

William Morello
Pediatric Nephrology, Dialysis and Transplant Unit, Fondazione IRCCS Ca' Granda Ospedale Maggiore Policlinico, Milan, Italy
Pediatric Nephrology, Dialysis and Transplant Unit, Fondazione Ca' Granda Istituto di Ricovero e Cura a Carattere Scientifico Ospedale Maggiore Policlinico, Milan, Italy

Marie-Louise Syren
Department of Clinical Sciences and Community Health, University of Milan, Milan, Italy

Valentina De Cosmi and Carlo Agostoni
Department of Clinical Sciences and Community Health, University of Milan, Milan, Italy
Pediatric Intermediate Care Unit, Fondazione IRCCS Ca' Granda Ospedale Maggiore Policlinico, Milan, Italy

Erika A. Demarco, Alfredo Berrettini and Gianantonio Manzoni
Pediatric Urology Unit, Fondazione IRCCS Ca' Granda Ospedale Maggiore Policlinico, Milan, Italy

Ai-Qian Zhang
Department of Obstetrics and Gynecology, The Third Xiangya Hospital of Central South University, Changsha, China

Fang-Mei Luo, Yue Sheng, Chen-Yu Wang and Yi Dong
Department of Cell Biology, The School of Life Sciences, Central South University, Changsha, China
Hunan Key Laboratory of Animal for Human Disease, School of Life Sciences, Central South University, Changsha, China

Yu-Xing Liu and Liangliang Fan
Department of Obstetrics and Gynecology, The Third Xiangya Hospital of Central South University, Changsha, China
Department of Cell Biology, The School of Life Sciences, Central South University, Changsha, China
Hunan Key Laboratory of Animal for Human Disease, School of Life Sciences, Central South University, Changsha, China
Department of Respiratory Medicine, Diagnosis and Treatment Center of Respiratory Disease, The Second Xiangya Hospital of Central South University, Changsha, China

Lv Liu
Department of Respiratory Medicine, Diagnosis and Treatment Center of Respiratory Disease, The Second Xiangya Hospital of Central South University, Changsha, China

Ling Bai
Department of Nephrology and Rheumatology, Children's Hospital of Xinjiang Uygur Autonomous Region, Urumqi, China

Jing Zhuang, Changrong Zhang and Hong Jiang
Division of Nephrology, Department of Internal Medicine, People's Hospital of Xinjiang Uygur Autonomous Region, Urumqi, China

Chen Lu
Division of Nephrology, Department of Internal Medicine, The First Affiliated Hospital of Xinjiang Medical University, Urumqi, China

Xuefei Tian
Section of Nephrology, Department of Internal Medicine, Yale University School of Medicine, New Haven, CT, United States

Ronith Chakraborty
Akron Nephrology Associates/Cleveland Clinic Akron General, Akron, OH, United States
Akron Nephrology Associates/Cleveland Clinic Akron General Medical Center, Akron, OH, United States

Cheryl Sanchez-Kazi
Department of Nephrology, Loma Linda University Children's Hospital, Loma Linda, CA, United States

Alejandro Quiroga
Department of Nephrology, Spectrum Health (Helen De Vos Children's Hospital), Grand Rapids, MI, United States

Robert Mathias
Department of Pediatrics, Nemours Children's Hospital, Orlando, FL, United States

Megan Lo
Department of Pediatrics, Children's Hospital of Richmond at VCU, Richmond, VA, United States

Julia Steinke
Division of Pediatric Nephrology, Dialysis and Transplantation, Helen Devos Children's Hospital and Clinics, Grand Rapids, MI, United States

Timothy Bunchman
Pediatric Nephrology and Transplantation, Children's Hospital of Richmond, Virginia Commonwealth University, Richmond, VA, United States

Joshua Zaritsky
Nemours, A.I. duPont Hospital for Children, Wilmington, DE, United States

Eugènia Serramontmany, Aurora Fernández-Polo, Laura Gómez- Ganda and Carme Cañete-Ramírez
Pharmacy Department, Vall d'Hebron University Hospital, Barcelona, Spain

Marina Muñoz and Gema Ariceta
Pediatric Nephrology Department, Vall d'Hebron University Hospital, Barcelona, Spain

María Morillo
Nursery Department, Vall d'Hebron University Hospital, Barcelona, Spain

Rui Ma, Dengyan Wu, Zhiqin He and Qian Chang
Department of Pediatric Nephrology, Lanzhou University Second Hospital, Lanzhou, China
Department of Nephrology, Gansu Children's Hospital, Lanzhou, China

Yonghong Yang
Department of Pediatric Nephrology, Lanzhou University Second Hospital, Lanzhou, China
Department of Nephrology, Gansu Children's Hospital, Lanzhou, China
Department of Pediatrics, Children's Hospital of Xi'an International Medical Center, Xi'an, China

Index

R

S

T

U

V

W

www.ingramcontent.com/pod-product-compliance
Lightning Source LLC
LaVergne TN
LVHW082152200926
848484LV00008B/2149